Progressive Tinnitus: Assessment and Management

Progressive Tinnitus: Assessment and Management

Editor: Jasmine Richards

AMERICAN
MEDICAL PUBLISHERS
www.americanmedicalpublishers.com

AMERICAN
MEDICAL PUBLISHERS
www.americanmedicalpublishers.com

Cataloging-in-Publication Data

Progressive tinnitus : assessment and management / edited by Jasmine Richards.
p. cm.
Includes bibliographical references and index.
ISBN 979-8-88740-395-3
1. Tinnitus. 2. Tinnitus--Diagnosis. 3. Tinnitus--Treatment. 4. Hearing disorders. I. Richards, Jasmine.
RF293.8 .P76 2023
617.8--dc23

American Medical Publishers,
41 Flatbush Avenue,
1st Floor, New York,
NY 11217, USA

ISBN 979-8-88740-395-3 (Hardback)

Contents

Preface

Hearing disorders are a type of disorder wherein the affected person is not able to perceive or process auditory information. Hearing disorders may lead to hearing loss which can be partial or complete, and may occur in one or both ears. There are various hearing disorders that include tinnitus, endaural phenomena, hyperacusis, presbycusis, etc. Tinnitus is a disorder characterized by sensitivity to sound when, in fact, there is no actual sound. This obstructs the normal functioning of the ear as the patient experiences sounds such as ringing, clicking, buzzing, or hissing. It often impedes concentration, leading to anxiety and depression. The management of tinnitus includes identification of the specific cause followed by the treatment. The primary treatments are classified into psychological, sound based interventions, and medications. These involve talk therapy, sound therapy, and hearing aids. Cognitive behavioral therapy (CBT) is the best supported treatment for this disorder. This book contains some path-breaking studies on tinnitus. It strives to provide a fair idea about this medical condition and to help develop a better understanding of the latest advances related to its assessment and management. Those in search of information to further their knowledge will be greatly assisted by this book.

This book is a result of research of several months to collate the most relevant data in the field.

When I was approached with the idea of this book and the proposal to edit it, I was overwhelmed. It gave me an opportunity to reach out to all those who share a common interest with me in this field. I had 3 main parameters for editing this text:

1. Accuracy – The data and information provided in this book should be up-to-date and valuable to the readers.

2. Structure – The data must be presented in a structured format for easy understanding and better grasping of the readers.

3. Universal Approach – This book not only targets students but also experts and innovators in the field, thus my aim was to present topics which are of use to all.

Thus, it took me a couple of months to finish the editing of this book.

I would like to make a special mention of my publisher who considered me worthy of this opportunity and also supported me throughout the editing process. I would also like to thank the editing team at the back-end who extended their help whenever required.

Editor

1

A Pilot Genome-Wide Association Study Identifies Potential Metabolic Pathways Involved in Tinnitus

Annick Gilles[1,2,3]*, *Guy Van Camp*[4], *Paul Van de Heyning*[1,2] *and Erik Fransen*[4,5]

[1] *Department of Translational Neuroscience, Faculty of Medicine and Health Sciences, University of Antwerp, Wilrijk, Belgium,* [2] *University Department of Otorhinolaryngology and Head and Neck Surgery, Antwerp University Hospital, Edegem, Belgium,* [3] *Department of Human and Social Welfare, University College Ghent, Ghent, Belgium,* [4] *Center for Medical Genetics, Antwerp University Hospital and University of Antwerp, Antwerp, Belgium,* [5] *StatUa Center for Statistics, University of Antwerp, Antwerp, Belgium*

Correspondence:
Annick Gilles
annick.gilles@uza.be

Tinnitus, the perception of an auditory phantom sound in the form of ringing, buzzing, roaring, or hissing in the absence of an external sound source, is perceived by ~15% of the population and 2.5% experiences a severely bothersome tinnitus. The contribution of genes on the development of tinnitus is still under debate. The current manuscript reports a pilot Genome Wide Association Study (GWAS) into tinnitus, in a small cohort of 167 independent tinnitus subjects, and 749 non-tinnitus controls, who were collected as part of a cross-sectional study. After genotyping, imputation, and quality checking, the association between the tinnitus phenotype and 4,000,000 single-nucleotide polymorphisms (SNPs) was tested followed by gene set enrichment analysis. None of the SNPs reached the threshold for genome-wide significance ($p < 5.0e{-}8$), with the most significant SNPs, situated outside coding genes, reaching a p-value of 3.4e–7. By using the Genetic Analysis of Complex Traits (GACT) software, the percentage of the variance explained by all SNPs in the GWAS was estimated to be 3.2%, indicating that additive genetic effects explain only a small fraction of the tinnitus phenotype. Despite the lack of genome-wide significant SNPs, which is, at least in part, due to the limited sample size of the current study, evidence was found for a genetic involvement in tinnitus. Gene set enrichment analysis showed several metabolic pathways to be significantly enriched with SNPs having a low p-value in the GWAS. These pathways are involved in oxidative stress, endoplasmatic reticulum (ER) stress, and serotonin reception mediated signaling. These results are a promising basis for further research into the genetic basis of tinnitus, including GWAS with larger sample sizes and considering tinnitus subtypes for which a greater genetic contribution is more likely.

Keywords: genome-wide association study, tinnitus, heritability, GWAS, phenotype, oxidative stress, serotonin, gene set enrichment analysis

INTRODUCTION

Tinnitus is the perception of a sound which can be perceived as hissing, ringing, buzzing, or roaring in the absence of an external sound source. It is therefore often referred to as an auditory phantom sound (Eggermont and Roberts, 2004). The prevalence of tinnitus in the adult population is ~15% (Seidman and Jacobson, 1996; Gilles et al., 2012, 2013), and in 2.5% of the population, the tinnitus causes significant burden (Axelsson and Ringdahl, 1989). The evolvement of incapacitating tinnitus may lead to social isolation, anxiety, depression, sleep disorders, and concentration issues severely affecting ones quality of life (Henry et al., 2005).

The causes of tinnitus have been extensively investigated over the years. Tinnitus appears as a symptom with increasing prevalence with age. Tinnitus appears to emerge from a complex interaction between aging, diseases, auditory malfunctions, and environmental stressors. In 50% of the cases, tinnitus is attributable to otologic malfunctions (hearing loss, noise trauma, Ménière disease, vestibular schwannoma, temporomandibular junction disorder, ototoxic medications, or substances etc.) (Gilles et al., 2014). In others, the tinnitus is a result of neurologic, metabolic, and/or psychogenic disorders (Crummer and Hassan, 2004). Environmental factors increasing the chances to develop tinnitus are recreational and work-related noise exposure (Sindhusake et al., 2003; Kim et al., 2015), smoking, sleep deprivation (Park et al., 2014; Schecklmann et al., 2015), stress (Nondahl et al., 2011), smaller households (Kim et al., 2015), and obesity (Gallus et al., 2015; Martines et al., 2015) whereas high household income and moderate alcohol consumption are considered to be inversely related to tinnitus occurrence (Nondahl et al., 2011; Gallus et al., 2015).

In contrast to the largely known environmental risk factors for tinnitus, less is known about the genes involved. Many genes have been put forward for possibly underlying tinnitus susceptibility but no consensus has been reached so far. An important complicating factor is the heterogeneity in tinnitus causes and types (Sand et al., 2010; Pawelczyk et al., 2012; Elgoyhen et al., 2014; Lopez-Escamez et al., 2016). In several monogenic disorders associated with secondary chronic tinnitus, such as neurofibromatosis type II, episodic ataxia type II, osteogenesis imperfecta type I and Fabry disease, causative genes have been identified. For an overview of monogenic diseases associated with secondary tinnitus and its associated mutated genes, we refer the reader to Sand et al. (2007). The role of genetics in the more common types of primary, chronic tinnitus in a healthy population, is under debate as data on primary chronic tinnitus heritability is very limited and family and/or twin studies are mostly lacking. The study of Kvestad et al. (2010) was the first large population-based family study to provide an estimation of the relative contribution of genetic effects on the susceptibility to tinnitus. The data were collected by use of a self-report questionnaire including questions concerning tinnitus characteristics (duration, distress, frequency) and first-degree family relationships. In total, a sample of 12,294 spouses, 27,607 parent-offspring, and 11,498 siblings was used for structural equation modeling. A heritability of 11% was obtained suggesting that the involvement of genetic factors in tinnitus is rather low (Kvestad et al., 2010).

It seems unlikely that families with hereditary tinnitus are under-reported in the literature given the large number of families reported with hereditary hearing loss. Therefore, the lack of reported families showing a Mendelian pattern of inheritance, probably indicates that primary chronic tinnitus is not a single-gene disorder but rather a complex trait, controlled by complex interactions between multiple genes and environmental risk factors. In recent years, much effort has been devoted to the genetic elucidation of the genes involved in complex traits. This showed that most complex traits and diseases are highly polygenic, involving the combined action of a multitude of genetic variants, each of which having small effect sizes. Odds ratios are typically smaller than 1.1, although variants with a larger effect size (odds ratios above 1.25) have been reported (Michailidou et al., 2015). For tinnitus, the previously estimated heritability of 11% suggests that only a small fraction of the variance is due to genetic variants. However, since the heritability represents the variance accounted for by the combined effect of several genes, it cannot be excluded that the number of involved genes is limited, and that one or more major genes account for most of the heritability. A recent study provides novel insights into the genetic contribution to tinnitus. This longitudinal study in a male twin cohort investigated the genetic contribution to tinnitus revealing a ratio of 40/60% for, respectively, genetic and environmental influences. These genetic influences for tinnitus were independent of those for hearing loss (Bogo et al., 2016). Genome-wide association studies (GWAS) are the method of choice to identify the genes involved in complex diseases. In a GWAS, genotypes from many single nucleotide polymorphisms (SNPs) throughout the entire genome (often 1 million or more) are determined and tested for association with the disease status. A strong association between a particular SNP can indicate a possible role of the variant (or the gene in which it resides) in the pathophysiology of the disease. To date, more than 2000 different disease-associated variants have been identified through GWAS analysis, providing many new insights into the pathophysiology of several diseases and traits (Welter et al., 2014).

The authors of the present manuscript previously carried out a GWAS on age-related hearing impairment (ARHI) for which a highly polygenic character of ARHI was shown, with presumably no major genes involved (Fransen et al., 2015). In the ARHI dataset, 18% of the participants reported to perceive tinnitus. The aim of the current study was to gain an insight into the genetic influence of SNPs on the tinnitus phenotype using the genome-wide SNP data from the previously collected ARHI dataset.

METHODS

Ethics Approval

The collection of the original ARHI dataset was approved by the ethics committee of the University Hospital Antwerp on October 22, 2002 (file #A02-055).

Sample Collection

The local city councils in southern Antwerp (Belgium) made population registries available by which a population-based sample could be obtained. It was requested that at least three out of the four grandparents originated from Belgium which made the population ethnically homogenous. All responding subjects underwent clinical examination, otoscopy, and completed a detailed questionnaire on medical history and exposure to environmental risk factors. A list of all questions and answers used in this study is available on request.

Strict exclusion criteria were applied to exclude persons having or having had a condition that possibly leads to hearing impairment. No phenotypic inclusion criteria were used for the sample collection. Subjects with ear diseases, possible monogenic forms of hearing impairment or other major pathologies with a possible influence on hearing, were excluded. The main goal was to study healthy subjects and therefore persons with multiple hospitalizations were excluded. The extensive, complete list of exclusion criteria was previously reported (Van Eyken et al., 2006) and is provided as Supplementary Information (Supplement 1).

Pure tone audiometry was measured in all participating subjects according to the current clinical standards (ISO 8253-1, 2010) using a two-channel Interacoustics AC-40 audiometer in a soundproof booth. Air conduction thresholds were measured at 125, 250, 500 Hz, 1, 2, 4, and 8 kHz. Bone conduction thresholds were measured within the range of 250 Hz and 4 kHz.

The phenotype of tinnitus was scored in a very basic fashion using the question "Nowadays, do you ever hear noises in your head or ear(s) (tinnitus) which usually last longer than 5 min?" No further phenotyping of tinnitus was performed as this was a retrospective study to initially identify genes involved in age-related hearing impairment (Fransen et al., 2015). Noise exposure was addressed through the question "Have you ever worked for more than a year in an environment where you had to shout to an individual standing at less than a meter from you."

Collection of the study subjects was cross-sectional with no enrichment for any phenotype. However, the selection of the genotyped samples was based upon audiometric criteria as discussed in Fransen et al. (2015). In brief, the pure-tone thresholds from 250, 500, 1000, 2000, 4000, and 8000 Hz on age, age^2, and age^3 were regressed, fitting separate models for males and females. Subsequently, principal component analysis was performed on the residuals. Principal component (PC) scores for PC1, PC2, and PC3 were calculated. Since the aim was to obtain a maximal statistical power to detect genes involved in hearing loss, the phenotypically most extreme individuals for the three PC scores were selected for genotyping.

Genotyping

DNA was extracted from blood samples using standard procedures. Genomic DNA concentrations were determined with PicoGreen (Invitrogen, Carlsbad, CA, USA). Additionally, the quality of the genomic DNA was assessed for each sample by gel electrophoresis. Five-hundred DNA samples were genotyped with the Illumina CNV370 quad chip, 1060 DNA samples using the Illumina HumanOmniExpress BeadChip (Illumina, Inc., San Diego, CA, USA).

Imputation and Filtering

Pre-imputation filtering was carried out to exclude SNPs with a minor allele frequency (MAF) below 1%, a *p*-value for Hardy-Weinberg equilibrium below 1.0e–6, a call rate below 95% across all samples and across all SNPs. Duplicate samples were identified using pi-hat analysis (pi-hat > 0.99). For each of these duplicates, the sample with the lowest genotyping call rate was removed.

Imputation was performed using the program impute2, version 2.1.2 (Howie et al., 2009) with the 1000 Genomes Phase 1 Interim panel (June 2011) as reference panel. Imputation resulted in a total of 11 626 570 SNPs. An additional post-imputation filtering was carried out using the same exclusion criteria as in the pre-imputation stage, and removing imputed SNPs with an Impute2 info metric below 0.5. Gene boundaries used for mapping SNPs onto genes are: 110 kb upstream to the most extreme gene transcript start position, and 40 kb downstream to the most extreme gene transcript end position, taking gene orientation into account.

Association Analysis

Association between the tinnitus status (affected or not affected) and the common variant genotypes (MAF > 0.01) was tested using the logistic regression option in the software package PLINK v1.07. An additive model was fitted taking the affection status as a dependent variable. This analysis tests for the main effect of a SNP on the tinnitus phenotype.

The effect of SNP genotype to noise sensitivity was tested using logistic regression by fitting a model with SNP genotype, noise exposure, and their interaction. Two significance tests were carried out on this model: first the significance on the interaction term (1df-test) was tested as well as the joint significance of the SNP genotype and the interaction term (2df-test).

Heritability Estimates

The cumulative effect of all genotyped SNPs on the phenotypic variance was estimated through variance component analysis using the genomic-relatedness-based restricted maximum-likelihood (GREML) method implemented in the Genetic Analysis of Complex Traits (GACT) software (Yang et al., 2011). All SNPs that passed the quality control were included. The Genetic Relationship Matrix was estimated correcting for incomplete Linkage Disequilibrium (LD) between genotyped and causative variants. The percentage of variance explained by the SNPs is obtained as the ratio of the genetic variance to the total variance.

The presence of genome-wide gender-specific effects was tested using a likelihood ratio test, comparing the models with and without a variance component for gene-sex interaction, as implemented in GACT.

Gene Set Enrichment Analysis

Gene set enrichment analysis was performed using the software package MAGENTA (Meta-Analysis Gene-set Enrichment of varianT Associations; Segre et al., 2010). This program first expresses the significance of a whole gene as a gene score, based upon the individual *p*-values of the SNPs within the gene, adjusting for confounders (gene size, number of SNPs within the gene, amount of LD, and number of recombination hotspots within the gene). Subsequently, gene scores are combined at the level of gene sets, whereby the *p*-values of a given gene set are generated by counting the fraction of the genes within that gene set that have a gene score above a predefined enrichment cut-off. As recommended by the authors, the 75th percentile of all observed gene scores was used as enrichment cut-offs to generate the *p*-values for the individual pathways. Correction for multiple testing was performed using the False Discovery Rate (FDR) method.

Analysis was performed using the *p*-values of the GWAS, using the three tests (main effects, interaction test, and joint test) as discussed earlier. SNPs were mapped to genes using Genome build36 (hg18), using gene sets from the following databases: Gene Ontology (April 2010), PANTHER (January 2010), Ingenuity (June 2008), KEGG (2010), Reactome and BioCarta.

RESULTS

Sample Collection

All individuals in this study were recruited through population registries in a residential suburb of Antwerp, Belgium. No enrichment for any phenotype was carried out, but strict exclusion criteria were applied to exclude individuals having or having had a disease with a possible influence on hearing. A detailed list with the exclusion criteria is provided as Supplementary Data (Supplement 1). All individuals were of Belgian ancestry. In total, 2161 individuals were randomly collected in a cross-sectional way. Of these, 1560 were selected for genotyping based upon audiometric data described in Fransen et al. (2015). Of these genotyped individuals, tinnitus information was available for 916 persons (456 females and 460 males), of which 167 (18%) were reporting episodes of tinnitus lasting longer than 5 min and the remaining 749 did not. The fraction of individuals with tinnitus was significantly different between males and females. Twenty-two percent of the males in the dataset reported tinnitus, against only 15% of the females ($p = 0.006$, chi-square test; odds ratio = 1.61 with 95% confidence interval 1.15–2.27). This difference may, at least in part, be due to a difference in noise exposure: 94 of the 167 tinnitus patients reported having worked in a noisy environment for more than a year. Only 13 of them were female, vs. 81 males ($p < 0.001$, chi-square test). **Table 1** provides an overview of the characteristics of the affected and non-affected individuals in this study.

TABLE 1 | Social-demographic factors of the study population.

	Affected by tinnitus	Control	*N*
Total population	167	749	916
Belgian ethnic origin	167 (100%)	749 (100%)	
Age range	55–65	55–65	
Mean age (st. deviation)	61.2 (3.1)	61.4 (3.1)	
Number of males (%)	100 (60%)	360 (48%)	460
Noise exposure data available	164 (98%)	733 (98%)	897
Noise exposure (%)	23 (14%)	71 (10%)	897

Association Testing

All association tests were carried out on the 916 individuals with a known tinnitus status, with the 167 tinnitus patients as cases and the 749 non-tinnitus individuals as controls.

Three types of statistical tests were performed to test the effect of the SNP genotypes on tinnitus. First, the main effect of the SNPs on the phenotype was tested, via the association between tinnitus, and the genotype without accounting for noise exposure. This highlights the SNPs that lead to an increased risk for tinnitus across both noise-exposed and non-exposed individuals. Results of this analysis are shown in the table "MainEffect" (Supplement 2). None of the SNPs reached the threshold for genome-wide significance ($p < 5.0e{-}8$). The most significant SNPs reach a *p*-value of 3.4e–7. Two genes contain SNPs with a *p*-value below 1.0e–5 (VDAC1 and NKTR). The significance of the SNPs is graphically shown in a Manhattan plot in **Figure 1**, where the *p*-value is plotted vs. the chromosomal location. The SNPs within a coding gene, with a *p*-value below 1.0e–5, are shown in green.

Since it is known that noise exposure is a risk factor for tinnitus, the interaction between the SNPs and noise exposure was analyzed. This analysis would identify SNPs having a different effect on the phenotype depending on noise exposure. For instance, it could identify SNPs that render an individual susceptible to tinnitus, following noise. These SNPs would not be identified in the first analysis, as their effect on the phenotype depends on noise exposure. *P*-values for this interaction were calculated in two ways: the significance of the interaction term and the joint test for genotype and interaction with noise In general, *p*-values for the joint test are more significant than those for the interaction test, but not as significant as the *p*-values for the main effects. Genic SNPs in three genes (VDAC1, NKTR, and COG3) reach a *p*-value below 1.0e–5 for the joint test, as highlighted in the Manhattan plots (**Figures 2, 3**).

Tables with results are provided as Supplementary Materials (Supplement 2). These tables have been sorted by *p*-value (most significant value on top), and show the SNPs with a *p*-value below 0.0001. The far right column ("ANNOT") shows the gene in which the SNP is located. If the SNP is further than 110 kb upstream the most extreme gene transcript start site of a coding gene, or more than 40 kb downstream to the most extreme gene transcript end position of a coding gene, this column is empty. For each of the three significance tests (main effects, interaction test and joint test), we present two tables. The first table shows all SNPs with a *p*-value below 1e–4, whereas the second one (extension "Genic") shows the SNPs within or close to a coding gene.

Pathway Analysis

To investigate if genes, belonging to certain metabolic pathways or biological processes, were enriched in SNPs with low *p*-values, gene set enrichment analysis (GSEA) was carried out using the MAGENTA package. The analysis was performed with the results from both the main effects test, the interaction test and the joint test. Upon FDR correction for multiple testing, a total of seven pathways were significantly enriched in low *p*-values. An overview of the significant pathways is provided in **Table 2**. A complete overview is provided in the Supplementary Materials (Supplement 3).

Using GACT software, the fraction of the phenotypic variance attributable to additive genetic effects was estimated. All genotyped SNPs passing quality control had a cumulative effect

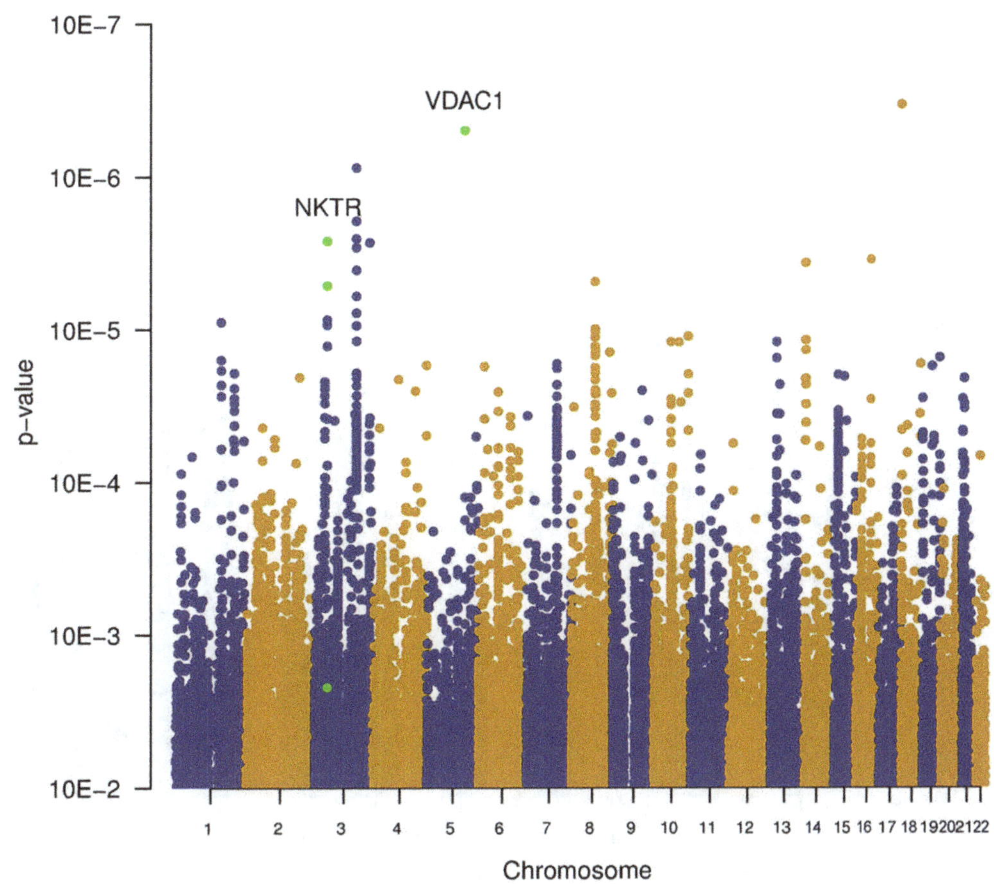

FIGURE 1 | Manhattan plot illustrating the main effect of the SNPs on the phenotype, tested via the association between tinnitus and the genotype without accounting for noise exposure. This highlights the SNPs that lead to an increased risk for tinnitus across both noise-exposed and non-exposed individuals. None of the SNPs reached the threshold for genome-wide significance ($p < 5e^{-8}$). The most significant SNPs reach a p-value of $3.4e^{-7}$. Two genes contain SNPs with a p-value below $1e^{-5}$ (VDAC1 and NKTR). These SNPs are indicated in green.

accounting for 3.2% of the phenotypic variance in the trait, with a 95% confidence interval ranging from 0 to 21%.

DISCUSSION AND CONCLUSIONS

To our knowledge, this is the first genome-wide association study on tinnitus phenotype ever performed, including 916 individuals aged between 55 and 65, consisting of 167 tinnitus cases and 749 controls. Although none of the SNPs reached the conventional threshold for genome-wide significance ($p < 5.0e-8$), and the proportion of the variance accounted for by all SNPs together is small, evidence was found for a genetic involvement in tinnitus through gene set enrichment analysis (GSEA). Throughout the three methods with which the SNPs were tested for association, seven pathways with a significant enrichment in significant SNPs emerged. On the basis of a literature search, we could not find an obvious link between tinnitus and the RAS pathway, vascular smooth muscle contraction, NDK Dynamin, and coenzyme A biosynthesis.

On the other hand, a beneficial effect of antidepressants on tinnitus has been suggested several times (Baldo et al., 2012; Beebe Palumbo et al., 2015), and this possibly involves serotonin (5HT) receptor mediated signaling pathways. Deniz et al. reported that one allelic variant of the serotonin transporter gene SLC6A4 was associated with the emotional distress associated with tinnitus (Deniz et al., 2010). Because the studies are small and often of limited quality, the results remain inconclusive at this time (Baldo et al., 2012). Moreover, since anxiety is associated with both serotonin and tinnitus (Lesch et al., 1996), it is unclear whether serotonin and tinnitus are directly associated or whether the apparent link between tinnitus and serotonin is attributable to anxiety as a confounder. The involvement of genetic variants in the serotonin mediated signaling pathways would provide a biological link between the action of antidepressants and the improvement of tinnitus (Deniz et al., 2010).

The most remarkable associations are those with endoplasmatic reticulum (ER) stress, and with the NRF2-mediated oxidative stress response. Oxidative stress plays an important role in the pathogenesis of noise-induced hearing loss and noise-induced tinnitus. Delmaghani et al. showed a direct molecular link between noise-induced hearing loss and an impaired oxidative stress defense, in a study on mice with

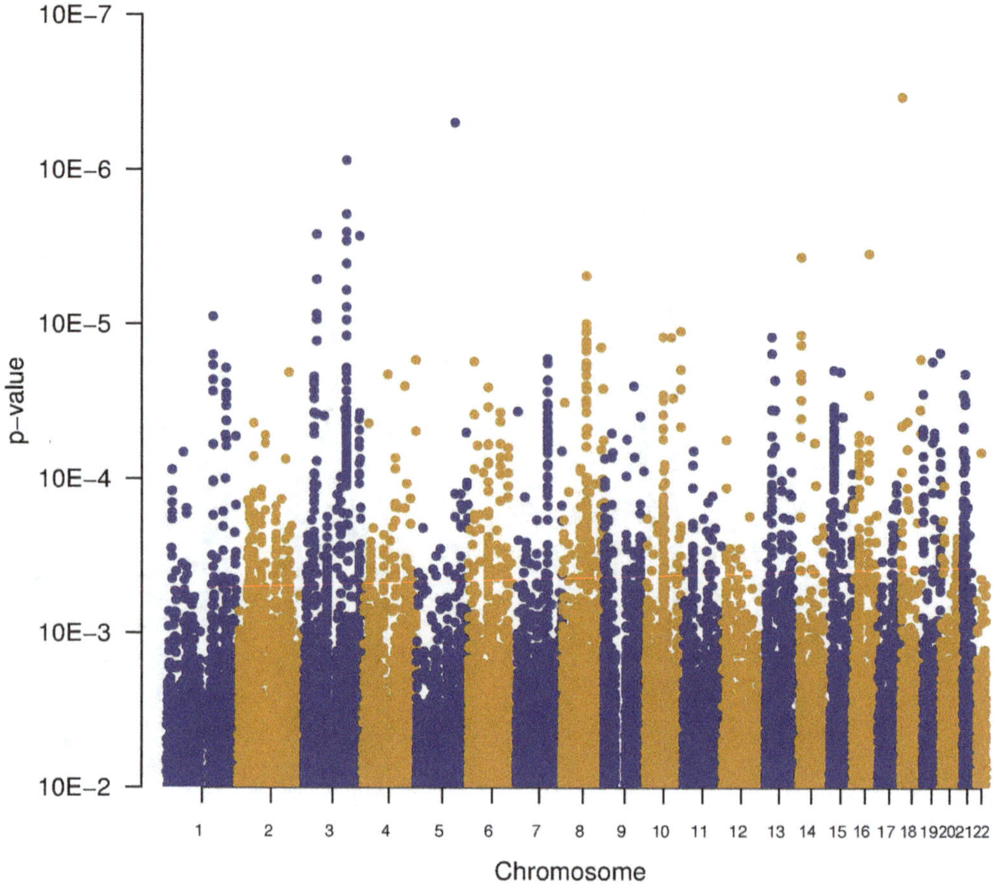

FIGURE 2 | Manhattan plot illustrating the interaction test between genotype and noise exposure. The *p*-values test if the effect of the SNP genotype on the phenotype is altered by noise exposure. This test could highlight SNPs making an individual susceptible to tinnitus, following noise exposure.

an inactivation of the Pejvakin (*Pjvk*) gene (Delmaghani et al., 2015). They showed that in regular animals, sensory cells in the inner hair respond to noise-induced oxidative stress by upregulating *Pjvk* expression. This in turns upregulates the number of peroxysomes, which defend the cell against reactive oxygen species by restoring the normal redox balance. In mice with an inactivated *Pjvk* gene, this defense mechanism against noise-induced oxidative stress was totally absent. Following noise exposure, levels of oxidative stress were significantly increased compared to normal animals, and hearing function sharply declined. A recent study showed that tinnitus patients express significantly higher total oxidant status and oxidative index levels compared to control subjects (Koç et al., 2016) which can possibly cause dysfunctions in the microcirculation of the inner ear (Neri et al., 2002, 2006). The exact role of oxidative stress in tinnitus is still under debate. However, Honkura et al. showed that NRF2 is an undeniably crucial player in the defense mechanism against noise-induced oxidative stress (Honkura et al., 2016). A significant association between an NRF2 SNP influencing expression and susceptibility for noise-induced hearing damage was shown in noise-exposed subjects. In particular a noise notch at 4 kHz was more prevalent in subjects with a low NRF2 gene expression resulting into lower antioxidant capacity. In the current study all subjects had age-related hearing impairment, which is the most common form of sensorineural hearing loss. Oxidative stress is known to play a vital role in the development of ARHI. Along the aging process progressive decline of mitochondrial function emerges resulting into increased ROS production which in turn elicits oxidative damage and dysfunction in various tissues (Wallace, 2005). With ARHI being the most frequent cause of tinnitus development, it can be argued that besides the increase in susceptibility to hearing loss, a low NRF2 expressor allele also contributes to tinnitus development.

The endoplasmatic reticulum (ER) overload response, also referred to as ER stress or the unfolding protein response (UPR), is an evolutionary conserved response of the ER to the accumulation of unfolded proteins in the ER lumen. Although the response is primarily aimed at re-establishing the normal ER function, prolonged ER stress results in cell death through apoptosis (Xu et al., 2005). Kalinec et al. showed that the previously reported ototoxicity of N-acetyl-para-aminophenol (APAP) acts through oxidative stress and the ER overload pathway in cells derived from mouse organ of Corti (Kalinec et al., 2014). ER stress has also been linked to hearing loss in cellular and animal models for noise induced and age related

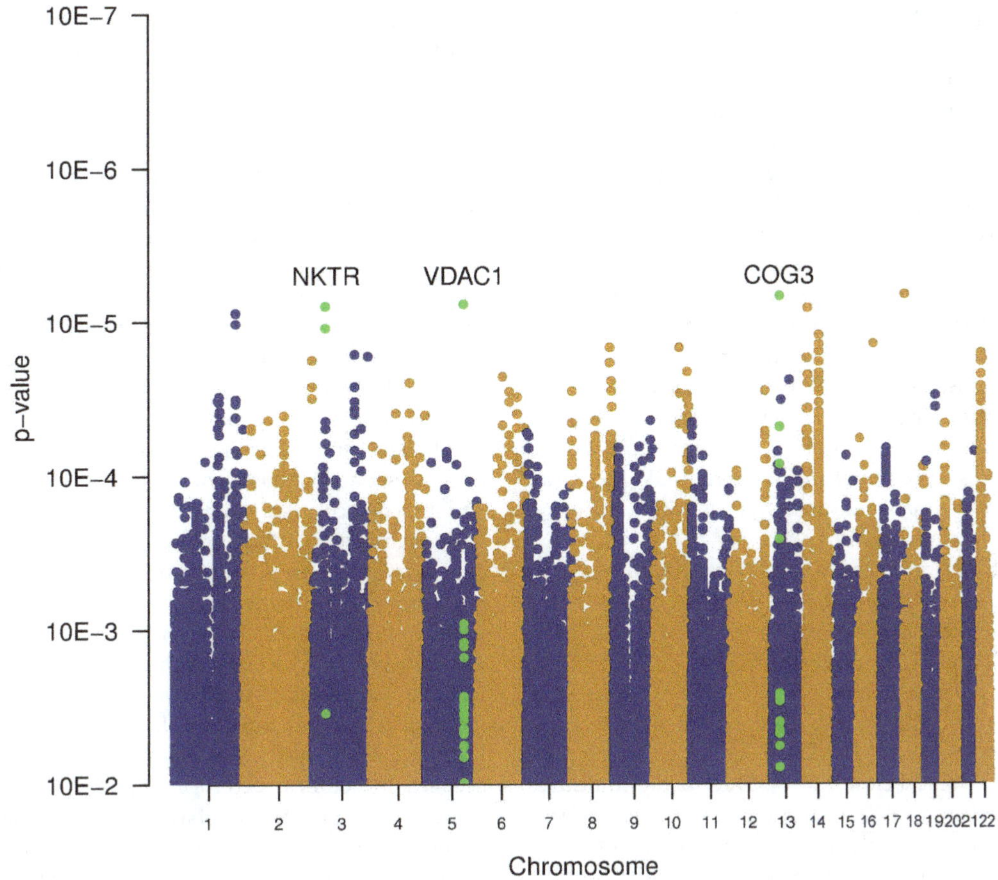

FIGURE 3 | Manhattan plot illustrating the joint test for genotype and interaction with noise. This test combines the significance of the main effect test (**Figure 1**) and the interaction test (**Figure 2**). Two genes contain SNPs with a p-value below 1e-5 (VDAC1 and NKTR). The SNPs within these genes are shown in green.

TABLE 2 | Results of Gene set enrichment analysis.

Pathway	Database	No. of genes above 75th percentile		*p*-value	
		Expected	Observed no.	Nominal	FDR-corrected
MAIN EFFECTS					
RAS	Panther	3	9	8.0 e–4	0.02
Vascular Smooth Muscle contraction	KEGG	26	43	1.0 e–4	0.03
INTERACTION TEST					
Coenzyme A biosynthesis	Panther	2	6	1.6 e–3	0.02
5HT2-type receptor mediated signaling pathway		2	6	1.4 e–3	0.03
NDK Dynamin	Biocarta	4	11	5.0 e–4	0.05
JOINT TEST					
NRF2-mediated oxidative stress response	Ingenuity	12	25	4.7 e–5	0.002
ER overload response	GOTERM	2	8	1.7 e–5	0.004

hearing loss (Van Rossom et al., 2015; Hu et al., 2016; Xue et al., 2016). ER stress was suggested to be the earliest molecular event leading to hearing loss (Hu et al., 2016), and progression could be delayed with an ER stress inhibitor.

The identification of pathways involved in tinnitus is a useful first step into a better understanding of the pathophysiology and the identification of possible drug targets. A further step would be the identification of individual SNPs associated with tinnitus, which would deepen our understanding how the symptom arises on a molecular basis. A potential follow-up study could therefore focus on genotyping SNPs in genes belonging to the pathways identified in the current study.

It is not surprising that the current study has not been able to find individual SNPs associated with tinnitus. First of all, this sample set was initially not optimized to study the genetic causes of tinnitus. It was collected as a cross-sectional study to investigate age-related hearing impairment, and no selective enrichment for tinnitus patients was carried out. The observed prevalence of 18% is in line with previously reported epidemiological studies (Axelsson and Ringdahl, 1989; Gilles et al., 2013). There was no matching for other tinnitus risk factors, although noise exposure was accounted for in the analysis stage. Hence, the current dataset had limited power to detect individual SNPs associated with tinnitus. A sensitivity analysis using the Genetic Power calculator (Purcell et al., 2003) showed that the current dataset holds 80% power to detect an allele with a genotype relative risk of 2, under an additive model, at a genome-wide significance level ($p < 5e{-}8$). Since no genome-wide significant SNPs were found in the current GWAS, it can be concluded that presumably, no major genes with a genotype relative risk of 2 or larger in tinnitus exist.

The finding of several pathways significantly enriched in significant SNPs, seems in contradiction with the lack of SNPs reaching genome-wide significance and the low heritability. The genetic signal, picked up using the GSEA, must therefore reside in the SNPs reaching a nominal, but not a genome-wide, significance level. For instance, for both the main effect test and the joint test, there are about 700 SNPs (both genic and non-genic) reaching a p-value below 1.0e–4. Due to the multitude of hypotheses tested in a GWAS, it is quite likely that a large part of these association signals represent false positives, but a fraction of the SNPs with low p-values will represent a genuine association signal. This is in line with previous studies into, amongst others, psychiatric diseases and age-related hearing loss, where the SNPs with a low p-value not reaching genome-wide significance, still hold substantial genetic information on the phenotype (International Schizophrenia Consortium et al., 2009; Fransen et al., 2015).

A very low heritability estimate was obtained through variance components analysis as implemented in GACT. This showed that the cumulative effect of all SNPs in the GWAS on the phenotype only explains 3.2% of the phenotypic variance in tinnitus. Several explanations are possible to reconcile this weak effect of genes with the presence of genetic signals through the GSEA. A first explanation is the inaccuracy of the current estimate due to the small sample size. The standard error of the estimate was 9.2%, which leads to a confidence interval for the heritability ranging from 0 to 21%. The previously reported heritability of 11% by Kvestad et al. (2010), falls within this 95% confidence interval. Moreover, the GCTA-GREML method implemented in GCTA only accounts for the additive genetic effects of the SNPs in the GWAS. The actual genetic effect may be larger due to, amongst other, rare SNPs that are not analyzed in a GWAS or SNP-SNP interactions. The combination of this very weak effect of all individual SNPs combined, with the significant results of the GSEA, seems to indicate that only a very limited number of SNPs are involved in tinnitus, but these SNPs seem to be confined in a small number of disease-associated pathways.

Although GWASs have been very successful in the identification of disease genes, the technique has its limitations. Most SNP variants genotyped in the current GWAS are common, typically with a minor allele frequency of at least 5%. The effects of low-frequency and rare SNPs are not captured. Novel techniques, such as next-generation sequencing, now allow to more thoroughly study the role of rare variants in complex diseases, and traits (Rivas et al., 2011; Gudmundsson et al., 2012). Moreover, intense research is being carried out on the role of non-coding variation in the genome. Since most SNPs identified in GWAS are located outside coding genes, and probably reside within regulatory regions, subtle alterations in gene expression level may be a major player in complex traits and diseases. However, there are very few non-coding SNPs for which the exact role in gene expression has already been elucidated.

The ideal study design, for a genetic study on tinnitus, would be a case-control dataset with an equal number of tinnitus cases and matched controls taking into account potential confounders such as anxiety, age, hearing loss, occupational/recreational noise exposure, and distress. Since most genetic effect sizes for complex traits are small, with the variance explained by a single SNP in the order of 0.1% of the phenotypic variance and genotype relative risks around 1.1, detecting such risk alleles is only feasible using massive sample sizes of 10,000 individuals, collected through large, international consortia. In addition, these studies should more carefully study the tinnitus phenotype and take into account the clinical heterogeneity of the trait. In the current study, the anamnesis was based upon one simple question in a questionnaire, without any distinction between the various subgroups of tinnitus. Tinnitus phenotype has proven to be very heterogeneous and, as such, the tinnitus phenotype in the present study was inevitably heterogeneous as well. Further improvement can be reached by construction of a standardized operation protocol to collect and phenotype tinnitus patients and controls. Limiting the tinnitus patients to certain subtypes, excluding for example somatic tinnitus for which a non-genetic etiology is likely (Lopez-Escamez et al., 2016), would increase the power of genetic studies into tinnitus.

So far no large GWAS into tinnitus has been carried out. The lack of large international studies into tinnitus genetics is possibly attributable to the general assumption that tinnitus is a symptom rather than a trait with few genetic factors involved. Interestingly, a recent longitudinal twin study (Bogo et al., 2016) estimated the proportion of additive genetic factors in tinnitus at 40%, which is substantially higher than the 11% previously estimated by Kvestad (Kvestad et al., 2010).Together with the results from the current study, the idea seems to emerge that the role of genetic factors in tinnitus is larger than initially assumed, and that the identification of SNPs involved in tinnitus is feasible if sufficiently large sample sets of well-characterized tinnitus and control subjects are collected.

AUTHOR CONTRIBUTIONS

AG wrote the manuscript, co-operated in the statistical analyses, and is the corresponding author. GV and PV were involved in the design of the study, the collecting of the original data, and reviewed the draft manuscript. EF performed statistical analyses and co-operated in writing the manuscript.

ACKNOWLEDGMENTS

The authors want to thank Geert van de Weyer for bioinformatics assistance. The current research was financially supported by a TOP-BOF scholarship of the University Antwerp.

REFERENCES

Axelsson, A., and Ringdahl, A. (1989). Tinnitus–a study of its prevalence and characteristics. *Br. J. Audiol.* 23, 53–62. doi: 10.3109/03005368909077819

Baldo, P., Doree, C., Molin, P., McFerran, D., and Cecco, S. (2012). Antidepressants for patients with tinnitus. *Cochrane Database Syst. Rev.* 12:CD003853. doi: 10.1002/14651858.CD003853.pub3

Beebe Palumbo, D., Joos, K., De Ridder, D., and Vanneste, S. (2015). The management and outcomes of pharmacological treatments for tinnitus. *Curr. Neuropharmacol.* 13, 692–700. doi: 10.2174/1570159X13666150415002743

Bogo, R., Farah, A., Karlsson, K. K., Pedersen, N. L., Svartengren, M., and Skjonsberg, A. (2016). Prevalence, incidence proportion, and heritability for tinnitus: a longitudinal twin study. *Ear Hear.* doi: 10.1097/AUD.0000000000000397. [Epub ahead of print].

Crummer, R. W., and Hassan, G. A. (2004). Diagnostic approach to tinnitus. *Am. Fam. Physician* 69, 120–126.

Delmaghani, S., Defourny, J., Aghaie, A., Beurg, M., Dulon, D., Thelen, N., et al. (2015). Hypervulnerability to sound exposure through impaired adaptive proliferation of peroxisomes. *Cell* 163, 894–906. doi: 10.1016/j.cell.2015.10.023

Deniz, M., Bayazit, Y. A., Celenk, F., Karabulut, H., Yilmaz, A., Gunduz, B., et al. (2010). Significance of serotonin transporter gene polymorphism in tinnitus. *Otol. Neurotol.* 31, 19–24. doi: 10.1097/MAO.0b013e3181c2dcbc

Eggermont, J. J., and Roberts, L. E. (2004). The neuroscience of tinnitus. *Trends Neurosci.* 27, 676–682. doi: 10.1016/j.tins.2004.08.010

Elgoyhen, A. B., Langguth, B., Nowak, W., Schecklmann, M., De Ridder, D., and Vanneste, S. (2014). Identifying tinnitus-related genes based on a side-effect network analysis. *CPT Pharmacometrics Syst. Pharmacol.* 3, e97. doi: 10.1038/psp.2013.75

Fransen, E., Bonneux, S., Corneveaux, J. J., Schrauwen, I., Di, B. F., White, C. H., et al. (2015). Genome-wide association analysis demonstrates the highly polygenic character of age-related hearing impairment. *Eur. J. Hum. Genet.* 23, 110–115. doi: 10.1038/ejhg.2014.56

Gallus, S., Lugo, A., Garavello, W., Bosetti, C., Santoro, E., Colombo, P., et al. (2015). Prevalence and determinants of tinnitus in the italian adult population. *Neuroepidemiology* 45, 12–19. doi: 10.1159/000431376

Gilles, A., De Ridder, D., Van Hal, G., Wouters, K., Kleine Punte, A., and Van de Heyning, P. (2012). Prevalence of leisure noise-induced tinnitus and the attitude toward noise in university students. *Otol. Neurotol.* 33, 899–906. doi: 10.1097/mao.0b013e31825d640a

Gilles, A., Goelen, S., and Van de Heyning, P. (2014). Tinnitus: a cross-sectional study on the audiologic characteristics. *Otol. Neurotol.* 35, 401–406. doi: 10.1097/MAO.0000000000000248

Gilles, A., Van Hal, G., De Ridder, D., Wouters, K., and Van de Heyning, P. (2013). Epidemiology of noise-induced tinnitus and the attitudes and beliefs towards noise and hearing protection in adolescents. *PLoS ONE* 8:e70297. doi: 10.1371/journal.pone.0070297

Gudmundsson, J., Sulem, P., Gudbjartsson, D. F., Masson, G., Agnarsson, B. A., Benediktsdottir, K. R., et al. (2012). A study based on whole-genome sequencing yields a rare variant at 8q24 associated with prostate cancer. *Nat. Genet.* 44, 1326–1329. doi: 10.1038/ng.2437

Henry, J. A., Dennis, K. C., and Schechter, M. A. (2005). General review of tinnitus: prevalence, mechanisms, effects, and management. *J. Speech Lang. Hear. Res.* 48, 1204–1235. doi: 10.1044/1092-4388(2005/084)

Honkura, Y., Matsuo, H., Murakami, S., Sakiyama, M., Mizutari, K., Shiotani, A., et al. (2016). NRF2 is a key target for prevention of noise-induced hearing loss by reducing oxidative damage of cochlea. *Sci. Rep.* 6:19329. doi: 10.1038/srep19329

Howie, B. N., Donnelly, P., and Marchini, J. (2009). A flexible and accurate genotype imputation method for the next generation of genome-wide association studies. *PLoS Genet.* 5:e1000529. doi: 10.1371/journal.pgen.1000529

Hu, J., Li, B., Apisa, L., Yu, H., Entenman, S., Xu, M., et al. (2016). ER stress inhibitor attenuates hearing loss and hair cell death in Cdh23erl/erl mutant mice. *Cell Death Dis.* 7, e2485. doi: 10.1038/cddis.2016.386

International Schizophrenia Consortium, Purcell, S. M., Wray, N. R., Stone, J. L., Visscher, P. M., O'Donovan, M. C., et al. (2009). Common polygenic variation contributes to risk of schizophrenia and bipolar disorder. *Nature* 460, 748–752. doi: 10.1038/nature08185

Kalinec, G. M., Thein, P., Parsa, A., Yorgason, J., Luxford, W., Urrutia, R., et al. (2014). Acetaminophen and NAPQI are toxic to auditory cells via oxidative and endoplasmic reticulum stress-dependent pathways. *Hear. Res.* 313, 26–37. doi: 10.1016/j.heares.2014.04.007

Kim, H. J., Lee, H. J., An, S. Y., Sim, S., Park, B., Kim, S. W., et al. (2015). Analysis of the prevalence and associated risk factors of tinnitus in adults. *PLoS ONE* 10:e0127578. doi: 10.1371/journal.pone.0127578

Koç, S., Akyuz, S., Somuk, B. T., Soyalic, H., Yilmaz, B., Taskin, A., et al. (2016). Paraoxonase activity and oxidative status in patients with tinnitus. *J. Audiol. Otol.* 20, 17–21. doi: 10.7874/jao.2016.20.1.17

Kvestad, E., Czajkowski, N., Engdahl, B., Hoffman, H. J., and Tambs, K. (2010). Low heritability of tinnitus: results from the second Nord-Trondelag health study. *Arch. Otolaryngol. Head Neck Surg.* 136, 178–182. doi: 10.1001/archoto.2009.220

Lesch, K. P., Bengel, D., Heils, A., Sabol, S. Z., Greenberg, B. D., Petri, S., et al. (1996). Association of anxiety-related traits with a polymorphism in the serotonin transporter gene regulatory region. *Science* 274, 1527–1531. doi: 10.1126/science.274.5292.1527

Lopez-Escamez, J. A., Bibas, T., Cima, R. F., Van de Heyning, P., Knipper, M., Mazurek, B., et al. (2016). Genetics of tinnitus: an emerging area for molecular diagnosis and drug development. *Front. Neurosci.* 10:377. doi: 10.3389/fnins.2016.00377

Martines, F., Sireci, F., Cannizzaro, E., Costanzo, R., Martines, E., Mucia, M., et al. (2015). Clinical observations and risk factors for tinnitus in a Sicilian cohort. *Eur. Arch. Otorhinolaryngol.* 272, 2719–2729. doi: 10.1007/s00405-014-3275-0

Michailidou, K., Beesley, J., Lindstrom, S., Canisius, S., Dennis, J., Lush, M. J., et al. (2015). Genome-wide association analysis of more than 120,000 individuals identifies 15 new susceptibility loci for breast cancer. *Nat. Genet.* 47, 373–380. doi: 10.1038/ng.3242

Neri, S., Mauceri, B., Cilio, D., Bordonaro, F., Messina, A., Malaguarnera, M., et al. (2002). Tinnitus and oxidative stress in a selected series of elderly patients. *Arch. Gerontol. Geriatr. Suppl.* 8, 219–223. doi: 10.1016/S0167-4943(02)00137-1

Neri, S., Signorelli, S., Pulvirenti, D., Mauceri, B., Cilio, D., Bordonaro, F., et al. (2006). Oxidative stress, nitric oxide, endothelial dysfunction and tinnitus. *Free Radic. Res.* 40, 615–618. doi: 10.1080/10715760600623825

Nondahl, D. M., Cruickshanks, K. J., Huang, G. H., Klein, B. E., Klein, R., Nieto, F. J., et al. (2011). Tinnitus and its risk factors in the Beaver Dam offspring study. *Int. J. Audiol.* 50, 313–320. doi: 10.3109/14992027.2010.551220

Park, B., Choi, H. G., Lee, H. J., An, S. Y., Kim, S. W., Lee, J. S., et al. (2014). Analysis of the prevalence of and risk factors for tinnitus in a young population. *Otol. Neurotol.* 35, 1218–1222. doi: 10.1097/mao.0000000000000472

Pawelczyk, M., Rajkowska, E., Kotylo, P., Dudarewicz, A., Van Camp, G., and Sliwinska-Kowalska, M. (2012). Analysis of inner ear potassium recycling genes as potential factors associated with tinnitus. *Int. J. Occup. Med. Environ. Health* 25, 356–364. doi: 10.2478/s13382-012-0061-3

Purcell, S., Cherny, S. S., and Sham, P. C. (2003). Genetic power calculator: design of linkage and association genetic mapping studies of complex traits. *Bioinformatics* 19, 149–150. doi: 10.1093/bioinformatics/19.1.149

Rivas, M. A., Beaudoin, M., Gardet, A., Stevens, C., Sharma, Y., Zhang, C. K., et al. (2011). Deep resequencing of GWAS loci identifies independent rare variants associated with inflammatory bowel disease. *Nat. Genet.* 43, 1066–1073. doi: 10.1038/ng.952

Sand, P. G., Langguth, B., Kleinjung, T., and Eichhammer, P. (2007). Genetics of chronic tinnitus. *Prog. Brain Res.* 166, 159–168. doi: 10.1016/S0079-6123(07)66014-2

Sand, P. G., Luettich, A., Kleinjung, T., Hajak, G., and Langguth, B. (2010). An examination of KCNE1 mutations and common variants in chronic tinnitus. *Genes* 1, 23–37. doi: 10.3390/genes1010023

Schecklmann, M., Pregler, M., Kreuzer, P. M., Poeppl, T. B., Lehner, A., Cronlein, T., et al. (2015). Psychophysiological associations between chronic tinnitus and sleep: a cross validation of tinnitus and insomnia questionnaires. *Biomed Res. Int.* 2015:461090. doi: 10.1155/2015/461090

Segre, A. V., DIAGRAM Consortium, MAGIC Investigators, Groop, L., Mootha, V. K., Daly, M. J., et al. (2010). Common inherited variation in mitochondrial genes is not enriched for associations with type 2 diabetes or related glycemic traits. *PLoS Genet.* 6:e1001058. doi: 10.1371/journal.pgen.1001058

Seidman, M. D., and Jacobson, G. P. (1996). Update on tinnitus. *Otolaryngol. Clin. North Am.* 29, 455–465.

Sindhusake, D., Golding, M., Newall, P., Rubin, G., Jakobsen, K., and Mitchell, P. (2003). Risk factors for tinnitus in a population of older adults: the blue mountains hearing study. *Ear Hear.* 24, 501–507. doi: 10.1097/01.AUD.0000100204.08771.3D

Van Eyken, E., Van Laer, L., Fransen, E., Topsakal, V., Lemkens, N., Laureys, W., et al. (2006). KCNQ4: a gene for age-related hearing impairment? *Hum. Mutat.* 27, 1007–1016. doi: 10.1002/humu.20375

Van Rossom, S., Op de Beeck, K., Hristovska, V., Winderickx, J., and Van Camp, G. (2015). The deafness gene DFNA5 induces programmed cell death through mitochondria and MAPK-related pathways. *Front. Cell. Neurosci.* 9:231. doi: 10.3389/fncel.2015.00231

Wallace, D. C. (2005). A mitochondrial paradigm of metabolic and degenerative diseases, aging, and cancer: a dawn for evolutionary medicine. *Annu. Rev. Genet.* 39, 359–407. doi: 10.1146/annurev.genet.39.110304.095751

Welter, D., MacArthur, J., Morales, J., Burdett, T., Hall, P., Junkins, H., et al. (2014). The NHGRI GWAS Catalog, a curated resource of SNP-trait associations. *Nucleic Acids Res.* 42, D1001–D1006. doi: 10.1093/nar/gkt1229

Xu, C., Bailly-Maitre, B., and Reed, J. C. (2005). Endoplasmic reticulum stress: cell life and death decisions. *J. Clin. Invest.* 115, 2656–2664. doi: 10.1172/JCI26373

Xue, Q., Li, C., Chen, J., Guo, H., Li, D., and Wu, X. (2016). The Protective effect of the endoplasmic reticulum stress-related factors BiP/GRP78 and CHOP/Gadd153 on noise-induced hearing loss in guinea pigs. *Noise Health* 18, 247–255. doi: 10.4103/1463-1741.192481

Yang, J., Lee, S. H., Goddard, M. E., and Visscher, P. M. (2011). GCTA: a tool for genome-wide complex trait analysis. *Am. J. Hum. Genet.* 88, 76–82. doi: 10.1016/j.ajhg.2010.11.011

2

Variable Effects of Acoustic Trauma on Behavioral and Neural Correlates of Tinnitus in Individual Animals

Ryan J. Longenecker* and Alexander V. Galazyuk

Department of Anatomy and Neurobiology, Northeast Ohio Medical University, Rootstown, OH, USA

***Correspondence:**
Ryan J. Longenecker
rlongenecker@neomed.edu

The etiology of tinnitus is known to be diverse in the human population. An appropriate animal model of tinnitus should incorporate this pathological diversity. Previous studies evaluating the effect of acoustic over exposure (AOE) have found that animals typically display increased spontaneous firing rates and bursting activity of auditory neurons, which often has been linked to behavioral evidence of tinnitus. However, only a subset of studies directly associated these neural correlates to individual animals. Furthermore, the vast majority of tinnitus studies were conducted on anesthetized animals. The goal of this study was to test for a possible relationship between tinnitus, hearing loss, hyperactivity and bursting activity in the auditory system of individual unanesthetized animals following AOE. Sixteen mice were unilaterally exposed to 116 dB SPL narrowband noise (centered at 12.5 kHz) for 1 h under ketamine/xylazine anesthesia. Gap-induced prepulse inhibition of the acoustic startle reflex (GPIAS) was used to assess behavioral evidence of tinnitus whereas hearing performance was evaluated by measurements of auditory brainstem response (ABR) thresholds and prepulse inhibition PPI audiometry. Following behavioral assessments, single neuron firing activity was recorded from the inferior colliculus (IC) of four awake animals and compared to recordings from four unexposed controls. We found that AOE increased spontaneous activity in all mice tested, independently of tinnitus behavior or severity of threshold shifts. Bursting activity did not increase in two animals identified as tinnitus positive (T+), but did so in a tinnitus negative (T−) animal with severe hearing loss (SHL). Hyperactivity does not appear to be a reliable biomarker of tinnitus. Our data suggest that multidisciplinary assessments on individual animals following AOE could offer a powerful experimental tool to investigate mechanisms of tinnitus.

Keywords: gap-induced prepulse inhibition of the acoustic startle reflex, prepulse audiometry, single unit recording, inferior colliculus, tinnitus, hearing loss

---

Abbreviations: AMPA, α-amino-3-hydroxy-5-methyl-4-isoxazolepropionic acid receptors; ANOVA, analysis of variance; AOE, acoustic over exposure; Arc, activity-regulated cytoskeletal immediate early gene; ASR, acoustic startle reflex; CV, coefficient of variation; GAP, Gap + Startle; GPIAS, gap-induced prepulse inhibition of the acoustic startle reflex; HB, high bursting activity; HL, Hearing Loss; IC, inferior colliculus; ISI, inter spike interval; ITI, inter trial interval; LB, low bursting activity; LSD, least significant difference *post hoc* test; mGluRs, metabotropic glutamate receptors; NB, no bursting activity; NMDA, N-methyl-D-aspartate receptors; NoHL, no hearing loss; PPI, prepulse inhibition; SHL, Severe Hearing Loss; SO, startle only; T+, tinnitus positive; T−, tinnitus negative.

INTRODUCTION

Tinnitus, the perception of sound in the absence of an external sound source, is often developed after acoustic over exposure (AOE; Hoffman and Reed, 2004; Møller, 2011; Baguley et al., 2013). Animal studies have shown that AOE leads to cochlear damage and subsequent threshold shifts (Liberman and Kiang, 1978; Kujawa and Liberman, 2009). Following this damage, the central auditory system increases its gain to compensate for the reduced sensorineural input from the cochlea, which can lead to tinnitus (Salvi et al., 2000; Schaette and McAlpine, 2011; Auerbach et al., 2014). In most clinical cases, there is a strong correlation between hearing loss and tinnitus (Lockwood et al., 2002), but interestingly, this is not always true, as some patients with clinically normal thresholds have tinnitus (Weisz et al., 2006; Job et al., 2007). Just as in humans (Hall et al., 2016), the extent of peripheral damage and central plasticity in individual animals of the AOE model differs greatly, leading to a heterogeneous population of hearing loss (HL) and/or tinnitus pathology (Longenecker and Galazyuk, 2011; Singer et al., 2013; Hickox and Liberman, 2014; Knipper et al., 2015).

Ever since the first animal model of tinnitus (Jastreboff et al., 1988), research has focused on being able to separate animals into T+ and T− groups to reach conclusions concerning the underlying pathology related to AOE. Following AOE animals typically demonstrate increased spontaneous firing, bursting, and neural synchrony at multiple levels of the central auditory system (see Roberts et al., 2010; Kaltenbach, 2011; Wang et al., 2011). Recordings form anesthetized animals have revealed coincidence of hyperactivity and increased burst firing in the cochlear nucleus (Kaltenbach and Afman, 2000; Chang et al., 2002; Brozoski and Bauer, 2005; Finlayson and Kaltenbach, 2009; Pilati et al., 2012), inferior colliculus (IC; Wang et al., 1996; Ma et al., 2006; Bauer et al., 2008; Coomber et al., 2014), medial geniculate body (Kalappa et al., 2014), and auditory cortex (Syka and Rybalko, 2000; Noreña and Eggermont, 2003). It is thought that hyperactivity could manifest as the phantom sound of tinnitus (Gerken, 1996; Salvi et al., 2000; Eggermont and Roberts, 2004). In contrast to many of these pioneer works, recent studies have found that hyperactivity is not always linked to tinnitus because only a fraction of animals in these studies exhibited behavioral signs of tinnitus after AOE (Ropp et al., 2014: Coomber et al., 2014). Similarly, increased bursting activity was elevated in the IC of all noise-exposed guinea pigs, but there was no difference found between T+ and T− groups (Coomber et al., 2014). However, excluding hyperactivity and increased bursting as neural correlates of tinnitus would be inappropriate because there is no compelling evidence that these abnormalities are absent in T+ animals. It is possible that more than one, or a specific combination of these neural correlates is required for tinnitus percept.

The vast majority of tinnitus studies have been conducted on anesthetized animals, which might alter experimental results and lead to erroneous conclusions. Ketamine, perhaps the most used anesthetic drug in animals, is known to affect many molecular targets which include: disrupting N-methyl-D-aspartate (NMDA) receptors, Ih currents, nicotinic acetyl-choline channels, nitric oxide, α-amino-3-hydroxy-5-methylisoxazole-4-propionic acid (AMPA) receptors, and metabotropic glutamate receptors (mGluRs; Sleigh et al., 2014). Ketamine also has long-term effects on suppression of many immediate early genes, NMDA receptor phosphorylation, and reduced astrocyte and microglial function (Sleigh et al., 2014). While awake recordings can be challenging, the data gathered from the relatively unaltered nervous system might elucidate new information about the neural correlates of tinnitus.

In the present study, we investigate the effects of AOE on behavioral hearing thresholds, auditory brainstem response (ABR) thresholds, and behavioral signs of tinnitus assessed by gap-induced prepulse inhibition of the acoustic startle reflex (GPIAS) on 16 CBA/CaJ mice. To investigate several suspected neural correlates of tinnitus in detail, we performed single unit recordings in 4 mice out of the 16 behaviorally tested mice. To eliminate a possible effect of anesthesia, all single unit recordings were performed in awake animals. We found that each of the four animals studied in depth demonstrated a unique phenotype following near-identical AOE. All of these mice showed some degree of increase spontaneous activity, while only one showed increased burst firing. While results should be considered in light of the small sample size presented here, future tinnitus studies might benefit from studying individual animals to elucidate the neural mechanisms of tinnitus.

MATERIALS AND METHODS

Subjects

A total of 20 male CBA/CBJ mice were used. Sixteen mice were used for the experimental group which included behavioral testing pre exposure and 3–4 months post exposure. Four mice from the experimental group were randomly selected for single unit recordings. The remaining four mice were also used for single unit recordings as controls (age-matched, without AOE). Mice were obtained from Jackson Laboratories, Bar Harbor, ME, USA and were approximately 12 weeks old with a mean weight of 27.5 g at the beginning of behavioral testing. Mice were housed in pairs within a colony room with a 12-h light–dark cycle at 25°C. Procedures used in this study were approved by the Institutional Animal Care and Use Committee at the Northeast Ohio Medical University.

Acoustic Trauma

Sixteen mice were anesthetized with an intraperitioneal injection of a ketamine/xylazine mixture (100/10 mg/kg). Mice were at least 5 months old at the time of exposure. An additional injection (50% of the initial dose) was given intramuscularly 30 min after the initial injection. Mice were exposed to a one octave band noise centered at 12.5 kHz (~8–17 kHz) unilaterally for 1 h. This noise was generated using a waveform generator (Wavetek model 395), amplified (Sherwood RX-4109) to 116 dB Sound Pressure Level (SPL), and played through a loudspeaker (Fostex FT17H). The output of the loudspeaker was calibrated with a 0.25-inch microphone (Brüel and Kjaer, 4135) and found to be ±4 dB between 10 and 60 kHz. The left external ear canal was obstructed with a cotton plug and a Kwik-Sil silicone elastomer plug (World Precision Instruments), a manipulation which typically reduces sound levels by 30–50 dB SPL (Turner et al., 2006; Ropp et al., 2014).

Auditory Brainstem Response (ABR) Thresholds

Mice were anesthetized with ketamine/xylazine. ABR thresholds were obtained by presenting tone bursts at 4, 12.5, 16, 20, 25 and 31.5 kHz at increasing sound intensities ranging from 10–80 dB SPL in 10 dB steps. Tones were 5 ms in duration, with 0.5 ms rise/fall time and delivered at the rate of 50/s. ABR thresholds were obtained before, directly following, and 3 months after acoustic trauma. Sterile stainless-steel electrodes were placed subdermally, one behind the right pinna of the sound exposed ear and the other along the vertex. The unexposed ear was obstructed with a cotton plug. Evoked potentials were averaged over 300 repetitions. These potentials were amplified (Dagan 2400A preamplifier), filtered (100–3,000 Hz bandpass), digitized (HEKA Elektronik), and stored on a computer hard drive. Thresholds, the smallest sound amplitude that evoked a visible ABR, were determined by visually examining the averaged ABR waveforms in response to every sound frequency presented at different sound levels.

Behavioral Assessments of Tinnitus and Hearing Loss

Prior to exposure, the 16 experimental mice were behaviorally tested with GPIAS and prepulse inhibition (PPI) to obtain baseline values for gap detection and hearing thresholds. Mice were assessed for tinnitus/threshold shifts 3 months after exposure. Four mice were randomly selected to highlight the importance of individual differences.

Acoustic Startle Hardware/Software

The equipment used to collect all acoustic startle reflex (ASR) data has been described in detail previously (Longenecker and Galazyuk, 2012). Briefly, commercial hardware/software equipment from Kinder Scientific, Inc. Poway, CA, USA was used. Each behavioral testing station was lined with anechoic foam to prevent sound reflection and wave cancelling sound echoes (Sonex foam from Pinta Acoustics, Minneapolis, MN, USA). Mice restrainers were open walled to allow for maximum sound penetration (Figure 3 in Longenecker and Galazyuk, 2012). Background sound levels within each testing chamber were calibrated with a 0.25-inch microphone (Brüel and Kjaer 4135) attached to a measuring amplifier (Brüel and Kjaer 2525) and found to be less than 40 dB SPL between 4 and 60 kHz. Startle waveforms were recorded using load-cell platforms which measure actual force changes during an animal's startle. Each load cell was calibrated with a 100 g weight which corresponds to 1 newton of force. Offline waveform analysis converted these forces into animals' center of mass displacement (in mm; Grimsley et al., 2015).

Startle Waveform Identification and Measurement

All waveforms collected during testing sessions were analyzed offline using a recently developed automatic method of startle waveform identification via a template matching paradigm (Grimsley et al., 2015). In this study, we used high-speed video recordings (1,000 frames/s) to visualize animal startles in order to identify stereotyped waveforms associated with a startle. This allowed us to develop custom software which automatically separates data into either startles or non-startle-related movements. Based on this separation, we have only included trials that resulted in successful startle responses in our data analysis. We also used a mathematical approach to normalize startle response magnitudes of individual animals to their body mass (Grimsley et al., 2015). This mathematical conversion allows legitimate comparisons between animals of different mass.

GPIAS for Tinnitus Assessment

The ability of mice to detect a gap of silence preceding the startle stimulus was determined using a startle stimulus presented alone (startle only: SO) and a startle stimulus paired with a gap (Gap + startle: GAP) both embedded into continuous background noise. The gap had a 20 ms duration and 1 ms rise/fall time. Background for all these trials was presented as a narrow band (1/3 octave) noise centered at six different frequencies (8, 10, 12.5, 16, 20 and 25 kHz). This background noise level was constant (65 dB SPL) throughout the session. The startle stimulus was presented at 105 dB SPL (white noise, 1 ms rise/fall, 20 ms duration). The gap was presented 100 ms before (onset to onset) the startle stimulus. The testing session started with an acclimation period lasting 3 min. Immediately afterwards, animals received five SO trials in order to habituate their startle responses to a steady state level. For each of six background frequencies, we presented five SO trials and five GAP trials. The SO and GAP trials were pseudo-randomized. The inter-trial intervals were also pseudo-randomized between 7 and 15 s. After we completed testing all six background frequencies, the entire session was repeated two more times. Thus, during this testing for each background frequency we obtained 15 data points for both the SO and GAP trials.

Tinnitus was classified in the same way as in previous studies (Longenecker and Galazyuk, 2011; Dehmel et al., 2012; Coomber et al., 2014). A two-way repeated measures analysis of variance (ANOVA) was applied to the behavioral data to determine whether there were any significant changes ($p < 0.05$) in gap detection levels before vs. 3 months after exposure. A Least Significant Difference (LSD) *post hoc* test was used to determine the specific frequency of any deficits. Importantly, this allowed each animal to act as its own control. Mice that exhibited a significant reduction in gap detection ability at one or two background frequencies after noise exposure were categorized as "tinnitus positive" (T+) animals while those that did not were assigned to a "tinnitus negative" (T−) group.

PPI Audiometry for Hearing Assessments

PPI audiometry was described in detail previously (Longenecker et al., 2016), and heavily relied on the advanced startle waveform analysis mentioned above (Grimsley et al., 2015). Hearing thresholds assessed by PPI audiometry were conducted at the same experimental epochs as GPIAS tests to ensure behavioral data were comparable and relevant. Testing sessions contained two types of stimuli. The SO stimulus was identical to the GPIAS tests except it was presented at 100 dB SPL. The second stimulus type consisted of a congruent startle stimulus preceded by a prepulse. Prepulse stimuli were 20 ms pure tones with a 1 ms rise/fall time presented at six different frequencies (4, 12.5, 16, 20, 25 and 31.5 kHz) 100 ms before the startle stimulus. Prepulses were presented pseudo-randomized by intensity (10–80 dB SPL, 10 dB step) for each sound frequency (each frequency was one block of testing; six blocks total). Each frequency/intensity combination was presented 39 times. SOs were pseudo-randomly mixed throughout each testing session. In each session, the magnitudes of the SOs were compared to the magnitudes of startles preceded by prepulses with various frequencies and intensities. A significant reduction in the magnitude of the startle response by the prepulse compared to the SO was defined as the prepulse detection threshold.

Identifying this threshold involved several steps. First, we examined the distribution of the raw startle magnitudes. Startle magnitude is known to be quite variable in mice, and indeed the startle magnitude typically was strongly positively skewed. This positive skew could allow aberrantly high values to obscure reliable changes in startle magnitude across stimulus parameters. Furthermore, a normal distribution of magnitudes is an assumption underlying the method for threshold determination that we use here. Thus we transformed the data (Tukey, 1977). A square root transform was found to best generate a normal distribution of startle responses within each trial type, as assessed using the Anderson-Darling test. This standard statistical transform reduces skew by enhancing the lesser and reducing the larger startle magnitudes. Second, for each animal, the transformed SO data was bootstrapped to determine 95% confidence intervals for the SO response magnitudes. Then we calculated medians of transformed magnitudes for each frequency and intensity, as the median value is a better measure of central tendency than the mean for skewed distributions. For each frequency, a detection function was calculated by fitting a cubic spline from the median transformed SO magnitude through the median transformed magnitudes for prepulses presented at various intensities. Detection threshold was defined as the sound level at which the fitted detection function crossed the lower 95% confidence interval.

Each animal was classified as having hearing loss (HL), severe hearing loss (SHL), or no hearing loss (NoHL) based on the number of frequencies at which PPI thresholds were elevated. HL was defined as at least a 30 dB threshold increase in at least two frequencies, while SHL was similarly defined, but with more than two frequencies affected. These classifications can be seen in **Figure 2**.

Electrophysiological Recordings

Surgery

Four mice from the control and four mice from the sound exposed groups were used for extracellular recordings. Each mouse was anesthetized using isoflurane (1.5–2.0%) prior to surgery. A midline incision of the skin over the cranium was made. The tissue overlying the skull then was removed and a small metal rod was glued to the skull using glass ionomer cement (3 M ESPE, Germany). Following 2 days of recovery, each mouse was trained to stay inside a small plastic tube, to be used as a holding device during recording sessions. The metal rod on the head of the mouse was secured to a small holder designed to restrain the head of the animal without causing distress, while the ears were unobstructed for free-field acoustic stimulation.

Extracellular IC Recordings

Recordings were made from both the ipsi- and contra-lateral IC (compared to the side of exposure) in awake mice inside a single-walled sound attenuating chamber (Industrial Acoustics Company, Inc., North Aurora, IL, USA). Throughout the recording session (2–3 h), the animal was offered water periodically and monitored for signs of discomfort. After a recording session, the exposed skull was covered with sterile bone wax and the animal was returned to its holding cage. Experiments were conducted every day for 6 days after which the animal was sacrificed with an IP injection of FatalPlus. No sedative drugs were used during recording sessions. If the animal showed any signs of discomfort, the recording session was terminated and the mouse was returned to its cage.

Recording electrodes were inserted through a small (50 μm) hole drilled in the skull and dura overlying the IC. Extracellular single-unit recordings were made with quartz glass micropipettes (10–20 MΩ impedance, 2–3 μm tip) filled with 0.5 M sodium acetate. The electrode was positioned into the drilled hole by means of a precision (1 μm) digital micromanipulator using a surgical microscope (Leica MZ9.5). The relative position of each electrode was monitored from the readouts of digital micrometers using a common reference point on the skull.

Extracellular recordings were limited to the central nucleus of the IC based on the depth of recordings. Vertical advancement of the electrode was made by a precision piezoelectric microdrive (Model 660, KOPF Instruments) from outside the sound-attenuating chamber. Recorded action potentials were amplified (Dagan 2400A preamplifier), monitored audio-visually on a digital oscilloscope (DL1640, YOKOGAWA), digitized and then stored on a computer hard drive using EPC-10 digital interface and PULSE software from HEKA Elektronik at a bandwidth of 100 kHz.

The search stimulus consisted of a train of tone bursts (20 ms duration, 5–50 kHz, 5 kHz step). This train was repeated while the recording electrode was advanced in 3 μm steps. To ensure that the sample of neurons we recorded was unbiased based on frequency tuning, the characteristic frequency of recorded neurons was assessed manually by presenting tone pips 100 ms in duration using a wide range of sound frequencies (4–50 kHz, 2 kHz step) and different sound levels (20, 40, 60 dB SPL). The spontaneous rate (SR) of neuronal firing was assessed during a 40 s recording (without stimulus). No sound-evoked recordings are reported.

RESULTS

Behavioral Signs of Tinnitus After Sound Exposure

Behavioral assessments using GPIAS methodology were conducted on 16 mice before vs. 3 months after sound exposure. Six of 16 mice developed significant gap detection deficits at frequencies between 12.5 and 25 kHz. Since gap detection deficits have been associated with tinnitus (see Galzyuk and Hébert, 2015), these mice constituted the T+ group. The remaining 10 mice did not show gap detection deficits and they were considered as T−. Data from two representative mice from each group are shown in **Figure 1**. Comparison of the gap detection performance before vs. 3 months after exposure with a repeated measures ANOVA indicated a significant effect of AOE in mouse #13 ($F_{(1,75)} = 666.11$, $p < 0.001$) and mouse #1 ($F_{(1,61)} = 661.73$, $p < 0.001$). A LSD *post hoc* test revealed a frequency-specific deficit at 20 kHz for mouse #13 ($p = 0.05$) and 16 kHz for mouse #1 ($p = 0.012$). Two representative mice from T− group (#10 and #12) did show significant overall differences in gap detection performance before vs. 3 months after exposure (mouse #10 ($F_{(1,57)} = 326.40$, $p > 0.001$); mouse #12 ($F_{(1,50)} = 435.22$, $p > 0.001$), but LSD *post hoc* tests did not reveal any frequency specific differences (**Figure 1**). When data from all six T+ mice were averaged, a significant effect of exposure was seen ($F_{(1,30)} = 1562.12$, $p < 0.000$). However, LSD *post hoc* tests did not determine any specific tinnitus frequencies, although the deficits at 16 kHz were close to significance ($p = 0.053$). The 10 animals determined to be T− did not show any significant gap detection deficits after exposure, but interestingly, did tend (not significant) to demonstrate improved gap detection performance at frequencies above the sound exposure.

Effect of Sound Exposure on Hearing Performance

Hearing thresholds assessed by PPI audiometry revealed inter-animal differences in the severity of threshold shifts in AOE mice (**Figure 2**), and each animal was classified based on the criteria explained above in "PPI Audiometry for Hearing Assessments" Section. Threshold elevations were seen in 13 of the 16 exposed mice. Six of these 16 mice showed narrowband frequency deficits. Examples of this type of deficit are shown in mouse #13 (at 25 kHz) and mouse #1 (at 16 kHz) in **Figure 2**. Seven out of 16 mice exhibited severe deficits spanning a wider frequency range. A representative mouse from this population (mouse #10) showed elevated thresholds from 12.5 kHz to 25 kHz (**Figure 2**). Finally, 3 out of 16 mice did not show PPI audiometric threshold changes after noise exposure (**Figure 2**, representative mouse #12). When animals were grouped together by T+ and T− classifications (as in **Figure 1**), differences in threshold elevations were observed (**Figure 2**). The T+ group demonstrated increased thresholds following sound exposure ($F_{(1,30)} = 316.56$, $p < 0.001$), LSD *post hoc* tests showed a significant threshold shift only at 16 kHz ($p = 0.01$). The T− group by comparison demonstrated further exaggerated thresholds after sound exposure ($F_{(1,54)} = 385.37$, $p < 0.001$). This group of mice, which comprised more animals with the "SHL" classification, showed significant threshold increases at 12.5 kHz ($p = 0.035$), 16 kHz ($p = 0.003$), 20 kHz ($p < 0.001$) and 25 kHz ($p < 0.001$).

ABRs were collected to serve as a control for PPI hearing assessments following sound exposure (**Figure 3**), however these measures were compared extensively in our previous work (Longenecker et al., 2016). Thresholds of the T+ group nearly returned to baseline levels 3 months following exposure, with an average increase across frequencies of 6.11 dB SPL ($F_{(1,30)} = 478.47$, $p < 0.001$). *Post hoc* LSD tests revealed that only 31.5 kHz significantly differed from control levels ($p = 0.021$), with a 13.33 dB SPL shift. These results contrasted ABR threshold shifts from the T− group, which as mentioned previously, encompassed more animals determined to have SHL measure by PPI. This group showed an average threshold increase of 7.33 dB SPL across frequencies after exposure ($F_{(1,54)} = 1366.24$, $p < 0.001$). Specific deficits were seen at 12.5 kHz ($p = 0.037$), 16 kHz ($p = 0.001$), 20 kHz ($p = 0.001$), and 25 kHz ($p = 0.001$). Not surprisingly, the range of frequencies showing a deficit with ABR (**Figure 3**) closely followed the deficits seen by PPI audiometry (**Figure 2**), although ABR deficits were not nearly as pronounced.

Increased Spontaneous Activity Following Sound Exposure

To determine how spontaneous firing rates of IC neurons changed for each behavioral AOE outcome single unit recordings were conducted in awake mice. Behavioral AOE outcomes included classifications for T+ and T− groups as well as the severity of hearing loss (based on number of elevated thresholds; 0 = NoHL; 1–2 = HL; 3–6 = SHL). Spontaneous activity from 118 neurons recorded in four control (unexposed) mice was compared to the activity of 384 neurons in the four exposed mice described above. In the exposed mice, the ipsi- and contra-lateral ICs were considered separately in an attempt to differentiate the possible effects of unilateral sound exposure. A one-way ANOVA was used to compare spontaneous firing rates of IC neurons between control and exposed (both ipsi and contra exposed IC's) mice ($F_{(500,8)} = 5.34$, $p < 0.001$; **Figure 4**). The Tukey HSD *post hoc* tests revealed significant increases in neural firing rates following sound trauma in the following IC's: #13contra ($p < 0.001$), #13ipsi ($p = 0.012$), #10contra ($p = 0.043$), #1ipsi ($p = 0.030$). Although not all statistically significant, seven

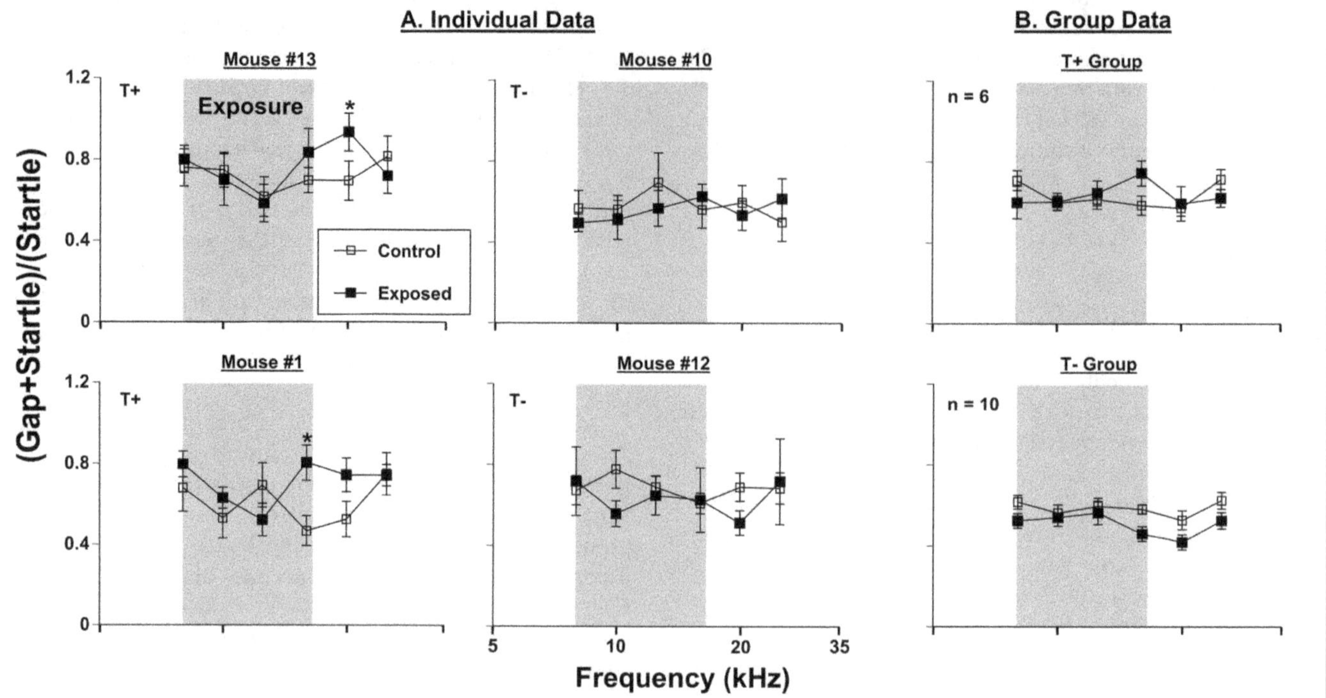

FIGURE 1 | Gap-induced prepulse inhibition of the acoustic startle reflex (GPIAS) assessment for tinnitus. (A) Four individual mice were tested before (control) and 3 months (exposed 3M) after sound exposure. **(B)** Group GPIAS data for T+ mice (n = 6) and T− mice (n = 10), in the same conditions as **(A)**. The narrow band exposure stimulus is represented by a gray box. Data are represented by ratio means and standard errors. Tinnitus was identified as a significant (*) difference between control and exposed conditions. Tinnitus positive and negative mice are labeled as (T+) and (T−), respectively.

out of eight ICs demonstrated increased mean spontaneous rates. Interestingly, mouse #10's ipsilateral IC demonstrated a non-significant slight decrease in activity compared to control rates (p = 1.00), however, the ipsi IC had significantly higher neural firing rates than the contralateral IC ($t_{(64)}$ = 6.23, $p < 0.001$).

Effect of Sound Exposure on Burst Firing in IC Neurons

To determine the effect of sound exposure on bursting activity in IC neurons, the spontaneous firing of 118 neurons from control (unexposed) mice and 384 neurons from exposed mice was analyzed and compared. These are the same pool of neurons that have been used for assessing spontaneous firing rate changes described above.

Bursting activity has been linked to tinnitus-like behavior in many studies (review by Wang et al., 2011). In our study, we adopted the following burst classifications from Bauer et al. (2008) to define a bursting event: (1) maximum allowable burst duration: 310 ms; (2) maximum ISI at burst start: 500 ms; (3) maximum within-burst ISI: 10 ms; (4) minimum interval between bursts: 50 ms; (5) minimum burst duration: 5 ms; and (6) minimum number of spikes comprising a burst: 2 ms. The distribution of burst firing neurons (**Figure 5**) was not bimodal as determined by the Kolmogorov-Smirnov test of normality ($D_{(178)}$ = 0.176, $p < 0.001$). However, if the data were separated into low bursting and high bursting units at the 35% mark, the two divisions became normally distributed (Low Bursting (LB): $D_{(53)}$ = 0.97, p = 0.09; High Bursting (HB): $D_{(48)}$ = 0.106, p = 0.20; **Figure 5**). Neurons with no bursting (NB) were not include in this distribution. Therefore, we developed a new classification system to further separate bursting activity into three categories: high bursting, low bursting, or non-bursting based on the percentage of total spikes within each bursting event (**Figure 5**).

The percentage of units exhibiting bursting activity was plotted based on the degree of bursting activity (**Figure 6**). In control, unexposed mice, 31% of neurons demonstrated bursting activity (24% LB, 7% HB), while 69% of the neurons did not show bursting activity. This observation is similar to the bursting rate distributions found in sound exposed guinea pigs (Coomber et al., 2014). The percentage of bursting neurons in mouse #13, #1, and #12 were similar to the control (unexposed) distribution. Furthermore, the differences between ipsi- and contralateral IC's were surprisingly small. In contrast, mouse #10 demonstrated a unique change in bursting activity following sound exposure. Eighty-three percentage of the neurons in the ipsilateral IC of this mouse showed some degree of bursting activity (55% LB, 28% HB). Interestingly, the contralateral IC of mouse #10 had only 19% of its neurons displaying bursting, which was the lowest value among all IC's tested.

To quantify changes in bursting activity, we applied the coefficient of variation (CV) analysis, a statistic that is derived by

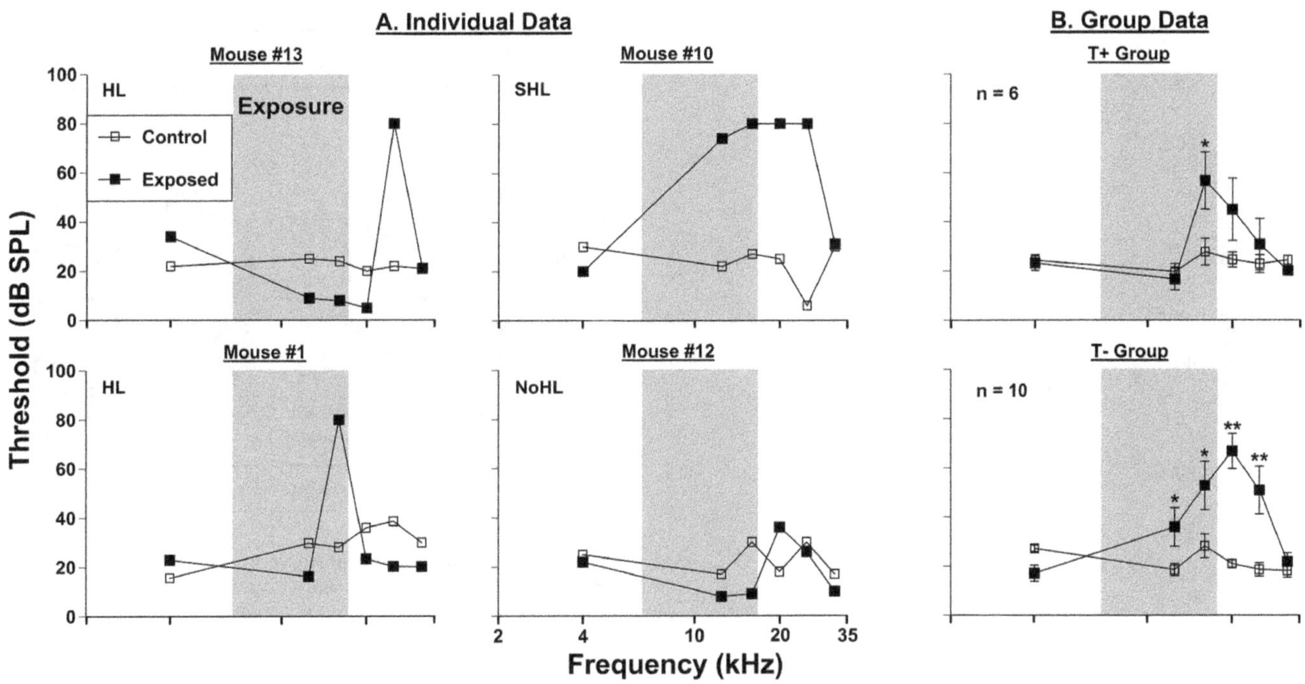

FIGURE 2 | Auditory thresholds assessed via prepulse inhibition (PPI) audiometry. (A) Four individual mice were tested before (control) and 3 months (exposed 3M) after sound exposure. **(B)** Group PPI data for T+ mice (n = 6) and T− mice (n = 10; from **Figure 1B**), in the same conditions as **(A)**. The narrow band exposure stimulus is represented by a gray box. Each animal was classified as having hearing loss (HL), severe hearing loss (SHL), or no hearing loss (NoHL) based on the number of frequencies at which PPI thresholds were elevated. Significant threshold shifts indicated with (*) at p = 0.05 level or (**) at p = 0.001 level.

normalizing the standard deviation of each unit's ISI distribution by its mean (Ma et al., 2006; Kalappa et al., 2014). Units with high CVs had more irregular ISIs, which suggests that they had more bursting activity (**Figure 7**). The normal physiological range for CVs has been reported as 0.5 to 1 in cortical neurons (Christodoulou and Bugmann, 2001), however recent studies have shown values of 1.2 or higher in the dorsal cochlear nucleus (DCN) following acoustic trauma (Pilati et al., 2012). Statistical comparisons of the mean distribution of CVs across each IC of four exposed mice were tested with a Wilcoxon Signed Rank Test to evaluate whether sound exposure changed the bursting patterns in IC neurons (**Figure 7**). Small but significant CV decreases were observed in the contra IC of mouse #13 ($Z = -2.67$, $p = 0.007$), mouse #1 ($Z = 2.15$, $p = 0.049$) and mouse #12 ($Z = 2.92$, $p = 0.003$). A much more significant CV increase was only observed for the ipsilateral IC for mouse #10 ($Z = -4.24$, $p < 0.001$), and a large significant decrease was found in the contralateral IC for mouse #10 ($Z = -3.06$, $p = 0.002$).

DISCUSSION

The important finding of this study was that despite identical sound exposure parameters, behavioral and neural assessments revealed a diverse set of pathologies among mice. Behavioral evidence of tinnitus was observed in just under half of mice exposed, which was often accompanied with some degree of threshold shifts measured by PPI audiometry. The burst firing rate in animals classified as T+ was not significantly different from the control animals. The bursting activity, however, greatly increased in one animal with significant PPI threshold shifts. Increases in spontaneous activity following sound exposure were observed regardless of behavioral evidence of tinnitus or hearing loss in the small sample of mice tested.

To this point, most animal model tinnitus studies have grouped T+ and T− animals together in order to explain differences in any number of physiological factors that change after AOE. While this is a reasonable approach to make conclusions about sample populations that underwent the identical experimental manipulations, it does not lend credence to the significant variability of peripheral, central auditory, emotional, and cognitive aspects of the human tinnitus population (Langers et al., 2012). Clinically, this sort of problem might be best addressed by increased data sharing and a systematic review of all clinical studies (Hall et al., 2016). However, in animal studies both group and individual results should be included in order to parse apart the various factors that could influence tinnitus manifestation. Below, we discuss the individual results of a small sample of mice that underwent several behavioral and electrophysiological evaluations.

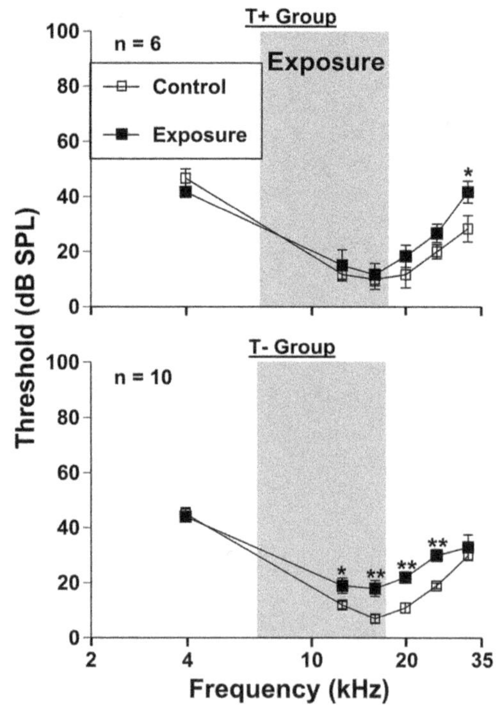

FIGURE 3 | Auditory thresholds assessed via auditory brainstem response (ABR) grouped by T + (*n* = 6) and T− (*n* = 10) animals (from Figure 1B). Mice were tested before (control) and 3 months (exposed 3M) after sound exposure. The narrow band exposure stimulus is represented by a gray box.

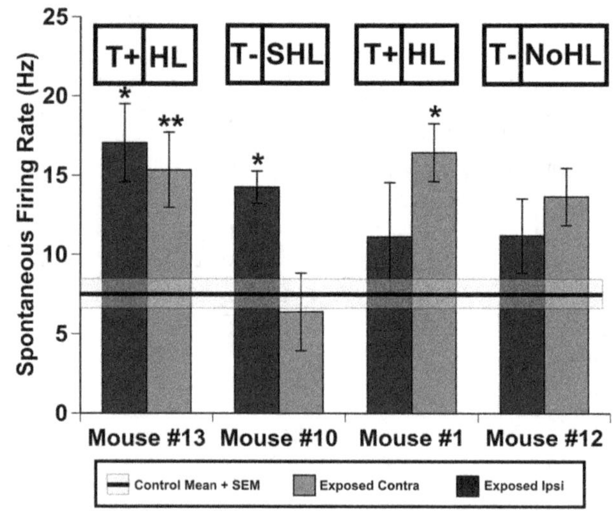

FIGURE 4 | Spontaneous firing of inferior colliculus (IC) neurons in four individual mice after sound exposure. Data represents means and standard errors of spontaneous rate (SR)s of contra- and ipsi-lateral ICs (relatively to the exposed ear) for each mouse. Signifcant differences (*0.05, **0.001) between each IC of exposed mice and averaged values across four control (unexposed) animals (black line = mean, shaded region = std. error). Tinnitus and hearing loss abbreviations are taken from **Figures 1**, **2** respectively.

Behavioral Data: Group vs. Individual Analysis

We found that 6 out of 16 mice developed GPIAS deficits consistent with behavioral evidence of tinnitus 3 months following AOE. This percentage of T+ animals fits within the range of other studies that report between 30% and 75% rates of tinnitus among animals tested (see Galzyuk and Hébert, 2015). The T+ group (n = 6) showed a non-significant, although close (p = 0.053), GPIAS deficit at 16 kHz, whereas the T− group (n = 10) did not show deficits at any frequencies, and in fact showed non-significant improvements in high frequency gap detection following AOE (**Figure 1**). It is not surprising that GPIAS results assessed in the T+ group did not show a significant deficit because the frequency of the gap detection deficit varies among mice, although usually manifests at, or above the center frequency of exposure (Longenecker and Galazyuk, 2011; Turner et al., 2012; Coomber et al., 2014; Ropp et al., 2014). Thus, 16 kHz would fall within this expected deficit range following an AOE with a 12.5 kHz centered noise. Indeed, all individual animal GPIAS deficits ranged from 16 kHz to 25 kHz, of which two examples can be seen in **Figure 1**.

PPI audiometry can provide behavioral thresholds in a matter of a couple hours compared with months of training for behavioral audiograms (Heffner et al., 2008; Radziwon et al., 2009). Because behavioral thresholds are considered the "gold standard" for auditory evaluations, it is important that they are used in conjunction with tinnitus assessments. With the same 16 mice tested for behavioral evidence of tinnitus, we found that thirteen showed increased behavioral thresholds when assessed by PPI audiometry 3 months after AOE. Of those 13 with increased thresholds, six showed narrowband frequency deficits restricted to one or two neighboring frequencies tested, while wide-band deficits were seen in seven mice. The animals with narrowband deficits, had PPI threshold increases within the same 16–25 kHz band as GPIAS deficits were usually seen. This finding does bring into question whether the animals with specific deficits (like mouse #1) have tinnitus. If GPIAS (**Figure 1**) and PPI deficits (**Figure 2**) match in frequency it is possible that the mouse could not hear the background noise during the GPIAS testing and thus showed a gap detection deficit at that frequency. Seven mice however showed broadband deficits, exemplified by mouse #10 (**Figure 2**). If the dramatic PPI audiometric threshold elevations are reflecting peripheral damage, it would imply that many of these animals could not hear well. Future experiments should identify the level of cochlear damage at which GPIAS could not be used for tinnitus assessment.

Thresholds assessed by ABRs were nearly identical for all animals before and 3 months after AOE (**Figure 3**), with only minor permanent threshold increases. Although this does not exclude "hidden hearing loss" as a result of deafferentation at the ribbon synapses of the cochlea (Schaette and McAlpine, 2011). ABR wave one amplitudes would better assess these changes (Kujawa and Liberman, 2009; Lin et al., 2011). In a

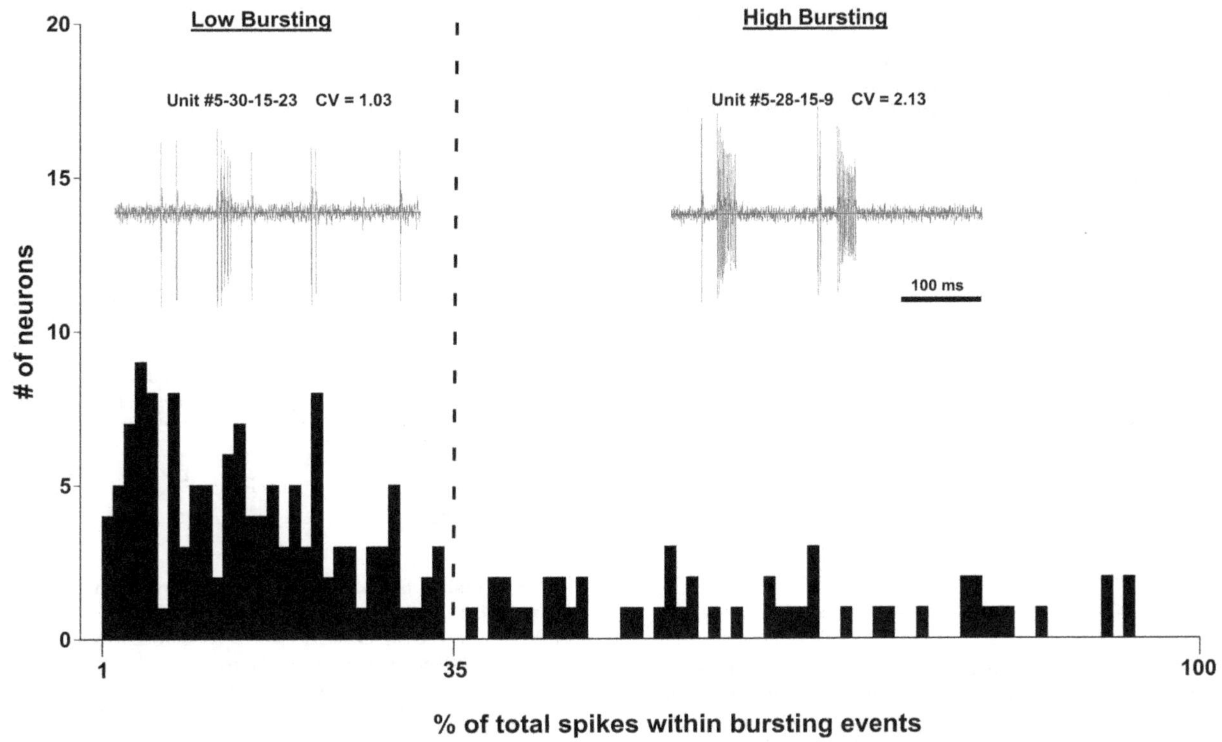

FIGURE 5 | Histogram of the percentage of spikes that occurred in bursting events of 502 IC neurons recorded from four control mice and four exposed mice. Units were separated into Low Bursting (LB) and High Bursting (HB) units using a 35% cutoff point (vertical dashed line) which was determined statistically. Examplar units for each bursting classification are shown in the upper part of the figure. Each unit includes its coefficient of varation (CV) which represents a measure of spike regularity. Higher CV values mean that a given neuron is bursting more.

mirror study with the same AOE parameters we found that wave one amplitudes were dramatically decreased, especially at suprathreshold levels, and more importantly, that these deficits corresponded to PPI audiometric deficits (Longenecker et al., 2016). Therefore, we expect that these animals also experience a decrease in ABR wave one amplitudes, signifying peripheral deafferentation (Kujawa and Liberman, 2015). Only small threshold shifts were seen at 31.5 kHz in the T+ group, which contrasted with the more significant deficits seen in the T− group between 12.5 and 25 kHz (**Figure 3**). This ABR data correlates well with PPI threshold data (**Figure 2**), which suggests that T− animals might have a tendency towards more wide spread peripheral and/or central damage (Roberts et al., 2012). A similar finding demonstrated that non-tinnitus rats had a higher expression of activity-regulated cytoskeletal (Arc) immediate early gene measured across the hippocampus, amygdala, and auditory cortex (Singer et al., 2013). This means more central plasticity occurred in animals with SHL, and more importantly that tinnitus generation might require a more focused peripheral/central damage.

Relationship Between Hyperactivity and Tinnitus

AOE causes peripheral damage that gradually leads to central plastic changes, possibly leading to tinnitus in some individuals, but not others. Possible reasons for this variability are discussed below. Regardless of the behavioral variability of tinnitus, some neural correlates have consistently been seen after AOE (see Eggermont, 2016), many in the IC (see Berger and Coomber, 2015). For several decades animal studies have suggested hyperactive neuronal activity is a neural correlate of tinnitus (see review by Eggermont, 2005, 2013). Our study demonstrated hyperactivity is developed in all mice regardless of behavioral evidence of tinnitus (**Figure 4**). A similar finding has been reported for rats (Ropp et al., 2014) and guinea pigs in IC neurons (Coomber et al., 2014) as well as in neurons of the auditory cortex (Engineer et al., 2011). Interestingly, mouse #10 in our study demonstrated decreased spontaneous activity in the ipsilateral IC. This is particularly interesting when considering the bursting activity in this ipsilateral IC was dramatically increased compared to all other exposed ICs tested as discussed below. This might suggest that increased bursting activity in the IC could be an alternative neural coding strategy following decreased peripheral input (see Roberts et al., 2010). When combining the behavioral data with the single unit recordings, the results of this study would suggest that hyperactivity should be considered as a generalized outcome of sound exposure rather than a specific neural correlate of tinnitus. Our study also suggests that there does not seem to be a specific effect of being T+ and symmetry of neural firing in contra/ipsi ICs following AOE. While both

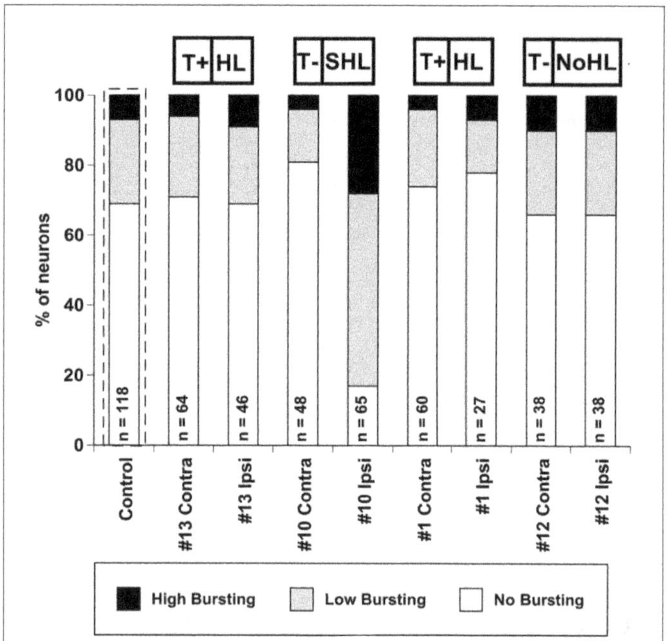

FIGURE 6 | Percent distribution of auditory neurons having different levels of bursting activity (high bursting, low bursting, and no bursting) in conta- and ipsilateral ICs of four exposed mice. The average distribution from four control (unexposed) mice is outlined by a dashed line. The number of neurons collected is labeled for each exposed IC (or all ICs for control). Tinnitus and hearing loss abbreviations are taken from **Figures 1**, **2** respectively.

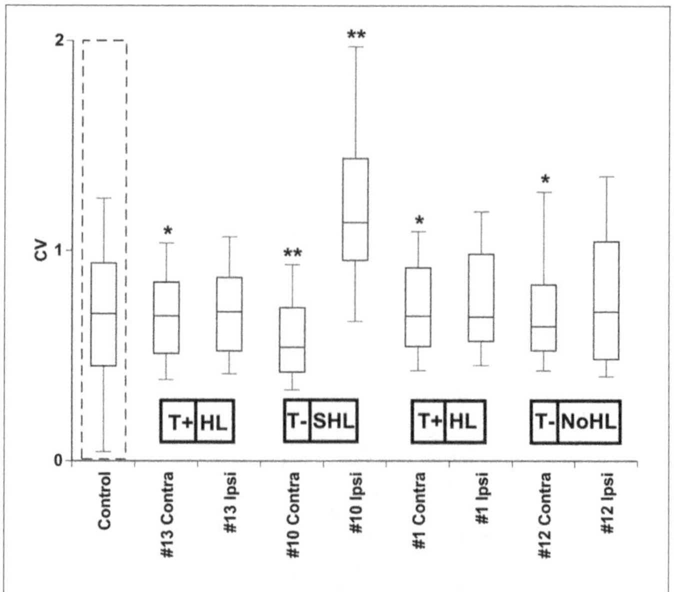

FIGURE 7 | Distribution of CVs across conta- and ipsilateral ICs of four exposed mice. The average CV from four control (unexposed) mice is outlined by a dashed line. Significant differences between control and each exposed IC was determined by a paired *t*-test (*0.05, **0.001). Tinnitus and hearing loss abbreviations are taken from **Figures 1**, **2** respectively.

the ipsi and contra ICs had significantly elevated neural activity for mouse #13 (T+ group), only the ipsi IC showed this effect in mouse #1 (T+ group; **Figure 4**). Mouse #10 which was T− and had SHL when measured with PPI audiometry, demonstrated a bias of hyperactivity skewed toward the contra IC. While the overall results of hyperactivity correlate well with previous studies on different model species (Coomber et al., 2014; Ropp et al., 2014), specific details of increased spontaneous activity laterality should be further studied before robust conclusions can be made.

Bursting Activity and Tinnitus

Many studies have implicated increased bursting activity as one of several possible neural correlates of tinnitus (e.g., Ma et al., 2006; Bauer et al., 2008). Although estimates of bursting are somewhat dependent on distinct definitions of what constitutes a burst, our results clearly suggest that bursting activity decreases in the vast majority of exposed mice (**Figures 6**, **7**) and does not correlate with behavioral evidence of tinnitus (**Figure 1**). There are several possible explanations for such discrepancy: (1) The effect of anesthesia. In our study extracellular recordings were conducted without the use of any anesthetics, whereas other studies were conducted on ketamine-anesthetized animals which is known to affect NMDA receptors, AMPA receptors, mGluRs, and most modulatory neurotransmitter systems which in turn might alter bursting activity (Sleigh et al., 2014). (2) The difference in timing after sound exposure. Studies assessing bursting activity have started physiological recordings a few days (Noreña and Eggermont, 2003; Finlayson and Kaltenbach, 2009), 2–3 months, (Ma et al., 2006; Coomber et al., 2014) up to a maximum of a 9 months (Bauer et al., 2008) after sound exposure. We began testing our mice at least 2 months following exposure. This matches previous behavioral (Turner et al., 2012; Longenecker et al., 2014) and physiological (Mulders and Robertson, 2011) timelines for tinnitus development. It is possible that bursting activity during the acute phase of tinnitus is very different from the chronic tinnitus. (3) The difference in sound exposure. In our study animals were exposed to a 12.5 kHz octave band noise for 1 h presented unilaterally at 116 dB SPL. Unfortunately, nearly every hearing loss/tinnitus study has adapted unique sound exposure parameters, leading to possible differential exposure effects (Galzyuk and Hébert, 2015). Thus, direct comparisons between studies are extremely tenuous, especially considering the difficulty of tinnitus assessment and internal confounds arising from various levels of hearing loss resulting from sound exposure. Any or all of these factors could explain differences in burst firing activity observed in this study.

A unique pattern of neuronal activity was observed in the one mouse with severe widespread threshold deficits. This was the only animal which showed decreased bursting contralaterally and significant increased bursting ipsilaterally (**Figure 6**). In line with this observation, the CV value and percentage of spikes within bursts were also increased in the ipsilateral IC while decreasing in the contralateral IC (**Figure 7**). These results appear paradoxical when considering the spontaneous firing rates mentioned above because the spontaneous firing rate contralaterally was much higher than control levels while the ipsilateral IC had somewhat decreased firing rates. This increased bursting activity without increasing the firing rate could represent an alternative neural strategy in compensating for the putative decreased peripheral signals. Further research is necessary to clarify neuronal mechanisms underlying changes in bursting activity following sound exposure.

Different Pathologies Following Acoustic Exposure

Perhaps the most significant question that is left unanswered in both the literature and this study is why some animals develop tinnitus after sound exposure and others do not. This phenomenon has been indirectly reported in the vast majority tinnitus related publications but has not been studied systematically. For example, most clinical cases reported a strong correlation between hearing loss and tinnitus (Weisz et al., 2006), whereas other studies described tinnitus cases where tinnitus patients demonstrated no audiometric deficits (Schmuziger et al., 2006; Job et al., 2007; Langers et al., 2012). The diversity of tinnitus pathologies seen in the current study and other animal studies (Longenecker and Galazyuk, 2011; Coomber et al., 2014; Hickox and Liberman, 2014; Ropp et al., 2014) could be explained by a number of phenotypic factors including differences in individual animals in stress levels, unintentional noise exposure, differential peripheral damage, or unique animal-specific maladaptive neuroplasticity pattern caused by sound exposure.

Possible Causes of Phenotypic Diversity

Stress is known to play an important role in many disease states clinically, including tinnitus (Hébert and Lupien, 2007). Some literature suggests that stress is also an important factor for the etiology of tinnitus in animals (Singer et al., 2013). Many common housing and handling procedures can cause an animal's stress levels to increase dramatically (for review see Balcombe et al., 2004). Stress is known to impair cognitive function (Arnsten, 2009), and thus it can alter the results of behavioral tests (Kaneto, 1997; Dawood et al., 2004; Graham et al., 2011). It has been shown that loud unexpected sounds can raise levels of stress-related hormones (Burow et al., 2005). Both restraint and social stress are common in laboratory animals (Stone and Quartermain, 1997; Ma et al., 2015). Simple handling of an animal, putting it in a new environment, and cage changes can also raise levels of stress in animals (Seggie and Brown, 1975; Duke et al., 2001). Interestingly, it was found that mice subjected to restraint stress had less dramatic permanent threshold shifts after noise exposure (Wang and Liberman, 2002). All animals in our study were subjected to restraint stress before exposure when they were placed into small restrainers during behavioral testing. Although all animals were tested the same number of times, the stress of restraint could vary between animals, leading to the differential pathologies we observed. Animals housed alone show much higher stress levels than animals housed in pairs or groups (Sharp et al., 2003). However, dominance struggles between pairs can cause a great deal of stress to the subordinate animal (Makinson et al., 2015). Any or all of these stressing factors could lead to a potential difference in the outcome of sound exposure, especially since it is known that sound exposure itself leads to increased levels of stress hormones (Kozlovsky et al., 2009).

Unintentional exposure to sound could occur in animal housing facilities (see Turner et al., 2007). A recent study recorded sounds from an animal care facility and found that weekday sound levels could easily reach the level of 70 dB SPL, but varied in intensity throughout the day (Liberman et al., 2014). Even if sound levels are not damaging, each animal would be subjected to different auditory experience which may lead to animal specific plastic changes over the length of a longitudinal study. CBA/CaJ mice conditioned to moderate levels of sound (81–89 dB SPL) before exposure demonstrated less permanent threshold shifts compared to mice that were just exposed (Yoshida and Liberman, 2000). Sound conditioning can also lead to permanent central changes as well (Turner et al., 2013). These changes can lead to changes in ABRs, prepulse behavioral measures, and startle reflex magnitudes (Turner and Willott, 1998). This suggests that an animal facility, if not closely monitored, could be greatly influencing an animal's auditory experience and thus the results of sound exposure. Specific to the conclusions of this study, it is important to consider that each mouse could be in a slightly different area in reference to given unintentional sound source, so it is likely that sound levels were not even for every animal. Animals can also be unintentionally exposed during transportation to and from a lab or in the lab itself. These discrepancies could explain why certain mice develop tinnitus, hearing loss, or show the absence of such maladies.

Additionally, the actual conditions of exposure for each animal might differ slightly resulting in various degrees of damage. Such factors could include the exact animal placement in relation to the sound source, the time of day the animal was exposed (Meltser et al., 2014), the exact amount of anesthetic that is absorbed into the blood, as well as all stress-related factors listed above. Even among heterogeneous genotypes of guinea pig and inbred strain mice the variability of ABR threshold shifts after unanesthetized AOE can be dramatic (Wang et al., 2002). Similarly, ABR and ASR amplitudes were shown to be quite variable between mice after AOE in a recent tinnitus assessment study (Hickox and Liberman, 2014). Current theories of how this peripheral damage leads to the manifestation of tinnitus is still debated. However, it is known that exposure to loud sounds leads to permanent damage to cochlear nerve fibers, even without direct damage to inner or outer hair cells (Kujawa and Liberman, 2009; Lin et al., 2011). This was confirmed in human work, which suggested that tinnitus in patients with clinically normal audiograms may be correlated with a peripheral neuropathy, which is typically patient specific (Schaette and McAlpine, 2011; Gu et al., 2012). The resulting decrease of central input leads to maladaptive up regulation of firing in the lower auditory brainstem (for review see Roberts et al., 2010). A recent study has suggested that rats behaviorally positive for tinnitus demonstrated the greatest degree of ribbon synapse degeneration at the cochlear nerve terminal (Singer et al., 2013). Regardless of what peripheral damage occurs, the strongest evidence of the manifestation of the tinnitus percept is explained by peripherally-driven central auditory plasticity.

Central neural plastic changes resulting from AOE have been abundantly studied (see Eggermont, 2016) but how these changes result in tinnitus remains poorly understood. We know that the exposure increases the rate of peripheral degradation, assessed by threshold (Kujawa and Liberman, 2006) and suprathreshold (Fernandez et al., 2015) ABR measures. Further, it is known that unilateral peripheral damage, like the AOE in this study, drives central plasticity more significantly than bilateral lesions (Rubio, 2006). Here we describe common neuronal changes associated with tinnitus, hyperactivity and bursting activity in the IC in animals assumed to have some degree of unilateral peripheral deafferentation. The conclusions here match other recent studies that suggest hyperactivity is not associated with tinnitus but sound exposure in general (Coomber et al., 2014; Ropp et al., 2014). Additionally, a new finding in this work, albeit with a low sample size, advocates that bursting activity (**Figures 6, 7**) is more prevalent animals with the most significant auditory threshold shifts (**Figure 2**), but less so in T+ animals, with less significant threshold shifts (**Figure 2**). Although this finding requires more validation, due to the low sample size.

In agreement with our findings, it was found that the activity-regulated cytoskeletal protein, Arc was downregulated in the amygdala, hippocampus, and auditory cortex in mice with behavioral evidence of tinnitus but upregulated in animals with possible hearing loss (Singer et al., 2013). A similar finding in the cochlear nucleus of rats demonstrated that GAP-43 (a synaptic plasticity associated protein) was upregulated in rats with SHL but not in rats with tinnitus (Kraus et al., 2011). This suggests that certain neural activity might be downregulated in tinnitus animals but upregulated in animals with greater degrees of hearing loss. Human imaging studies have found neural plastic changes in many brain regions (see review by Simonetti and Oiticica, 2015). Most studies find that tinnitus patients show increased cerebral gray matter in the auditory pathways, and a decreased cerebral gray matter outside the auditory pathways (i.e., Limbic system, cerebellum, basal ganglia) in comparison to non-tinnitus controls. Although comparing changes in neuronal signatures between humans and animal models of tinnitus is difficult, future studies should work towards more relatable comparisons.

AUTHOR CONTRIBUTIONS

RJL: planned and conducted all experiments and manuscript production; AVG: planned experiments and manuscript production.

ACKNOWLEDGMENTS

Parts of this work were published in "Differential Pathologies Resulting from Sound Exposure: Tinnitus vs Hearing Loss," a dissertation submitted to Kent State University in partial fulfillment of the requirements of the degree of doctor of philosophy. This research was supported by grant R01 DC011330 to AVG and 1F31 DC013498-01A1 to RJL from the National Institute on Deafness and Other Communication Disorders of the US Public Health Service. The authors also thank Olga Galazyuk for developing software that allowed off-line data analysis and statistical evaluation.

REFERENCES

Arnsten, A. F. T. (2009). Stress signaling pathways that impair prefrontal cortex structure and function. *Nat. Rev. Neurosci.* 10, 410–422. doi: 10.1038/nrn2648

Auerbach, B. D., Rodrigues, P. V., and Salvi, R. J. (2014). Central gain control in tinnitus and hyperacusis. *Front. Neurol.* 5:206. doi: 10.3389/fneur.2014.00206

Baguley, D., McFerran, D., and Hall, D. (2013). Tinnitus. *Lancet* 382, 1600–1607. doi: 10.1016/S0140-6736(13)60142-7

Balcombe, J. P., Bernard, N. D., and Sandusky, C. (2004). Laboratory routines cause animal stress. *Contemp. Top. Lab. Anim. Sci.* 43, 42–51.

Bauer, C. A., Turner, J. G., Caspary, D. M., Myers, K. S., and Brozoski, T. J. (2008). Tinnitus and inferior colliculus activity in chinchillas related to three distinct patterns of cochlear trauma. *J. Neurosci. Res.* 88, 2564–2578. doi: 10.1002/jnr.21699

Berger, J. I., and Coomber, B. (2015). Tinnitus-related changes in the inferior colliculus. *Front. Neurol.* 6:61. doi: 10.3389/fneur.2015.00061

Brozoski, T. J., and Bauer, C. A. (2005). The effect of dorsal cochlear nucleus ablation on tinnitus in rats. *Hear. Res.* 206, 227–236. doi: 10.1016/j.heares.2004.12.013

Burow, A., Day, H. E. W., and Campeau, S. (2005). A detailed characterization of loud noise stress: intensity analysis of hypothalamo–pituitary–adrenocortical axis and brain activation. *Brain Res.* 1062, 63–73. doi: 10.1016/j.brainres.2005.09.031

Chang, H., Chen, K., Kaltenbach, J. A., Zhang, J., and Godfrey, D. A. (2002). Effects of acoustic trauma on dorsal cochlear nucleus neuron activity in slices. *Hear. Res.* 164, 59–68. doi: 10.1016/s0378-5955(01)00410-5

Christodoulou, C., and Bugmann, G. (2001). Coefficient of variation vs. mean interspike interval curves: What do they tell us about the brain? *Neurocomputing* 38, 1141–1149. doi: 10.1016/s0925-2312(01)00480-5

Coomber, B., Berger, J. I., Kowalkowski, V. L., Shackleton, T. M., Palmer, A. R., and Wallace, M. N. (2014). Neural changes accompanying tinnitus following unilateral acoustic trauma in the guinea pig. *Eur. J. Neurosci.* 40, 2427–2441 doi: 10.1111/ejn.12580

Dawood, M. Y., Lumley, L. A., Robison, C. L., Saviolakis, G. A., and Meyerhoff, J. L. (2004). Accelerated Barnes maze test in mice for assessment of stress effects on memory. *Ann. N Y Acad. Sci.* 1032, 304–307. doi: 10.1196/annals.1314.047

Dehmel, S., Eisinger, D., and Shore, S. E. (2012). Gap prepulse inhibition and auditory brainstem-evoked potentials as objective measures for tinnitus in guinea pigs. *Front. Syst. Neurosci.* 6:42. doi: 10.3389/fnsys.2012.00042

Duke, J. L., Zammit, T. G., and Lawson, D. M. (2001). The effects of routine cage-changing on cardiovascular and behavioral parameters in male Sprague-Dawley rats. *Contemp. Top. Lab. Anim. Sci.* 40, 17–20.

Eggermont, J. J., and Roberts, L. E. (2004). The neuroscience of tinnitus. *Trends Neurosci.* 27, 676–682. doi: 10.1016/j.tins.2004.08.010

Eggermont, J. J. (2005). Tinnitus: neurobiological substrates. *Drug Discov. Today* 10, 1283–1290. doi: 10.1016/s1359-6446(05)03542-7

Eggermont, J. J. (2013). Hearing loss, hyperacusis, or tinnitus: what is modeled in animal research? *Hear. Res.* 295, 140–149 doi: 10.1016/j.heares.2012.01.005

Eggermont, J. J. (2016). Acquired hearing loss and brain plastisity. *Hear. Res.* 1–15. doi: 10.1016/j.heares.2016.05.008

Engineer, N. D., Riley, J. R., Seale, J. D., Vrana, W. A., Shetake, J. A., Sudanagunta, S. P., et al. (2011). Reversing pathological neural activity using targeted plasticity. *Nature* 470, 101–104. doi: 10.1038/nature09656

Fernandez, K. A., Jeffers, P. W. C., Lall, K., Liberman, M. C., and Kujawa, S. G. (2015). Aging after noise exposure: Acceration of cochlear synaptopathy in "recovered" ears. *J. Neurosci.* 35, 7509–7520. doi: 10.1523/JNEUROSCI.5138-14.2015

Finlayson, P. G., and Kaltenbach, J. A. (2009). Alterations in the spontaneous discharge patterns of single units in the dorsal cochlear nucleus following intense sound exposure. *Hear. Res.* 256, 104–117. doi: 10.1016/j.heares.2009.07.006

Galzyuk, A., and Hébert, S. (2015). Gap-prepulse inhibition of the acoustic startle reflex (GPIAS) for tinnitus assessment: current status and future directions. *Front. Neurol.* 6:88. doi: 10.3389/fneur.2015.00088

Gerken, G. M. (1996). Central tinnitus and lateral inhibition: an audiotry brainstem model. *Hear. Res.* 97, 75–83. doi: 10.1016/s0378-5955(96)80009-8

Graham, L. K., Yoon, T., and Kim, J. J. (2011). Stress impairs optimal behavior in a water foraging choice task in rats. *Learn Mem.* 17, 1–4 doi: 10.1101/lm.1605510

Grimsley, C. A., Longenecker, R. J., Rosen, M. J., Young, J. W., Grimsley, J. M., and Galazyuk, A. V. (2015). An improved approach to separating startle data from noise. *J. Neurosci. Methods* 253, 206–217. doi: 10.1016/j.jneumeth.2015.07.001

Gu, J. W., Herrmann, B. S., Levine, R. A., and Melcher, J. R. (2012). Brainstem auditory evoked potentials suggest a role for the ventral cochlear nucleus in tinnitus. *J. Assoc. Res. Otolaryngol.* 13, 819–833. doi: 10.1007/s10162-012-0344-1

Hall, D. A., Haider, H., Szczepek, A. J., Lau, P., Rabau, S., Jones-Diette, J., et al. (2016). Systemic review of outcome domains and instruments used in clincial trials of tinnitus treatments in adults. *Trials* 17:120. doi: 10.1186/s13063-016-1399-9

Hébert, S., and Lupien, S. J. (2007). The sound of stress: Blunted cortisol reactivity to psychosocial stress in tinnitus sufferers. *Neuros. Lett.* 411, 138–142. doi: 10.1016/j.neulet.2006.10.028

Heffner, H. E., Koay, G., and Heffner, R. S. (2008). Comparison of behavioral and auditory brainstem response measures of threshold shift in rats exposed to loud sound. *J. Acoust. Soc. Am.* 124, 1093–1104 doi: 10.1121/1.2949518

Hickox, A. E., and Liberman, M. C. (2014). Is noise-induced cochlear neuropathy key to the generation of hyperacusis or tinnitus? *J. Neurophysiol.* 111, 552–564. doi: 10.1152/jn.00184.2013

Hoffman, H. J., and Reed, G. W. (2004). "Epidemiology of tinnitus," in *Tinnitus Theory and Management* ed. J. Snow (Hamilton, ON: BC Decker), 16–41.

Jastreboff, P. J., Brennan, J. F., Coleman, J. K., and Sasaki, C. T. (1988). Phantom audiotry sensation in rats: An animal model for tinnitus. *Behav. Neurosci.* 102, 811–822. doi: 10.1037/0735-7044.102.6.811

Job, A., Raynal, M., and Kossowski, M. (2007). Susceptiblity to tinnitus revealed at 2 kHz range by bilateral lower DPOAEs in normal hearing subjects with noise exposure. *Audiol Neurotol.* 12, 137–144. doi: 10.1159/000099025

Kalappa, B. I., Brozoski, T. J., Turner, J. G., and Caspary, D. M. (2014). Single unit hyperactivity and bursting in the auditory thalamus of awake rats directly correlates with behavioral evidence of tinnitus. *J. Physiol.* 592, 5065–5078. doi: 10.1113/jphysiol.2014.278572

Kaltenbach, J. A., and Afman, C. E. (2000). Hyperactivity in the dorsal cochlear nucleus after intense sound exposure and its resemblance to tone-evoked activity: a physiological model for tinnitus. *Hear. Res.* 140, 165–172 doi: 10.1016/s0378-5955(99)00197-5

Kaltenbach, J. A. (2011). Tinnitus: Models and mechanisms. *Hear. Res.* 276, 52–60. doi: 10.1016/j.heares.2010.12.003

Kaneto, H. (1997). Learning/memory processes under stress conditions. *Behav. Brain Res.* 83, 71–74. doi: 10.1016/s0166-4328(97)86048-2

Knipper, M., Panford-Walsh, R., Singer, W., Rüttiger, L., and Zimmermann, U. (2015). Specific synaptopathies diversify brain responses and hearing disorders: you lose the gain from early life. *Cell Tissue Res.* 361, 77–93. doi: 10.1007/s00441-015-2168-x

Kozlovsky, N., Matar, M. A., Kaplan, Z., Zohar, J., and Cohen, H. (2009). A distinct pattern of intracellular glucocorticoid-related responses is associated with extreme behaviroal response to stress in an animal model of post-traumatic stress disorder. *Eur. Neuropsychopharm.* 19, 759–771. doi: 10.1016/j.euroneuro.2009.04.009

Kraus, K. S., Ding, D., Jiang, H., Lobarinas, E., Sun, W., and Salvi, J. R. (2011). Relationship between noise-induced hearing-loss, persistent tinnitus and growthassociated protein-43 expression in the rat cochlear nucleus: Does synaptic plasticity in ventral cochlear nucleus suppress tinnitus? *Neuroscience* 194, 309–325 doi: 10.1016/j.neuroscience.2011.07.056

Kujawa, S. G., and Liberman, M. C. (2006). Acceration of age-related hearing loss by early noise exposure: evidence of a misspent youth. *J. Neurosci.* 26, 2115–2123. doi: 10.1523/JNEUROSCI.4985-05.2006

Kujawa, S. G., and Liberman, M. C. (2009). Adding insult to injury: cochlear nerve degeneration after "temporary" noise-induced hearing loss. *J. Neurosci.* 29, 14077–14085 doi: 10.1523/JNEUROSCI.2845-09.2009

Kujawa, S. G., and Liberman, M. C. (2015). Synaptopathy in the noise-exposed and aging cochlea: Primary neural degeneration in aquired sensorineural hearing loss. *Hear. Res.* 330, 191–199. doi: 10.1016/j.heares.2015.02.009

Langers, D. R. M., de Kleine, E., and van Dijk, P. (2012). Tinnitus does not require macroscopic tonotopic map reorganization. *Front Syst Neurosci.* 6:2. doi: 10.3389/fnsys.2012.00002

Liberman, M. C., and Kiang, N. Y. S. (1978). Acoustic trauma in cats. Cochlear pathlogy and auditory-nerve activity. *Acta. Otolaryngol Suppl.* 358, 1–63.

Liberman, M. C., Liberman, L. D., and Maison, S. F. (2014). Efferent feedback slows cochlear aging. *J Neurosci.* 34, 4599–4607. doi: 10.1523/JNEUROSCI.4923-13.2014

Lin, H. W., Furman, A. C., Kujawa, S. G., and Liberman, M. C. (2011). Primary neural degeneration in the guinea pig cochlea after reversible noise-induced threshold shift. *J. Assoc. Res. Otolaryngol.* 12, 605–616. doi: 10.1007/s10162-011-0277-0

Lockwood, A. H., Salvi, R. J., and Burkard, R. F. (2002). Tinnitus. *N. Engl. J. Med.* 347, 904–910. doi: 10.1056/NEJMra013395

Longenecker, R. J., and Galazyuk, A. V. (2011). Development of tinnitus in CBA/CaJ mice following sound exposure. *J. Assoc. Res. Otolaryngol.* 12, 647–658 doi: 10.1007/s10162-011-0276-1

Longenecker, R. J., and Galazyuk, A. V. (2012). Methodological optimization of tinnitus assessment using prepulse inhibition of the acoustic startle reflex. *Brain Res.* 1485, 54–62 doi: 10.1016/j.brainres.2012.02.067

Longenecker, R. J., Chonko, K. T., Maricich, S. M., and Galazyuk, A. V. (2014). Age effects on tinnitus and hearing loss in CBA/CaJ mice following sound exposure. *Springerplus* 3, 542–554. doi: 10.1186/2193-1801-3-542

Longenecker, R. J. (2015). *Differential Pathologies Resulting from Sound Exposure: Tinnitus vs. Hearing Loss.* Kent, OH: Kent State University (Dissertation).

Longenecker, R. J., Alghamdi, F., Rosen, M. J., and Galazyuk, A. V. (2016). Prepulse inhibition of the acoustic startle reflex vs. auditory brainstem response for hearing assessment. *Hear. Res.* 339, 80–93. doi: 10.1016/j.heares.2016.06.006

Ma, W.-L. D., Hidaka, H., and May, B. J. (2006). Spontaneous activity in the inferior colliculus of CBA/J mice after manipulations that induce tinnitus. *Hear. Res.* 212, 9–21 doi: 10.1016/j.heares.2005.10.003

Ma, Z., Wang, G., Cui, L., and Wang, Q. (2015). Myricetin attenuates depressant-like behavior in mice subjected to repeated restraint stress. *Int. J. Mol. Sci.* 16, 28377–28385. doi: 10.3390/ijms161226102

Makinson, R., Lundgren, K. H., Seroogy, K. B., and Herman, J. P. (2015). Chronic social subordination stress modulates glutamic acid decarboxylase (GAD) 67 mRNA expression in central stress circuits. *Physiol. Behav.* 146, 7–15. doi: 10.1016/j.physbeh.2015.04.025

Meltser, I., Cederroth, C. R., Basinou, V., Savelyev, S., Lundkvist, G. S., and Canlon, B. (2014). TrkB-mediated protection against ciradian sensitivity to noise trauma in the murine cochlea. *Curr. Biol.* 24, 658–663. doi: 10.1016/j.cub.2014.01.047

Møller, A. R. (2011). "Epidemiology of tinnitus in adults," in *Textbook of Tinnitus.* New York, NY: Springer Science + Business Media, LLC

Mulders, W. H. A. M., and Robertson, D. (2011). Progressive Centralization of midbrain hyperacitivty after acoustic trauma. *Neurosci.* 192, 1–17. doi: 10.1016/j.neuroscience.2011.06.046

Noreña, A.J., and Eggermont, J. J. (2003). Changes in spontaneous neural activity immediately after an acoustic trauma: implications for neural correlates of tinnitus. *Hear. Res.* 183, 137–153 doi: 10.1016/s0378-5955(03)00225-9

Pilati, N., Large, C., Forsythe, I. D., and Hamann, M. (2012). Acoustic over-exposure triggers burst firing in dorsal cochlear nucleus fusiform cells. *Hear. Res.* 283, 98–106. doi: 10.1016/j.heares.2011.10.008

Pilati, N., Ison, M. J., Barker, M., Mulheran, M., Large, C. H., Forsythe, I. D., et al. (2012). Mechanisms contributing to central excitability changes during hearing loss. *Proc. Natl. Acad. Sci. U S A* 109, 8292–8297. doi: 10.1073/pnas.1116981109

Radziwon, K. E., June, K. M., Stolzberg, D. J., Xu-Friedman, M. A., Salvi, R. J., and Dent, M. L. (2009). Behaviorally measured audiograms and gap detection thresholds in CBA/CaJ mice. *J. Comp. Physiol. A. Neuroethol. Sens. Neural. Behav. Physiol.* 195, 961–969. doi: 10.1007/s00359-009-0472-1

Roberts, L. E., Eggermont, J. J., Caspary, D. M., Shore, S. E., Melcher, J. R., and Kaltenbach, J. A. (2010). Ringing ears: The neuroscience of tinnitus. *J. Neurosci.* 30, 14972–14979. doi: 10.1523/JNEUROSCI.4028-10.2010

Roberts, L. E., Bosnyak, D. J., and Thompson, D.C. (2012). Neural plasticity expressed in central auditory structures with and without tinnitus. *Front. Syst. Neurosci.* 6:40. doi: 10.3389/fnsys.2012.00040

Ropp, T.-J. F., Tiedemann, K. L., Young, E. D., and May, B. J. (2014). Effects of unilateral acoustic trauma on tinnitus-related spontaneous activity in the inferior colliculus. *J. Assoc. Res. Otolaryngol.* 15, 1007–1022. doi: 10.1007/s10162-014-0488-2

Rubio, M. E. (2006). Redistribution of synaptic AMPA receptors at glutamatergic synapses in the dorsal cochlear nucleus as an early response to cochlear ablation in rats. *Hear. Res.* 216–217, 154–167. doi: 10.1016/j.heares.2006.03.007

Salvi, R. J., Wang, J., and Ding, D. (2000). Audiotry plasticity and hyperactivity following cochlear damage. *Hear. Res.* 147, 261–274. doi: 10.1016/s0378-5955(00)00136-2

Schaette, R., and McAlpine, D. (2011). Tinnitus with a normal audiogram: physiological evidence for hidden hearing loss and computational model. *J. Neurosci.* 31, 13452–13457. doi: 10.1523/JNEUROSCI.2156-11.2011

Schmuziger, N., Fostiropoulos, K., and Probst, R. (2006). Long-term assessment of auditory changes resulting from a single noise exposure associated with nonoccupational activities. *Int. J. Audiol.* 45, 46–54. doi: 10.1080/14992020500377089

Seggie, J. A., and Brown, G. M. (1975). Stress response patterns of plasma corticosterone, prolactin, and growth hormone in the rat, following handling or exposure to novel environment. *Can. J. Physiol. Pharmacol.* 53, 629–637.

Sharp, J., Zammit, T., Azar, T., and Lawson, D. (2003). Stress-like responses to common procedures in individually and group-housed female rats. *Contemp. Top. Lab. Anim. Sci.* 42, 9–18.

Simonetti, P., and Oiticica, J. (2015). Tinnitus neural mechanisms and structural changes in the brain: The contribution of neuroimaging research. *Int. Arch. Otorhinolaryngol.* 19, 259–265. doi: 10.1055/s-0035-1548671

Singer, W., Zuccotti, A., Jaumann, M., Lee, S. C., Panford-Walsh, R., Xiong, H., et al. (2013). Noise-induced inner hair cell ribbon loss disturbs central arc mobilization: a novel molecular paradigm for understanding tinnitus. *Mol. Neurobiol.* 47, 261–279. doi: 10.1007/s12035-012-8372-8

Sleigh, J., Harvey, M., Voss, L., and Denny, B. (2014). Ketamine—More mechanisms of action than just NMDA blockade. *Curr. Anaesth. Crit. Care* 4, 76–81. doi: 10.1016/j.tacc.2014.03.002

Stone, E. A., and Quartermain, D. (1997). Greater behavioral effects of stress in immature as compared to mature male mice. *Physiol. Behav.* 63, 143–145. doi: 10.1016/s0031-9384(97)00366-1

Syka, J., and Rybalko, N. (2000). Threshold shifts and enhancement of cortical evoked responses after noise exposure in rats. *Hear. Res.* 139, 59–68. doi: 10.1016/s0378-5955(99)00175-6

Tukey, J. W. (1977). *Exploratory Data Analysis.* Boston, MA: Addison-Wesley Publishing Company.

Turner, J. G., Brozoski, T. J., Bauer, C. A., Parrish, J. L., Myers, K., Hughes, L. F., et al. (2006). Gap detection deficits in rats with tinnitus: a potential novel screening tool. Behav. *Neurosci.* 120, 188–195. doi: 10.1037/0735-7044.120.1.188

Turner, J. G., Bauer, C. A., and Rybak, L. P. (2007). Noise in animal facilities: why it matters. *J. Am. Assoc. Lab. Anim. Sci.* 46, 10–13.

Turner, J. G., Larsen, D., Hughes, L., Moechars, D., and Shore, S. (2012). Time course of tinnitus development following noise exposure in mice. *J. Neurosci. Res.* 90, 1480–1488. doi: 10.1002/jnr.22827

Turner, J. G., Parrish, J. L., Zuiderveld, L., Darr, S., Hughes, L. F., Caspary, D. M., et al. (2013). Acoustic experience alters the aged auditory system. *Ear Hear.* 34, 151–159. doi: 10.1097/AUD.0b013e318269ca5b

Turner, J. G., and Willott, J. F. (1998). Exposure to an augmented acoustic environment alters auditory function in hearing-impaired DBA/2J mice. *Hear. Res.* 118, 101–113. doi: 10.1016/s0378-5955(98)00024-0

Wang, Y., and Liberman, M. C. (2002). Restraint stress and protection from acoustic injury in mice. *Hear. Res.* 165, 96–102. doi: 10.1016/s0378-5955(02)00289-7

Wang, J., Salvi, R. J., and Powers, N. (1996). Plasticity of response properties of inferior colliculus neurons following acute cochlear damage. *J. Neurophysiol.* 75, 171–183.

Wang, Y., Hirose, K., and Liberman, M. C. (2002). Dynamics of noise-induced cellular injury and repair in the mouse cochlea. *J. Assoc. Res. Otolaryngol.* 3, 248–268. doi: 10.1007/s101620020028

Wang, H., Brozoski, T. J., and Caspary, D. M. (2011). Inhibitory neurotransmition in animal models of tinnitus: Maladaptive plasticity. *Hear. Res.* 279, 111–117. doi: 10.1016/j.heares.2011.04.004

Weisz, N., Hartmann, T., Dohrmann, K., Schlee, W., and Noreña, A. (2006). High-frequency tinnitus without hearing loss does not mean absence of deafferentation. *Hear. Res.* 222, 108–114. doi: 10.1016/j.heares.2006.09.003

Yoshida, N., and Liberman, M. C. (2000). Sound conditioning reduces noise-induced permanent threshold shift in mice. *Hear. Res.* 148, 213–219. doi: 10.1016/s0378-5955(00)00161-1

3

Analysis of Audiometric Differences of Patients with and without Tinnitus in a Large Clinical Database

Dominik Gollnast[1†], Konstantin Tziridis[1†], Patrick Krauss[1,2], Achim Schilling[1,2], Ulrich Hoppe[3] and Holger Schulze[1]*

[1] Experimental Otolaryngology, Department of Otorhinolaryngology, Head and Neck Surgery, Friedrich Alexander University Erlangen-Nürnberg (FAU), Erlangen, Germany, [2] Department of Physics, Center for Medical Physics and Technology, Biophysics Group, Friedrich-Alexander University Erlangen-Nürnberg (FAU), Erlangen, Germany, [3] Audiology, Department of Otorhinolaryngology, Head and Neck Surgery, Friedrich Alexander University Erlangen-Nürnberg (FAU), Erlangen, Germany

Correspondence:
Konstantin Tziridis
konstantin.tziridis@uk-erlangen.de

†These authors have contributed equally to this work.

Human hearing loss (HL) and comorbidities like tinnitus pose serious problems for people's daily life, which in most severe cases may lead to social isolation, depression, and suicide. Here, we investigate the relationship between hearing deficits and tinnitus. To this end, we conducted a retrospective study on anonymized pure tone and speech audiometric data from patients of the ENT hospital Erlangen in which we compare audiometric data between patients with and without tinnitus. Overall data from 37,661 patients with sensorineural (SHL) or conductive HL (CHL) with (T, 9.5%) or without (NT, 90.5%) a tinnitus percept in different age groups and with different tinnitus pitches were included in this study. The results of the pure tone audiometry comparisons showed significant differences in T patients compared to NT patients. In young patients, we generally found lower hearing thresholds in T compared to NT patients. In adult patients, differences were more heterogeneous: hearing thresholds in T patients were lower in low frequency ranges, while they were higher at high frequencies. Furthermore, lower thresholds were more often found in CHL patients and could rarely be detected in SHL patients. In speech audiometry, only CHL patients with high-pitched tinnitus showed lower thresholds compared to NT patients' thresholds. The results of this study may point to a biologically plausible functional benefit on hearing thresholds in HL tinnitus patients. We hypothesize that the physiological mechanism of stochastic resonance counteracts HL by adding neuronal noise to the system. This neuronal noise may induce changes in the auditory pathway and finally—as a side effect of threshold improvement—lead to the development of a tinnitus percept. We propose a general model of changed hearing thresholds in T patients, being either decreased or increased compared to NT patients.

Keywords: human, pure tone audiometry, speech audiometry, sensorineural hearing loss, conductive hearing loss, tinnitus model

INTRODUCTION

Hearing is crucial for audio-verbal communication in humans and by that essential for social interactions. Consequently, hearing impairment pose serious problems for the people's daily life, which in most severe cases may lead to social isolation, depression, and suicide (1, 2). The fact that our western societies face increasing noise exposure in daily routine, work, and spare time adds to the problem and results in continuously increasing numbers of people suffering from hearing impairments. Studies in the United States revealed about 9% of the general population being affected by hearing deficits in 2000 (3)—with an overrepresentation of 15% in children (4)—and an increase of cases over 10 years when assessed with more advanced testing procedures (5).

In general, factors leading to this high prevalence of hearing impairments are diverse. Consequently, the cause for hearing impairment may be located within different anatomical structures. Hearing disorders may have their origin in outer or middle ear, causing conductive hearing loss (CHL), or sensorineural structures (starting in the cochlea and including all structures along the auditory pathway), causing sensorineural hearing impairments. Of course patients can also suffer from a combination of conductive and sensorineural hearing loss (HL), either with unilateral or bilateral impairments. Probably, the most common cause for sensorineural hearing impairments is noise-induced HL (NIHL), which can lead to a number of secondary symptoms like tinnitus [for review, see Ref. (6)], depression (7), or hyperacusis (8). With increasing HL over time, the capability of speech discrimination is affected, generating difficulties in everyday life communication (9). As Cruickshanks and colleagues (10) demonstrated that the risk of HL is increased by almost 90% every 5 years, the demographic changes in most industrialized western countries will make age-dependent HL even more relevant in the future.

Tinnitus is a widespread, but poorly understood symptom often seen in HL patients. The prevalence in the general population is assumed to be at around 10–15% (11). Men seem to be more often affected then women up to the age of 75, when prevalence is about equal for both genders (12). About 1–2% of the tinnitus patients state their quality of life being significantly decreased by their phantom percept (13). Although HL and the prevalence of tinnitus are increasing with age (14), it is still under debate if age-related HL or age-related changes in physiological processes in the central and peripheral auditory system are the source of the increasing prevalence of tinnitus (15).

Population studies revealed that individuals with tinnitus on average suffer from stronger HL in high frequencies; patients with low-pitched tinnitus (below 1,500 Hz) show stronger low frequency HL than patients with middle- or high-pitched tinnitus [e.g., Ref. (16–19)]. In any case, the question remains why in some patients with HL subjective tinnitus is developing at all. In a recent study (20), we put forward a model for the physiological improvement of hearing thresholds, which as side effect also explains the development of tinnitus. The model is based on the idea that the auditory system tries to compensate for a HL by means of stochastic resonance (SR) at the receptor level. SR refers to the phenomenon that weak signals that are subthreshold for a given sensor still can be detected and transmitted by that sensor if noise (internal or external) is added to the sensor input, both in technical and physiological systems (21–24). We further assume that HL leads to an unequal distribution of spectral input into the auditory system, with a reduced input from the affected spectral ranges. Our model proposes that the impaired hearing thresholds within those frequency channels may be improved again (at least to a certain degree) by means of SR. Obviously, for SR to work, internal noise has to be generated within the auditory system and fed back to the receptor level (20). We propose that this internal noise is reflected in neuronal hyperactivity. If the HL is permanent, the neuronal hyperactivity that enables SR to compensate for increased thresholds may subsequently cause neuronal plasticity along the auditory pathway and finally may lead to the development of a phantom percept, i.e., subjective tinnitus. In that sense, the model views tinnitus as a side effect of a mechanism within the auditory system that seeks to optimize signal transmission at the receptor level. If this model would be true, we would expect that, in tinnitus patients, initial HL should be compensated to a certain degree, resulting in overall better hearing thresholds in tinnitus patients compared to non-tinnitus patients with comparable damage in the auditory system.

In this retrospective study, we search for data in support of this hypothesis by performing a fine-grained analysis of the audiometric data of over 37,000 patients with different forms of HL, and with or without a tinnitus percept.

MATERIALS AND METHODS

We performed a retrospective study on anonymized audiometric data from patients with HL who came to the ENT hospital in Erlangen for medical examination. Therefore, no declaration of consent was required by German law. All data were collected between the years 2000 and 2015, HL patients who complained about experiencing pure-tone tinnitus percepts were classified as tinnitus patients (group T) and patients without complains about any form of tinnitus were classified as non-tinnitus patients (group NT). Patients with other forms of tinnitus (e.g., noise-like tinnitus) were not included in this study. Applied audiometric methods were pure-tone and speech audiometry for multisyllabic numbers. Data from 37,661 patients (74,976 ears) including all groups of age [median (25, 75% quantil): 42 (21, 58)] were investigated. Patients were not characterized by their gender or by former or current pathologies not affecting hearing.

Testing Procedures

Standardized audiometric testing instruments of an audiological clinic were used for this study. All devices fulfilled the necessary requirements according to ISO 8253-1 and 8253-3. The following audiometric methods were performed: pure-tone audiometry: air conduction hearing level thresholds were measured for both ears separately for every patient. Analyzed frequencies were 250; 500; 750; 1,000; 1,500; 2,000; 3,000; 4,000; 6,000; and 8,000 Hz and HL was calculated (range: −10–130 dB). Speech Audiometry: using the Freiburger test, multisyllabic numbers were presented to each ear separately. For these data, acoustic levels at 50% understanding were calculated and used for further analysis (range: 0–120 dB). Audibility was directly linked to the acoustic level (range: 0–100%). The Freiburg multisyllabic numbers were used since it belongs to our standard procedure to determine the level of 50% understanding. This value usually correlates with the hearing threshold in the low frequency region and is less affected by high-frequency HL. We did not use the monosyllabic words since monosyllabic perception is usually measured at higher levels.

Tinnitus characteristics were determined in terms of signal type and signal level measured in decibel HL by comparison of the internal tinnitus with external sound from the audiometer. Three types of signals were possible: broadband noise, narrow band noise (1/3 octave bandwidth), and pure tones between 0.25 and 8 kHz. Tinnitus loudness was determined by increasing the signal level above hearing threshold slowly in steps of 1 dB and asked the subjects for a comparison with their tinnitus percept.

Data Preprocessing and Statistical Analysis

Data preprocessing was performed with a custom-made Matlab 2008 program (MathWorks, MA, USA). For statistical analysis Statistica 2007 (StatSoft. Inc., OK, USA) was used. Patients were classified within the preprocessing into groups based on their audiometric data: mild to medium symmetric sensorineural HL in adults [SHL, mean air-bone–gap ≤5 dB across all frequencies, HL difference between both ears <20 dB, maximal HL ≤40 dB; number of ears: n(T) = 4,390, n(NT) = 26,142], symmetric CHL in adults [CHL, mean air-bone gap >5 dB across all frequencies, HL difference between both ears <20 dB, maximal HL ≤40 dB; n(T) = 2,538, n(NT) = 24,726], and a group of children and adolescents under 18 years with symmetric HL [HL difference between both ears <20 dB, maximal HL ≤40 dB; n(T) = 234, n(NT) = 16,946] without further subdivision in SHL or CHL patients.

Furthermore, adult subjects were grouped by age: young adults 18–39 years [SHL: n(T) = 1,418, n(NT) = 8,540; CHL: n(T) = 630, n(NT) = 7,642], elder adults 40–60 years [SHL: n(T) = 2,164; n(NT) = 11,236; CHL: n(T) = 1,182; n(NT) = 9,254], and seniors >60 years [SHL: n(T) = 808; n(NT) = 6,366; CHL: n(T) = 726; n(NT) = 7,830]. The subjective pure-tone tinnitus frequencies were grouped by pitch: low-pitched [<1,000 Hz; n(SHL) = 507; n(CHL) = 387], medium-pitched [1,000–4,000 Hz; n(SHL) = 875; n(CHL) = 662], and high-pitched [>4,000 Hz; n(SHL) = 3,008; n(CHL) = 1,489].

In pure tone audiometry, we aimed to quantify the potential threshold decrease or increase tinnitus may have on hearing thresholds in each single tested hearing frequency. To this end, the difference of mean HL in each frequency was calculated for each age and tinnitus pitch group and its age matched NT patients (mean HL difference, where positive values indicate a threshold decrease, negative values indicate an increase of hearing thresholds by tinnitus in decibel) and compared by multifactorial ANOVAs. Generally, for statistical population analysis, parametrical tests like Students t-test and multifactorial ANOVAs were used. Tukey *post hoc* tests enabled detailed analysis within the ANOVAs. Additionally, we compared the paired pure tone and speech audiometry data of 2,548 patients in which both audiometric methods were allied by multiple linear regressions and 2-factorial ANOVA (Figure S1 in Supplementary Material).

RESULTS

Pure-Tone Audiometry in Patients with and without Tinnitus Percepts

Hearing Thresholds of Children and Adolescents

The HL of young patients without (NT) and with reports of tinnitus (T) was compared. To rule out any age bias due to audiometric limitations in infants, we tested first if any difference in hearing thresholds of very young children (aged 1–9 years) and adolescents (aged 10–17 years) could be found. Neither in NT (t-test, mean ± SD: children 20.5 ± 17.3 dB, adolescents 19.2 ± 21.6 dB, $p = 0.15$) nor in T patients group (t-test: children 16.0 ± 12.6 dB, adolescents 14.3 ± 19.8 dB, $p = 0.17$) any significant differences were found. Therefore, all subjects were pooled and HL was analyzed by a 2-factorial ANOVA with the factors frequency and group.

Figure 1A depicts this variance analysis. The upper panel shows an increase of mean HL toward higher frequencies in all patients (**Figure 1A**, upper panel). Interestingly, young people with tinnitus generally suffered less from HL than non-tinnitus patients (**Figure 1A**, inset), overall showing about 5 dB lower mean hearing thresholds. They were especially less affected at frequencies below 4,000 Hz and above 6,000 Hz (**Figure 1A**, lower panel, Tukey *post hoc* tests, always $p < 0.05$). In **Figure 1B**, the mean HL difference of NT and T patients is given as a function of frequency. Each green bar indicates the significant difference (tested by single sample t-tests) of the HL at a given stimulation frequency. Again, all frequencies except 4 and 6 kHz show significantly positive values indicating lower hearing thresholds in T compared to NT patients.

Note that this young patients group is not representative for patients affected by tinnitus in the "general population" where usually only adults are considered (1, 25). For that reason, further analyses were focused on adult groups with SHL and CHL. In these patients, we were able to analyze a significantly larger number of patients' ears.

Hearing Thresholds in Adults with and without Tinnitus

In a first overview, NT and T patients' audiograms separated for their cause of HL (sensorineural or conductive) were analyzed by 2-factorial ANOVAs with the factors frequency and group as depicted in **Figures 2A,C** and further illustrated by the HL difference in **Figures 2B,D**, respectively.

In adult patients, we generally found that T patients' thresholds in lower frequency ranges were lower compared to NT patients, while in other frequency ranges there was no difference or, especially above 2 kHz, those patients showed higher thresholds compared to NT patients: a detailed analysis revealed that for both groups, SHL (**Figure 2A**, upper panel) and CHL (**Figure 2C**, upper panel), HL significantly increased from low to high frequencies. HL in general was higher for CHL patients (30.9 ± 20.0 dB) than for subjects suffering from SHL (18.3 ± 16.7 dB; t-test, $p < 0.001$).

In patients with SHL, the analysis revealed the opposite result seen in young patients, namely mean thresholds across all

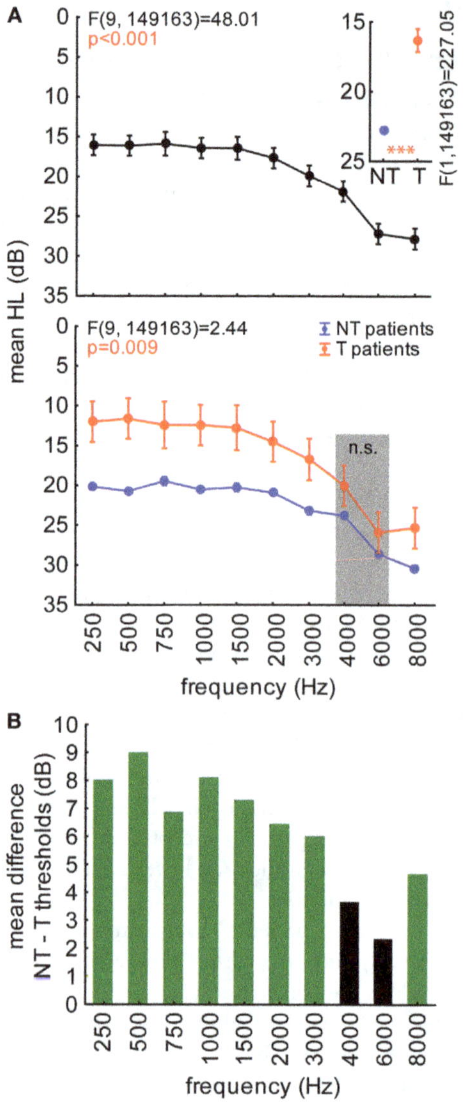

FIGURE 1 | Hearing loss (HL in decibel) in young patients (aged 1–17 years) with and without tinnitus. (A) Results of a 2-factorial ANOVA on HL with factors frequency (upper panel) and patient group (inset), interaction plot at the bottom. Symbols depict mean values; whiskers give 95% confidence intervals. Asterisks depict significance value of the 1-factorial ANOVA part: ***$p < 0.001$. Gray-shaded area indicates two frequencies not significantly different between groups (Tukey *post hoc* tests). **(B)** Mean differences between the HL of NT [blue in **(A)**] and T patients [red in **(A)**] quantifying the threshold difference referred to as mean HL difference, where positive values indicate lower, negative values higher hearing thresholds in decibel. Values significantly different from 0 are colored green (single sided *t*-tests).

frequencies being higher in patients with tinnitus compared to patients without such a mispercept by roughly 1 dB (**Figure 2A**, inset). In the interaction of both factors, it became clear (Tukey *post hoc* tests, $p < 0.001$) that T patients only showed significantly higher thresholds compared to NT patients at frequencies above 2 kHz (**Figure 2A**, lower panel). This result is further illustrated in **Figure 2B** showing the mean HL difference, which also revealed a significant threshold increase at frequencies above 2 kHz for SHL patients with tinnitus.

In patients with CHL, the analysis of the factor group showed no significant difference between T and NT patients when thresholds were averaged across all frequencies (**Figure 2C**, inset). Nevertheless, the interaction analysis (**Figure 2C**, lower panel) revealed significantly lower thresholds in T patients for frequencies below 750 Hz but higher thresholds compared to NT patients in the range of 3–4 kHz (Tukey *post hoc* tests, $p < 0.05$), which was further supported by the HL difference analysis (**Figure 2D**).

Next, we analyzed different aspects of our patient cohort to outline some additional characteristics of the threshold differences between T and NT patients. First, we focused on the age dependency of thresholds as a function of the existence of a tinnitus percept: SHL patients of all ages showed higher hearing thresholds when affected by tinnitus, while CHL patients with tinnitus only showed such higher thresholds in the age group of 40–60 years. This was assessed by 3-factorial ANOVAs with the factors frequency, age and group as depicted in **Figures 3A,C**. Lower hearing thresholds in T patients only reached significance when analyzed across frequency ranges (low = < 1 kHz, mid = < 4 kHz, high = ≥ 4 kHz; green shaded areas in **Figures 3A,C**) but could be further identified when analyzed by HL differences for specific age groups (**Figures 3B,D**).

Patients with SHL (**Figure 3A**) replicated the results shown in **Figure 2** averaged over all three age groups when factors frequency, group, or the corresponding interaction were analyzed. For the factor age [(F2, 291,140) = 11,515.0, $p < 0.001$], we found lower HL in 18- to 39-year-old adults (12.0 ± 0.2 dB) compared to 40- to 60-year-old adults (19.6 ± 0.15 dB) and adults above 60 years (30.4 ± 0.2 dB). The interaction of age and frequency is given in the upper left panel of **Figure 3A** and the interaction of age and group in the right upper panel. There, T patients showed generally higher thresholds than NT patients (Tukey *post hoc* tests), which is carved out in the three-way interaction in the lower part of **Figure 3A**: in SHL, Tinnitus patients' higher frequencies showed significantly larger thresholds than those of non-tinnitus patients (cf. red shaded areas; statistical tests were performed separately for every stimulation frequency). When 2-factorial ANOVAs [factors frequency range (low, mid, high) and group] were performed, significantly lower hearing thresholds in T patients could be detected for low frequencies in the above 60 years group only (green shaded area in **Figure 3A**). The HL difference (**Figure 3B**) for the three different age groups showed corresponding frequency ranges affected, with higher values at high frequency ranges of the tinnitus patients and lower values at 750 Hz in the above 60 years tinnitus patients.

In CHL patients (**Figure 3C**), we found a similar age-dependent HL as above [F(2, 262,589) = 5,794.5, $p < 0.001$; 18- to 39-year-old adults: 18.7 ± 0.15 dB, 40- to 60-year-old adults: 31.7 ± 0.3 dB, adults above 60 years: 46.5 ± 0.4 dB]. Again, a significant interaction of age and frequency as well as age and group was found (**Figure 3C**, upper panels). Across all frequencies, CHL T patients' hearing thresholds differed by age, as we found higher threshold in 40- to 60-year-old adults but lower threshold in 18- to 39-year-old adults. No overall significant differences were seen in adults above 60 years (Tukey *post hoc*

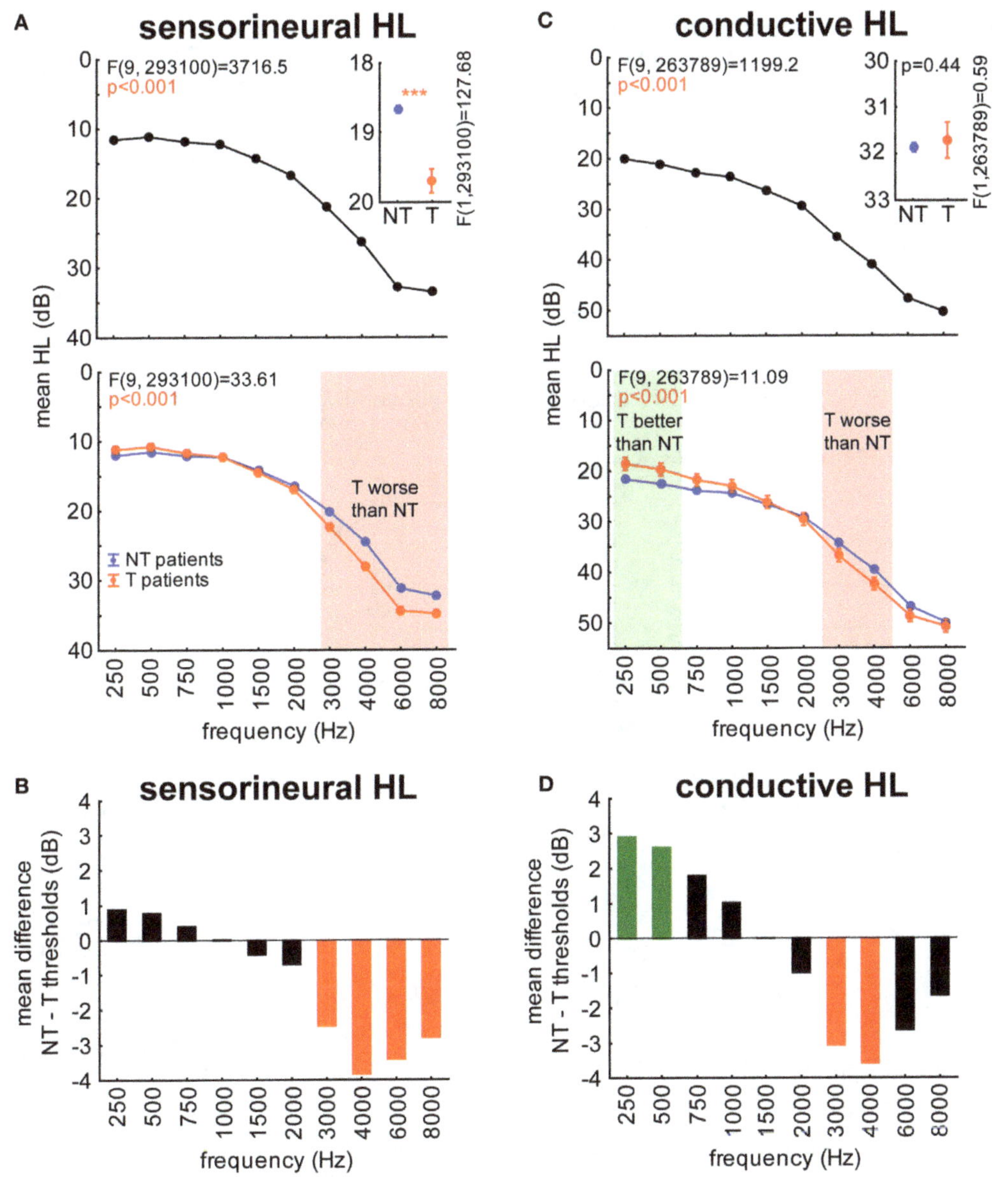

FIGURE 2 | Hearing loss (HL in decibel) in sensorineural (A,B) and conductive HL (C,D) patients. Symbols as in **Figure 1**. **(A,C)** Red areas indicate frequencies where T patients exhibit higher hearing thresholds compared to NT patients, the green area indicates frequencies where T patients show lower thresholds than NT patients (Tukey *post hoc* tests). **(B,D)** Red bars indicate significantly higher thresholds, green bars significantly lower thresholds.

tests; **Figure 3C**, upper right panel). In the three-way interaction (**Figure 3C**, lower panel) higher thresholds in T patients were found at frequencies above 1 kHz in 40- to 60-year-old adults (cf. red shaded area, statistical tests were performed separately for every stimulation frequency), while significantly lower hearing thresholds in T patients could be detected at low frequencies in 18- to 39-year-old adults and the adults above 60 years of age only [2-factorial ANOVAs for frequency ranges (low, mid, and high) and group, green shaded area in **Figure 3C**]. Correspondingly, in the analyses of HL differences (**Figure 3D**) of CHL patients, we found significantly lower values for low frequency thresholds in 18- to 39-year-old adults and adults above 60 years of age with tinnitus while 40- to 60-year-old adults with tinnitus showed significantly higher values in the mid- to high-frequency range.

From **Figures 2** and **3**, it became clear that potential effects of the perception of tinnitus on hearing thresholds follow a frequency-specific pattern: in T compared to NT patients, lower thresholds were only observed in the low-frequency range while higher thresholds were exclusively seen in the high-frequency range. As pitches of tonal tinnitus percepts most frequently are located in the high-frequency range, we hypothesized that the higher hearing thresholds in T patients may be due to masking of the perception of tones in that frequency range. To test this hypothesis, we analyzed if there is a relation between the perceived

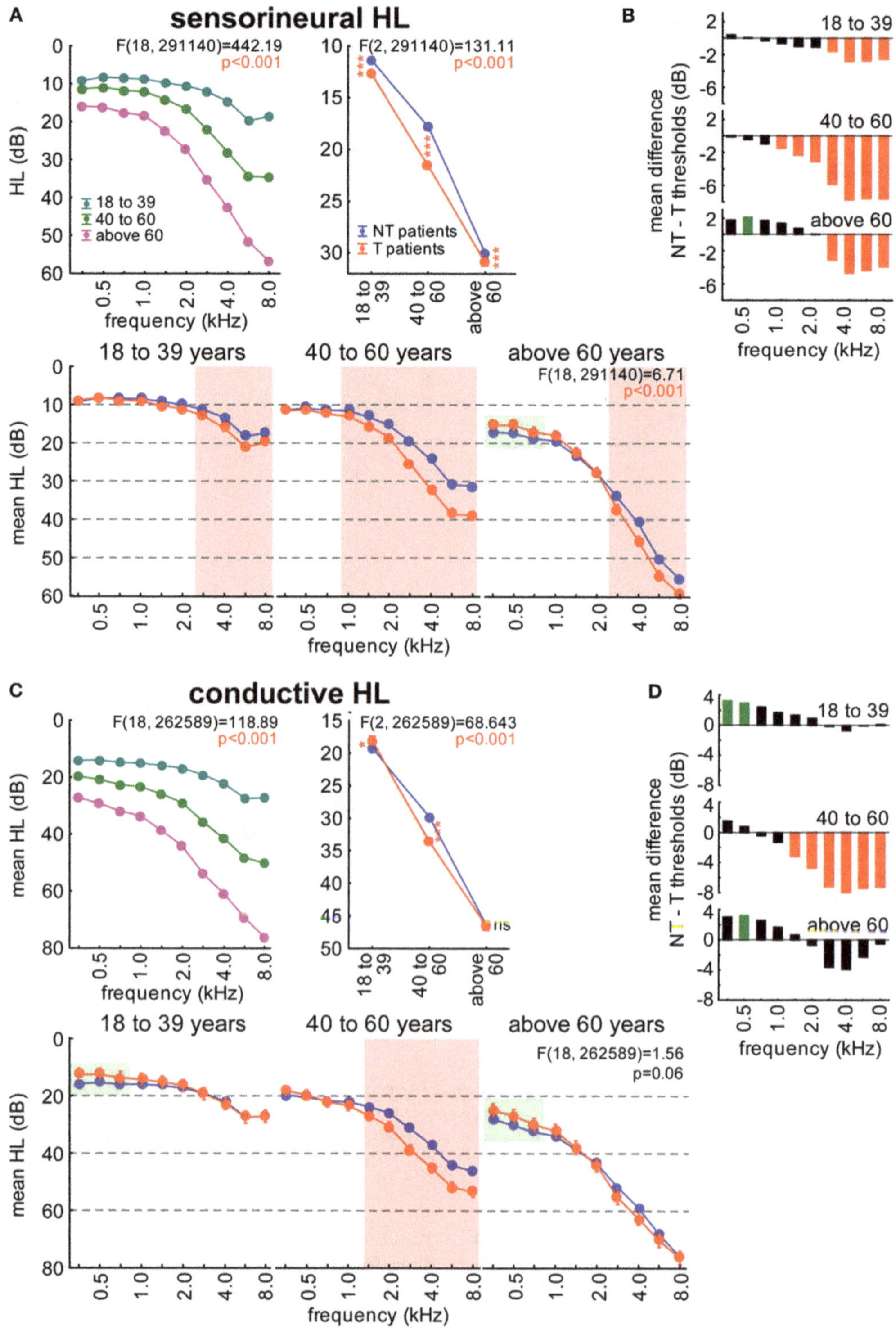

FIGURE 3 | **Age dependency of hearing loss (HL in decibel) in sensorineural (A,B) and conductive HL (C,D) patients. (A,C)** show the interaction plots of the 3-factorial ANOVAs of HL with factors age, patient group, and frequency. Asterisks depict significance levels of the Tukey *post hoc* tests in the interaction plot of age X patient group: ns, not significant, $^{*}p < 0.05$, $^{***}p < 0.001$. Red shaded areas indicate frequencies with T patients exhibiting higher hearing thresholds compared to NT patients (Tukey *post hoc* tests separately for each frequency). Green shaded areas indicate frequency ranges (low: <1 kHz, mid: <4 kHz, high: ≥4 kHz) with T patients exhibiting lower hearing thresholds compared to NT patients (2-factorial ANOVAs for frequency ranges and patient groups). **(B,D)** give the mean HL difference of NT and T patients with red bars indicating significantly higher thresholds, green bars significantly lower thresholds in T patients compared to NT patients.

tinnitus pitch and the hearing thresholds of patients by 2-factorial ANOVAs with the factors frequency and perceived tinnitus pitch (NT, low, medium, and high tinnitus pitch). The results of these analyses are depicted in **Figure 4**. We found higher thresholds in SHL T patients rather being independent of tinnitus pitch. Lower threshold in CHL T patients on the other hand were most prominent in patients with high-pitched tinnitus percepts.

In detail, in SHL patients' data (**Figure 4A**, center panel), we found higher thresholds in T compared to the NT patients being most prominent but frequency unspecific in low-pitch tinnitus patients (Tukey *post hoc* tests), but also significant in the medium and high-pitch tinnitus patients, especially for frequencies above 2 kHz (**Figure 4B**). In CHL patients, a somewhat different picture emerged (**Figure 4C**). While low- and medium-pitch tinnitus patients showed generally higher thresholds than NT patients when averaged across all stimulation frequencies, the high-pitch tinnitus patients did show lower thresholds compared to the NT patients' thresholds (**Figure 4C**, center panel). This difference (**Figure 4D**) was most prominent for frequencies below 1,500 Hz in high-pitched T groups, while the higher values in tinnitus patients with medium-pitched tinnitus frequencies started at 1,500 Hz and reached up to the highest tested frequency of 8 kHz (Tukey *post hoc* tests). For low-pitched T patients, thresholds were again generally higher compared to NT patients.

In summary, the results of the pure tone audiometry comparisons showed significant differences in hearing thresholds of T compared to NT patients in both directions. In young patients with tinnitus, we generally found significantly lower thresholds almost independent of stimulation frequency (**Figure 1**) or perceived tinnitus pitch (not shown). In adult patients (**Figures 2–4**), data were more heterogeneous: in T compared to NT patients, lower hearing thresholds were found at low frequencies only, while higher thresholds were generally found at high frequencies. Furthermore, lower thresholds in T patients were more often found in CHL patients and could rarely be detected in SHL patients.

Differences in Speech Audiometry between Patients with and without Tinnitus

In order to examine the potential differences in speech comprehension between both patient groups, we analyzed the results of the Freiburger test, which examines the intelligibility of multisyllabic numbers. **Figure 5** shows the 2-factorial ANOVA of the speech reception thresholds with factors age group and tinnitus pitch group, tested for the two major patients groups separately.

Variance analysis of speech audiometry in SHL patients (**Figure 5A**) showed the expected dependency of speech reception thresholds on age (left panel), but in addition, a stronger impairment of speech intelligibility in patients with low tinnitus pitch in comparison to all other groups (Tukey *post hoc* tests), the medium and high tinnitus frequency perceivers were not significantly different in their understanding of numbers compared to each other and to the NT patients. We did find a significant interaction of both factors (age group and tinnitus pitch), with Tukey *post hoc* tests revealing stronger impairments in adults above 39 years of age and with tinnitus pitches below 1 kHz (**Figure 6**, right panel).

In CHL patients (**Figure 5B**), we found a comparable age dependency of the speech reception thresholds (**Figure 5B**, left panel) as in SHL patients as well as a decrease of speech intelligibility in low-pitch tinnitus patients. In contrast to SHL patients, CHL high-pitched tinnitus patients showed an increase of speech intelligibility thresholds of 7 dB compared to NT patients' thresholds (**Figure 5B**, middle panel). No interaction of both factors was found, indicating a threshold decrease in high-pitched tinnitus patients at all ages (**Figure 5B**, right panel).

To control for any direct effect of the individual hearing threshold on speech reception threshold, we analyzed the relation of both thresholds by multiple linear regressions, center of gravity comparisons, and a 2-factorial ANOVA of the individual threshold differences of the two, pooled across all patients. The results of these analyses are depicted in Figure S1 in Supplementary Material and show no qualitative differences between the age or tinnitus groups in the first two analyses. Nevertheless, the differences between low and medium-pitched tinnitus patients and high-pitched tinnitus and NT patients emerge in the 2-factorial ANOVA and further support the finding, that low/medium pitch tinnitus patients show a different pattern of threshold loss compared to high-pitched tinnitus and NT patients, namely a lower distance between speech reception and pure tone thresholds.

Analysis of Tinnitus Loudness

The subjective tinnitus loudness perceived by the patients of the two groups relative to their hearing thresholds turned out to be not a good predictor of speech intelligibility. An analysis of this relative tinnitus loudness by a 3-factorial ANOVA with the factors age group, HL group, and tinnitus pitch is given in **Figure 6**. The tinnitus perception was loudest in 40- to 60-year-old adults (**Figure 6**, upper left panel, Tukey *post hoc* tests, always $p < 0.001$) and in the SHL patients (**Figure 6**, upper center panel), particularly in the high-frequency pitched pure tone tinnitus percepts (**Figure 6**, upper right panel, Tukey *post hoc* tests, always $p < 0.001$). No interaction of age and HL group indicated a parallel shift of tinnitus loudness (**Figure 6**, center left panel). Furthermore, we found significant interactions of age and pitch (**Figure 6**, center panel) with a decrease of tinnitus loudness with age for low frequencies and increase for high frequencies. We also found a significant interaction of pitch and HL group (**Figure 6**, center right panel) with louder low-pitched tinnitus percepts in SHL patients (tukey *post hoc* test, $p < 0.001$) and louder high-pitched tinnitus in CHL patients (tukey *post hoc* test, $p < 0.01$). Most interestingly, the lack of a significant three-way interaction (**Figure 6**, bottom panel) indicated that the identified differences of tinnitus loudness dependency on age and pitch seemed to be similar in both HL groups.

DISCUSSION

Hearing Thresholds in Patients with and without Tinnitus

In this retrospective study, we compared audiometric data of a total of more than 37,000 patients (74,976 ears) with sensorineural

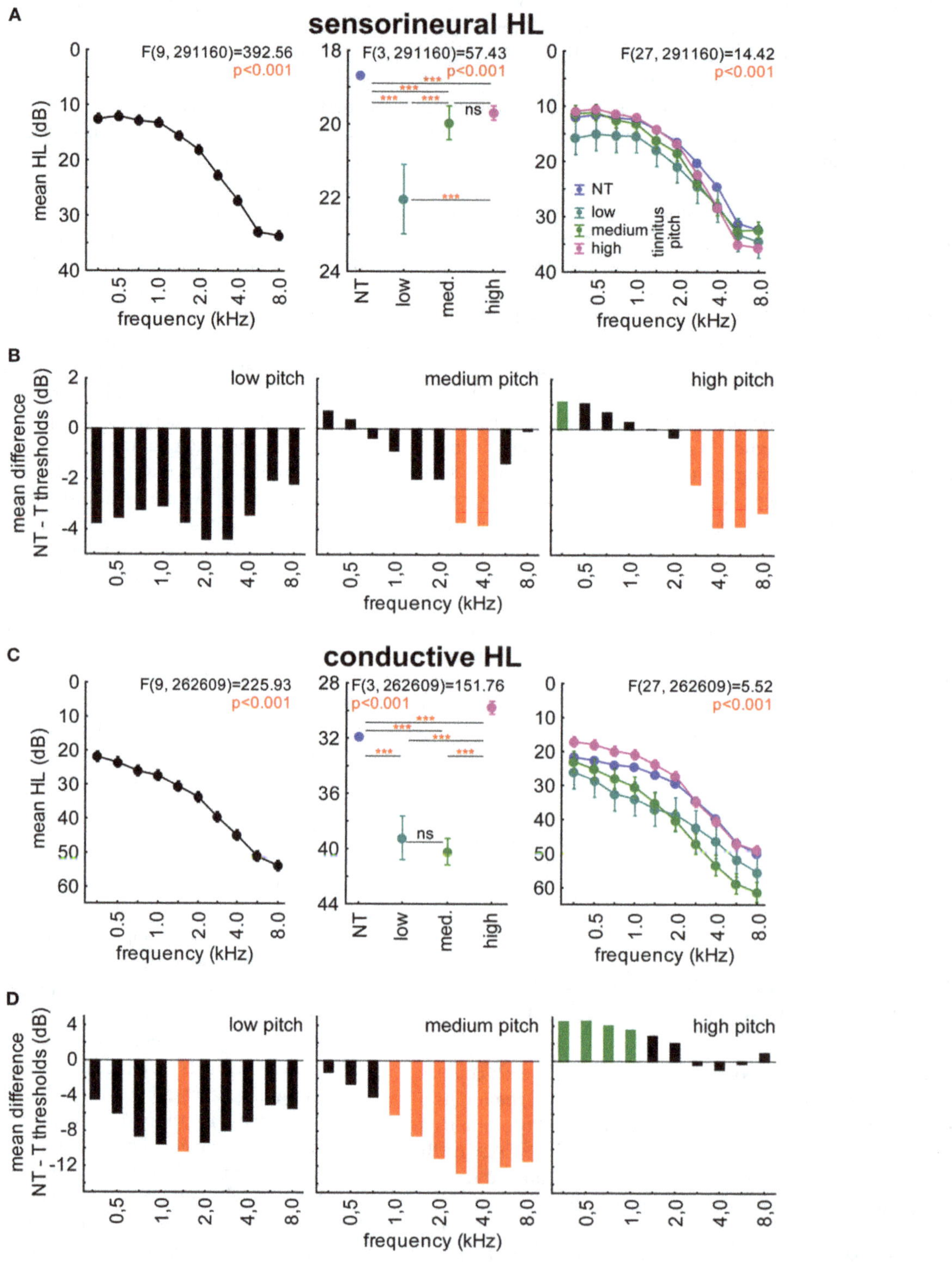

FIGURE 4 | **Relation between hearing loss in (HL in decibel) and tinnitus pitch in sensorineural (A,B) and conductive HL (C,D) patients. (A,C)** show the results of the 2-factorial ANOVAs of HL with factors frequency and perceived tinnitus pitch (including NT patients) in the two patient groups. Asterisks depict significance levels of the Tukey *post hoc* tests: ns, not significant; $^{***}p < 0.001$. **(B,D)** The threshold difference between T and NT patients is given, with red bars indicating significantly higher thresholds, green bars significantly lower thresholds in T patients compared to NT patients.

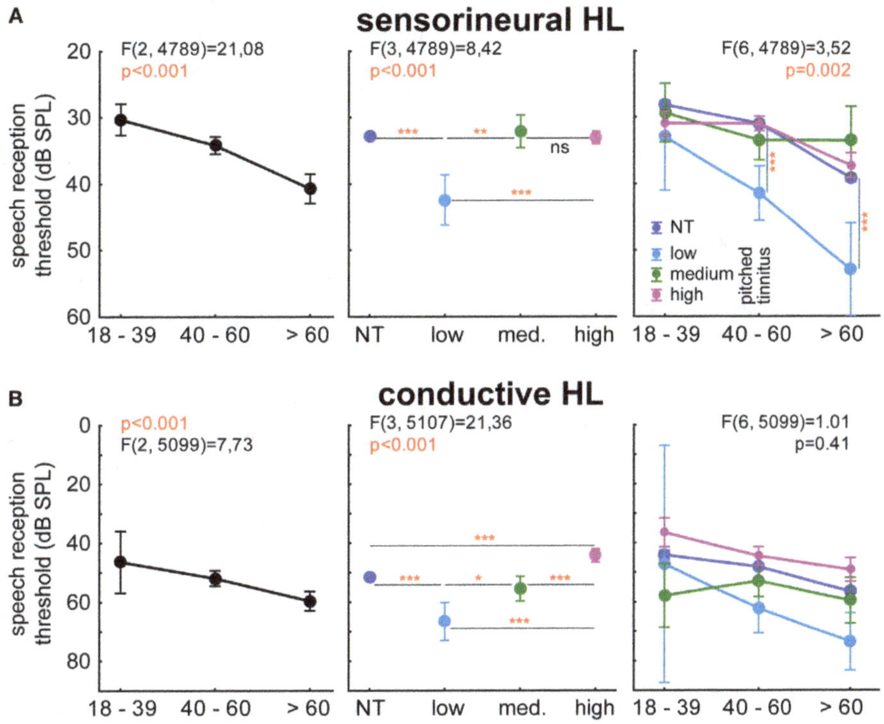

FIGURE 5 | Speech reception thresholds (decibel SPL) of sensorineural (A) and conductive HL (B) patients in the Freiburger speech intelligibility test (multisyllable numbers). 2-factorial ANOVAs of the 50% threshold with the factors age and perceived tinnitus pitch (including NT patients). Asterisks depict significance levels of the Tukey *post hoc* tests: *$p < 0.05$, *$p < 0.01$, ***$p < 0.001$.

or CHL with or without tinnitus. We hypothesize that tinnitus is an epiphenomenon of a neuronal process normalizing impaired hearing thresholds. The audiometric results and tinnitus frequency distributions of tinnitus patients of different age groups are in line with the literature [e.g., Ref. (17, 26, 27)] even though the sample groups investigated there were much smaller than in our patient cohort. Also, the hearing thresholds of non-tinnitus patients are comparable to other cohorts (28, 29). Only few studies compared both patient groups directly (30, 31) and found either no change or a worsening of speech perception in tinnitus patients. To our knowledge, no peer reviewed study compared the pure tone hearing thresholds of both patient groups the way we did.

Here, we report specific differences in hearing thresholds between T and NT patients that may be interpreted as gains or losses in patients with tinnitus compared to non-tinnitus patients. These differences emerged on the population level of over 37,000 patients and in the paired analysis of a smaller subpopulation of roughly 2,500 patients in both pure tone and speech audiometry that seemed to follow a certain systematic (**Figure 7**, center panel): in T compared to NT adults, lower thresholds were seen in the low frequency range only, while higher thresholds were observed the high frequency range. In addition, lower thresholds were more often seen in CHL patients, while in SHL patients, higher thresholds predominated. Finally, the individually perceived tinnitus pitch seemed to be correlated with systematic alterations to the differences in hearing thresholds (**Figure 4**), which obviously are more complex than the simple masking we had first hypothesized to explain threshold increasing effects (see Hearing Thresholds in Adults with and without Tinnitus). In the case of paired data (Figure S1 in Supplementary Material), it becomes clear additionally that the most frequent (high) tinnitus pitch leads to the strongest improvement in speech intelligibility. Children and adolescents did not seem to follow this systematic, as only lower thresholds were seen there (**Figure 1**).

Based on our observations, we here put forward a model of tinnitus impact on hearing thresholds as shown in **Figure 7**: the basic feature of the model (**Figure 7**, center panel) is that thresholds in the low frequency range are lowered in tinnitus patients, i.e., in the range where HL is typically mild (**Figure 7**, center panel, green shaded area). Here, high frequency thresholds are higher in tinnitus patients, i.e., in the range where HL is typically more severe (**Figure 7**, center panel, red shaded area). This general scheme of hearing threshold change in tinnitus patients may be shifted by two main factors: sensorineural HL can shift the threshold function down (**Figure 7**, upper row)—CHL (**Figure 7**, lower row) has no effect on the function, while tinnitus pitch may shift the function along the abscissa (**Figure 7**, columns), resulting in a larger frequency range of lower thresholds (green shaded areas) for high-pitched tinnitus and a larger frequency range of higher thresholds (red shaded areas) for low-pitched tinnitus.

This model qualitatively reproduces the results of our retrospective data analysis (see **Figures 2B,D** and **4B,D**). Interestingly,

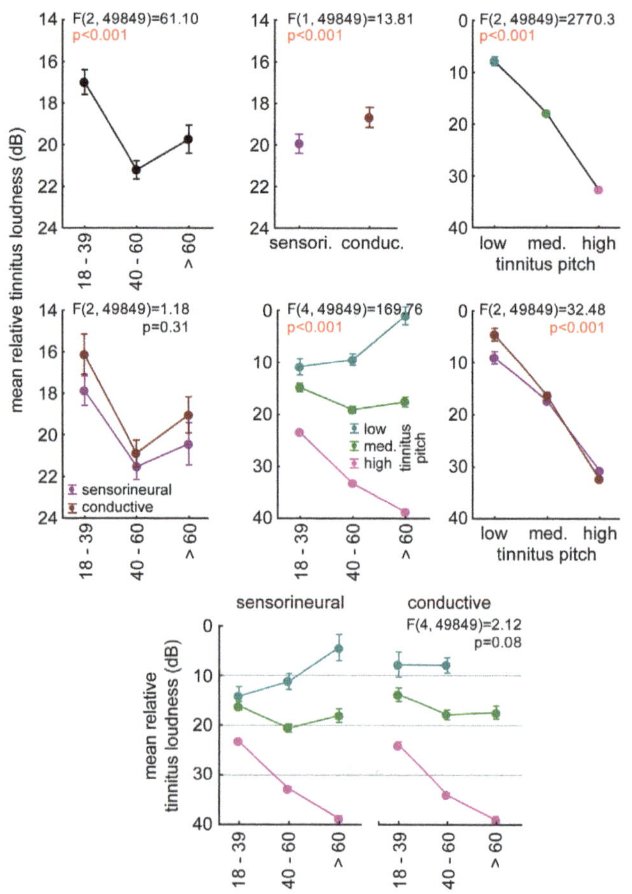

FIGURE 6 | Relation between mean relative tinnitus loudness (dB) and age, tinnitus pitch, and hearing loss (HL). The individual tinnitus loudness was calculated relative to the threshold at that frequency. Results of the 3-factorial ANOVA of tinnitus loudness relative to hearing threshold with the three factors described above. The upper three panels represent the 1-factorial part of the ANOVA results (age, HL, tinnitus pitch), the center line panels show the 2-factorial ANOVA interaction plots (age vs. HL, age vs. tinnitus pitch, tinnitus pitch vs. age), and the bottom line panel shows the interaction plot of all three factors.

when analyzing the relative frequency of the different tinnitus–threshold-interaction types postulated here (percent values in panels of **Figure 7**), it became obvious that interaction types with predominantly higher hearing thresholds are less frequent (adding up to 25.5%) than those types with lower thresholds (adding up to 74.4%). As these lower thresholds were exclusively observed for pure tone measurements in the low frequency range, we here put forward the hypothesis that *the biological function of the neuronal mechanism that finally also leads to tinnitus is to improve speech perception in the case of hearing loss.* This seems to work particularly well for high-pitched tinnitus which was encountered in about 2/3 of the patients (64.9%). In other words, patients suffering from tinnitus might be affected by this phantom percept as a side effect of their auditory system compensating for HL (cf. below).

Models of Tinnitus Development

Recent tinnitus models (32–37) all postulate damage to the peripheral receptor epithelium to be etiologic for the development of tinnitus. In response to the decreased input into the auditory system caused by such damage, one class of models further suggest an increased neuronal gain to provide homeostatic plasticity, while other suggest misbalanced lateral inhibition or a failure of a compensatory mechanism as the source of the phantom percept. Both types of models lack explanatory power since the potential biological function of homeostatic plasticity (in terms of information processing) or misbalanced lateral inhibition remains unclear.

To overcome these conceptual problems, we have recently put forward a model for tinnitus-related development of neuronal hyperactivity that is based on SR to restore hearing thresholds after HL (20). SR refers to the phenomenon that weak signals that are sub-threshold for a given sensor still can be detected and transmitted by that sensor if noise is added to the sensor input (21–24). In that way, SR serves to lift signals above a given hearing threshold and most probably is a mechanism that already works in the healthy system (38–40). One could interpret earlier results in a way that SR (while not mentioned explicitly) may also counteract increased hearing thresholds (17, 41). In this interpretation, tinnitus would be a (condoned) side effect of threshold restoration (42). In this context, recent studies have shown that patients with tinnitus show poorer listening performance in noise than patients without tinnitus (30). This is in line with our results, as the researchers focused mainly on sensorineural HL patients with and without tinnitus where we find comparable effects in our large patient cohort.

The analysis of audiometric patient data presented here are perfectly in line with the view of our model: first, the decreasing effects of SR on hearing threshold predicted by our model were observed in all adolescents and child HL patients with tinnitus as well as 65% of the adult HL patients with tinnitus. Second, threshold decreasing effects in tinnitus patients were observed in the low frequency range where HL is mild, that is, in a range where SR should be more effective as the amount of internal noise to be added to the signal to lift it above threshold must not be too high. Third, the threshold decreasing effects were most frequently observed in CHL tinnitus patients and were rather uncommon in SHL patients, which is in line with the idea that an intact neuronal system (as in CHL) more likely is able to compensate for HL by means of a neuronal SR mechanism than a damaged system (as in SHL). Note that still not all CHL patients may show lower thresholds, as patients suffering from CHL and SHL would be classified as CHL based on the diagnostic criteria (mean air-bone gap >5 dB; see Materials and Methods) and, therefore, may reduce the effect in the group. Finally, our model seems biologically plausible in that tinnitus development is condoned as a side effect of threshold restoration, as it particularly improves the speech intelligibility (improved thresholds in the speech relevant frequency range, most frequent (high) tinnitus pitch leads to strongest improvement of speech intelligibility), and communication by speech is crucial for social interaction and communication between

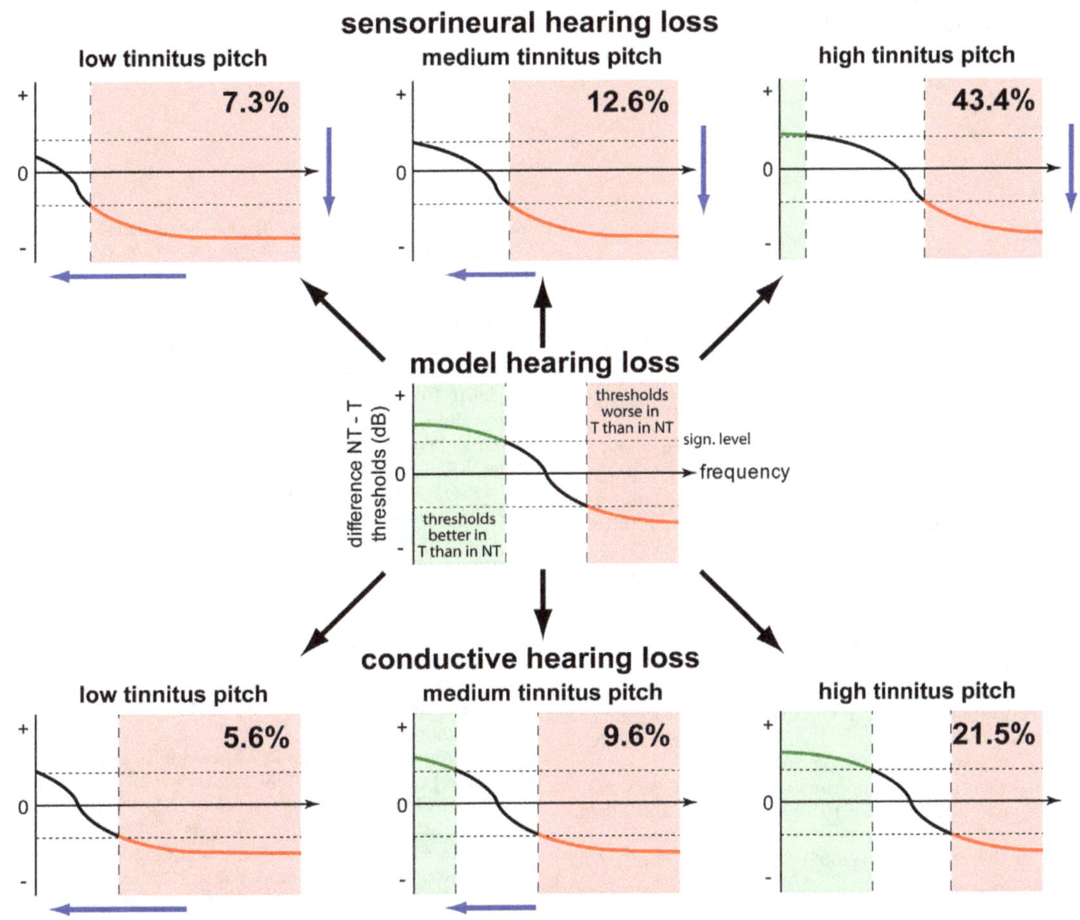

FIGURE 7 | Model of decreasing (green) or increasing (red) effects of tinnitus on hearing thresholds. In the center panel, the general effect of tinnitus on hearing threshold is given. Tinnitus is beneficial for thresholds in the low frequency range and detrimental in the high frequency range. The horizontal broken lines symbolize the significance levels. Two main factors alter this relationship by shifting the function either down (SHL) or left (tinnitus pitch). For more explanation, refer to the text.

humans (2, 25, 43). This view is supported by the fact that high pitch tinnitus patients show the largest distance of speech and corresponding pure tone thresholds, which are even higher than those of NT patients. An alternative interpretation of the data presented here is that steeper audiogram slopes due to better hearing thresholds at low frequencies and worse hearing thresholds at high frequencies are more likely to lead to the development of tinnitus (17).

One drawback of this retrospective study is the lack of information on etiology, comorbidities or medication of the 37,000 patients pooled together here. As tinnitus is only a symptom resulting from different diseases, its specific characteristic may differ from case to case. The fact that our analysis still yielded highly systematic results further strengthens our interpretation of the functional benefit of tinnitus on hearing thresholds.

In conclusion, we think that within an evolutionary frame of reference it makes perfectly sense to optimize hearing and information extraction ability on the cost of generating a phantom percept off the frequencies of interest, i.e., high-pitched tinnitus. Why some patients suffer from low or medium-pitched tinnitus remains unclear and may have different reasons than the threshold decreasing high pitch tinnitus. Another open question why only a minority of CHL patients is developing a tinnitus percept has to be addressed in a more detailed, possibly prospective, follow-up study.

AUTHOR CONTRIBUTIONS

DG analyzed the data and wrote a part of the manuscript. KT wrote a part of the manuscript, interpreted the data, and performed the statistical analysis. PK and AS provided assistance in the statistical analysis and interpretation of the data. UH provided the data. HS wrote a part of the manuscript.

FUNDING

The present work was performed in fulfillment of the requirements for obtaining the degree “Dr. med. dent.” at the Friedrich-Alexander University Erlangen-Nürnberg (FAU). PK was supported by the Dr. Willmar Schwabe GmbH & Co., KG, Karlsruhe, Germany. AS was supported by the Interdisciplinary Center for Clinical Research (IZKF, Project E15). We acknowledge support by Deutsche Forschungsgemeinschaft and Friedrich-Alexander-Universität Erlangen-Nürnberg (FAU) within the funding program Open Access Publishing.

REFERENCES

Coles R. Epidemiology of tinnitus: (2) demographic and clinical features. *J Laryngol Otol* (1984) 98:195–202. doi:10.1017/S1755146300090466

Lewis JE, Stephens SD, Mckenna L. Tinnitus and suicide. *Clin Otolaryngol Allied Sci* (1994) 19:50–4. doi:10.1111/j.1365-2273.1994.tb01147.x

Ruben RJ. Redefining the survival of the fittest: communication disor- ders in the 21st century. *Laryngoscope* (2000) 110:241–5. doi:10.1097/ 00005537-200002010-00010

Niskar AS, Kieszak SM, Holmes AE, Esteban E, Rubin C, Brody DJ. Estimated prevalence of noise-induced hearing threshold shifts among children 6 to 19 years of age: the Third National Health and Nutrition Examination Survey, 1988-1994, United States. *Pediatrics* (2001) 108:40–3. doi:10.1542/peds.108.1.40

Holube I, Fredelake S, Vlaming M, Kollmeier B. Development and analysis of an International Speech Test Signal (ISTS). *Int J Audiol* (2010) 49:891–903. doi:10.3109/14992027.2010.506889

Daniel E. Noise and hearing loss: a review. *J Sch Health* (2007) 77:225–31. doi:10.1111/j.1746-1561.2007.00197.x

Li CM, Zhang XZ, Hoffman HJ, Cotch MF, Themann CL, Wilson MR. Hearing impairment associated with depression in US Adults, National Health and Nutrition Examination Survey 2005-2010. *JAMA Otolaryngol Head Neck Surg* (2014) 140:293–302. doi:10.1001/jamaoto.2014.42

Katzenell U, Segal S. Hyperacusis: review and clinical guidelines. *Otol Neurotol* (2001)22:321–6;discussion326-327.doi:10.1097/00129492-200105000-00009

Gates GA, Mills JH. Presbycusis. *Lancet* (2005) 366:1111–20. doi:10.1016/S0140-6736(05)67423-5

Cruickshanks KJ, Wiley TL, Tweed TS, Klein BE, Klein R, Mares-Perlman JA, et al. Prevalence of hearing loss in older adults in Beaver Dam, Wisconsin. The Epidemiology of Hearing Loss Study. *Am J Epidemiol* (1998) 148:879–86. doi:10.1093/oxfordjournals.aje.a009713

Baguley D, Mcferran D, Hall D. Tinnitus. *Lancet* (2013) 382:1600–7. doi:10.1016/S0140-6736(13)60142-7

Hoffman HJ, Reed GW. Epidemiology of tinnitus. In: Snow JB, editor. *Theory and Management*. Hamilton: BC Decker (2004). p. 24–7.

Hebert S, Canlon B, Hasson D, Magnusson Hanson LL, Westerlund H, Theorell T. Tinnitus severity is reduced with reduction of depressive mood – a prospective population study in Sweden. *PLoS One* (2012) 7:e37733. doi:10.1371/journal.pone.0037733

Lockwood AH, Salvi RJ, Burkard RF. Tinnitus. *NEngl J Med* (2002) 347:904–10. doi:10.1056/NEJMra013395

Møller AR. Epidemiology of tinnitus in adults. 1st ed. In: Møller AR, Langguth B, De Ridder D, Kleinjung T, editors. *Textbook of Tinnitus*. New York: Springer (2011). p. 29–37.

Henry JA, Meikle M, Gilbert A. Audiometric correlates of tinnitus pitch: insights from the Tinnitus Data Registry. In: Hazell J, editor. *Proceedings of the Sixth International Tinnitus Seminar*. London: The Tinnitus and Hyperacusis Centre (1999). p. 51–7.

König O, Schaette R, Kempter R, Gross M. Course of hearing loss and occur- rence of tinnitus. *Hear Res* (2006) 221:59–64. doi:10.1016/j.heares.2006.07.007

Moore BC, Vinay, Sandhya. The relationship between tinnitus pitch and the edge frequency of the audiogram in individuals with hearing impairment and tonal tinnitus. *Hear Res* (2010) 261:51–6. doi:10.1016/j.heares.2010.01.003

Sereda M, Hall DA, Bosnyak DJ, Edmondson-Jones M, Roberts LE, Adjamian P, et al. Re-examining the relationship between audiometric profile and tinnitus pitch. *Int J Audiol* (2011) 50:303–12. doi:10.3109/14992027.2010.551221

Krauss P, Tziridis K, Metzner C, Schilling A, Hoppe U, Schulze H. Stochastic resonance controlled upregulation of internal noise after hearing loss as a putative cause of tinnitus-related neuronal hyperactivity. *Front Neurosci* (2016) 10:597. doi:10.3389/fnins.2016.00597

Benzi R, Sutera A, Vulpiani A. The mechanism of stochastic resonance. *J Phys A Math Gen* (1981) 14:L453. doi:10.1088/0305-4470/14/11/006

Collins JJ, Imhoff TT, Grigg P. Noise-enhanced information transmission in rat SA1 cutaneous mechanoreceptors via aperiodic stochastic resonance. *J Neurophysiol* (1996) 76:642–5.

Levin JE, Miller JP. Broadband neural encoding in the cricket cercal sensory system enhanced by stochastic resonance. *Nature* (1996) 380:165–8. doi:10.1038/380165a0

Gammaitoni L, Hänggi P, Jung P, Marchesoni F. Stochastic resonance. *Rev Mod Phys* (1998) 70:223. doi:10.1103/RevModPhys.70.223

Coles RR. Epidemiology of tinnitus: (1) prevalence. *J Laryngol Otol Suppl* (1984) 9:7–15. doi:10.1017/S1755146300090041

Axelsson A, Sandh A. Tinnitus in noise-induced hearing loss. *Br J Audiol* (1985) 19:271–6. doi:10.3109/03005368509078983

Savastano M. Tinnitus with or without hearing loss: are its characteristics different? *Eur Arch Otorhinolaryngol* (2008) 265:1295–300. doi:10.1007/s00405-008-0630-z

Nadol JB Jr. Hearing loss. *N Engl J Med* (1993) 329:1092–102. doi:10.1056/NEJM199310073291507

Schreiber BE, Agrup C, Haskard DO, Luxon LM. Sudden sensorineural hearing loss. *Lancet* (2010) 375:1203–11. doi:10.1016/S0140-6736(09)62071-7

Moon I, Won J, Kang H, Kim D, An Y, Shim H. Influence of tinnitus on auditory spectral and temporal resolution and speech perception in tinnitus patients. *J Neurosci* (2015) 35:14260–9. doi:10.1523/JNEUROSCI.5091-14.2015

Gilles A, Schlee W, Rabau S, Wouters K, Fransen E, Van De Heyning P. Decreased speech-in-noise understanding in young adults with tinnitus. *Front Neurosci* (2016) 10:288. doi:10.3389/fnins.2016.00288

Gerken GM. Central tinnitus and lateral inhibition: an auditory brainstem model. *Hear Res* (1996) 97:75–83. doi:10.1016/S0378-5955(96)80009-8

Eggermont JJ. Central tinnitus. *Auris Nasus Larynx* (2003) 30(Suppl):S7–12. doi:10.1016/S0385-8146(02)00122-0

Eggermont JJ, Roberts LE. The neuroscience of tinnitus. *Trends Neurosci* (2004) 27:676–82. doi:10.1016/j.tins.2004.08.010

Schaette R, McAlpine D. Tinnitus with a normal audiogram: physiological evidence for hidden hearing loss and computational model. *J Neurosci* (2011) 31:13452–7. doi:10.1523/JNEUROSCI.2156-11.2011

Knipper M, Van Dijk P, Nunes I, Ruttiger L, Zimmermann U. Advances in the neurobiology of hearing disorders: recent developments regarding the basis of tinnitus and hyperacusis. *Prog Neurobiol* (2013) 111:17–33. doi:10.1016/j.pneurobio.2013.08.002

Ruttiger L, Singer W, Panford-Walsh R, Matsumoto M, Lee SC, Zuccotti A, et al. The reduced cochlear output and the failure to adapt the central auditory response causes tinnitus in noise exposed rats. *PLoS One* (2013) 8:e57247. doi:10.1371/journal.pone.0057247

Zeng F-G, Fu Q-J, Morse R. Human hearing enhanced by noise. *Brain Res* (2000) 869:251–5. doi:10.1016/S0006-8993(00)02475-6

Long Z-C, Shao F, Zhang Y-P, Qin Y-G. Noise-enhanced hearing sensitivity. *Phys Lett A* (2004) 323:434–8. doi:10.1016/j.physleta.2004.02.019

Ries DT. The influence of noise type and level upon stochastic resonance in humanaudition. *Hear Res* (2007) 228:136–43. doi:10.1016/j.heares.2007.01.027

Hebert S, Fournier P, Norena A. The auditory sensitivity is increased in tinnitus ears. *J Neurosci* (2013) 33:2356–64. doi:10.1523/JNEUROSCI.3461-12.2013

Parra LC, Pearlmutter BA. Illusory percepts from auditory adaptation. *J Acoust Soc Am* (2007) 121:1632–41. doi:10.1121/1.2431346

Langguth B, Landgrebe M, Kleinjung T, Sand GP, Hajak G. Tinnitus and depression. *World J Biol Psychiatry* (2011) 12:489–500. doi:10.3109/15622975.2011.575178

4

Speech Comprehension Difficulties in Chronic Tinnitus and its Relation to Hyperacusis

Veronika Vielsmeier[1,2], Peter M. Kreuzer[2,3], Frank Haubner[1], Thomas Steffens[1,2], Philipp R. O. Semmler[1,2], Tobias Kleinjung[4], Winfried Schlee[2,3], Berthold Langguth[2,3] and Martin Schecklmann[2,3]*

[1] Department of Otorhinolaryngology, University of Regensburg, Regensburg, Germany, [2] Interdisciplinary Tinnitus Center of the University of Regensburg, Regensburg, Germany, [3] Department of Psychiatry and Psychotherapy, University of Regensburg, Regensburg, Germany, [4] Department of Otorhinolaryngology, University of Zurich, Switzerland

Correspondence:
Veronika Vielsmeier
veronika.vielsmeier@ukr.de

Objective: Many tinnitus patients complain about difficulties regarding speech comprehension. In spite of the high clinical relevance little is known about underlying mechanisms and predisposing factors. Here, we performed an exploratory investigation in a large sample of tinnitus patients to (1) estimate the prevalence of speech comprehension difficulties among tinnitus patients, to (2) compare subjective reports of speech comprehension difficulties with behavioral measurements in a standardized speech comprehension test and to (3) explore underlying mechanisms by analyzing the relationship between speech comprehension difficulties and peripheral hearing function (pure tone audiogram), as well as with co-morbid hyperacusis as a central auditory processing disorder.

Subjects and Methods: Speech comprehension was assessed in 361 tinnitus patients presenting between 07/2012 and 08/2014 at the Interdisciplinary Tinnitus Clinic at the University of Regensburg. The assessment included standard audiological assessments (pure tone audiometry, tinnitus pitch, and loudness matching), the Goettingen sentence test (in quiet) for speech audiometric evaluation, two questions about hyperacusis, and two questions about speech comprehension in quiet and noisy environments ("How would you rate your ability to understand speech?"; "How would you rate your ability to follow a conversation when multiple people are speaking simultaneously?").

Results: Subjectively-reported speech comprehension deficits are frequent among tinnitus patients, especially in noisy environments (cocktail party situation). 74.2% of all investigated patients showed disturbed speech comprehension (indicated by values above 21.5 dB SPL in the Goettingen sentence test). Subjective speech comprehension complaints (both for general and in noisy environment) were correlated with hearing level and with audiologically-assessed speech comprehension ability. In contrast, co-morbid hyperacusis was only correlated with speech comprehension difficulties in noisy environments, but not with speech comprehension difficulties in general.

Conclusion: Speech comprehension deficits are frequent among tinnitus patients. Whereas speech comprehension deficits in quiet environments are primarily due to peripheral hearing loss, speech comprehension deficits in noisy environments are related to both peripheral hearing loss and dysfunctional central auditory processing. Disturbed speech comprehension in noisy environments might be modulated by a central inhibitory deficit. In addition, attentional and cognitive aspects may play a role.

Keywords: chronic tinnitus, speech perception problems, Goettingen sentence test, hearing loss, hyperacusis

INTRODUCTION

Subjective tinnitus is the perception of sound in the absence of a corresponding acoustic signal (Baguley et al., 2013). Hearing loss is a recognized risk factor for tinnitus (Hoffmann and Reed, 2004). It is assumed that tinnitus is generated by plastic changes in the central nervous system as a reaction to reduced auditory input similar to mechanisms associated with phantom perceptions after limb amputation (De Ridder et al., 2011). Accordingly, the majority of tinnitus patients show elevated hearing thresholds in the standard pure tone audiogram (Norena et al., 2002). And many tinnitus patients with normal or nearly normal hearing thresholds in the pure tone audiogram exhibit cochlear damage (Shore et al., 2016). Hair cell loss at frequencies between the tested frequencies ("dead regions") (Weisz et al., 2006) or at high frequencies (Vielsmeier et al., 2015) have been observed in tinnitus patients with normal standard audiograms. There is also evidence for damage of high-threshold auditory nerve fibers in tinnitus patients with normal standard audiograms (Schaette and McAlpine, 2011). Speech comprehension difficulties are frequently reported by tinnitus patients (Tyler and Baker, 1983; Newman et al., 1994), even by those with normal pure tone audiograms. Particular difficulties in following a conversation are reported in situations when multiple people are speaking simultaneously, e.g., in a classical "cocktail party situation" (Jones and Litovsky, 2008).

Speech comprehension difficulties are for many tinnitus patients among the leading causes for their tinnitus-related handicap and therefore clinically, highly relevant. In contrast, knowledge about prevalence, assessment, pathogenetic mechanisms, and management of speech comprehension impairment in tinnitus patients is still very limited. Only few studies have addressed specifically impaired speech comprehension abilities in tinnitus patients. An early study demonstrated that 13 out of 25 normal hearing patients with tinnitus have deficits in at least one out of several conducted speech comprehension tests (Goldstein and Shulman, 1999). The investigation of a large sample of 495 workers who suffered from tinnitus showed speech intelligibility deficits as compared to workers without tinnitus (Soalheiro et al., 2012). A small study investigating 20 Chinese speaking patients with tinnitus revealed that speech comprehension was impaired as compared to a control group, particularly in noisy environments (Huang et al., 2007). Another study revealed that masking of tinnitus by sound improved speech comprehension (Ryu et al., 2012). An improvement of speech comprehension in noise was also observed in patients with unilateral cochlear implants when tinnitus loudness was reduced by activation of cochlear implants (Mertens et al., 2013a) or in patients whose tinnitus was successfully suppressed by rTMS treatment (Barwood et al., 2013). Wearing hearing aids over a time of 3 months showed amelioration of the performance in two speech comprehension tests for elderly patients (Araujo and Iório, 2016). Speech comprehension was worse in patients with tinnitus at the beginning of the trial, improved in patients with and without tinnitus during the trial, but speech comprehension abilities remained reduced in all evaluated parameters at the end of the treatment.

These findings suggest that tinnitus and impaired speech comprehension in noise share a common pathophysiological substrate in the central auditory pathways, a notion supported by a recent study demonstrating that ears with and without tinnitus did not differ in auditory spectral and temporal resolution abilities, but in speech comprehension in noise (Moon et al., 2015). It seems also likely that speech comprehension deficits among tinnitus patients are not solely explainable by cochlear damage, as speech comprehension deficits are also reported by patients with normal audiograms.

One of the most common comorbidities with a prevalence of 40–55% in chronic tinnitus is hyperacusis (Schecklmann et al., 2014). Hyperacusis is in general defined as abnormal intolerance to sounds. For this work we define hyperacusis as stated in the Tinnitus Sample Case History Questionnaire (TSCHQ) from the TRI (Tinnitus Research Initiative) database (refer to the methods; Schecklmann et al., 2014, 2015). Two studies investigated the relationship between hyperacusis and speech comprehension: Ten patients with auditory processing disorder, but normal audiogram, showed elevated hyperacusis scores and worse transient evoked otoacoustic emission suppression test results in contrast to 12 age-matched controls (Spyridakou et al., 2012). Strong correlations were found for a speech in babble test targeting the right ear and self-described speech in noise understanding, and also for a transient evoked otoacoustic emission suppression test targeting the right ear and hyperacusis. Nineteen normal-hearing patients with tinnitus and hyperacusis showed similar performance in speech comprehension in silence but lower performance in a communication scenario in contrast to 23 normal hearing subjects without hearing complaints (Hennig et al., 2012). The authors speculated that the common pathophysiologic substrate of tinnitus, hyperacusis, and speech comprehension (in noise) may be a dysfunction in the medial olivary cochlear system. This is an efferent inhibitory system from the primary auditory cortex along the auditory pathway to the outer and inner hair cells of the cochlea with the function to filter out irrelevant noise (Harkrider and Bowers, 2009).

In summary, the available data suggest that both peripheral and central auditory dysfunction is involved in speech comprehension difficulties in tinnitus (and hyperacusis) patients. However, most available data come from small and heterogeneous samples and there is only very limited information about how many tinnitus patients suffer from speech comprehension difficulties in quiet and in noisy environments, and how these communication difficulties relate to audiometric findings and to tinnitus characteristics. Moreover no established standard exists for the clinical assessment of speech comprehension difficulties. The mechanisms of this phenomenon are still incompletely understood and no specific evidence-based treatments exist.

The primary aim of the present work was to investigate how many patients with tinnitus suffer from subjective speech comprehension in quiet and in noisy environments. The second aim was to investigate how subjective impairments in speech comprehension relate to audiological findings in the standard audiogram and in a validated sentence comprehension test. The third aim was to explore the relationship between speech comprehension difficulties and co-morbid hyperacusis.

MATERIALS AND METHODS

Subjects/Sample

All patients presenting with subjective chronic tinnitus at the Interdisciplinary Tinnitus Center at the University of Regensburg (Regensburg, Germany, a tertiary referral center) between July, 1st 2012 and August, 31th 2014 were invited to participate in this exploratory prospective study.

Assessment

All patients completed various tinnitus questionnaires including the Tinnitus Sample Case History Questionnaire (TSCHQ; Langguth et al., 2007) and the German version of the Tinnitus Questionnaire (TQ; Goebel and Hiller, 1994; range: 0–84 with higher scores presenting higher distress), underwent microscopy of the ear and received an audiological examination including pure tone audiometry (125–8000 Hz), stapedius reflex testing, and tympanometry.

In addition to this standard assessment, speech comprehension was prospectively assessed by a specific German sentence test ["Goettingen Satztest" (Kollmeier and Wesselkamp, 1997)] and by asking two subjective questions about speech comprehension impairment.

The Goettingen sentence test was chosen as it reflects a realistic comprehension situation and has a high ecological validity (Kollmeier and Wesselkamp, 1997; Arweiler-Harbeck et al., 2011; May-Mederake and Shehata-Dieler, 2013). This test was performed in silence via air conduction by using headphones. A total of 20 sentences were presented starting at 35 dB SPL. Based on the results given by the patient the loudness was elevated or reduced accordingly in the upcoming sentences. The result is expressed as the 50% perception-threshold in dB and can range from 0 to 100 dB SPL.

Subjective speech comprehension impairment was assessed by the following two questions: "How would you rate your ability to understand speech? (German: Wieviele Probleme haben Sie, Sprache zu verstehen?)" and "How would you rate your ability to follow a conversation when multiple people are speaking simultaneously (e.g., in restaurant situation)? [German: Wieviele Probleme haben Sie, Gesprächen zu folgen, wenn mehrere Personen gleichzeitig sprechen (z.B. in einer Gaststätte)?]" on a scale ranging between 0 and 5 points (0, no problems; 1, minimal problems; 2, minor problems; 3, moderate problems; 4, significant problems; 5, massive problems; German: 0, keine Probleme; 1, sehr wenig Probleme; 2, wenig Probleme; 3, mäßig; 4, starke Probleme; 5, sehr starke Probleme). Patients gave written informed consent that data were gathered and analyzed for the Tinnitus Research Initiative Database which was approved by the Ethics Committee of the University Hospital of Regensburg (Germany; reference number 08/046).

For descriptive analyses, "normal" was defined by the cut-off criterion that the hearing thresholds at all frequencies measured in the standard pure tone audiogram (125, 250, 500 Hz, 1, 2, 4, 6, 8 kHz) were equal or below 20 dB hearing loss. The mean value over all frequencies (125, 250, 500 Hz, 1, 2, 4, 6, 8 kHz) and both ears was calculated for each patient. Patients with normal or disturbed speech comprehension in accordance to the Goettingen sentence test were determined by the cut-off criterion $\leq$ 21.5 dB SPL.

Moreover we explored whether tolerability of loud sounds (hyperacusis) was related to subjectively perceived speech comprehension deficits. For this purpose, we used two questions ["Do you have a problem tolerating sounds because they often seem much too loud? That is, do you often find sounds too loud or hurtful, which other people around you find quite comfortable?" (answers: never, rarely, sometimes, usually, always; rated with 1, 2, 3, 4, 5, respectively); "Do sounds cause you pain or physical discomfort?" (answers: no, yes, I don't know; rated with 0, 1, 2, respectively)], that have recently been validated as useful screening questions for hyperacusis (Schecklmann et al., 2015). Notably, these questions focus particularly on symptoms of fear/pain-related hyperacusis and do not diagnosis hyperacusis comprehensively.

Data were collected within the framework of the Tinnitus Research Initiative Database (Landgrebe et al., 2010).

Statistical Analysis

For statistical analyses, we initially present descriptive data and the number of patients with speech comprehension problems. Speech comprehension ratings are also shown compared to normal values for the audiogram and Goettingen test results. To evaluate possible factors contributing to subjective speech comprehension deficits (dependent variables) we analyzed possible associations by using Pearson correlation coefficients for metric variables (hearing level, Goettingen Satztest, and hyperacusis question 1 with speech comprehension questions 1 and 2) and Student t-tests for independent samples for dichotomous variables (patients with yes vs. no answers in hyperacusis question 2 with respect to speech comprehension questions 1 and 2). For these analyses, we firstly used the average hearing level and the Goettingen test score. We assumed that these audiologic variables were related to the subjectively perceived deficit in speech comprehension. To assess the influence of sound tolerability on speech comprehension we correlated the answers for the question "Do you have a problem tolerating sounds because they often seem much too loud? That is, do you often find sounds too loud or hurtful, which other people around you find quite comfortable?" and "Do sounds cause you pain or physical discomfort?" with the speech comprehension scores and compared the speech comprehension scores between patients who experienced physical discomfort or pain to sounds and those who did not (**Table 1**). All association analyses were repeated with the Tinnitus severity (Tinnitus Questionnaire Score) as co-variate by using partial correlations for the Pearson correlations and analyses of covariance for the Student *t*-test. Spearmen correlations revealed the same results. As partial correlations are only possible for parametric tests we provide results of the Pearson correlations. The significance threshold was set to 5%. No corrections for multiple comparisons were performed because of the explorative character of the study. Strength of correlations was indicated as small (r = 0.1), medium (r = 0.3), and high (r = 0.5). Effect sizes for Student *t*-tests were indicated by Cohen's d with 0.2 as small, 0.5 as medium and 0.8 as large effect size. Statistical analyses were performed with SPSS (SPSS Inc., USA, version 22).

RESULTS

Complete data sets (audiogram, Goettingen sentence test, speech comprehension questions) were available from 361 patients. One hundred and thirty-one (36.3%) were female, 51 (14.1%) reported right-sided tinnitus, 92 (25.5%) left-sided tinnitus, and 216 (59.8%) tinnitus in both ears or within the head. Age was 52.4 ± 12.5 (mean ± SD) years, tinnitus distress was 39.8 ± 17.3 as indicated by the tinnitus questionnaire (Hiller and Goebel, 1992; Goebel and Hiller, 1994; Hiller et al., 1994), and tinnitus duration was 93.8 ± 97.0 months. 296 (82%) patients had hearing loss (>20 dB HL in one or more frequencies of the standard audiogram) and 268 (74.2%) showed disturbed speech comprehension as indicated by values above 21.5 dB SPL in the Goettingen sentence test. One hundred and fifty-two (42.1%) patients reported problems with speech comprehension in general (score of at least one in question 1) and 288 (79.8%) problems with speech comprehension when multiple people were speaking simultaneously (speech comprehension in group conversation or noisy environment; score of at least one in question 2). For detailed distribution of answers to the two questions see **Figure 1**. As can be seen in **Figure 2** there is a quite

TABLE 1 | (A) Association of variables of audiometry, Goettingen sentence test, and hyperacusis with subjective speech comprehension.

	General speech comprehension problems (0–5)	Speech comprehension problems in noisy environment (0–5)
Average hearing loss (dB HL) (n = 361)	r = 0.474; p < 0.001	r = 0.517; p < 0.001
Goettingen sentence test (dB SPL) (n = 361)	r = 0.351; p < 0.001	r = 0.387; p < 0.001
Do you have a problem tolerating sounds because they often seem much too loud? That is, do you often find too loud or hurtful sounds which other people around you find quite comfortable? (n = 349)	r = 0.071; p = 0.188	r = 0.268; p < 0.001
Do sounds cause you pain or physical discomfort? (yes: n = 188; no = 126)	yes: 0.96 ± 1.25; no: 0.83 ± 1.17; t = 0.982; df = 312; p = 0.327; d = 0.107	yes: 2.66 ± 1.54; no: 2.10 ± 1.62; t = 3.140; df = 312; p = 0.002; d = 0.354

r, Pearson correlations coefficient; t, Student t-test; xx ± xx, mean ± sd.

TABLE 1 | (B) Association of variables of audiometry, Goettingen sentence test, and hyperacusis with subjective speech comprehension with the tinnitus questionnaire as covariate.

	General speech comprehension problems (0–5)	Speech comprehension problems in noisy environment (0–5)
Average hearing loss (dB HL) (n = 344)	r = 0.443; p < 0.001	r = 0.467; p < 0.001
Goettingen sentence test (dB SPL) (n = 344)	r = 0.310; p < 0.001	r = 0.330; p < 0.001
Do you have a problem tolerating sounds because they often seem much too loud? That is, do you often find too loud or hurtful sounds which other people around you find quite comfortable? (n = 344)	r = –0.025; p = 0.644	r = 0.167; p = 0.002
Do sounds cause you pain or physical discomfort? (yes: n = 186; no = 125)	yes: 0.97 ± 1.25; no: 0.82 ± 1.17; F = 0.296; df = 1308; p = 0.645	yes: 2.66 ± 1.55; no: 2.07 ± 1.61; F = 1.685; df = 1308; p = 0.195

r, Pearson correlations coefficient; F, analysis of covariance; xx ± xx, mean ± sd.

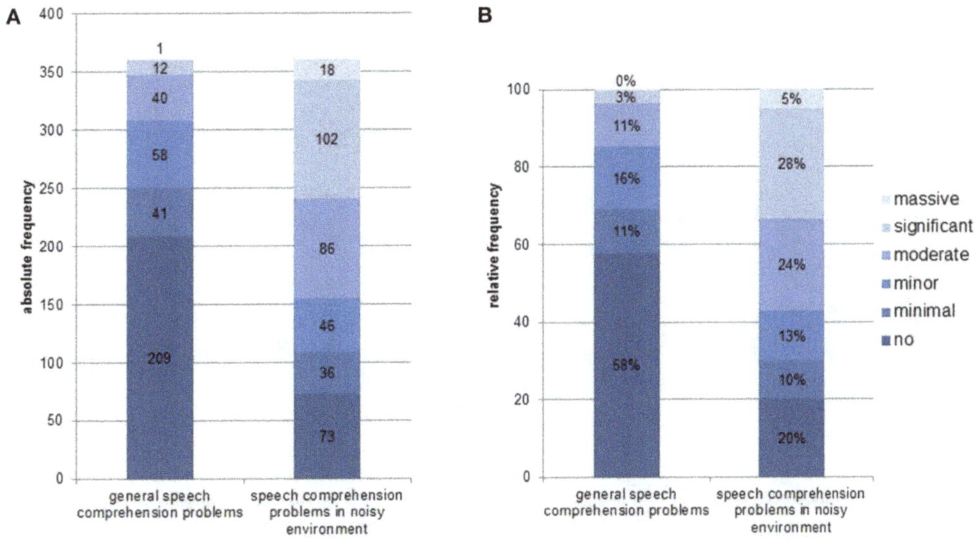

FIGURE 1 | Distribution of answers from the speech comprehension questions ["How would you rate your ability to understand speech?" and "How would you rate your ability to follow a conversation when multiple people are speaking simultaneously (e.g., in restaurant situation)? on a scale ranging between 0, no problems; 1, minimal problems; 2, minor problems; 3, moderate problems; 4, significant problems; to 5, massive problems]. **(A)** Absolute frequency of distribution; **(B)** Relative frequency of distribution.

good overlap of audiometry results or results from the Goettingen sentence test with subjective ratings of speech comprehension. This is also evident by correlating these variables showing significant positive correlations of the mean audiogram and the comprehension test with subjective speech comprehension in general and in noisy environment with medium to high correlations coefficients (**Table 1A**).

Moreover we assessed the influence of co-morbid hyperacusis (low tolerability of loud sounds) on speech comprehension (**Table 1A**). Patients with hyperacusis (Schecklmann et al., 2015) showed an association with speech comprehension problems in noisy environments (negligible effects sizes), but not in quiet environments (small effect sizes correlation coefficient). For the first hyperacusis question, patients reporting greater problems with sound tolerance showed greater problems with speech comprehension in noisy environments and vice versa. For hyperacusis question two, patients with discomfort to sounds report significant higher speech comprehension deficits in noisy environments in contrast to patients without discomfort to sounds.

All correlations in **Table 1A** were also repeated with the Tinnitus severity (Tinnitus Questionnaire Score) as co-variate. Apart from the correlation between the categorical hyperacousis question "Do sounds cause you pain or physical discomfort?" and the speech comprehension in noise score, which lost significance after inclusion of the TQ score as co-variate, results remained unchanged (**Table 1B**), indicating that the main findings are not driven by global tinnitus severity.

DISCUSSION

The study of speech comprehension difficulties in a large sample of tinnitus patients revealed several main findings. First, with a prevalence of about 40%, subjectively-reported speech comprehension deficits are frequent among tinnitus patients. This number substantially increased when patients were asked about speech comprehension in noisy environments (cocktail party situation) where almost 80% of all investigated tinnitus patients reported difficulties. We are aware that there may be a selection bias as the sample comes from a tertiary referral clinic. However, our sample is much larger than previously investigated samples (Huang et al., 2007) and consisted of unselected patients who consecutively presented because of tinnitus in our clinic. Moreover, there are similar reports of high prevalence of speech intelligibility deficits in workers with exposure to noise and tinnitus (Soalheiro et al., 2012). A further aspect that was not considered in this study is the potential influence of tinnitus-related cognitive or attentional impairment on speech comprehension difficulties. Therefore population-based studies and studies involving cognitive testing will be needed for a valid estimation of the prevalence of speech comprehension difficulties among tinnitus patients. Future studies should also consider the use of more specific diagnostic tests for the presence of hyperacusis beyond the screening questions used in this study. In order to identify the relevance of tinnitus in the interplay between hearing loss and speech comprehension, future research should also include people without tinnitus.

Subjectively-reported speech comprehension difficulties were correlated with the Goettingen sentence test scores. The highly-significant correlation between the subjective perception reports and the behavioral audiological measurements with the Goettingen sentence test provides some validation for the speech comprehension-related questions used for this study. On the other hand, the score in the Goettingen sentence test only explained about 12% of the variance (r^2) of the subjective

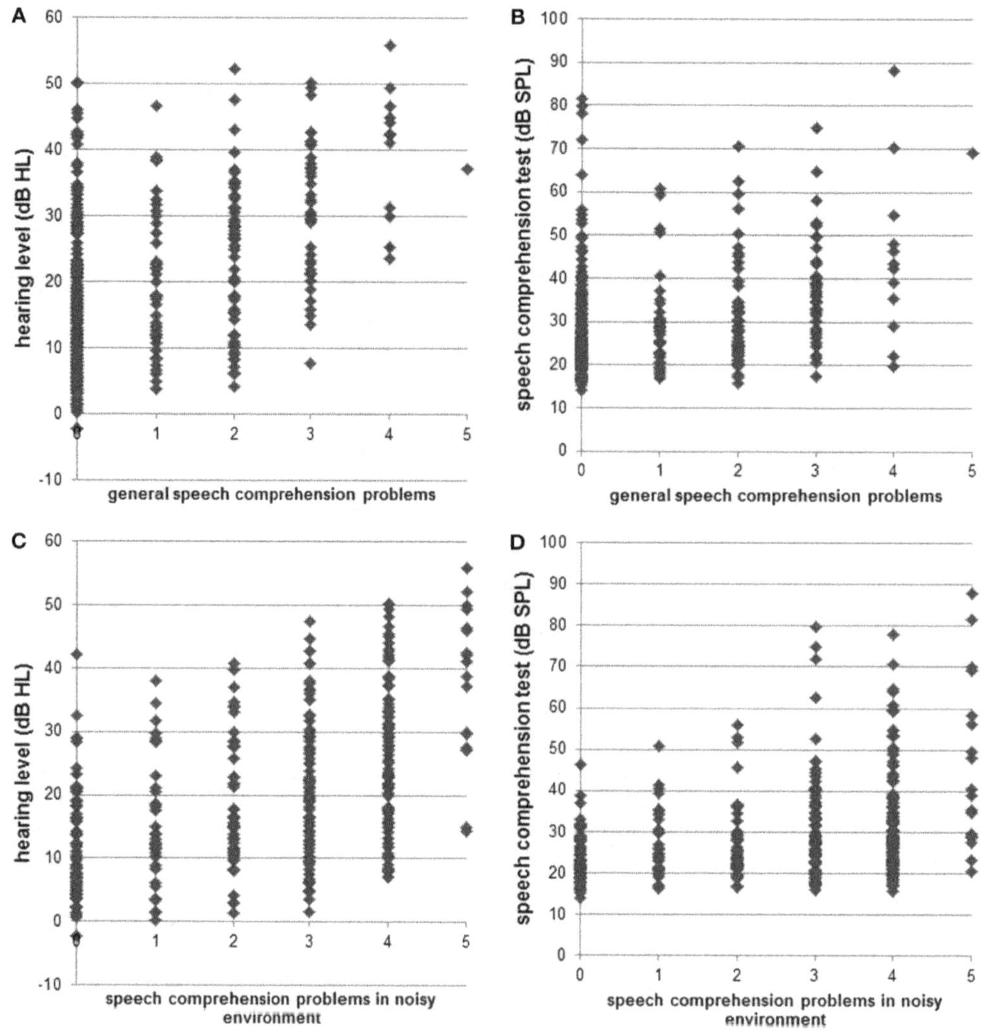

FIGURE 2 | Scatter plots indicate single subject data for hearing status [pure tone audiogram; (A): $r = 0.474$; **(C):** $r = 0.517$] and speech comprehension status [results from Goettingen sentence test; **(B):** $r = 0.351$, **(D):** $r = 0.387$] compared to the subjective speech comprehension report in quiet and in noisy environments, respectively.

speech comprehension impairment. This suggests that the two measurements reflect different aspects and arguing for the usefulness of both subjective and behavioral assessment of speech comprehension.

As most people with tinnitus have some form of cochlear damage, both hearing impairment and tinnitus can contribute to impaired speech comprehension in tinnitus patients (Tyler and Baker, 1983). Here, we found a high correlation between audiometrically-determined hearing threshold shifts and the subjectively-perceived speech comprehension difficulties. This clearly suggests that the degree of cochlear damage has a significant impact of speech comprehension difficulties—both in general (per question 1) and in "cocktail party" situations (per question 2). On the other hand, both our data and previous studies show that there are also tinnitus patients with normal hearing who complain about speech comprehension deficits (Goldstein and Shulman, 1999; Soalheiro et al., 2012) highlighting the role of non-peripheral modulating factors of speech comprehension deficits.

We also investigated the relationship between co-morbid hyperacusis and speech comprehension difficulties. Answers to the two screening questions for hyperacusis (Schecklmann et al., 2015) were significantly related to speech comprehension in the cocktail party situation, but not to speech comprehension in general. As hyperacusis is presumably due to increased central gain as a consequence of deficient central inhibitory mechanisms (Brotherton et al., 2015), our findings suggest that this inhibitory dysfunction of the auditory pathway has a specific impact on speech comprehension difficulties in the cocktail party situation.

According to current knowledge, a central inhibitory deficit is occurring both in tinnitus and hyperacusis, but is especially pronounced in hyperacusis (Noreña, 2011; Hébert et al., 2013). This central inhibitory deficit seems to be particularly relevant for speech comprehension deficits in noisy environments. One could speculate that speech comprehension in cocktail party situations requires functional inhibitory systems in the neural auditory pathways to actively filter out irrelevant sounds and this function is impaired in tinnitus patients and particularly in tinnitus patients with hyperacusis. This "Central Inhibitory Deficit"—hypothesis would fit with the reported improvement of speech-in-noise perception after successful tinnitus reduction (Barwood et al., 2013; Mertens et al., 2013b).

The medial olivary cochlear system is involved in the auditory efferent system originating in the auditory cortex with connections to the inner and outer hair cells (Hennig et al., 2012). This filter system for peripheral input (Harkrider and Bowers, 2009) takes part in the processing of interaural time differences for sound localization (Myoga et al., 2014), which is necessary for conversation in noisy environment. Moreover, the medial olivary cochlear system has anti-masking functions to adjust cochlear amplification in situations of listening to speech-in-noise (Bidelman and Bhagat, 2015). This might be involved in hyperacusis as shown by decreased distortion-product otoacoustic emissions, as elicited by noise presented to the contralateral ear in patients with tinnitus and low sound level tolerance (Knudson et al., 2014).

Previously, an association between otoacoustic emissions and hyperacusis (but not with hearing in noise) was found (Spyridakou et al., 2012). This study showed elevated hyperacusis scores and reduced otoacoustic emissions of 10 patients with auditory processing disorder but normal hearing in contrast to 12 age-matched controls. Nineteen normal-hearing patients with tinnitus and hyperacusis showed similar performance in speech comprehension in silence, but lower performance in a communication scenario in contrast to 23 normal hearing subjects without hearing complaints (Hennig et al., 2012). In conclusion, a central inhibitory deficit (e.g., an impairment of the medial olivary cochlear system) might represent the common pathophysiologic substrate of tinnitus, hyperacusis, and speech comprehension (in noise) (Hennig et al., 2012).

Electroencephalographic studies have demonstrated that auditory alpha oscillations, which are reduced in tinnitus patients, are critically involved in speech comprehension(Weisz et al., 2011), suggesting that reduced alpha oscillations in the temporal cortex could represent a neuronal correlate of deficient central inhibitory activity in the auditory system, which can manifest as tinnitus and as deficient speech-in-noise comprehension.

In summary, our data suggest that speech comprehension difficulties occur frequently among tinnitus patients and are caused by both peripheral hearing loss and deficient central inhibitory mechanisms. The latter are probably important for speech comprehension difficulties in noisy environments.

The presented work has several implications for clinical management and research. First, our data indicate that speech comprehension difficulties occur frequently among tinnitus patients and should be regularly explored in clinical routine. Second, the proposed screening questions can be used for a simple and easily feasible standardized assessment of speech comprehension difficulties in tinnitus patients. Third, our data also suggest that it would be worthwhile to investigate whether improvement of tinnitus severity and hyperacousis, e.g., by cognitive behavioral therapy, might also improve speech comprehension in noise. Fourth, the effects of hearing aids and specific forms of hearing training should be evaluated in clinical trials.

AUTHOR CONTRIBUTIONS

VV and BL: conception, acquisition, interpretation, manuscript. PK and FH: acquisition, manuscript. TS and WS: interpretation, analysis, manuscript. PS: acquisition, interpretation, manuscript. TK: conception, interpretation, manuscript. MS: acquisition, interpretation, analysis, manuscript.

REFERENCES

Araujo, T. M., and Iório, M. C. M. (2016). Effects of sound amplification in self-perception of tinnitus and hearing loss in the elderly. *Braz. J. Otorhinolaryngol.* 82, 289–296. doi: 10.1016/j.bjorl.2015.05.010

Arweiler-Harbeck, D., Janeschik, S., Lang, S., and Bagus, H. (2011). Suitability of auditory speech sound evaluation (A§E®) in German cochlear implant patients. *Eur. Arch. Otorhinolaryngol.* 268, 1259–1266. doi: 10.1007/s00405-011-1505-2

Baguley, D., McFerran, D., and Hall, D. (2013). Tinnitus. *Lancet* 382, 1600–1607. doi: 10.1016/S0140-6736(13)60142-7

Barwood, C. H., Wilson, W. J., Malicka, A. N., McPherson, B., Lloyd, D., Munt, K., et al. (2013). The effect of rTMS on auditory processing in adults with chronic, bilateral tinnitus: a placebo-controlled pilot study. *Brain Stimul.* 6, 752–759. doi: 10.1016/j.brs.2013.01.015

Bidelman, G. M., and Bhagat, S. P. (2015). Right-ear advantage drives the link between olivocochlear efferent 'antimasking' and speech-in-noise listening benefits. *Neuroreport* 26, 483–487. doi: 10.1097/WNR.0000000000000376

Brotherton, H., Plack, C. J., Maslin, M., Schaette, R., and Munro, K. J. (2015). Pump up the volume: could excessive neural gain explain tinnitus and hyperacusis? *Audiol. Neurootol.* 20, 273–282. doi: 10.1159/000430459

De Ridder, D., Elgoyhen, A. B., Romo, R., and Langguth, B. (2011). Phantom percepts: tinnitus and pain as persisting aversive memory networks. *Proc. Natl. Acad. Sci. U.S.A.* 108, 8075–8080. doi: 10.1073/pnas.1018466108

Goebel, G., and Hiller, W. (1994). [The tinnitus questionnaire. A standard instrument for grading the degree of tinnitus. Results of a multicenter study with the tinnitus questionnaire]. *HNO* 42, 166–172. German.

Goldstein, B., and Shulman, A. (1999). Central auditory speech test findings in individuals with subjective idiopathic tinnitus. *Int. Tinnitus J.* 5, 16–19.

Harkrider, A. W., and Bowers, C. D. (2009). Evidence for a cortically mediated release from inhibition in the human cochlea. *J. Am. Acad. Audiol.* 20, 208–215. doi: 10.3766/jaaa.20.3.7

Hébert, S., Fournier, P., and Noreña, A. (2013). The auditory sensitivity is increased in tinnitus ears. *J. Neurosci.* 33, 2356–2364. doi: 10.1523/JNEUROSCI.3461-12.2013

Hennig, T. R., Costa, M. J., Rossi, A. G., and Moraes, A. B. (2012). Auditory rehabilitation effects on the temporal ordering ability in elderly hearing aids users. *J. Soc. Bras. Fonoaudiol.* 24, 26–33. doi: 10.1590/S2179-64912012000100006

Hiller, W., and Goebel, G. (1992). A psychometric study of complaints in chronic tinnitus. *J. Psychosom. Res.* 36, 337–348.

Hiller, W., Goebel, G., and Rief, W. (1994). Reliability of self-rated tinnitus distress and association with psychological symptom patterns. *Br. J. Clin. Psychol.* 33 (Pt 2), 231–239.

Hoffmann, H. J., and Reed, G. W. (2004). "Epidemiology of tinnitus," in *Tinnitus: Theory and Management*, ed J. Snow (London: BC Decker), 16–41.

Huang, C. Y., Lee, H. H., Chung, K. C., Chen, H. C., Shen, Y. J., and Wu, J. L. (2007). Relationships among speech perception, self-rated tinnitus loudness and disability in tinnitus patients with normal pure-tone thresholds of hearing. *ORL J. Otorhinolaryngol. Relat. Spec.* 69, 25–29. doi: 10.1159/000096713

Jones, G. L., and Litovsky, R. Y. (2008). Role of masker predictability in the cocktail party problem. *J. Acoust. Soc. Am.* 124, 3818–3830. doi: 10.1121/1.2996336

Knudson, I. M., Shera, C. A., and Melcher, J. R. (2014). Increased contralateral suppression of otoacoustic emissions indicates a hyperresponsive medial olivocochlear system in humans with tinnitus and hyperacusis. *J. Neurophysiol.* 112, 3197–3208. doi: 10.1152/jn.00576.2014

Kollmeier, B., and Wesselkamp, M. (1997). Development and evaluation of a German sentence test for objective and subjective speech intelligibility assessment. *J. Acoust. Soc. Am.* 102, 2412–2421.

Landgrebe, M., Zeman, F., Koller, M., Eberl, Y., Mohr, M., Reiter, J., et al. (2010). The Tinnitus Research Initiative (TRI) database: a new approach for delineation of tinnitus subtypes and generation of predictors for treatment outcome. *BMC Med. Inform. Decis. Mak.* 10:42. doi: 10.1186/1472-6947-10-42

Langguth, B., Goodey, R., Azevedo, A., Bjorne, A., Cacace, A., Crocetti, A., et al. (2007). Consensus for tinnitus patient assessment and treatment outcome measurement: Tinnitus Research Initiative meeting, Regensburg, July 2006. *Prog. Brain Res.* 166, 525–536. doi: 10.1016/S0079-6123(07)66050-6

May-Mederake, B., and Shehata-Dieler, W. (2013). A case study assessing the auditory and speech development of four children implanted with cochlear implants by the chronological age of 12 months. *Case Rep. Otolaryngol.* 2013:359218. doi: 10.1155/2013/359218

Mertens, G., Kleine Punte, A., De Ridder, D., and Van de Heyning, P. (2013b). Tinnitus in a single-sided deaf ear reduces speech reception in the nontinnitus ear. *Otol. Neurotol.* 34, 662–666. doi: 10.1097/MAO.0b013e31828779f0

Mertens, G., Punte, A. K., and Van de Heyning, P. (2013a). Self-assessment of hearing disabilities in cochlear implant users using the SSQ and the reduced SSQ5 version. *Otol. Neurotol.* 34, 1622–1629. doi: 10.1097/MAO.0b013e31829ce980

Moon, I. J., Won, J. H., Kang, H. W., Kim, D. H., An, Y. H., and Shim, H. J. (2015). Influence of tinnitus on auditory spectral and temporal resolution and speech perception in tinnitus patients. *J. Neurosci.* 35, 14260–14269. doi: 10.1523/JNEUROSCI.5091-14.2015

Myoga, M. H., Lehnert, S., Leibold, C., Felmy, F., and Grothe, B. (2014). Glycinergic inhibition tunes coincidence detection in the auditory brainstem. *Nat. Commun.* 5, 3790. doi: 10.1038/ncomms4790

Newman, C. W., Wharton, J. A., Shivapuja, B. G., and Jacobson, G. P. (1994). Relationships among psychoacoustic judgments, speech understanding ability and self-perceived handicap in tinnitus subjects. *Audiology* 33, 47–60.

Noreña, A. J. (2011). An integrative model of tinnitus based on a central gain controlling neural sensitivity. *Neurosci. Biobehav. Rev.* 35, 1089–1109. doi: 10.1016/j.neubiorev.2010.11.003

Norena, A., Micheyl, C., Chéry-Croze, S., and Collet, L. (2002). Psychoacoustic characterization of the tinnitus spectrum: implications for the underlying mechanisms of tinnitus. *Audiol. Neurootol.* 7, 358–369. doi: 10.1159/000066156

Ryu, I. S., Ahn, J. H., Lim, H. W., Joo, K. Y., and Chung, J. W. (2012). Evaluation of masking effects on speech perception in patients with unilateral chronic tinnitus using the hearing in noise test. *Otol. Neurotol.* 33, 1472–1476. doi: 10.1097/MAO.0b013e31826dbcc4

Schaette, R., and McAlpine, D. (2011). Tinnitus with a normal audiogram: physiological evidence for hidden hearing loss and computational model. *J. Neurosci.* 31, 13452–13457. doi: 10.1523/JNEUROSCI.2156-11.2011

Schecklmann, M., Landgrebe, M., Langguth, B., and TRI Database Study Group. (2014). Phenotypic characteristics of hyperacusis in tinnitus. *PLoS ONE* 9:e86944. doi: 10.1371/journal.pone.0086944

Schecklmann, M., Lehner, A., Schlee, W., Vielsmeier, V., Landgrebe, M., and Langguth, B. (2015). Validation of screening questions for hyperacusis in chronic tinnitus. *Biomed. Res. Int.* 2015:191479. doi: 10.1155/2015/191479

Shore, S. E., Roberts, L. E., and Langguth, B. (2016). Maladaptive plasticity in tinnitus–triggers, mechanisms and treatment. *Nat. Rev. Neurol.* 12, 150–160. doi: 10.1038/nrneurol.2016.12

Soalheiro, M., Rocha, L., do Vale, D. F., Fontes, V., Valente, D., and Teixeira, L. R. (2012). Speech recognition index of workers with tinnitus exposed to environmental or occupational noise: a comparative study. *J. Occup. Med. Toxicol.* 7:26. doi: 10.1186/1745-6673-7-26

Spyridakou, C., Luxon, L. M., and Bamiou, D. E. (2012). Patient-reported speech in noise difficulties and hyperacusis symptoms and correlation with test results. *Laryngoscope* 122, 1609–1614. doi: 10.1002/lary.23337

Tyler, R. S., and Baker, L. J. (1983). Difficulties experienced by tinnitus sufferers. *J. Speech Hear. Disord.* 48, 150–154.

Vielsmeier, V., Lehner, A., Strutz, J., Steffens, T., Kreuzer, P. M., Schecklmann, M., et al. (2015). The relevance of the high frequency audiometry in tinnitus patients with normal hearing in conventional pure-tone-audiometry. *Biomed. Res. Int.* 2015:302515. doi: 10.1155/2015/302515

Weisz, N., Hartmann, T., Dohrmann, K., Schlee, W., and Norena, A. (2006). High-frequency tinnitus without hearing loss does not mean absence of deafferentation. *Hear. Res.* 222, 108–114. doi: 10.1016/j.heares.2006.09.003

Weisz, N., Hartmann, T., Müller, N., Lorenz, I., and Obleser, J. (2011). Alpha rhythms in audition: cognitive and clinical perspectives. *Front. Psychol.* 2:73. doi: 10.3389/fpsyg.2011.00073

5

Transition from Acute to Chronic Tinnitus: Predictors for the Development of Chronic Distressing Tinnitus

Elisabeth Wallhäusser-Franke[1], Roberto D'Amelio[2], Anna Glauner[1], Wolfgang Delb[1†], Jérôme J. Servais[3], Karl Hörmann[1,3] and Ines Repik[3]*

[1] Otorhinolaryngology, Phoniatrics and Audiology, Medical Faculty Mannheim, Heidelberg University, Mannheim, Germany, [2] Department of Internal Medicine IV and Neurocenter, Saarland University Medical Center, Saarland University, Homburg, Germany, [3] Otorhinolaryngology, University Medical Centre Mannheim, Mannheim, Germany

***Correspondence:**
Elisabeth Wallhäusser-Franke
elisabeth.wallhaeusser-franke@medma.uni-heidelberg.de

Background: Acute tinnitus and its transition to chronic tinnitus are poorly investigated, and factors associated with amelioration *versus* exacerbation are largely unknown. Aims of this study were to identify early predictors for the future development of tinnitus severity.

Method: Patients with tinnitus of no longer than 4 weeks presenting at an otolaryngologist filled out questionnaires at inclusion (T1), as well as 3 (T3), and 6 months (T4) after tinnitus onset. 6 weeks after onset, an interview was conducted over the phone (T2). An audiogram was taken at T1, perceived tinnitus loudness, and tinnitus-related distress were assessed separately and repeatedly together with oversensitivity to external sounds and the levels of depression and anxiety. Furthermore, coping strategies with illness were recorded.

Results: Complete remission until T4 was observed in 11% of the 47 participants, while voiced complaints at onset were stable in the majority. In the subgroup with a relevant level of depression at T1, tinnitus-related distress worsened in 30% until T4. For unilateral tinnitus, perceived loudness in the chronic condition correlated strongly with hearing loss at 2 kHz on the tinnitus ear, while a similar correlation was not found for tinnitus located to both ears or within the head.

Conclusion: Results suggest early manifestation of tinnitus complaints, and stress the importance of screening all patients presenting with acute tinnitus for levels of depression and tinnitus-related distress. Furthermore, hearing levels should be monitored, and use of hearing aids should be considered to reduce tinnitus loudness after having ascertained that sound sensitivity is within normal range.

Keywords: recent-onset tinnitus, prospective study, acute-chronic transition, hearing impairment, depression, anxiety, coping with illness

INTRODUCTION

Subjective tinnitus is an acoustic perception which is not caused by an external sound source, but by aberrant activation within the auditory system (1). This type of tinnitus is rather common, and because of its subjective nature, characteristics of the tinnitus are mostly derived from patients' reports. Tinnitus is usually associated with hearing loss (HL) as detected by pure tone audiometry, but the perceived severity bears only weak to moderate relations with hearing thresholds and other psycho-acoustically determined features of the tinnitus, while high tinnitus-related distress is often associated with poor mental well-being (2–4). As tinnitus may severely impair life quality of affected individuals, it is crucial to identify factors that are predictive for the development of disabling tinnitus before it becomes a chronic condition.

There exists a multitude of cross-sectional studies on factors associated with chronic tinnitus (e.g., this Frontiers Topic), whereas only few studies have attempted to assess participants with acute tinnitus (5–7) including a study that investigated tinnitus patients one year after their first visit to a clinic if they entered the clinic within 6 months of tinnitus onset (8). Therefore, time course as well as mechanisms involved in the transition from the acute to the chronic condition are unknown, and factors predisposing for the development of a chronic, disabling, or decompensated tinnitus are mostly inferred from retrospective reports. Furthermore, studies on acute tinnitus usually were concerned with tinnitus following sudden HL (6, 7) or acute acoustic trauma (9), which appear to be distinct as indicated by high remission rates which may reach 70% (10). High remission rates concomitant with an incidence of HL are likely related to partial recovery of hearing function in the first weeks after a temporary threshold shift (11), but not all patients can relate tinnitus onset to worsening of their hearing. Therefore, remission rates may be lower and it may not be advantageous to wait for spontaneous remission but take action early on to prevent the development of a chronic disabling tinnitus.

Across many cross-sectional studies on chronic tinnitus, psychiatric comorbidity in particular depression is the most frequent condition for those with severe tinnitus (3, 4, 12, 13). Therefore, it has been suggested that pre-existent psychiatric comorbidity may foster decompensation (5), a notion that is corroborated by the few studies with early interventions, which suggest that psychological interventions may prevent the development of disabling tinnitus to some extent (5, 14–16). In contrast, tinnitus related to acute worsening of hearing thresholds may be susceptible to pharmacological interventions (17, 18). However, effectiveness of all these interventions is challenged because of unknown remission rates.

We set out to investigate the development of acute tinnitus within the 6 months after its first appearance, i.e., during transition from the acute to the chronic condition (19). As tinnitus is a phenomenon associated with the ears, patients experiencing it for the first time are likely to seek help by an otolaryngologist, at least in a country where the general health system allows them to do so without extra cost. Therefore, we aimed to investigate the history of tinnitus in patients seen by otolaryngologists within 4 weeks after tinnitus onset. Concerned with these patients the otolaryngologist has to decide on the type of treatment that is suitable for the particular patient knowing that some may lose their tinnitus and that most will not bother with it in the long run, while a low percentage will develop a distressing tinnitus that severely affects their quality of life. Because early interventions may prevent the acute symptoms to become a chronic disabling condition (5, 14–18), it is crucial to find out early which patients are at risk to develop a disabling chronic tinnitus, and which interventions may be suitable for the individual patient. To our knowledge, the present study represents the first attempt to assess in detail the characteristics of this tinnitus population including spontaneous recovery.

Factors to be investigated in relation to tinnitus were derived from the literature on chronic tinnitus and from our experience with acute tinnitus patients (5, 14). Particular focus on the instruments used was their applicability by otolaryngologists. In addition to pure tone audiometry, self-report measures on subjectively perceived tinnitus loudness and tinnitus-related distress were used in conjunction with screening instruments for the levels of depression and anxiety and a questionnaire on coping with illness.

Aims of the study are to

(1) describe characteristics of acute tinnitus patients that seek medical help from otolaryngologists.
(2) describe the time course of transition from the acute to the chronic condition.
(3) find out whether a high level of depression at tinnitus onset promotes development of a decompensated chronic tinnitus, and whether individuals at risk can be identified early on.
(4) identify maladaptive ways of coping with tinnitus,
(5) describe factors associated with spontaneous remission.

Preliminary data based on 28 participants have been published already (20).

MATERIALS AND METHODS

Procedure

Between 6/2013 and 4/2016, all first-time presenters with tinnitus at the Ear, Nose and Throat Clinic of the University Medical Centre Mannheim and at 4 participating ENT practices in the region (see acknowledgements) were asked if they were willing to participate in the study. All willing to participate and meeting inclusion criteria were informed about aims and time required for the study. Inclusion criteria were first time tinnitus of no longer than 4 weeks, age above 18, and sufficient command of German. Exclusion criteria were neurological diseases and simultaneous psychological therapies. Participants were informed that in case they were developing distressing tinnitus, they would be assisted to contact a specialized outpatient care for tinnitus patients at the Central Institute of Mental Health, Mannheim. After completion of the study, those who wished a feedback were informed about their level of tinnitus-related distress. Study design and procedures were approved by the Ethics Committee II of Heidelberg University at the Medical Faculty Mannheim.

After giving written informed consent, the audiogram that was routinely taken was archived with the study documents. In addition, study participants filled out a comprehensive paper and pencil questionnaire with the instruments outlined below, and they gave the exact date when they first noticed their tinnitus (T1). Questionnaires were collected at a regular basis by the authors. A telephone interview was conducted 6 weeks after the recorded date of tinnitus onset (T2). During this assessment participants could ask tinnitus-related questions. Hence, this interview can be seen as additional counseling which was received by each of the participants. At T2, the interviewer remembered each participant that two more questionnaires were going to be sent within 3 (T3) and 6 (T4) months after tinnitus onset. Questionnaires were accompanied by pre-stamped return envelopes. Patients who had not answered within 2 weeks after sending these questionnaires were contacted by phone, and asked to return the filled-in questionnaire.

Instruments

At T1, demographic information was collected, and participants were asked about date and circumstances of tinnitus onset. At all assessments, they answered questions regarding tinnitus laterality and character, aggravation, or alleviation in relation to first appearance and previous treatments. In addition, the self-report measures described below were administered.

Audiometry

At T1, a pure tone audiogram was taken separately for each ear according to general procedures in otolaryngology practices in Germany for the standard frequencies between 0.25 and 8 kHz. When no response to stimulation was evoked, the measurement was considered to be impossible, and for calculation, a value of 100 dB was used.

Outcome-Variables on Tinnitus Severity

Since clinically there appear to be significant differences between patients who focus on sensory aspects of the tinnitus and those who focus on functional disability and handicap (4, 21), we used separate measures for those two aspects. Tinnitus loudness as perceived by the participant (T-NRS) was recorded at T1, T3, and T4 on a Numeric Rating Scale [NRS (21)] with the anchors "heard only during silence" (0) and "louder than all other sounds" (10).

Tinnitus-related distress was assessed with the 12-item Tinnitus Questionnaire [Mini-TQ12 (22)]. According to Zeman et al. (23), the Mini-TQ12 shows satisfying psychometric results and is sensitive to changes in tinnitus severity. For the Mini-TQ12, each of 12 items may be answered with "true," "partially true," and "not true," scored as 2, 1, and 0, respectively. Tinnitus-related distress is the sum of points given to the 12 items and ranges from 0 (no distress) to 24 (maximal distress). According to Hiller and Goebel (22), 4 grades are discerned with grade 1 (0–7) representing no or mild distress and grade 2 (8–12) representing moderate distress. The range of 0–12 is also classified as compensated tinnitus, while decompensated tinnitus includes grades 3 (distressing tinnitus: 13–18), and 4 (severely distressing tinnitus: 19–24). In order to prevent a potential aggravation when asking for specific tinnitus-related consequences on life at T1, the Mini-TQ12 was used at T2, i.e., 6 weeks after tinnitus onset, for the first time and then again at T3 and T4. During the telephone interview at T2, the twelve Mini-TQ12 items were read to the participant together with the response options. Questions were repeated as needed.

As a second instrument to address tinnitus-related distress, we employed the Sheehan Disability Scale (SDS, 24) at T1, T3, and T4. In contrast to the Mini-TQ12, the SDS circumvents the potential risk of tinnitus aggravation. It assesses functional impairment in work/school (SDS1), social (SDS2), and family life (SDS3) on three 10 point visual analog scales that present numeric and verbal descriptive anchors in addition. There is no cutoff but scores of ≥5 on any of the scales; and high scores in general are associated with significant functional impairment. A SDS total sum score was not calculated, because not all participants worked and therefore not all reported a SDS1 score. The SDS was validated and shown to be sensitive to treatment-related changes in a variety of conditions (24–27) but has not been used in relation to tinnitus before.

Outcome Predictors

Outcome predictors were chosen according to the literature on chronic tinnitus and according to our experience with acute and chronic tinnitus patients.

Depression and Anxiety

Depression and anxiety are common comorbidities of disabling tinnitus (3, 4). Levels were assessed at T1, T3, and T4, with the freely available PHQ9 scale for depression and the GAD7 scale for generalized anxiety disorder (GAD) [(28), German (29)]. Both scales have been validated in primary care populations [PHQ9 (30); GAD7 (31)], there exist normative data for Germany (29, 32), and the scales have been used in tinnitus studies (4, 33). GAD is the most frequent anxiety disorder in primary care, and the GAD7 is sensitive also to other common forms of anxiety (29). Subjects were asked how often, during the past 2 weeks, they have been bothered, and response options for both scales were "not at all," "several days," "more than half the days," "nearly every day" scored as 0, 1, 2, and 3, respectively. PHQ9 scores range from 0 to 24, and GAD7 scores range from 0 to 21. In both scales, lower score points indicate favorable conditions, while sum scores ≥10 indicate potential problems in these fields, and scores of 15 or above in the PHQ9 scale are classified as Major Depression.

Coping with Illness

The way people cope with their tinnitus was shown to be related to adjustment to the tinnitus (34), and it may be improved by psychological interventions (5, 14, 35). Coping strategies with illness were assessed with the German-language Freiburg Questionnaire of Coping with Illness (FKV: 36) at T1, T3, and T4. This 35-item questionnaire covers the following coping strategies in 5 subscales: depressive coping, active problem-oriented coping, distraction and self-affirmation, religiousness and search for meaning, and trivialization and wishful thinking. Answers are scored on 5-point Likert scales with higher scores indicating a higher intensity of coping in a particular domain. Mean scores in subscales are used for analysis. The questionnaire has good internal consistency with a Cronbach's α of 0.68 and 0.77 for single scales (36) and has been used in relation to tinnitus (37).

Oversensitivity to External Sounds

As tinnitus is often associated with diminished sound-level tolerance or hyperacusis (38), oversensitivity to external sound was assessed on a 0–10 NRS (Hyper-NRS) with the extremes "normal" (0) and "extremely sensitive" (10) at T1, T3, and T4.

Statistics

Descriptive statistics, and tests for statistical significance were performed with SPSS version 24 (SPSS/IBM, Chicago, IL, USA). Changes of the tinnitus variables, sound sensitivity, and mental health factors during the study were monitored, and differences were tested for statistical significance with the Global Linear Model for repeated measures and Bonferroni corrected *post Hoc* tests in the case of normal distribution, or with non-parametric Friedman and *post hoc* Wilcoxon tests if the variables were not normally distributed. A *p* value below 0.05 was considered to be statistical significant, and a *p* below 0.01 was considered as statistically highly significant. Bivariate correlations were performed between predictor variables at T1 and outcome variables at T4. Since this was an exploratory study, bivariate *p*-values of correlations are presented along with an indication which *p*-levels achieve the Bonferroni-corrected significance level. Because 54 bivariate correlations were performed, the Bonferroni-corrected *p*-value to reach statistical significance was 0.0009. Step-wise regression analyses were performed separately for each of the 5 outcome variables. Predictor variables with significant correlations, or correlations reaching a Pearson correlation coefficient above 0.300 and an uncorrected *p*-value below 0.05 with an outcome variable were included in the final step-wise regression analysis for this outcome.

Participant Characteristics

Fifty-seven participants were included in the study, three were excluded because the time interval between tinnitus onset and T1 was longer than 4 weeks, and one participant was excluded for taking part in a psychotherapeutical tinnitus intervention in a tinnitus clinic during the study interval. Six participants dropped out, one obviously after his tinnitus was not present at T2 anymore and the others without notice, leaving 47 (82.5%) with complete data that contributed to the results. Their sociodemographic data are given in **Table 1**. Most lived in a long-term partnership, education standard was high and no one used a hearing aid.

TABLE 1 | Sociodemographic factors at T1.

	Persisting tinnitus (*N* = 41)	Remitting (*N* = 5) or fluctuating (*N* = 1) tinnitus
Sex (m/f)	53.2%/46.8%	83.3%/16.7%
Age in years [mean (SD)]	41.4 (15.6)	41.0 (14.8)
Range	21–79	23–61
Cohabitation		
Single	8.5%	
Cohabitating	91.5%	100%
Highest educational achievement		
None	2.1%	–
Basic	8.5%	33.3%
Middle	19.1%	–
University entrance	27.6%	33.3%
University degree	42.6%	33.3%
Occupational activities		
Working	74.5%	83.3%
Scholastic	10.6%	16.7%
Working in own household	6.4%	
Retired	6.4%	
Inability to work	4.3%	
Not working because of tinnitus	0%	
Other chronic health conditions		
No/yes/no statement	68.3%/29.3%/2.4%	66.7%/33.3%

TABLE 2 | Comparison of subgroups with persisting and remitting tinnitus.

Assessment at T1/T2	Persisting tinnitus (*N* = 41)	Remitting tinnitus (*N* = 6)
T-NRS	3.95 ± 1.66	3.17 ± 1.72
Mini-TQ12	8.32 ± 5.76	No tinnitus
Sheehan Disability Scale (SDS)1	3.82 ± 2.43	2.00 ± 2.0
SDS2	3.38 ± 2.15	2.00 ± 1.5
SDS3	3.60 ± 2.23	2.00 ± 2.10
Hyper-NRS	4.66 ± 2.77	3.00 ± 1.50
PHQ9	7.24 ± 4.76	3.83 ± 1.60
GAD7	5.66 ± 3.85	3.00 ± 2.50
Audiogram mean right ear	17.74 ± 9.65	15.77 ± 4.25
Audiogram mean left ear	19.51 ± 9.44	14.13 ± 2.22

Means and SDs are shown.

RESULTS

Potential underlying causes of the tinnitus were unknown to most participants. Tinnitus onset was associated with a reduction of hearing ability that was noticeable to the patient in 24%. Some presented with vertigo which was not the major complaint, however, and no one was diagnosed with Meniere's. Two participants had an ear infection. Of note is that most of the study participants did not have a very loud or very distressing tinnitus when seeking medical advice (**Table 2**).

Tinnitus Therapies during the Study

Therapies were prescribed by the ENT-physician and were independent of study participation except for psychological/psychotherapeutic therapies that let to exclusion. Of the six participants with remitting tinnitus, one took an antibiotic for middle ear infections, another two received corticosteroid infusions, and one took medication enhancing blood flow, while two did not undergo a tinnitus-specific therapy.

Of the 41 participants with persisting tinnitus, 23 underwent a tinnitus-specific therapy until T2, and an additional 2 participants had received a tinnitus-specific therapy until T4. Fourteen received corticosteroids *via* infusions or orally, 9 took a Gingko preparation, 4 were prescribed Arlevert or Dusodril and one received an antibiotic for middle ear infections. Two underwent acupuncture and 2 received physical therapy. No one was prescribed a hearing aid. Nine participants used several therapies in combination. Tinnitus onset appeared suddenly more often in the group that underwent a tinnitus-specific therapy (84%) as compared to those without (56%). Averages of T-NRS, SDS1-3, PHQ9, and GAD7 scores at T1 were higher in the group that underwent a tinnitus-specific therapy. Group differences and most importantly group differences in the reductions of tinnitus complaints between T1 and T4 did not reach statistical significance, however. Therefore, data of both groups were pooled.

Tinnitus Remission

Complete remission of the tinnitus until T4 occurred in 5 study participants, and tinnitus was absent at T2 and T3 in another one but returned until T4. One presented with a middle ear infection at T1 that was treated successfully with an antibiotic and the tinnitus had vanished until T2. Two reported sudden HL, they were treated with steroid infusions, their hearing recovered and the tinnitus was gone before T2. Reasons for remission in the others are unknown as well as for the fluctuation of tinnitus in another one for whom the tinnitus had reappeared at T4. Further characteristics of the group with tinnitus remission are shown in **Tables 1–3** and in **Figure 1**. Although average age was similar to the group with persisting tinnitus, maximum age was lower, tinnitus onset was more often associated with a noticeable HL, and a higher percentage localized their tinnitus to one ear as opposed to both ears or within the head (**Table 3**). Whereas perceived tinnitus loudness was similar to the group with persisting tinnitus, tinnitus-related distress and oversensitivity to sound were lower (**Table 2**), coinciding with personal statements regarding changes in tinnitus loudness and distress between onset and T1. No one with remitting tinnitus reported an increase in tinnitus loudness or distress. Most notable were also the lower levels of depression and anxiety (**Table 2**).

TABLE 3 | Comparison of tinnitus characteristics between groups with persisting and remitting tinnitus.

Tinnitus characteristics at T1	Persisting tinnitus (N = 41)	Remitting (N = 5) or fluctuating (N = 1) tinnitus
Days between onset and T1		
Mean ± SD	14.9 ± 8.5	7.7 ± 10.7
Range	1–28	2–29
Sudden onset	30 (73.2%)	3 (50%)
Subtle onset	11 (26.3%)	3 (50%)
Onset		
Associated with hearing loss (HL)	7 (17.1%)	3 (50%)
Not associated with HL	34 (82.9%)	3 (50%)
Permanent	28 (68.3%)	4 (66.7%)
Intermittent	13 (31.7%)	2 (33.3%)
Localization		
Right ear	10 (24.4%)	4 (66.7%)
Left ear	16 (39.0%)	1 (16.7%)
Both ears	10 (24.4%)	1 (16.7%)
Within head	5 (12.2%)	1 (16.7%)[a]
Change in perceived loudness between onset and T1		
None	28 (68.3%)	2 (33.3%)
Less loud	4 (9.8%)	4 (66.7%)
Louder	7 (17.1%)	0
No statement	2 (4.9%)	
Change in tinnitus-related distress between onset and T1		
None	19 (46.3%)	2 (33.3%)
Less distressing	3 (7.3%)	1 (16.7%)
More distressing	11 (26.8%)	
No statement	8 (19.5%)	3 (50%)

Differences between these groups exist for localization of the tinnitus, a higher frequency of sudden onset, a higher percentage with no change or increasing loudness and distress between onset and T1.

[a]*Same participant that experienced tinnitus on both ears.*

As data on tinnitus variables was not available for all time points for participants with remitting tinnitus, the following analyses on the progression on tinnitus loudness and distress was performed with the remaining 41 with persisting tinnitus until T4.

Acute Condition

For 73% with persisting tinnitus, the tinnitus had started suddenly whereas it began gradually in the remaining 27%, and 68% reported permanent tinnitus (**Figure 2**). Tinnitus onset coincided with notable HL in 17%, 26 localized tinnitus to either left (16) or right ear (10), whereas 15 heard it on both ears (10) or within the head (5). The tinnitus sound was characterized as whistling (49%), hissing (10%), complex (34%), or other (7%). Between onset and T1, tinnitus loudness had augmented in 17% and lessened in 10%, while tinnitus-related distress had worsened in 27% and lessened in 7%. T-NRS at T1 was 5 or less in 76%, and SDS scores were 5 or below in all scales in 63% of the study participants, while 15% reported a score above 5 in all scales. At T2, 30% presented with a decompensated tinnitus indicated by a sum score of 13 or above in the Mini-TQ12.

Hearing Loss

Audiograms were available from 39 participants. In 9 thresholds did not exceed 20 dB in any of the measured frequencies, 20 had mild to moderate HL exceeding 20 dB, 9 presented with severe HL exceeding 50 dB in at least one frequency on one ear, and one presented with single sided deafness. In unilateral tinnitus, HL was more pronounced at the tinnitus ear, and HL differences were smaller for frequencies below 2 kHz but larger for frequencies above 6 kHz as compared to bilateral tinnitus (**Figure 1**).

Change of Tinnitus Complaints during Study Period

Almost 90% of the study participants developed a chronic tinnitus. At each assessment, participants were asked whether their tinnitus had changed since onset, and until T4 about half experienced stable loudness and distress, while increases were reported by 7 and 15%, respectively (**Table 4**). Localization and sound quality remained essentially constant, but time of awareness lessened considerably from 68% with permanent tinnitus at T1 to 29% at T4.

In contrast, average T-NRS did not change significantly during the study period (mean ± SD: T1: 3.95 ± 1.66/T4: 3.44 ± 1.98), and therefore, initial reports at least of those who retain their tinnitus are likely to reflect perceived loudness in the chronic state. There exists no estimate for a significant clinical change for the NRS-loudness estimate, but one can assume that a change of 3 points or 27% on the 0–10 NRS represents a noticeable change. Applying this criterion, two participants experienced significant worsening of tinnitus loudness between T1 and T4, while it lessened significantly in 6 and remained stable in a majority of 80.5%. In contrast, subjective reports (**Table 4**) indicated 3/18 with noticeably increased/decreased loudness. Thus 12 participants thought that their tinnitus loudness had decreased since tinnitus onset despite indicating a reduction of less than 3 on the T-NRS scale, and one experienced an increase

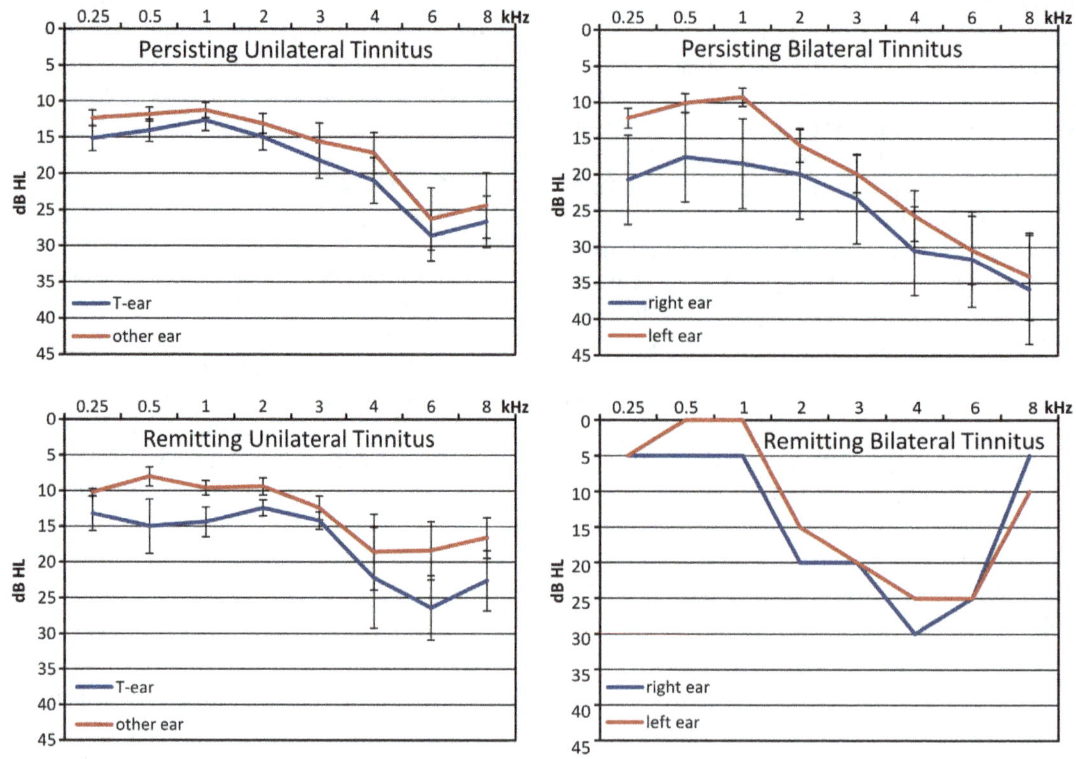

FIGURE 1 | Pure Tone Audiograms for groups with persisting and remitting, unilateral and bilateral tinnitus: shown are means with respective standard errors. Unilateral tinnitus: tinnitus heard from one ear, bilateral tinnitus: tinnitus heard on both ears or within the head. An audiogram was not available from one individual with persisting unilateral tinnitus and from another one with persisting bilateral tinnitus.

in tinnitus loudness despite a difference of less than 3 points on the T-NRS scale. Therefore, a change of 3 points appears to be a rather conservative measure for a relevant change of tinnitus loudness.

Reduction of tinnitus-related distress was statistically significant with both assessment instruments, the SDS and the Mini-TQ12. Between T1 and T4, SDS1 reduced from 3.82 ± 2.43 to 2.69 ± 2.56 (χ^2 = 11.642; p = 0.003**); SDS2 reduced from 3.38 ± 2.15 to 2.29 ± 2.45 (χ^2 = 16.487; p = 0.004**), and SDS3 reduced from 3.60 ± 2.23 to 2.37 ± 2.46 (χ^2 = 13.795; p = 0.001**). Average scores in the Mini-TQ12 were 8.32 ± 5.76 at T2 and 6.80 ± 5.65 at T4 (F = 4.425; p = 0.015*). *Posthoc* tests with Bonferroni correction revealed that for the 3 SDS scales reductions between T1 and T3 and between T1 and T4 were highly significant, and for the Mini-TQ12 a significant decrease was present between T2 and T4. Average reductions between first and last assessment were small, however (SDS1: 1.2 ± 1.92; SDS2: 1.05 ± 2.10; SDS3: 1.20 ± 2.09, Mini-TQ12: 1.63 ± 3.55). As for the T-NRS scale, a reduction of 3 points in the SDS scales may be seen as a clinically relevant difference. According to this criterion, tinnitus complaints remained stable in 80% (SDS1), 73% (SDS2), and 75% (SDS3), while reduction of complaints between T1 and T4 was reported by 20%/25%/23% and worsening was reported by one individual for each of the SDS2 and SDS3 scales. According to the literature, a reduction of at least 5 points or 21% on the 0–24 point Mini-TQ12 may be seen as a criterion for a relevant decrease on this 24 point scale (20, 39). According to this criterion, the Mini-TQ12 score worsened significantly in 10% and ameliorated in 20%, while responses to the question whether tinnitus-related distress had changed since onset were improvement for 37%, and worsening for 15% (**Table 4**).

All instruments indicate, that tinnitus-related distress is stable for the majority within a short time interval following onset, and although average reductions were statistically significant, clinically relevant changes were seen only in few individuals. Regarding a detection of relevant changes, assessments with the SDS scales were the most conservative measure. Also, a 5 point increase in the Mini-TQ12 appears to be a rather conservative criterion for a relevant change, but it constituted a more sensitive instrument for the detection of change in tinnitus-related distress than the SDS scales, and measures derived from this questionnaire can be compared across studies.

Predictors of Chronic Tinnitus Severity

In order to find potential predictors for chronic tinnitus-related distress at T4, bivariate correlations were calculated for all predictor variables at T1 with the outcome variables at T4. For unilateral tinnitus, HL at 2 kHz on the tinnitus ear showed a strong correlation with T-NRS at T4 (r = 0.626; p = 0.001), while this was

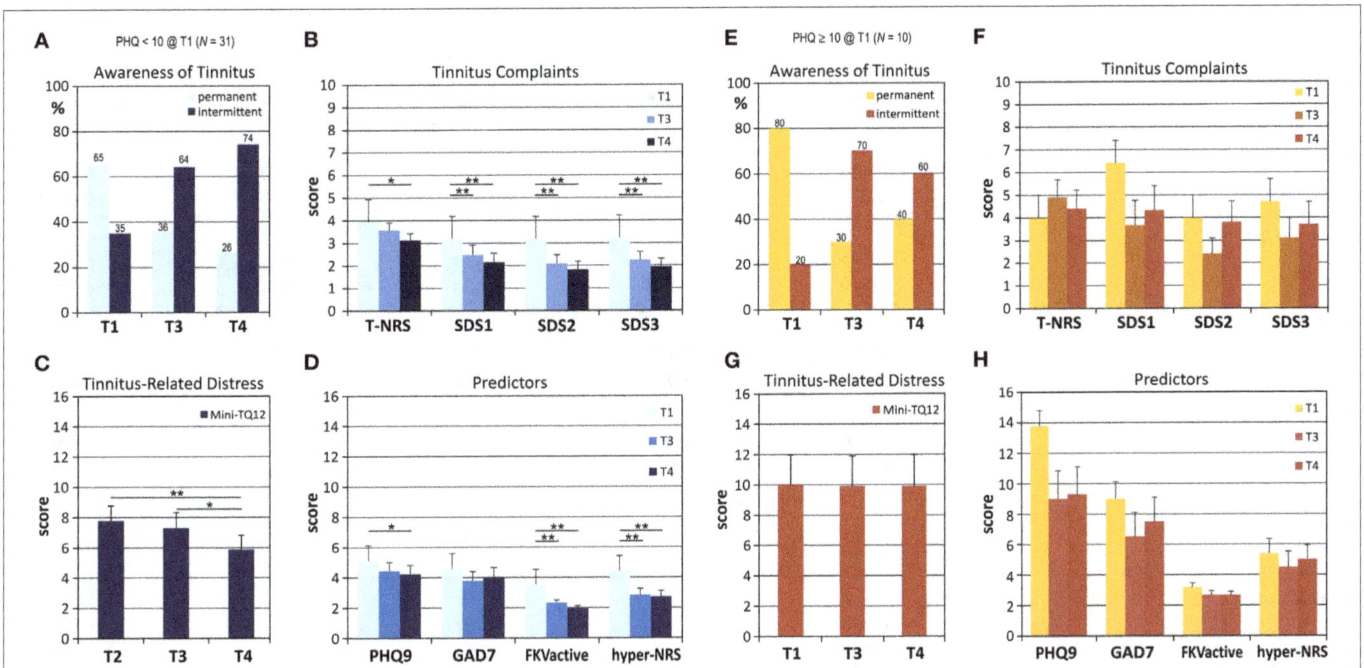

FIGURE 2 | Development of tinnitus complaints and variables that were identified as predictors for future tinnitus intensity for the group with low to moderate levels of depression [**(A–D)**, blue columns], and the group with high levels of depression, [**(E–H)**, orange-red bars]. Means and respective SEs are shown. **(A,E)** Awareness of the tinnitus, **(B,F)** perceived tinnitus loudness (T-NRS), and distress as assessed by the Sheehan scales (SDS), and **(C,G)** with the Mini-TQ12. **(D,H)** Predictor variables are levels of depression (PHQ9) and anxiety (GAD7), active coping with illness (FKVactive) and oversensitivity to sound (hyper-NRS). Values for all tinnitus measures dropped in the group with low PHQ9 scores at T1 with all reductions reaching statistical significance, while there was no significant decrease for these factors in the group with high depression levels. Also, scores of all predictor variables dropped significantly in the former while any reduction observed in the latter group did not reach statistical significance between assessments. $^*p < 0.05$; $^{**}p < 0.01$.

TABLE 4 | Response to question whether tinnitus had changed since onset.

		Change since onset			
		T1	**T2**	**T3**	**T4**
Perceived Loudness	None	28 (68.3%)	17 (41.5%)	20 (48.8%)	20 (48.8%)
	More	7 (17.1%)	3 (7.3%)	3 (7.3%)	3 (7.3%)
	Less	4 (9.8%)	19 (46.3%)	18 (43.9%)	18 (43.9%)
	No statement	2 (4.9%)	2 (4.9%)	–	–
Perceived distress	None	19 (46.3%)	15 (36.6%)	23 (56.1%)	20 (48.8%)
	More	11 (26.8%)	4 (9.8%)	4 (9.8%)	6 (14.6%)
	Less	3 (7.3%)	19 (46.3%)	11 (26.8%)	15 (36.6%)
	No statement	8 (19.5%)	3 (7.3%)	3 (7.3%)	–
Change in hearing if tinnitus onset was associated with hearing impairment	None		21 (51.2%)	12 (29.3%)	10 (24.4%)
	Better		7 (17.1%)	4 (9.8%)	2 (4.9%)
	Worse		2 (4.9%)	–	1 (2.4%)
	No statement		11 (26.8%)	25 (61%)	28 (68.3%)

not evident for the whole sample if HL was averaged across ears for those with bilateral tinnitus or tinnitus localized to the head. Bivariate correlations did not reach the Bonferroni-corrected p-level for significance ($p = 0.0009$) except for the correlations between the SDS scales at T1 and T4, and for the Mini-TQ12 at T2 and T4, (**Table 5**). These findings indicated that tinnitus complaints shortly after onset are potential predictors for the severity of chronic complaints. Furthermore, PHQ9, GAD7, hyper-NRS, FKVactive, and FKVdistraction at T1 exhibited correlation levels with outcome variables at T4 (**Table 5**) that were strong enough to be considered for the regression analysis.

Separate stepwise regression analyses for each of the outcome variables and the predictors with sufficiently strong correlations showed that the level of complaints at T1 in each scale was a good predictor for scores in that scale at T4. Mini-TQ12 scores at T4 were explained to 70% by the factors Mini-TQ12 at T2 and PHQ9 at T1. For Tinnitus loudness, the factors T-NRS, FKVactive, and PHQ9 all at T1 explained 50% of the variance. Scores in the

TABLE 5 | Pearson correlation coefficients (r) for bivariate correlations between predictor variables at T1 and outcome variables at T4 are shown together with p-values.

Predictors	Outcomes				
	T4-T-NRS	T4-SDS1	T4-SDS2	T4-SDS3	T4-Mini-TQ12
Same variable at T1 or T2, respectively					
r	**0.488**	**0.730**	**0.595**	**0.610**	**0.807**
p	**0.001**	**<0.0001***	**<0.0001***	**<0.0001***	**<0.0001***
T1 hyper-NRS					
r	0.252	**0.425**	**0.324**	**0.331**	**0.355**
p	0.112	**0.010**	**0.039**	**0.035**	**0.023**
T1 PHQ9					
r	**0.342**	**0.396**	**0.371**	**0.347**	**0.459**
p	**0.029**	**0.017**	**0.017**	**0.026**	**0.003**
T1 GAD7					
r	**0.366**	**0.352**	**0.366**	**0.360**	**0.466**
p	**0.019**	**0.035**	**0.019**	**0.021**	**0.002**
T1 FKVdepressive					
r	0.051	0.047	−0.18	0.044	0.221
p	0.757	0.787	0.913	0.786	0.170
T1 FKVactive					
r	**0.424**	**0.397**	**0.407**	**0.424**	**0.378**
p	**0.006**	**0.018**	**0.009***	**0.006**	**0.016**
T1 FKVdistraction					
r	**0.390**	**0.381**	0.306	**0.321**	0.231
p	**0.013**	**0.024**	0.055	**0.043**	0.152
T1 FKV search for meaning					
r	0.104	0.177	−0.030	0.041	0.066
p	0.521	0.309	0.852	0.801	0.687
T1 FKV trivialization					
r	0.203	0.074	0.037	0.043	0.212
p	0.208	0.673	0.821	0.793	0.189

*As this was an exploratory study, variables with a p-value below 0.05 and a correlation coefficient r above 0.300 (bold letters) were included in the step-wise regression analysis for the respective outcome variable. The Bonferroni-corrected p-value indicating statistical significance was *p = 0.0009.*

TABLE 6 | Results of step-wise regression analysis.

Predictor at T1	Outcome at T4				
	T-NRS	SDS1	SDS2	SDS3	Mini-TQ12
Explained variance	50%	53%	35%	49%	70%
R^2/adj R^2	0.497/0.455	0.527/0.509	0.354/0.337	0.485/0.457	0.695/0.678
F	11.841	30.026	20.819	21.483	42.111
Same variable at T1/T2					
Stand. beta$_{in}$	0.444	0.726	0.595	0.540	0.734
p	0.001**	<0.001**	<0.001**	<0.001**	<0.001**
T1 PHQ9					
Stand. beta$_{in}$	0.283				0.218
p	0.024*				0.030*
T1 FKVactive					
Stand. beta$_{in}$	0.376			0.350	
p	0.003**			0.007**	

*Stepwise linear regression analysis was performed separately for each of the outcome variables. Variables included in the analysis were those with sufficient bivariate correlations of r > 0.300 and a p < 0.05 with the respective outcome in the bivariate analyses as shown in **Table 5**. For the regression analysis significant predictors (*p < 0.05; **p < 0.01) together with the standardized beta values are shown for each of the outcome variables.*

SDS1 scale at T4 were explained to 53% the SDS1 score at T1, whereas the SDS2 score at T4 was explained by 35% by the SDS2 score at T1, and the SDS3 score at T4 was explained by 49% by the SDS3 score and the FKVactive score at T1 (**Table 6**). Thus, tinnitus-related distress can be foreseen in the acute state, and best predictors were the Mini-TQ12 and the PHQ9.

Groups with High versus Low Depression Scores

One of our initial hypotheses was that a high level of depression at tinnitus onset promotes development of a decompensated chronic tinnitus. We therefore compared the group with low level of depression, i.e., a PHQ9 score below 10 at T1 ($N = 31$) and the group with conspicuous levels of depression at T1 ($N = 10$), and found that a high level of depression around tinnitus onset allows a distinction between problematic and unproblematic tinnitus at T4. Tinnitus symptoms were lower and reduced significantly during the study interval in the group with low depression scores at T1, while they remained unchanged for the group with PHQ9 scores of 10 or above (**Figure 2**). In addition, GAD7 scores and hypersensitivity to external sounds was more pronounced in the latter group, and members of the group with high depression scores were more likely to undergo a tinnitus-specific therapy during the study interval (70%) compared to the group with an inconspicuous PHQ9 score (58%).

DISCUSSION

Aim of the present study was to describe the transition from acute to chronic tinnitus, identify factors associated with remission of the tinnitus and to identify predictors for the development of chronic disabling tinnitus. To our knowledge, this is the first study that aims to investigate individuals with a first episode of tinnitus who seek medical help from private practices of otolaryngologists. Former studies investigated tinnitus sufferers that were hospitalized for the treatment of sudden HL (6, 7), took part in a psychological therapy for acute tinnitus (14), or army personal developing tinnitus shortly after exposure to high noise levels (9).

Study Sample

The characteristics of our study sample suggest that patients seeking help from otolaryngologists for acute tinnitus are not necessarily the ones with high tinnitus-related distress or loud tinnitus as indicated by the rather moderate averages of these measures in comparison to those assessed with the same instruments in a large number of subjects with chronic tinnitus (4: T-NRS: 6.0 ± 2.5; Mini-TQ12: 10.4 ± 6.4). Averages are comparable, however, to those found by earlier studies with acute tinnitus patients (5, 6, 17). The authors of one study (17) assume that tinnitus questionnaires may underestimate tinnitus-related distress in acute patients because they were developed for the chronic condition. Alternatives which are not mutually exclusive are that patients with high tinnitus-related distress consult other specialists, or that tinnitus-related distress increases over time. Another observation was that not many patients consult an otolaryngologist early after tinnitus onset. This is in line with a former report, stating that the majority seeks medical help only years after tinnitus onset [(40); Lockwood et al. (41)], and with the results of a recent review on the literature (12). Of note is also that average scores of depression and anxiety are similar to those found with the same instruments for a large sample with chronic tinnitus [(4): PHQ9: 7.1 ± 5.5; GAD7: 6.0 ± 4.8] which is considerably higher than in the German normative samples [(32): PHQ9: 2.9 ± 3.5; 29: GAD7: 3.0 ± 3.4].

In the present sample, average age is 41.4 ± 15.6 years in the group with persisting tinnitus and 41.0 ± 14.8 years in the group with remitting tinnitus. This is lower than in a sample with tinnitus following sudden HL [(6): 47.3 years, range 19–78], but comparable to the average of a large group with chronic tinnitus who retrospectively reported age at tinnitus onset to be 42.4 ± 13.5 years (42). In that report, study participants with later tinnitus onset experienced a more distressing tinnitus right from the beginning (42). Whereas in a preliminary analysis of the present study with the data of 28 participants (20), we also found a significant correlation of moderate strength between age at tinnitus onset and tinnitus-related distress, we could not confirm this finding for the Mini-TQ12, the instrument used by Schlee et al. (42), in this larger sample, but found a stronger correlation between age at onset and tinnitus-related distress as assessed by the SDS2 and SDS3 scales at T4. In addition, we found strong correlations between age at onset and HL at frequencies of 3 kHz and above (r: 0.384–0.718). While prevalence of HL increases with age, it may go undetected by the affected individuals (43) and it is not known whether the sample investigated by Schlee et al. (42) had hearing levels within the normal range at tinnitus onset. HL increases the risk for developing tinnitus, and tinnitus-related distress may be augmented by the distress the participant experiences because of the accompanying HL (42).

Tinnitus Onset, Remission, and Transition to Chronic Condition

Remission rate was about 11% in the current study, it occurred more often in individuals who developed tinnitus concomitant with a noticeable HL, and remission usually occurred during the first weeks after onset, resembling the time course of recovery of hearing after incidences of acute HL (7, 11). The majority of our sample did not experience worsening of hearing concomitant with tinnitus onset, but this percentage is higher in the group with complete remission. Higher remission rates are commonly reported in studies with tinnitus in response to acute auditory insults (9), likely because of recovery after acute acoustic insult (11). Furthermore, hearing recovery appears to be age- and frequency dependent, as it is more complete in younger individuals and at frequencies below and above 4 kHz (44). As acute temporary threshold shifts are known to recover to some extent resulting in a less severe permanent threshold shift (11), tinnitus remission is more likely if its appearance is associated with acute worsening of hearing level. In animal models, threshold shifts of up to about 50 dB immediately after a single-noise exposure may recover completely, and recovery has been reported for periods extending up to 3 weeks. But even with complete recovery of hearing threshold large numbers of synapses between hair cells and primary afferent neurons may be lost resulting in hearing deficits that are not necessarily detected by audiometry (11).

Recovery in hearing seems to precede decreases in tinnitus loudness or tinnitus remission (45), and complete remission sets in earlier, i.e., by day 7, and benefits a significantly higher share of patients with mild-moderate HL as compared to those with more profound HL in whom remission was observed in a period of up to 30 days. Also, hearing impairment and tinnitus in response to an ear infection tend to recover completely (46). Interestingly, the ones with remitting tinnitus in our sample indicated at T1 that loudness or annoyance of their tinnitus had decreased since onset suggesting a gradual recovery of hearing thresholds and reduction of tinnitus severity soon after tinnitus onset. Mühlmeier et al. (7) report that tinnitus remission lagged complete hearing recovery, and that complete hearing recovery and complete tinnitus remission were not independent of each other confirming the association between both factors. Taken together, data suggest that remission can be expected with substantial recovery of hearing threshold, for instance after incidences of sudden HL or acoustic trauma while remission is not to be expected if tinnitus onset was not associated with a recent incidence of HL.

Most pronounced was the reduction of tinnitus awareness between T1 and T3. It did not necessarily result in a less distressing tinnitus, however. 59% retained the level of tinnitus-related distress experienced at T2 until T4, while some habituated as indicated by lower distress 6 months after onset. About 10% reported significant worsening of tinnitus-related distress during the study. Hence, tinnitus-related distress reported in the acute condition is likely to be representative for the chronic condition. This finding is corroborated by the results of the regression analysis. Similarly, perceived loudness of the tinnitus was stable between T1 and T4 in most of the study participants, which is no surprise since for most tinnitus onset was not related to worsening of the hearing. Taken together, tinnitus remission occurred early, but the tinnitus remained in 90%, and tinnitus complaints did not change in the majority. Therefore, initial complaints about high tinnitus-related distress and perceived loudness require immediate therapeutic action.

The time course of transition from the acute to the chronic condition is not entirely clear. Whereas, some define duration of up to 3 months as subacute and a tinnitus lasting at least 6 months as being chronic (12), others assume the chronic condition is reached already after 3 months (19). Assessments in the present study were chosen to investigate these time intervals and together with studies on spontaneous remission after sudden HL (7) indicate that chronification of the tinnitus is taking place during the first days or weeks after onset. This is nicely shown by an interventional study (18) reporting that adults with unilateral tinnitus who are treated with intratympanic dexamethasone or saline both together with oral gingko biloba, the latter thought to be a placebo treatment, reduced awareness of the tinnitus within a month of tinnitus onset, and also led to reductions of tinnitus loudness and annoyance within the following 4 weeks irrespective of the treatment. In contrast, Holgers et al. (8) report that between the first consultation which took place during the first 6 months after tinnitus onset and the endpoint of the study one year later, tinnitus symptoms decreased in 75% of the study participants, whereas the rest had symptoms that did not decrease over time.

Hearing Loss As a Predictive Factor

Hearing loss has been identified as the most relevant etiologic factor and as the probable trigger for tinnitus, although non-auditory factors may ameliorate or worsen the tinnitus (47). In the present sample 25% of those with unilateral tinnitus and 20% with bilateral tinnitus did not have an overt HL in the standard audiogram indicated by thresholds not exceeding 20 dB at any frequency. For those with unilateral tinnitus, thresholds in the affected ear were worse for the tinnitus ear which is in line with findings for patients with idiopathic sensorineural HL (48). Noteworthy, in our sample is the high correlation between HL at 2 kHz and future tinnitus loudness which has not been described before. In accordance, Mühlmeier et al. (7) report that tinnitus loudness 3 months after tinnitus onset was statistically significantly correlated with the level of PTA both at baseline and at 3 months.

Reasons why a tinnitus was heard despite normal hearing thresholds might be due to HL in frequencies above 8 kHz as seen in a recent study in patients suffering from acute tinnitus (49). Furthermore, tinnitus in normal hearing subjects may be due to cochlear pathologies undetected by the audiogram (11), or to a less well functioning efferent auditory system (50).

Depression and Anxiety As Predictive Factors

Variables with notable correlations with future tinnitus severity were the levels of depression and anxiety at T1. In the group with high levels of depression at T1, tinnitus loudness and distress did not diminish with time, but even augmented in most of those fulfilling the criterion for Major Depression. High levels of depression have been associated with chronic disabling tinnitus (4). Holgers et al. (8) report that above all symptoms of depression and anxiety together with HL and physical immobility are predictors for severity of the tinnitus, and high depression levels were not observed in any one of their patients that showed tinnitus remission.

In our sample, we find significant reductions of tinnitus-related distress, loudness, and the level of depressive symptoms only in the group with low levels of depression at T1, while neither factor reduced during the study interval if PHQ9 scores at T1 indicated conspicuous problems with depression. In addition, we found a significant correlation between tinnitus-related distress at onset and chronic tinnitus-related distress. This supports the notion, that high levels of tinnitus-related distress in particular in combination with high levels of depressive symptoms are indicators for the potential development of incapacitating tinnitus. Therefore, it is indicated to assess tinnitus-related distress in acute tinnitus patients, and this should always be accompanied by screening of the level of depression. As an additional measure, the level of anxiety could be assessed, as levels of depression and anxiety show strong correlations and it was found that during transition, for instance in the course of chronification, levels of anxiety show a stronger correlation with tinnitus symptoms than indicators of depression [(8, 17, 51)—this Frontiers Topic].

Data indicate the importance of interventions already during the acute phase of tinnitus, as previously suggested (14). Effects of such interventions should be more pronounced in acute tinnitus associated with high levels of depression. Therefore, we consider early psychological/psychotherapeutic intervention to be important to prevent the development of a decompensated chronic tinnitus that severely impairs life quality of affected individuals.

Active Coping with Tinnitus Is Maladaptive

Results of the regression analysis indicate that active coping is maladaptive in regard to tinnitus. Active coping with the tinnitus reduces significantly in the group with an inconspicuous level of depression at T1, while no reduction is found in the group with high levels of depression. It therefore appears that those with psychological problems tend to adhere to this strategy.

Limitations

Some limitations of the study should be named. As in the other few longitudinal studies, the number of participants is low. Furthermore, because measures on tinnitus-loudness and distress are not available on a large-scale for the acute condition, it cannot be decided, whether our sample is representative for the acute tinnitus population, but these measures may rather serve as a start to describe acute tinnitus patients.

Only few individuals appear to consult an otolaryngologist shortly after noticing the appearance of a tinnitus (40), and nowadays acute tinnitus patients may better be contacted via internet sources as suggested by a recent publication [(52), this Frontiers Topic]. An alternative which is not mutually exclusive is that perceived tinnitus loudness and tinnitus-related distress are mild at first but may increase over the life span. An increase of tinnitus loudness is likely because with advancing age most suffer from presbyacusis, and it has been shown that tinnitus loudness rather increases with age. An increase of tinnitus-related distress is not self-explicable as many of those with long-existing tinnitus report adjustment to the tinnitus and experience a decrease of tinnitus-related distress (4). It may be possible, however, that tinnitus-related distress increases for instance in individuals with high levels of depression or anxiety.

Because perceived tinnitus loudness and tinnitus-related distress were both low to moderate at T1/T2 reductions of tinnitus loudness and distress may not have been detected. We used the GAD7 for screening anxiety as it is a short freely available and validated instrument for screening GAD and was reported to perform almost as well for detecting other types of common anxiety disorders (29). A very recent publication of the same group (53) suggests that the first four items discriminate better than the last three items with respect to latent anxiety, and therefore suggest to use a 2item GAD version (GAD2) which will be even more time-economic. Nonetheless, we decided to report the sum scores of the GAD7 as they have been reported for a normative sample (29) and in former tinnitus studies (4, 33) but suggest to monitor the literature regarding further developments.

CONCLUSION

(1) Patients that present with acute tinnitus at otolaryngology practices are not a homogenous group in which psychological aspects are important to predict future progression of the tinnitus. Therefore, mental health should be assessed early on, for instance with the readily available PHQ9 and GAD7 questionnaires used in this study.
(2) If levels of depression or anxiety are elevated, patients should be referred to specialists treating these conditions.
(3) Results support early manifestation of tinnitus-related distress, and that development of disabling tinnitus is fostered by poor mental health.

Therefore, we suggest to screen depression symptoms and tinnitus-related distress of all tinnitus patients presenting with acute or subacute tinnitus, and to refer them to specialist evaluation and therapy if indicated. Furthermore, we suggest to consider provision with hearing prostheses, although it has to be assured first that a potentially existing oversensitivity to sounds, has reversed when using hearing aids.

ETHICS STATEMENT

Study design and procedures were approved by the Ethics Committee II of Heidelberg University at the Medical Faculty Mannheim (2013-541N-MA).

AUTHOR CONTRIBUTIONS

EW-F designed the study, collected part of the data, analyzed the data, and wrote the manuscript. RD interpretation of data, AG collected and analyzed part of the data, WD designed the study, JS critical review, KH critical review, IR recruitment and interpretation of data.

ACKNOWLEDGMENTS

The authors thank the participating ENT practices: Dr. Hülse University Clinic Mannheim, Dr. Kyrberg, Ludwigshafen; Dr. Raje, Heppenheim; Dr. Schubotz-Mitgau, Heppenheim and Dr. Zickler, Pfungstadt, Dr. S. Hetjen of the Medical Faculty Mannheim for statistical advice, and all study participants for their time and effort. The authors acknowledge financial support of the Deutsche Forschungsgemeinschaft and Ruprecht-Karls-Universität Heidelberg within the funding program Open Access Publishing.

REFERENCES

Eggermont JJ, Roberts LE. The neuroscience of tinnitus: understanding abnormal and normal auditory perception. *Front Syst Neurosci* (2012) 6:53. doi:10.3389/fnsys.2012.00053

Hiller W, Goebel G. Factors influencing tinnitus loudness and annoyance. *Arch Otolaryngol Head Neck Surg* (2006) 132:1323–30. doi:10.1001/archotol.132.12.1323

Langguth B, Kreuzer PM, Kleinjung T, De Ridder D. Tinnitus: causes and clinical management. *Lancet Neurol* (2013) 12:920–30. doi:10.1016/S1474-4422(13)70160-1

Wallhäusser-Franke E, Brade J, Balkenhol T, D'Amelio R, Seegmüller A, Delb W. Tinnitus: distinguishing between subjectively perceived loudness and tinnitus-related distress. *PLoS One* (2012) 7:e34583. doi:10.1371/journal.pone.0034583
D'Amelio R, Archonti C, Scholz S, Falkai P, Plinkert PK, Delb W. Psychological distress associated with acute tinnitus. *HNO* (2004) 52:599–603. doi:10.1007/s00106-003-0944-5
Langenbach M, Olderog M, Michel O, Albus C, Köhle K. Psychosocial and personality predictors of tinnitus-related distress. *Gen Hosp Psychiatry* (2005) 27:73–7. doi:10.1016/j.genhosppsych.2004.08.008
Mühlmeier G, Baguley D, Cox T, Suckfüll M, Meyer T. Characteristics and spontaneous recovery of tinnitus related to idiopathic sudden sensorineural hearing loss. *Otol Neurotol* (2016) 37:634–41. doi:10.1097/MAO.0000000000001081
Holgers KM, Zöger S, Svedlund K. Predictive factors for development of severe tinnitus suffering – further characterisation. *Int J Audiol* (2005) 44:584–92. doi:10.1080/14992020500190235
Bonfort G, Billot D, Trendel D, Salf E, Lindas P, Barberot JP. Acute acoustic trauma, a retrospective analysis about 225 military cases. *Rev Laryngol Otol Rhinol (Bord)* (2014) 135:25–31.
Weinaug P. Spontaneous remission in sudden deafness. *HNO* (1984) 32:346–51.
Ryan AF, Kujawa SG, Hammill T, Le Prell C, Kil J. Temporary and permanent noise-induced threshold shifts: a review of basic and clinical observations. *Otol Neurotol* (2016) 37:e271–5. doi:10.1097/MAO.0000000000001071
Altissimi G, Salviati M, Turchetta R, Orlando MP, Greco A, De Vincentiis M, et al. When alarm bells ring: emergency tinnitus. *Eur Rev Med Pharmacol Sci* (2016) 20:2955–73.
Dobie RA. Depression and tinnitus. *Otolaryngol Clin North Am* (2004) 36:383–8. doi:10.1016/S0030-6665(02)00168-8
Delb W, D'Amelio R, Boisten CJ, Plinkert PK. Evaluation of the tinnitus retraining therapy as combined with a cognitive behavioral group therapy. *HNO* (2002) 50:997–1004. doi:10.1007/s00106-002-0645-5
Gerhards F, Brehmer D. Distraction and relaxation training in acute tinnitus: effects of a complement to otorhinolaryngological treatment. *HNO* (2010) 58:488–96. doi:10.1007/s00106-009-2019-8
Nyenhuis N, Zastrutzki S, Weise C, Jäger B, Kröner-Herwig B. The efficacy of minimal contact interventions for acute tinnitus: a randomised controlled study. *Cogn Behav Ther* (2013) 42:127–38. doi:10.1080/16506073.2012.655305
Schildt A, Tönnies S, Böttcher S. Inpatient infusion treatment for acute tinnitus with and without adjuvant psychotherapeutic intervention. A com- parison of psychological effectivenes. *HNO* (2006) 54:781–91. doi:10.1007/ s00106-006-1447-y
Shim HJ, Lee ES, An YH, Kim DH. Comparison of long-term outcome of intratympanic dexamethasone therapy between acute noise-induced tinnitus and acute idiopathic tinnitus. *J Int Adv Otol* (2017) 13:53–60. doi:10.5152/ iao.2016.2632
Zenner HP, Delb W, Kröner-Herwig B, Jäger B, Peroz I, Hesse G, et al. On the interdisciplinary S3 guidelines for the treatment of chronic idiopathic tinnitus. *HNO* (2015) 63:419–27. doi:10.1007/s00106-015-0011-z
Wallhäusser-Franke E, Repik I, Delb W, Glauner A, Hörmann K. Long-term development of acute tinnitus. *Laryngorhinootologie* (2015) 94:759–69. doi:10.1055/s-0035-1550039
Meikle MB, Stewart BJ, Griest SE, Henry JA. Tinnitus outcomes assessment. *Trends Amplif* (2008) 12:223–35. doi:10.1177/1084713808319943
Hiller W, Goebel G. Rapid assessment of tinnitus-related psychological distress using the mini-TQ. *Int J Audiol* (2004) 43:600–4. doi:10.1080/14992020400050077
Zeman F, Koller M, Schecklmann M, Langguth B, Landgrebe M. Tinnitus assessment by means of standardized self-report questionnaires: psychometric properties of the tinnitus questionnaire (TQ), the tinnitus handicap inventory (THI), and their short versions in an international and multi-lingual sample. *Health Qual Life Outcomes* (2012) 10:128. doi:10.1186/1477-7525-10-128
Sheehan KH, Sheehan DV. Assessing treatment effects in clinical trials with the Discan metric of the Sheehan Disability Scale. *Int Clin Psychopharmacol* (2008) 23:70–83. doi:10.1097/YIC.0b013e3282f2b4d6
Arbuckle R, Frye MA, Brecher M, Paulsson B, Rajagopalan K, Palmer S, et al. The psychometric validation of the Sheehan Disability Scale (SDS) in patients with bipolar disorder. *Psychiatry Res* (2009) 165:163–74. doi:10.1016/ j.psychres.2007.11.018
Coles T, Coon C, DeMuro C, McLeod L, Gnanasakthy A. Psychometric evaluation of the Sheehan Disability Scale in adult patients with attention-deficit/hyperactivity disorder. *Neuropsychiatr Dis Treat* (2014) 10:887–95. doi:10.2147/NDT.S55220
Luciano JV, Bertsch J, Salvador-Carulla L, Tomás JM, Fernández A, Pinto-Meza A, et al. Factor structure, internal consistency and construct validity of the Sheehan Disability Scale in a Spanish primary care sam- ple. *J Eval Clin Pract* (2010) 16:895–901. doi:10.1111/j.1365-2753.2009. 01211.x
Kroenke K, Spitzer RL, Williams JB, Löwe B. The patient health question- naire somatic, anxiety, and depressive symptom scales: a systematic review. *Gen Hosp Psychiatry* (2010) 32:345–59. doi:10.1016/j.genhosppsych.2010. 03.006
Löwe B, Spitzer RL, Williams JBW, Mussell M, Schellberg D, Kroenke K. Depression, anxiety and somatization in primary care: syndrome overlap and functional impairment. *Gen Hosp Psychiatry* (2008) 30:191–9. doi:10.1016/ j.genhosppsych.2008.01.001
Kroenke K, Spitzer RL, Williams JB. The PHQ-9: validity of a brief depression severity measure. *J Gen Intern Med* (2001) 16:606–13. doi:10.1046/j.1525-1497.2001.016009606.x
Spitzer RL, Kroenke K, Williams JB. Validation and utility of a self-report version of PRIME-MD: the PHQ primary care study. *JAMA* (1999) 282: 1737–44. doi:10.1001/jama.282.18.1737
Kocalevent RD, Hinz A, Brähler E. Standardization of the depression screener patient health questionnaire (PHQ-9) in the general population. *Gen Hosp Psychiatry* (2013) 35:551–5. doi:10.1016/j.genhosppsych.2013. 04.006
Brüggemann P, Szczepek AJ, Klee K, Gräbel S, Mazurek B, Olze H. In patients undergoing cochlear implantation, psychological burden affects tinnitus and the overall outcome of auditory rehabilitation. *Front Hum Neurosci* (2017) 11:226. doi:10.3389/fnhum.2017.00226
Budd RJ, Pugh R. Tinnitus coping style and its relationship to tinnitus severity and emotional distress. *J Psychosom Res* (1996) 641:327–35. doi:10.1016/S0022-3999(96)00171-7
Henry JA, Thielman EJ, Zaugg TL, Kaelin C, Schmidt CJ, Griest S, et al. Randomized controlled trial in clinical settings to evaluate effectiveness of coping skills education used with progressive tinnitus management. *J Speech Lang Hear Res* (2017) 60:1378–97. doi:10.1044/2016_JSLHR-H-16-0126
Muthny FA. *Freiburger Fragebogen zur Krankheitsverarbeitung (FKV) Manual.* Weinheim, Germany: Beltz Test (1989).
Konzag TA, Rübler D, Bloching M, Bandemer-Greulich U, Fikentscher E, Frommer J. Counselling versus a self-help manual for tinnitus outpatients: a comparison of effectiveness. *HNO* (2006) 54:599–604. doi:10.1007/s00106-005-1350-y
Schecklmann M, Landgrebe M, Langguth B; TRI Database Study Group. Phenotypic characteristics of hyperacusis in tinnitus. *PLoS One* (2014) 9(1):e86944. doi:10.1371/journal.pone.0086944.e86944
Hall D. Interpreting treatment-related changes using the tinnitus question- naire in Argstatter H, Grapp M, Plinkert PK, Bolay HV. Heidelberg neuro- music therapy for chronic-tonal tinnitus – treatment outline and psychomet- ric evaluation. Int Tinnitus J (2012) 17:31-41. *Int Tinnitus J* (2017) 20:73–5. doi:10.5935/0946-5448.20160014
Bhatt JM, Lin HW, Bhattacharyya N. Prevalence, severity, exposures and treatment patterns of tinnitus in the United States. *JAMA Otolaryngol Head Neck Surg* (2016) 142:959–65. doi:10.1001/jamaoto.2016.1700
Henry JA, Dennis KC, Schechter MA. General review of tinnitus: prevalence, mechanisms, effects, and management. *J Speech Lang Hear Res* (2005) 48: 1204–35. doi:10.1044/1092-4388(2005/084)
Schlee W, Kleinjung T, Hiller W, Goebel G, Kolassa IT, Langguth B. Does tinnitus distress depend on age of onset? *PLoS One* (2011) 6(11):e27379. doi:10.1371/journal.pone.0027379
Moser S, Luxenberger W, Freidl W. Perception of hearing problems in the older population. *HNO* (2017) 65:671–9. doi:10.1007/s00106-017-0334-z
Harada H, Ichikawa D, Imamura A. Course of hearing recovery according to frequency in patients with acute acoustic sensorineural hearing loss. *Int Tinnitus J* (2008) 14:83–8.
Ishida IM, Sugiura M, Teranishi M, Katayama N, Nakashima T. Otoacoustic emissions, ear fullness and tinnitus in the recovery course of sudden deafness. *Auris Nasus Larynx* (2008) 35:41–6. doi:10.1016/j.anl.2007.04.003

Park JH, Park SJ, Kim YH, Park MH. Sensorineural hearing loss: a complication of acute otitis media in adults. *Eur Arch Otorhinolaryngol* (2014) 271:1879–84. doi:10.1007/s00405-013-2675-x

Langguth B, Landgrebe M, Schlee W, Schecklmann M, Vielsmeier V, Steffens T, et al. Different patterns of hearing loss among tinnitus patients: a latent class analysis of a large sample. *Front Neurol* (2017) 20:46. doi:10.3389/fneur.2017.00046

Lee HY, Choi MS, Chang DS, Kim AY, Cho CS. Acute-onset tinnitus is associated with contralateral hearing in sudden deafness. *Audiol Neurootol* (2015) 20(6):370–5. doi:10.1159/000438919

Sakata T, Ueno T, Takase H, Shiraishi K, Nakagawa T. Acute idiopathic sensorineural hearing impairment at frequency exceeding 8 kHz. *Acta Otolaryngol* (2010) 130:1141–6. doi:10.3109/00016481003664793

Riga M, Papadas T, Werner JA, Dalchow CV. A clinical study of the efferent auditory system in patients with normal hearing who have acute tinnitus. *Otol Neurotol* (2007) 28:185–90. doi:10.1097/MAO.0b013e31802e2a14

Servais JJ, Hörmann K, Wallhäusser-Franke E. Unilateral cochlear implantation reduces tinnitus loudness in bimodal hearing: a prospective study. *Front Neurol* (2017) 8:60. doi:10.3389/fneur.2017.00060

Probst T, Pryss RC, Langguth B, Spiliopoulou M, Landgrebe M, Vesala M, et al. Outpatient tinnitus clinic, self-help web platform, or mobile application to recruit tinnitus study samples? *Front Aging Neurosci* (2017) 21:113. doi:10.3389/fnagi.2017.00113

Jordan P, Shedden-Mora MC, LoÈwe B. Psychometric analysis of the generalized anxiety disorder scale (GAD-7) in primary care using modern item response theory. *PLoS One* (2017) 12:e0182162. doi:10.1371/journal.pone.0182162

6

Targeting Heterogeneous Findings in Neuronal Oscillations in Tinnitus: Analyzing MEG Novices and Mental Health Comorbidities

Pia Lau, Andreas Wollbrink, Robert Wunderlich, Alva Engell, Alwina Löhe, Markus Junghöfer and Christo Pantev**

Institute for Biomagnetism and Biosignalanalysis, University Hospital of Münster, Münster, Germany

Correspondence:
Pia Lau
pia.lau@uni-muenster.de
Christo Pantev
pantev@uni-muenster.de

Tinnitus is a prevalent phenomenon and bothersome for people affected by it. Its occurrence and maintenance have a clear neuroscientific tie and one aspect are differences in the neuronal oscillatory pattern, especially in auditory cortical areas. As studies in this field come to different results, the aim of this study was to analyze a large number of participants to achieve more stable results. Furthermore, we expanded our analysis to two variables of potential influence, namely being a novice to neuroscientific measurements and the exclusion of psychological comorbidities. Oscillatory brain activity of 88 subjects (46 with a chronic tinnitus percept, 42 without) measured in resting state by MEG was investigated. In the analysis based on the whole group, in sensor space increased activity in the delta frequency band was found in tinnitus patients. Analyzing the subgroup of novices, a significant difference in the theta band emerged additionally to the delta band difference (sensor space). Localizing the origin of the activity, we found a difference in theta and gamma band for the auditory regions for the whole group and the same significant difference in the subgroup of novices. However, no differences in oscillatory activity were observed between tinnitus and control groups once subjects with mental health comorbidity were excluded. Against the background of previous studies, the study at hand underlines the fragility of the results in the field of neuronal cortical oscillations in tinnitus. It supports the body of research arguing for low frequency oscillations and gamma band activity as markers associated with tinnitus.

Keywords: tinnitus, neuronal oscillations, spectral analysis, magnetencephalography, auditory cortex

INTRODUCTION

Tinnitus is a phantom auditory percept, which exists unrelated to any external source. It is – at least temporarily – familiar to up to 30% of the population and affects up to 14% as a chronic condition (Axelsson and Ringdahl, 1989; Sindhusake et al., 2003). Next to its perception as being annoying, between 1 and 3% of all people report a meaningful decrease in quality of life through the tinnitus, which can be expressed for example in sleeping disorders or depressed mood (Dobie, 2003). Hearing loss is strongly associated with tinnitus and triggering underlying maladaptive subcortical and cortical processes such as hypersynchronicity, hyperactivity, and burst firing (Shore et al., 2016). Markers of ongoing cortical activity are neuronal oscillations which represent the "rhythmic fluctuations in the excitability of neurons or populations of neurons" (Cohen, 2014).

Several studies in the past focused on neuronal oscillations in tinnitus (see Zobay et al., 2015) and tried to establish theories based on their results. Weisz et al. (2005) found an increase in delta and a decrease in alpha frequency band over temporal regions, nicely fitting into the established framework of alpha as a mechanism of an inhibitory balancing rhythm (Jensen and Mazaheri, 2010). A lack of alpha power – especially in the temporal regions where the auditory cortex is located – might thus represent a lack of inhibition in these areas. This might correspond to the above mentioned hyperactivity and increased spontaneous firing rate of the auditory cortex. Additional support for the idea of alpha oscillations as a key mechanism for tinnitus comes from research on comparable phenomena such as auditory hallucinations: Müller et al. (2014) for instance presented popular melodies to their subjects. In short gaps in the music, which were filled with pink noise, subjects who reported that they had the impression the melody would continue, showed decreased levels of alpha activity compared to those who did not report that the melody continued for them. Leske et al. (2014) demonstrated that the strength of the illusionary percept of the Zwicker tone negatively correlated with alpha frequency band power. Therefore, both studies show some form of reduced alpha activity in auditory areas if an auditory illusion is present. Recent neurofeedback studies further support this framework (Hartmann et al., 2014): if tinnitus patients were able to alternate, e.g., increase the power of alpha oscillations in their temporal areas of their brain, their tinnitus percept was altered as well, as it got more quiet. Despite its appealing and intuitive character of the findings in the alpha power band, results are not conclusive, as there are studies which do not report any anomalies in the alpha spectrum of tinnitus patients (Adjamian et al., 2012).

Two other prominent models explaining the role of neuronal oscillations in tinnitus make assumptions about theta/delta and gamma oscillations. One model thereby focuses on thalamocortical dysrhythmia (TCD, Llinas et al., 1999; Adjamian et al., 2012; De Ridder et al., 2015). A disrupted communication between the thalamus and cortical areas, that results in symptomatology, is the central idea of this model. This pathological communication is thought to be expressed in an increase in the theta and gamma activity (Llinas et al., 1999; Adjamian et al., 2012; De Ridder et al., 2015). The other model focuses on predictive coding, a current trend in neuroscience. This approach assumes that the brain is constantly producing predictions of the input and if those predictions are violated a prediction error is encoded. Sedley et al. (2016) state that spontaneous activity in the sub-cortical auditory pathway, the so-called tinnitus precursor, is existent but usually neglected in favor of the concept "silence." Tinnitus emerges, if the prediction and the precursor converge. This means, the concept or prediction of silence is abandoned. This occurs, if the precursor gains precision and lastly replaces the prediction "silence." Another option is, that the precursor codes a more intense tinnitus than the prediction would forecast. So in both cases, no-tinnitus and (less intense) tinnitus, the model would anticipate a prediction error, as there is a discrepancy between the prediction (silence or less intense tinnitus) and the precursor. This prediction error reflects a suppression of the tinnitus. Following this hypothesis, in case of tinnitus the prediction error would be reduced as prediction and precursor match. Their model also covers the specific prediction of neuronal oscillations: low frequencies as theta or delta and gamma oscillations, representing the incident of prediction errors, are expected. There is also some support for these suppositions in the research body of tinnitus, yet the results are still quite heterogeneous (Zobay et al., 2015). Taken together, results of previous studies offered heterogeneous results, which can be divided in evidence favoring the model of an importance of alpha oscillations, as well as models based on TCD or predictive coding, which underline the importance of low frequency oscillations.

Possible reasons for this heterogeneity in the different studies are hard to trace. They could represent systematic changes between the compared groups, yet influences through many other factors are likely, which may smear or veil the true effects. An overview of additional technical factors and aspects regarding data handling and data analysis of oscillatory brain activity, which could affect the results, are covered in a paper by Gross et al. (2013). Besides these technical and analyses-specific aspects pointed out in that paper, also biological factors [e.g., arousal level, hearing loss (Adjamian et al., 2012), the menstrual cycle (Brötzner et al., 2014)] as well as psychological variables (instruction, state of mind, mental health status) may affect neuronal oscillations. Additionally, sample sizes are varying between studies and are often considered to be too small (cf. Adjamian, 2014). In general the question was raised, if healthy subjects and patients have the same experience with the performed measurements. Experienced participants (e.g., persons who participated in multiple experiments) might show less arousal, less vigilance, than unexperienced participants leading to differential oscillatory resting state activity such as reduced alpha. A need to quantify those possible differences was acclaimed (Diaz et al., 2013). This question is of special importance for the research on neural oscillation in tinnitus, as tinnitus patients are often novices to the MEG and the healthy controls often function as control subjects on a regular basis for different studies and therefore they are no novices to the MEG measurement any more.

Of course, those confounding variables are always present in neuroscientific research. It is typically assumed that those variables are equally distributed between the groups and therefore their veiling effect is canceled out. However, in resting state measurements they may be more influential, as the measured signal is more subtle than for example evoked brain activity. Past research has shown, that there is powerful and meaningful output arising from this mode of measurement (resting state) in basic as well as clinical research (e.g., see Başar and Güntekin, 2008). Electrophysiological resting state measurements in tinnitus might be even more interesting to look at as these measurements are with high ecological validity as they are typically recorded in rather quiet surroundings without external activity/stimulation (e.g., no external source, permanently present).

Another important factor, which might add to the heterogeneity of the results in the research on tinnitus, are psychological comorbidities. Those are high in tinnitus patients (Zirke et al., 2010) and some comorbidities are known to have oscillatory correlates (e.g., for Depression: Jiang et al., 2016, for bipolar disorder: Degabriele and Lagopoulos, 2009). In tinnitus research is a focus on identifying underlying neural circuits of tinnitus distress and depression. For the former correlates in high alpha and beta band have been found, especially in right frontal areas, and for the latter in some studies alpha band correlations, here more left frontal lateralized; both constructs have a presumed neuronal overlap in parahippocampal areas (Vanneste et al., 2010; Joos et al., 2012; Meyer et al., 2017). Thus, another aim of the study at hand was to evaluate the impact of comorbid psychological disorders or rather the effect left, if psychological comorbidities in the sample are ruled out. In clinical research, conducting a DSM (Diagnostic and statistical Manual of Mental Disorders) based semi-structured interview covering psychological disorders (SKID, German version, Wittchen et al., 1997) is considered to be the gold standard for detecting and assessing mental health. Therefore, we screened a subgroup of tinnitus patients as well as healthy controls for psychological comorbidities with this instrument in order to detect any mental health disorders.

Taken the current body of research, we tried to shed more light onto the neuronal oscillations in tinnitus based on (a) a sufficiently large sample size (b) by approximation of potential confounding variables of being a novice in the measuring procedure and (c) by ruling out any mental health comorbidity.

MATERIALS AND METHODS

Subjects

Fifty-nine participants having chronic tinnitus were recruited and measured. Due to artifacts (e.g., eye blinks, muscle artifacts), 13 dropped out, leaving 46 participants (mean age ± standard deviation: 41.59 ± 9.92 years; 46% female) in the tinnitus group for data analysis. Fifty-seven healthy controls were recruited, in 15 cases the data did not meet our requirements for analysis (i.e., 90 artifact-free trials) so we conducted our analysis with 42 healthy control participants without tinnitus (39.52 ± 12.05 years; 62% female). There was no significant group difference regarding age and gender ($p > 0.05$). The study protocol was approved by the ethics committee of the Department of Psychology of the University of Münster and was conducted according to the Declaration of Helsinki. Each participant signed informed consent prior to the investigation. Recruitment was conducted through advertisements in local newspapers, flyers in public places, doctor's offices (ENT) and our homepage.

Subgroup of Novices

Twenty-nine subjects with a chronic tinnitus perception (mean age ± standard deviation: 39.00 ± 10.69 years; 48% female) and 26 healthy control participants without any tinnitus perception (42.65 ± 11.95 years; 62% female) were analyzed as a subgroup. All subjects participated for the first time in a MEG measurement. There was no significant group difference regarding age and gender ($p > 0.05$) between these subgroups.

Subgroup of Psychological Comorbidity Free Subjects

Out of the whole sample 40 subjects (20 per group) were screened for psychological disorders with the SKID. Two participants of the tinnitus group fulfilled the criteria of a mental health disorder (Major depressive Episode, Alcohol Abuse) and were therefore excluded from analysis. The other drop-outs ($n = 10$) were eliminated as their artifact free number of epochs was not sufficient. So 14 subjects with tinnitus (44.36 ± 13.45 years; 50% female) and 14 subjects without tinnitus (42.86 ± 10.26 years; 43% female) having no psychological disorder were analyzed. There was no significant group difference regarding age and gender ($p > 0.05$). For a graphical overview of the different groups analyzed in this paper see **Figure 1**.

Procedures

Five minutes resting state MEG recordings were collected by means of a 275 channel whole-head MEG system (OMEGA 2005 WC, CTF Systems, Inc., Port Coquitlam, BC, Canada) with first order axial gradiometers placed in a magnetically shielded and acoustically quiet room. The participants sat upright in a comfortable position; head position was supported through cotton pad stabilization in the dewar and constantly monitored. During data acquisition participants were instructed to look at a black screen with their eyes open [52 cm × 40 cm (WxH)] at a distance of 90 cm and 'to relax doing nothing.' A continuous data stream was acquired and digitally sampled at a rate of 600 Hz. The 5 min recordings of resting state were always performed prior to further MEG acquisitions used for other studies (Stein et al., 2014; Wunderlich et al., 2015; Domschke et al., 2016; Zwanzger et al., 2016).

Preprocessing and Data Analysis

Sensor Space

The recorded data were analyzed using the FieldTrip toolbox (Oostenveld et al., 2011) under Matlab (The MathWorks, Natick, MA, United States, Version R2013b). An independent component analysis by means of "runica algorithm" (Makeig et al., 1997) was performed in order to identify the strongest components corresponding to ocular, cardiac, and muscle artifacts. Based on their statistical performance, the individual independent components for each subject were rejected from the data in an automated procedure (Dammers et al., 2008). The continuous data stream was then segmented into 150 epochs of 2 s each. A 50 Hz notch filter (plus its harmonics) was applied to eliminate disturbances by the electric power supply. In order to analyze relevant brain waves, an offline 4th order Butterworth low-pass filter (cut-off frequency of 45 Hz) was applied to the data that were DC offset corrected based on the whole epoch length. Additionally, trials containing channels with a signal range larger than 2.5 pT were regarded as artifact-contaminated and excluded. Ninety of the remaining trials were randomly chosen for further analysis. Participants with a residual trial number below 90 were excluded. To account for intra-individual head positions during the MEG measurements, the data was projected onto a common sensor space (Knösche et al., 2002). Axial gradiometer recorded data were further transformed to planar gradiometers by taking the norm of the first spatial derivatives in polar and azimuthal directions for each sensor (Knösche and Bastiaansen, 2002). This was done for a better interpretation of the location of the activation picked up by the coils.

In the following, a spectral analysis was performed by means of a fast Fourier transformation (FFT) between DC and 30 Hz after applying a Hanning window to each epoch. Then, for each subject the power spectral density averaged across epochs was normalized by the individual overall spectral power (power spectral density averaged across all channels and frequencies).

Source Space

As most models have a prediction of neuronal activity in the auditory cortex (Zobay et al., 2015), we restricted the source space analysis to this area. To analyze the neuronal activity in the estimation of the auditory areas, the Brain Electrical Source Analysis software (BESA Research 6.0, Megis Software) was used. The recorded data was imported into BESA. In order to circumvent referring to data being processed by FieldTrip routines for the sensor space analysis, the data preprocessing has been repeated for the source space analysis using almost the same steps in BESA. Thereby we followed the FieldTrip approach described above as closely as possible. To eliminate artifact activity as eye blinks, movements or cardiac activity from the brain activity, an ICA was calculated as implemented in BESA (Lee et al., 1999). Independent component analysis using an extended infomax algorithm for mixed subgaussian and supergaussian sources was used (Lee and Lewicki, 2002) and identified artifact contaminated components were subtracted from the raw data. Data was again cut into epochs of 2 s and 1 Hz high pass and 180 Hz low pass filters were applied to the data. Trials with an amplitude range over 2.5 pT at any MEG sensor were regarded as contaminated and rejected.

Based on a source montage template for auditory brain regions (three temporal sources in the left and three symmetric sources in the right hemisphere; see also **Supplementary Figure S1**), we reconstructed the source strength waveforms (cf. Scherg et al., 2002) using BESA. This auditory source montage is based on literature on auditory activity (an overview of the exact procedure is provided in Scherg et al., 2002). Afterward a FFT frequency analysis was calculated for each source comprising the source montage. The obtained normalized power spectrum was exported to SPSS (IBM SPSS Statistics for Macintosh, Version 24.0) for further statistical analysis.

Statistical Analysis

Sensor Space

To check for group differences (tinnitus vs. no tinnitus) in the *a priori* defined frequency bands {delta [1–4 Hz], theta [5–7 Hz], alpha [8–12 Hz] (low alpha [8–10 Hz] and high alpha [10–12 Hz]), beta [13–30 Hz], gamma [31–45 Hz]}, non-parametric statistical tests were calculated. Cluster-based statistics were calculated to determine significance probabilities based on a permutation distribution (Monte Carlo). For each frequency band 1000 permutations were drawn. The Monte Carlo p-values were set to $p < 0.025$ on sensor and $p < 0.05$ on cluster level and the used statistic for the permuting were an independent t- tests.

These analyses were done for the whole group comparison (1), the subgroups of novices (2) and psychological comorbidity-free subjects (3) (all: tinnitus vs. no tinnitus).

Source Space

The spectral components of the temporal source montage extracted from the BESA analysis were averaged over the six individual sources in the auditory area for each frequency band and normalized (over all auditory sources and frequencies). Using a one-way ANOVA in SPSS we compared the frequency bands. As we tested for seven frequency bands, all p-values were Bonferroni-corrected for seven comparisons.

RESULTS

Sensor Space

All Participants

Visual inspection of the spectral power resembles the power distribution reported by Weisz et al. (2005), indicating an overall reduced alpha power in the tinnitus group and a slight increase at delta frequencies (cf. **Figure 2**) compared to the control group. A significant difference in the delta frequency band ($p = 0.048$) was located at a right fronto-temporal area (cf. **Figure 2**). In spite of its visual appearance, groups did not differ in the alpha band (8–12 Hz, $p = 0.18$) nor in the alpha sub-bands (low alpha; 8–10 Hz, $p = 0.178$, high alpha; 10–12 Hz, $p = 0.247$).

Groups did also not differ in the other frequency band (theta, beta, gamma; all $p > 0.05$). To explain the discrepancy between the visualized data (the plot, see **Figure 2**) and the statistics, we

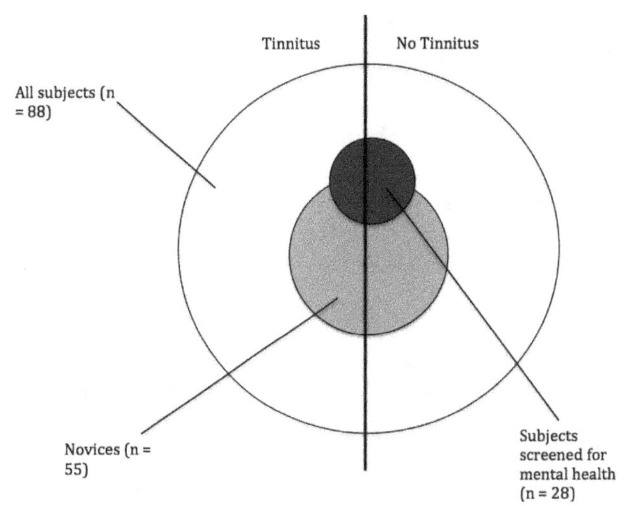

FIGURE 1 | Scheme of the organization of the subjects.

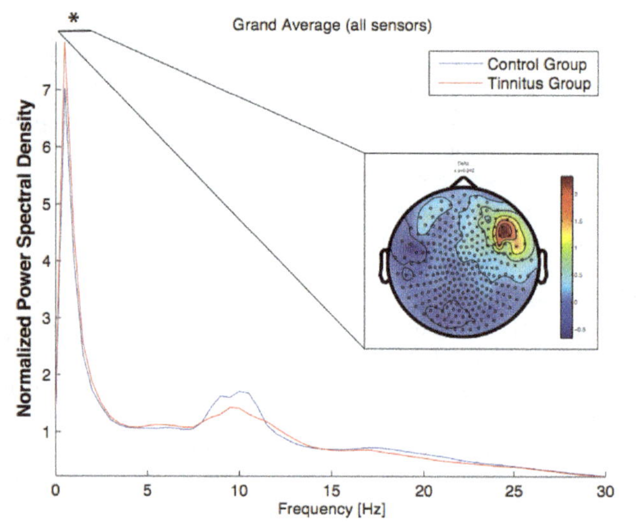

FIGURE 2 | Power spectral density across all sensors for the tinnitus group (blue line) and the control group (red line). The power spectral density was averaged across all epochs and was normalized by the overall spectral power (channels × frequency bins). The significant difference (*) in the delta band is depicted as topographic plot (tinnitus minus controls). The circles ('o') mark a sensor, the cross ('x') stands for a sensor, where a significant difference was found between the groups. The spectrum was cut off at 30 Hz to highlight the relevant frequency bands.

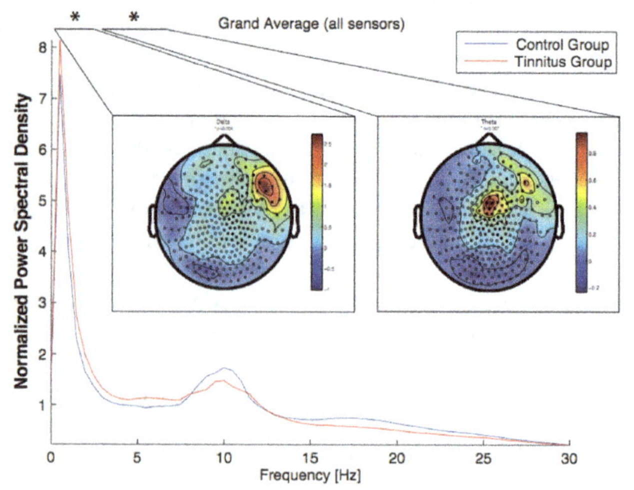

FIGURE 3 | Power spectral density across all sensors for the *Novices* group (tinnitus subjects: blue line; control group: red line). The power spectral density was averaged across all epochs and was normalized by the overall spectral power (channels × frequency bins). The significant difference (*) in the delta and the theta band is depicted as topographic plot (tinnitus minus controls). The circles ('o') mark a sensor, the star ('*') stands for a sensor, where a significant difference was found between the groups. The spectrum was cut off at 30 Hz to highlight the relevant frequency bands.

did a *post hoc* analysis of the alpha power, which displayed a considerable variance of the alpha power values in the patient group and therefore impeding the statistics to become significant.

Novices Only

Again, per visual inspection, the alpha frequency power in the novices (tinnitus vs. no tinnitus) appears to be different compared to those of the group of all subjects, yet this could not be affirmed through our statistical analysis. In the analysis of the MEG-Novices (tinnitus vs. no tinnitus) we found a significant difference in the delta (1–4 Hz, $p < 0.01$) and theta (4–8 Hz, $p < 0.01$, see **Figure 3**) frequency band. Again, all other frequency bands did not differ significantly between tinnitus subjects and healthy controls ($p > 0.05$).

Psychological Comorbidity Free Subjects Only

No significant differences between the group of mentally healthy tinnitus subjects and subjects without tinnitus occurred in the oscillatory resting state activity using the permutation testing on sensor level ($p > 0.05$, see **Figure 4**).

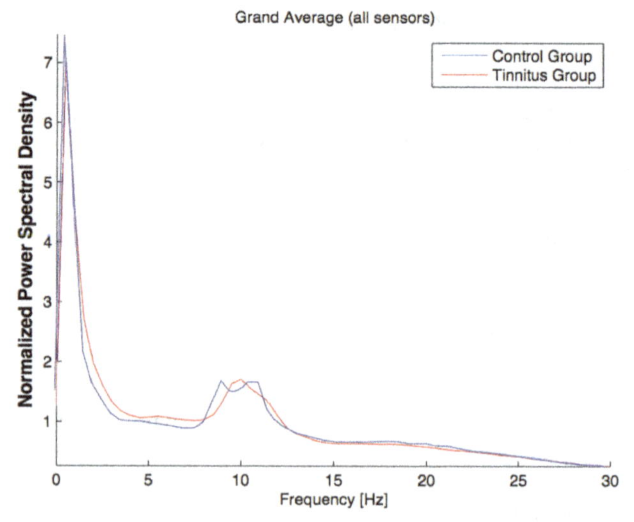

FIGURE 4 | Power spectral density across all sensors for the *Psychologically Healthy* group (tinnitus subjects: blue line; control group: red line). The power spectral density was averaged across all epochs and was normalized by the overall spectral power (channels × frequency bins). The spectrum was cut off at 30 Hz to highlight the relevant frequency bands.

Source Space

All Participants

When comparing the complete tinnitus group against the healthy controls using the BESA source reconstruction of oscillatory activity in the auditory areas, we find a significant difference in the theta and gamma band [one-way ANOVA with group as factor; theta: $F(1,86) = 8.403$, $p = 0.005$; gamma: $F(1,86) = 9.408$, $p = 0.003$, see **Figure 5**]. No significant difference emerged in the other frequency bands [$F(1,86) < 1.603$, $p > 0.209$].

Novices Only

A significant difference resulted in the theta and gamma band in the temporally located sources [theta: $F(1,53) = 18.026$, $p < 0.001$; gamma: $F(1,53) = 10.760$, $p = 0.002$; see **Figure 6**]. The other frequency bands did not differ significantly ($p > 0.05$).

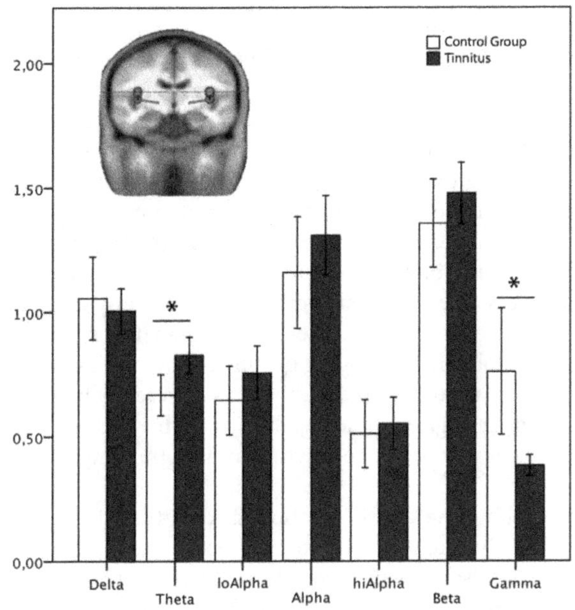

FIGURE 5 | Normalized power spectrum of the source waveforms, reconstructed in auditory areas. *Marks a significant difference between the groups. The dipoles (blue: left, red: right side) in the head scheme show exemplarily four of six locations of the source montage. The same locations and orientations were used for both groups. LoAlpha = low alpha frequency range (8–10 Hz); hiAlpha = High alpha frequency range (10–12 Hz). Error bars symbolize ±2 standard errors.

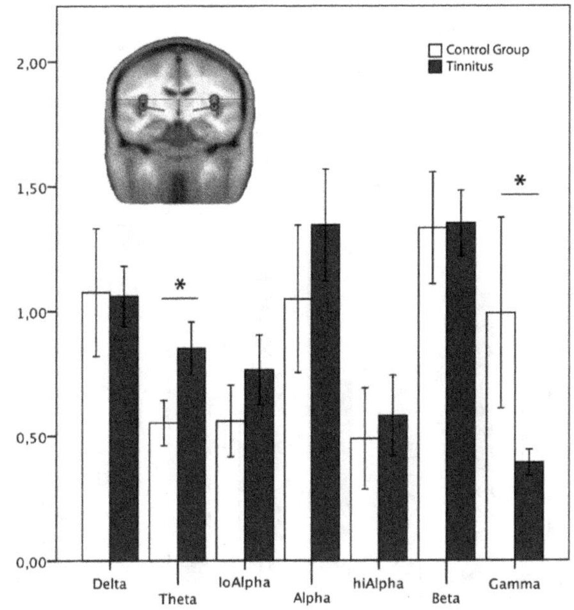

FIGURE 6 | Normalized power spectrum of the source waveforms, reconstructed in auditory areas for the group of *Novices* only. * Marks a significant difference between the groups. The dipoles (blue: left, red: right side) in the head scheme show exemplarily four of six locations of the source montage. The same locations and orientations were used for both groups. LoAlpha = low alpha frequency range (8–10 Hz); hiAlpha = high alpha frequency range (10–12 Hz). Error bars symbolize ±2 standard errors.

Psychological Comorbidity Free Subjects Only

There was no significant difference for any of the frequency bands between the control and the experimental group for the group, in which psychological disorders were measured and excluded [$F(1,26) < 2.587$; $p > 0.05$, see **Figure 7**].

DISCUSSION

To the best of our knowledge, this is the first study investigating the neural oscillations of a sample comprising 88 subjects with and without tinnitus. Due to this large sample size, results of the current study can be assumed to be valuable with regard to questions concerning the role of neural oscillations in tinnitus.

Encompassing the whole group of participants, we found an increase in the delta spectrum in sensor space in the right frontal–temporal area of the coils. This means we found differences in the slow wave power of delta between the tinnitus and the control group in the directly picked up signal, the sensor space. The depicted activity here could correspond to auditory areas, but other sources are also imaginable. When localizing the origin of the signal within the brain, the analysis in source space, we found a difference when focusing on the auditory cortical areas for theta, another slow wave frequency. Sensor and source space findings agree in the coinciding occurrence of low oscillatory frequencies. Besides this, we found a difference in high frequency activity, namely a significant reduction in gamma band in source space, which is not detectable in our sensor space analysis.

Following the goal to rule out one confounding factor by restricting the analysis to subjects from both groups who were in MEG for the first time, the novices, we saw similar results: again, we found the difference in delta activity in sensor space, but additionally also in the theta frequency band. Furthermore, in source space we found a significant difference in the theta and gamma band in areas associated with auditory processing.

When analyzing the subgroup of subjects, who had been screened for psychological disorders and had been adjudged to be without mental health comorbidity, we did not find any difference between the groups of tinnitus subjects and healthy controls neither in sensor nor in source space.

According to Zobay et al. (2015), the TCD model would rather predict differences in the theta than the delta band. Yet, delta and theta frequencies are thought to be originating from the same source and are often treated equally (Pierzycki et al., 2016). The increase in slow wave activity (delta/theta) is in line with the TCD as well as the predictive coding model and previous findings (Weisz et al., 2005; Adjamian, 2014; De Ridder et al., 2015; Sedley et al., 2016). And, according to these models, we would also have expected changes in the gamma activity. With respect to the model of De Ridder et al. (2015) one would expect an increase in gamma power, whereas the integrative model of Sedley et al. (2016) would be predict a gamma decrease in the tinnitus population. In our sample we found a reduction in gamma band activity in the tinnitus group. So, these findings would be in line with the theoretical assumptions of Sedley et al. (2016)

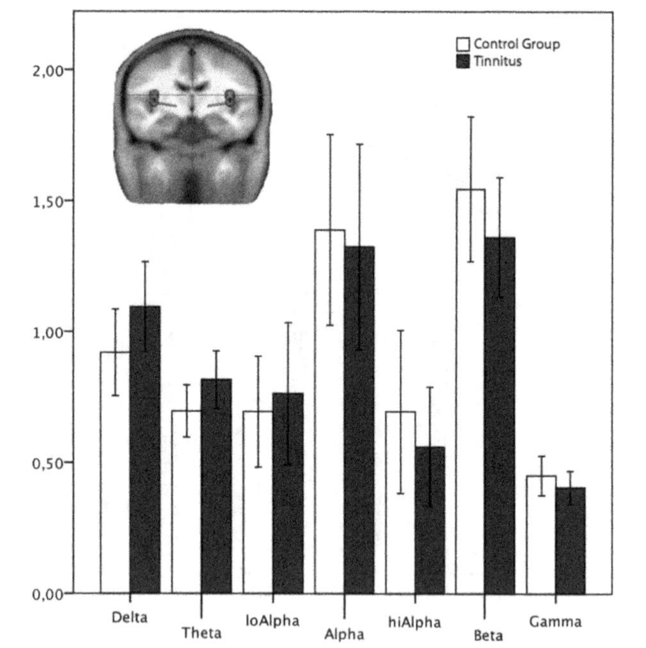

FIGURE 7 | Normalized power spectrum of the source waveforms, reconstructed in auditory areas for the group of *psychologically healthy*. The dipoles (blue: left, red: right side) in the head scheme show exemplarily four of six locations of the source montage. The same locations and orientations were used for both groups. LoAlpha, low alpha frequency range (8–10 Hz); hiAlpha, high alpha frequency range (10–12 Hz). Error bars symbolize ±2 standard errors.

that the mismatch in tinnitus patients is reduced. As described above, here prediction ('tinnitus') and the precursor would be consistent and therefore no mismatch would be elicited. Evidence for this assumptions is derived from intracranial measurements in a single-case study (Sedley et al., 2015) as well as a group study (Sedley et al., 2012), where residual inhibition was used to manipulate the tinnitus. Additionally, a decrease in gamma activity was reported by Müller et al. (2013) after they used rTMS stimulation and was associated with an increase in tinnitus loudness. But gamma activity in general might be difficult to measure: research from other fields of domains, e.g., in the visual field (Muthukumaraswamy et al., 2010), has shown, how unpredictable and therefore problematic it is to trace gamma oscillations. Furthermore, gamma networks seem to be less reliable, too (Jin et al., 2011), which adds up to the intricacy of analyzing gamma activity. This might also explain, why we found the gamma results in source space only. In source space we have a better signal to noise ratio and therefore were more prone to pick up subtle signals as presumably the gamma band.

A priori we defined our source of interest in the auditory areas and therefore limited out analysis to the estimation of this region. An analysis with less beforehand defined restrictions or even network analysis, could possibly add insight to the findings of this paper. Especially, a replication of the findings of the gamma activity would be needed to validate our results. As shown in this paper, calculating both analysis (sensor and source space) is fruitful, as they show overlapping, yet not redundant results, which can trigger more comprehension.

To shed light on possible confounders which influence the neuronal activity we examined the factor of "being a novice." Next to a different result in sensor space (finding a difference in theta and delta band), we saw in source space the same results as for the whole group. A comparison between novices and non-novices within the two groups (looking at tinnitus novices vs. tinnitus non-novices and the same for the control group) also would have been interesting; unfortunately these analyses were not possible as the two groups differed significantly in their age. In our sample, the novices were older than the non-novices. Students are our main resource of subjects and the novices were specifically recruited in the public and covered a broader age range. Concluding, our findings hint that this factor ("being a novice") does not seem to have a meaningful impact on the results.

If we follow the above mentioned idea, that the more you control for confounders, the more precise are the results, this effect should also have been visible in the second subgroup, the group of mentally healthy participants. Conversely, this did not appear. As effects are expected to be subtle (Adjamian, 2014), the most probable reason for that might be the sample size of this subgroup (14 per group). This might have been too small to see a significant effect. Another possibility is, that, if you carefully control for mental health comorbidities, some oscillatory effects between the groups (tinnitus and non-tinnitus) disappear. Psychological disorders do reflect in the neuronal firing pattern and might account for some variance between the groups if comparing a tinnitus group against a group of non-tinnitus sufferers. The connection between tinnitus and psychological disorders is complex and its direction (e.g., causality, mediation, vulnerability) unclear. It is likely that comorbid psychological disorders might interfere with tinnitus perception, as postulated, e.g., for somatoform disorders (Signal Filter-Modell according to Rief and Barsky) (Voderholzer and Hohagen, 2017). Here, the assumption is, that attentional processes, anxieties and depressive mood influence the cortical perception of the bodily symptoms. Next to this enhancement of bodily symptoms (the tinnitus correlate would most likely be tinnitus loudness), Zirke et al. (2010) state, that psychological comorbid disorders might hinder the habituation to the tinnitus itself. Furthermore, it is likely that the mental health status might also influence the overall distress perceived through the tinnitus. Handing out a questionnaire covering, e.g., the depressive symptomatic, is a good tool to estimate symptoms, yet these do not cover the full spectrum of mental health and are more a clue, not a tool to diagnose a person. Therefore the approach of this paper, performing the structured interviews covering the majority of psychological disorders, like the SKID or the CIDI (see Zirke et al., 2013), could be a step into the future to surely be aware of all mental health disorders in the participant group. The question, which oscillatory pattern between the two groups remains, if we control for as many confounders as possible, is yet to be answered.

Next to the two factors analyzed in this paper, many others may contribute to the heterogeneity within the measurement of neural oscillations. One step evolving from this issue is the development and handing out of questionnaires covering, e.g., cognitive states. Diaz et al. (2013) define the resting state "as a multi-faceted cognitive construct" and developed a questionnaire to quantify these cognitions. Seven dimensions were identified which were present during resting state measurements: discontinuity of mind, theory of mind, self, planning, sleepiness, comfort, and somatic awareness. Quantifying patient-control differences in the cognitive states might be a helpful tool for future measurements, to control more possible confounders and conduct measurements, which narrow down the true underlying difference of symptoms of tinnitus. To address this issue, other fields started projects of gathering multi-center data and meta data sharing in order to increase replicability and validity of the data (see Kafkafi et al., 2016).

One overall attempt to deal with the heterogeneity in tinnitus findings, is to define subtypes of tinnitus. TINNET (a European project on Tinnitus http://tinnet.tinnitusresearch.net) is aiming at quantifying and analyzing all aspects and facets of tinnitus and hopes to break down the heterogeneity. A workgroup of this project suggested guidelines for M/EEG measurements in tinnitus[1]. Those should make sure a better comparability of results between different labs and studies. The guideline advocates, next to other factors, the measurement of tinnitus distress, hearing loss, hyperacusis, and a resting state questionnaire. Taking them into consideration as confounders would have been helpful to rule out possible explanations. We think having quantified those factors would have helped to come to a more comprehensive and target-oriented interpretation of our results.

Another option to control for the heterogeneous characteristics in tinnitus research is to use a between-subjects-design with using tinnitus subjects only. Control group and tinnitus group may differ substantially in factors as, e.g., hearing loss or hyperacusis. With comparing subgroups within the group of tinnitus could therefore yield in more homogenous and more comparable groups. In this study we chose a comparison of tinnitus-experiencing subjects to subjects without tinnitus because we wanted to keep the comparability with other studies in the field (Weisz et al., 2005; Adjamian et al., 2012) and controlled that key aspects, as age and gender, are distributed equally in both groups.

Taken together, this study ruled out criticism of a too small sample size in the neuronal oscillations research in tinnitus. We were able to show that an analysis based on a sufficient sample size supports the significance of slow oscillatory frequencies and gamma band activity in the neuroscientific conceptualization of tinnitus. Yet, our data does not support a single model only. Targeting the heterogeneity of tinnitus on different levels, e.g., as focusing subtyping of tinnitus or, as done here, controlling more confounding variables, seems to be a necessary step to understand this phenomenon. To control the naiveté in studies is an approach to narrow down a manifold set of confounders (here: vigilance, arousal, stimulation due unfamiliarity to the situation). However, in our analysis of novices only, results did not hint toward a reduced variance in the sample and therefore to clearer results. Next to controlling factors forcefully (with excluding anyone who had experience in experiments beforehand or with a psychological comorbidity), quantifying the experience during the experiment is another option. This could, most likely, be done with questionnaires to assess those variable and take them into statistical analysis or at least into consideration when interpreting the findings. Controlling mental health comorbidities is, derived from the literature, clearly a worthy, yet very resource consuming approach. The lack of a statistical difference between the second subgroup in our study (*psychologically healthy*), could either show that whether or not those variables are controlled in a tinnitus sample, differences do disappear or that our sample size, thinned out through a relatively high drop-out rate and the time and a certain professional training demanding screening procedure, was too small to produce meaningful differences.

To sum up, we agree with previously published papers that neuronal oscillations in tinnitus are presently no distinctly defined biomarker (Pierzycki et al., 2016) and future research is needed to test the theoretically postulated models for tinnitus (e.g., TCD, predictive coding). Our study could contribute with highlighting the need of a thorough assessment of mental health in tinnitus studies and the rather minor importance of the factor 'being a novice' to the measurement. Overall, we could demonstrate a support for low neuronal frequencies as well as high frequencies to be connected with the percept of tinnitus.

AUTHOR CONTRIBUTIONS

PL, RW, AE, AL, and MJ recruited the participants. PL and AW developed and performed the data analysis. PL, AW, AE, RW, AL, and CP wrote the manuscript. All authors approved the final version of the manuscript.

FUNDING

This research was supported by the Deutsche Forschungsgesellschaft (PA 392/14-1) and Interdisziplinäres Zentrum für Klinische Forschung Münster (IZKF), Medical Faculty, University of Münster, Germany (Project No. CRA05).

ACKNOWLEDGMENTS

We are grateful to Karin Berning, Hildegard Deitermann, Ute Trompeter, Martin Winkels, Anna Shushakova, Miriam Miesen, the Audiometry Department and all our participants for their support.

SUPPLEMENTARY MATERIAL

FIGURE S1 | Location of the AEP montage by BESA covering the auditory areas.

[1]http://tinnet.tinnitusresearch.net/images/pdf/WG3/Standardisation_Report_V5.pdf

REFERENCES

Adjamian, P. (2014). The application of electro- and magneto-encephalography in tinnitus research – methods and interpretations. *Front. Neurol.* 5:228. doi: 10.3389/fneur.2014.00228

Adjamian, P., Sereda, M., Zobay, O., Hall, D. A., and Palmer, A. R. (2012). Neuromagnetic indicators of tinnitus and tinnitus masking in patients with and without hearing loss. *J. Assoc. Res. Otolaryngol.* 13, 715–731. doi: 10.1007/s10162-012-0340-5

Axelsson, A., and Ringdahl, A. (1989). Tinnitus—a study of its prevalence and characteristics. *Br. J. Audiol.* 23, 53–62. doi: 10.3109/0300536890 9077819

Başar, E., and Güntekin, B. (2008). A review of brain oscillations in cognitive disorders and the role of neurotransmitters. *Brain Res.* 1235, 172–193. doi: 10.1016/j.brainres.2008.06.103

Brötzner, C. P., Klimesch, W., Doppelmayr, M., Zauner, A., and Kerschbaum, H. H. (2014). Resting state alpha frequency is associated with menstrual cycle phase, estradiol and use of oral contraceptives. *Brain Res.* 1577, 36–44. doi: 10.1016/j.brainres.2014.06.034

Cohen, M. X. (2014). *Analyzing Neural Time Series Data*. Boston, MA: Institute of Technology.

Dammers, J., Schiek, M., Boers, F., Silex, C., Zvyagintsev, M., Pietrzyk, U., et al. (2008). Integration of amplitude and phase statistics for complete artifact removal in independent components of neuromagnetic recordings. *IEEE Trans. Biomed. Eng.* 55, 2353–2362. doi: 10.1109/TBME.2008.92 6677

De Ridder, D., Vanneste, S., Langguth, B., and Llinas, R. (2015). Thalamocortical dysrhythmia: a theoretical update in tinnitus. *Front. Neurol.* 6:124. doi: 10.3389/fneur.2015.00124

Degabriele, R., and Lagopoulos, J. (2009). A review of EEG and ERP studies in bipolar disorder: review article. *Acta Neuropsychiatr.* 21, 58–66. doi: 10.1111/j.1601-5215.2009.00359.x

Diaz, B. A., Van Der Sluis, S., Moens, S., Benjamins, J. S., Migliorati, F., Stoffers, D., et al. (2013). The Amsterdam Resting-State questionnaire reveals multiple phenotypes of resting-state cognition. *Front. Hum. Neurosci.* 7:446. doi: 10.3389/fnhum.2013.00446

Dobie, R. A. (2003). Depression and tinnitus. *Otolaryngol. Clin. North Am.* 36, 383–388. doi: 10.1016/S0030-6665(02)00168-8

Domschke, K., Zwanzger, P., Rehbein, M. A., Steinberg, C., Knoke, K., Dobel, C., et al. (2016). Magnetoencephalographic correlates of emotional processing in major depression before and after pharmacological treatment. *Int. J. Neuropsychopharmacol.* 19:pyv093. doi: 10.1093/ijnp/pyv093

Gross, J., Baillet, S., Barnes, G. R., Henson, R. N., Hillebrand, A., Jensen, O., et al. (2013). Good practice for conducting and reporting MEG research. *Neuroimage* 65, 349–363. doi: 10.1016/j.neuroimage.2012.10.001

Hartmann, T., Lorenz, I., Müller, N., Langguth, B., and Weisz, N. (2014). The effects of neurofeedback on oscillatory processes related to tinnitus. *Brain Topogr.* 27, 149–157. doi: 10.1007/s10548-013-0295-9

Jensen, O., and Mazaheri, A. (2010). Shaping functional architecture by oscillatory alpha activity: gating by inhibition. *Front. Hum. Neurosci.* 4:186. doi: 10.3389/fnhum.2010.00186

Jiang, H., Popov, T., Jylänki, P., Bi, K., Yao, Z., Lu, Q., et al. (2016). Predictability of Depression severity based on posterior alpha oscillations. *Clin. Neurophysiol.* 127, 2108–2114. doi: 10.1016/j.clinph.2015.12.018

Jin, S.-H., Seol, J., Kim, J. S., and Chung, C. K. (2011). How reliable are the functional connectivity networks of meg in resting States? *J. Neurophysiol.* 106, 2888–2895. doi: 10.1152/jn.00335.2011

Joos, K., vanneste, S., and de Ridder, D. (2012). Disentangling depression and distress networks in the tinnitus brain. *PLoS One* 7:e40544. doi: 10.1371/journal.pone.0040544

Kafkafi, N., Agassi, J., Chesler, E. J., Crabbe, J. C., Crusio, W. E., Eilam, D., et al. (2016). Reproducibility and replicability of rodent phenotyping in preclinical studies. *Neurosci. Biobehav. Rev.* (in press). doi: 10.1016/j.neubiorev.2018.01.003

Knösche, T. R., and Bastiaansen, M. C. (2002). On the time resolution of event-related desynchronization: a simulation study. *Clin. Neurophysiol.* 113, 754–763. doi: 10.1016/S1388-2457(02)00055-X

Knösche, T. R., Lattner, S., Maess, B., Schauer, M., and Friederici, A. D. (2002). Early parallel processing of auditory word and voice information. *Neuroimage* 17, 1493–1503. doi: 10.1006/nimg.2002.1262

Lee, T. W., Girolami, M., and Sejnowski, T. J. (1999). Independent component analysis using an extended infomax algorithm for mixed subgaussian and supergaussian sources. *Neural. Comput.* 11, 417–441. doi: 10.1162/089976699300016719

Lee, T. W., and Lewicki, M. S. (2002). Unsupervised image classification, segmentation, and enhancement using ica mixture models. *IEEE Trans. Image Process.* 11, 270–279. doi: 10.1109/83.988960

Leske, S., Tse, A., Oosterhof, N. N., Hartmann, T., Müller, N., Keil, J., et al. (2014). NeuroImage the strength of alpha and beta oscillations parametrically scale with the strength of an illusory auditory percept. *Neuroimage* 88, 69–78. doi: 10.1016/j.neuroimage.2013.11.014

Llinas, R. R., Ribary, U., Jeanmonod, D., Kronberg, E., and Mitra, P. P. (1999). Thalamocortical dysrhythmia: a neurological and neuropsychiatric syndrome characterized by magnetoencephalography. *Proc. Natl. Acad. Sci. U.S.A.* 96, 15222–15227. doi: 10.1073/pnas.96.26.15222

Makeig, S., Jung, T. P., Bell, A. J., Ghahremani, D., and Sejnowski, T. J. (1997). Blind separation of auditory event-related brain responses into independent components. *Proc. Natl. Acad. Sci. U.S.A.* 94, 10979–10984. doi: 10.1073/pnas.94.20.10979

Meyer, M., Neff, P., Grest, A., Hemsley, C., Weidt, S., and Kleinjung, T. (2017). EEG oscillatory power dissociates between distress- and depression-related psychopathology in subjective tinnitus. *Brain Res.* 1663, 194–204. doi: 10.1016/j.brainres.2017.03.007

Müller, N., Leske, S., Hartmann, T., Szebényi, S., and Weisz, N. (2014). Listen to yourself: the medial prefrontal cortex modulates auditory alpha power during speech preparation. *Cereb. Cortex* 25, 4029–4037. doi: 10.1093/cercor/bhu117

Müller, N., Lorenz, I., Langguth, B., and Weisz, N. (2013). rTMS induced tinnitus relief is related to an increase in auditory cortical alpha activity. *PLoS One* 8:e55557. doi: 10.1371/journal.pone.0055557

Muthukumaraswamy, S. D., Singh, K. D., Swettenham, J. B., and Jones, D. K. (2010). Visual gamma oscillations and evoked responses: variability, repeatability and structural MRI correlates. *Neuroimage* 49, 3349–3357. doi: 10.1016/j.neuroimage.2009.11.045

Oostenveld, R., Fries, P., Maris, E., and Schoffelen, J. M. (2011). FieldTrip: open source software for advanced analysis of MEG, EEG, and invasive electrophysiological data. *Comput. Intell. Neurosci.* 2011:156869. doi: 10.1155/2011/156869

Pierzycki, R. H., McNamara, A. J., Hoare, D. J., and Hall, D. A. (2016). Whole scalp resting state eeg of oscillatory brain activity shows no parametric relationship with psychoacoustic and psychosocial assessment of tinnitus: a repeated measures study. *Hear. Res.* 331, 101–108. doi: 10.1016/j.heares.2015.11.003

Scherg, M., Ille, N., Bornfleth, H., and Berg, P. (2002). Advanced tools for digital EEG review: virtual source montages, whole-head mapping, correlation, and phase analysis. *J. Clin. Neurophysiol.* 19, 91–112. doi: 10.1097/00004691-200203000-00001

Sedley, W., Friston, K. J., Gander, P. E., Kumar, S., Griffiths, T. D., Shargorodsky, J., et al. (2016). An integrative tinnitus model based on sensory precision. *Trends Neurosci.* 39, 799–812. doi: 10.1016/j.tins.2016.10.004

Sedley, W., Gander, P. E., Kumar, S., Oya, H., Kovach, C. K., Nourski, K. V., et al. (2015). Intracranial mapping of a cortical tinnitus system using residual inhibition. *Curr. Biol.* 25, 1208–1214. doi: 10.1016/j.cub.2015.02.075

Sedley, W., Teki, S., Kumar, S., Barnes, G. R., Bamiou, D. E., and Griffiths, T. D. (2012). Single-Subject oscillatory gamma responses in tinnitus. *Brain* 135, 3089–3100. doi: 10.1093/brain/aws220

Shore, S. E., Roberts, L. E., and Langguth, B. (2016). Maladaptive plasticity in tinnitus–triggers, mechanisms and treatment. *Nat. Rev. Neurol.* 12, 150–160. doi: 10.1038/nrneurol.2016.12

Sindhusake, D., Mitchell, P., Newall, P., Golding, M., Rochtchina, E., and Rubin, G. (2003). Prevalence and characteristics of tinnitus in older adults: the blue mountains hearing study: prevalencia y características del acúfeno en adultos mayores: el estudio de audición blue mountains. *Int. J. Audiol.* 42, 289–294. doi: 10.3109/14992020309078348

Stein, A., Engell, A., Junghoefer, M., Wunderlich, R., Lau, P., Wollbrink, A., et al. (2014). Inhibition-Induced plasticity in tinnitus patients after repetitive exposure to tailor-made notched music. *Clin. Neurophysiol.* 126, 1007–1015. doi: 10.1016/j.clinph.2014.08.017

Vanneste, S., Plazier, M., Van der Loo, E., Van de Heyning, P., Congedo, M., and De Ridder, D. (2010). The neural correlates of tinnitus-related distress. *Neuroimage* 52, 470–480. doi: 10.1016/j.neuroimage.2010.04.029

Voderholzer, U., and Hohagen, F. (2017). *Therapie Psychischer Erkrankungen.* Zurich: Urban & Fische.

Weisz, N., Moratti, S., Meinzer, M., Dohrmann, K., and Elbert, T. (2005). Tinnitus perception and distress is related to abnormal spontaneous brain activity as measured by magnetoencephalography. *PLoS Med.* 2:e153. doi: 10.1371/journal.pmed.0020153

Wittchen, H. U., Zaudig, M., and Fydrich, T. (1997). *Strukturiertes Klinisches Interview Für DSM-IV, Hogrefe. Göttingen, Germany.* Available at: http://scholar.google.com/scholar?hl_=en&btnG=Search&q=intitle:Strukturiertes+Klinisches+Interview+f?r+DSM-IV#6

Wunderlich, R., Lau, P., Stein, A., Engell, A., Wollbrink, A., Rudack, C., et al. (2015). Impact of spectral notch width on neurophysiological plasticity and clinical effectiveness of the tailor-made notched music training. *PLoS One* 10:e0138595. doi: 10.1371/journal.pone.0138595

Zirke, N., Goebel, G., and Mazurek, B. (2010). Tinnitus und psychische komorbiditäten. *HNO* 58, 726–732. doi: 10.1007/s00106-009-2050-9

Zirke, N. C., Seydel, D., Arsoy, B. F., Klapp, H., Haupt, A. J., Szczepek, H., et al. (2013). Analysis of mental disorders in tinnitus patients performed with composite international diagnostic interview. *Qual. Life Res.* 22, 2095–2104. doi: 10.1007/s11136-012-0338-9

Zobay, O., Palmer, A. R., Hall, D. A., Sereda, M., and Adjamian, P. (2015). Source space estimation of oscillatory power and brain connectivity in tinnitus. *PLoS One* 10:e0120123. doi: 10.1371/journal.pone.0120123

Zwanzger, P., Klahn, A. L., Arolt, V., Ruland, T., Zavorotnyy, M., Sälzer, J., et al. (2016). Impact of electroconvulsive therapy on magnetoencephalographic correlates of dysfunctional emotional processing in major depression. *Eur. Neuropsychopharmacol.* 26, 684–692. doi: 10.1016/j.euroneuro.2016.02.005.

7

Salivary Stress-Related Responses in Tinnitus: A Preliminary Study in Young Male Subjects with Tinnitus

Ola A. Alsalman[1], Denise Tucker[2] and Sven Vanneste[1]*

[1] Lab for Clinical and Integrative Neuroscience, School of Behavioral and Brain Sciences, The University of Texas at Dallas, Dallas, TX, USA, [2] Department of Communication Sciences and Disorders, University of North Carolina at Greensboro, Greensboro, NC, USA

***Correspondence:**
Ola A. Alsalman
ola.alsalman@utdallas.edu

Objective: This preliminary study examined if baseline measures of stress-related biomarkers as measured by salivary secretions of specific autonomic [measured by salivary α-amylase (sAA)], endocrine (measured by salivary cortisol), and immune (measured by salivary neopterin) responses are greater in male subjects with tinnitus in response to an induced-stress task.

Method: Twenty male subjects with no significant hearing loss, 10 with tinnitus, and 10 without tinnitus were enrolled in this study.Salivary secretions were collected before and after the induced stress task at four different time intervals.

Results: sAA levels were lower in the tinnitus group in comparison to subjects without tinnitus, suggesting impaired sympathetic activity in the subjects with tinnitus although these levels remained stable throughout the stress experiment.While no significant effects could be obtained for salivary cortisol or neopterin, salivary neopterin levels were trending toward significance over all measurements. Behavioral measures of stress were found to correlate negatively with measures of sAA and salivary neopterin.

Conclusion: The results of this study suggest impaired stress-related sAA mechanisms in male subjects with tinnitus, as evidenced by the different stress reactions induced in the endocrine system (as measured by salivary cortisol) and the immune system (as measured by salivary neopterin).

Keywords: tinnitus, stress-related responses, salivary alpha amylase, salivary cortisol, salivary neopterin

INTRODUCTION

Tinnitus is a sound that is perceived in the absence of an external acoustic stimulus (Jastreboff and Hazell, 1993). The complexity in identifying the underlying mechanism of tinnitus generation is in part related to the subjective nature of this condition, along with the cascade of associated emotional and psychological reactions accompanying its occurrence. Patients with chronic tinnitus can experience a disabling sense of depression, anxiety, stress, and sleep difficulties (Halford and Anderson, 1991; Folmer et al., 1999; Folmer and Griest, 2000; Shargorodsky et al., 2010).

Stress is widely acknowledged as a predisposing and precipitating factor in different neurological and psychiatric illnesses. While acute stress promotes adaptation, prolonged stress over time leads to wear-and-tear on the body—so called the allostatic load, which comprises the negative physiological and psychological effects of stress. Stress induces secretion of corticotropin-releasing hormone from the hypothalamus, which stimulates the secretion of adrenocorticotropin from the pituitary gland. That release of adrenocorticotropin to blood causes the adrenal gland to secrete stress hormones, such as cortisol (Hebert and Lupien, 2007). In addition, several studies have indicated that the sympathetic nervous system (SNS) plays an important role in stress (Cohen and Khalaila, 2014; Lupis et al., 2014; McKune et al., 2014; Carnuta et al., 2015; Het et al., 2015). Given that secretions from salivary glands are modulated by direct sympathetic innervations, salivary α-amylase (sAA) is proposed to be a surrogate marker of SNS activity, with changes in sAA reflecting sympathetic influences on salivary glands.

Reaction to acute stress is not only limited to activity that involves the activation of sympathetic and endocrine systems, but can also be observed in the immune system (Fuchs et al., 1993a; Moynihan, 2003). In the course of an immune response, a whole spectrum of active substances is generated, one of them being neopterin. Neopterin is released into the body by the kidneys and produced by monocytes/macrophages after stimulation by the cytokine interferon-γ (Widner et al., 2002). Both animal and human research has demonstrated that an acute stressor does change neopterin levels (Breinekova et al., 2007; Lindsay et al., 2015). Particularly, stress is found to impact hormonal regulatory function, causing immune cells to become insensitive to hormones and consequently resulting in suppression of immune system responses, triggering increased susceptibility to diseases (Cohen et al., 1991; van West and Maes, 2001).

Taken as a whole, alteration of individual physiological status as a result of a stressor is generally accepted as an underlying mechanism for stress generation (Chrousos and Gold, 1992; Chrousos, 2000; Tsigos and Chrousos, 2002; Kudielka and Wust, 2010). This mechanism involves activation of both the hypothalamic-pituitary-axis (HPA) and SNS. Given that there is a clear association between stress and tinnitus (Hinton et al., 2006; Shargorodsky et al., 2010; Nondahl et al., 2011; Kim et al., 2015), similar HPA and SNS salivary reactions can be expected in subjects with tinnitus.

With this in mind, the aim of this preliminary study is to examine autonomic, immune, and endocrine stress-related markers in male subjects with tinnitus in comparison to healthy controls (i.e., subjects without tinnitus). We wanted to examine if the concentrations of circulating sAA and salivary cortisol in male subjects with tinnitus differ from healthy controls. In addition, since increase in immune system function can lead to deregulation of the endocrine and immune systems, we also looked at salivary neopterin as an immune system marker in relation to tinnitus. As such, we hypothesized that salivary stress related markers could be used to distinguish stress influences and variations between the two groups.

MATERIALS AND METHODS

Participants

Male subjects were invited to participate in a research study by posting flyers at the University of North Carolina at Greensboro (UNCG) campus and surrounding areas. Subjects were excluded if they were smokers, had any dental work within the 48 h prior to sample collection, were prescribed or currently taking any medications for depression, anxiety, stress, bipolar disorder, epilepsy, thyroid dysfunction, schizophrenia, or insomnia, or any other neurological diseases. Because of monthly hormonal fluctuation (specifically cortisol) due to the menstrual cycle, only males were included in this study. In addition, due to the hormonal changes, which accompany increased age, the age limits were set from 18 to 35 years.

In total, 16 male subjects with tinnitus and 20 male subjects without tinnitus applied to participate in the study. However, 6 male subjects with tinnitus and 10 male subjects without tinnitus were excluded because they did not fit the inclusion criteria. Twenty male subjects with no significant hearing loss, 10 with tinnitus (mean age: 23.9 years; $Sd = 3.78$) and 10 without tinnitus (mean age: 23.6 years; $Sd = 4.47$), were enrolled in this study. All research involved in this study was approved by the authors' Institutional Review Board (The university of North Carolina at Greensboro IRB #12-0223), and all subjects gave signed informed consent prior to enrollment. All clinical investigation was conducted according to the principles expressed in the Declaration of Helsinki. Informed consent, written or oral, was obtained from the participants.

Questionnaires and Audiometric Testing

Male subjects with tinnitus completed all questionnaires, while those without tinnitus only filled in four out of the six questionnaires (tinnitus medical history intake questionnaire and tinnitus severity index excluded). All questionnaires were mailed out to subjects prior to their scheduled lab visit. In addition, audiometric testing was administrated to determine subjects hearing level. Subjects with tinnitus had their tinnitus pitch and loudness match measured.

Stress Test

To induce stress, we adapted the mental arithmetic task, part of the the Trier Social Stress Test (TSST), which has proven to be effective in inducing physiological changes in response to stress (Kirschbaum et al., 1993). After collecting the baseline measure, subjects were asked to perfrom a mental arthmetic task, by counting backwards, starting at 5000, in intervals of seven, for up to 5 min.

Clinical Assessment

The neuromeric rating scale (NRS) and saliva collections were assessed before beginning the stress task as well as 5, 30, and 60 min after inducing stress.

Numeric Rating Scale (NRS) of Acute Stress

Numeric Rating Scale (NRS) of acute stress was assessed subjectively by asking subjects to rate how stressed they were before collecting each of the four saliva samples on a scale from 0 (=no stress) to 10 (=extremely stressed).

Saliva Collection

Commercial collection aids were used from the Salimetrics laboratory (Salimetrics, LLC, USA). All samples were measured using a kinetic kit. The collection aid was used to collect unstimulated saliva samples via a passive drool method. All saliva samples obtained were stored in a 2 ml cryovials, and immediately stored in an $-80°$C laboratory freezer. Collected saliva sample were de-identified, and subjects were assigned a number that was used in the saliva testing and in subsequent psychometric scores analysis. Prior to saliva collections, all subjects were instructed to avoid food, dental surgery, sugary drinks, alcohol, caffeine, nicotine, acidic drinks, and excessive napping or exercising on scheduled lab visits, for at least an hour before collecting the saliva samples. In addition, subjects' were instructed not to brush their teeth within 45 min prior to sample collection in order to avoid any risk of lowering pH levels and influencing bacterial growth. Due to the sensitive nature of some of the targeted biomarkers and to minimize possible influence of circadian rhythm, all collection procedures took place at the same time of day: 6:00 p.m.

Flow Rate Correction

If correction for saliva flow rate is not made, there will be variation in the concentration per volume unit from subject-to-subject. This variation could cause problems in statistical analysis that might make it difficult to reveal a biomarker-behavior-relationship.

The correction method explained below enabled us to correct for sAA concentration per minute for each trial result:

$$\textit{Flow rate (ml/min)} = \textit{((saliva (ml)/(time (min)))} \tag{1}$$

There was no need to correct sAA activity for flow rate since the alpha amylase levels were not correlated with flow rate at each measurement.

Saliva Processing

Upon completion of the collection procedures, a total of 80 saliva samples were packed in dry ice and sent to the Salimetrics laboratory (Salimetrics, LLC, USA) for analysis. Salivary cortisol and neopterin were measured in duplicates, while sAA was measured in singulate.

Statistics

All parameters, along with each subject's demographic and psychometric data, were analyzed using descriptive statistics. A Mann–Whitney test was conducted to determine whether there was a difference in the Pittsburgh sleep quality index (PSQI) and the perceived stress scale (PSS) between subjects, with and without tinnitus. In addition, Spearman's Rho correlation was computed to determine associations between baseline measures of PSS and NRS.

To test if there is a significant difference between sAA, salivary cortisol and salivary neopterin between subjects, with and without tinnitus at baseline, a Mann–Whitney test was conducted. In addition Spearman's Rho correlation was computed to determine associations between PSS and baseline measures of sAA, salivary cortisol, and salivary neopterin, respectively.

A Kruskal–Wallis test was applied using the values of the different time intervals (baseline and post-test) as the test variables, and the groups, control vs. tinnitus, as the grouping variables, for each of the three stress-related markers (sAA, salivary cortisol, and salivary neopterin) to examine any significant effect. When significance value was obtained a follow-up with Mann–Whitney test was conducted. To avoid type I error a Bonferroni correction was made adjusting the p-value by dividing 0.05/(# comparison). Effect size was computed manually using the following formula:

$$r = Z/\sqrt{(N)} \tag{2}$$

Similarly, a Kruskal–Wallis test was conducted to examine any evidence of difference on each of the three biomarkers for the follow-up measures at 30 and 60 min. When significance value was obtained a follow-up with Mann–Whitney test was conducted.

We applied a Mann–Whitney test to determine whether there was a difference in flow rate measures for sAA at baseline, 5, 30, and 60 min post-test. In addition, Spearman's Rho was conducted between flow rate and sAA at baseline, and 5, 30, and 60 min.

To confirm the experimental validation of the stress test we applied a Kruskal–Wallis test using values of NRS of the different time intervals as the test variables, and the groups, control vs. tinnitus, as the grouping variables. A similar analysis was applied for post-measurements.

To look for the association or dissociation between sAA and salivary cortisol, we calculated area under the curve (AUC) (Pruessner et al., 2003; Ali and Pruessner, 2012). AUC, with respect to ground, was first calculated for sAA, cortisol, and neopterin using the trapezoid formula described previously (Pruessner et al., 2003):

$$AUC = \sum_{i=1}^{n-1} \frac{\left(m_{(i+1)} + m_i\right) \cdot t_i}{2}$$

m = measurements

t = denoting the distance (time) between the measurements

This score incorporates information regarding both baseline and reactivity individually for sAA and cortisol within one score. We then divided the AUC of sAA by the AUC of salivary cortisol to derive an overall ratio (Ali and Pruessner, 2012), representing the variable of amylase over cortisol based on the individual AUC variables, which we named AOC. This variable can be thought of as the variation in sAA levels after correcting for variations in salivary cortisol. Complimentarily, the ratio variable cortisol over amylase (COA) was calculated by dividing the AUC of salivary cortisol by the AUC of sAA. This variable can be thought of as the variation of cortisol corrected for the variation in amylase. We also divided the AUC of sAA and the AUC of salivary neopterin to derive an overall ratio variable of amylase over neopterin (AON) as well as the AUC of salivary neopterin by the AUC of sAA (NOA). In addition, we also divided the AUC of salivary cortisol and the AUC of salivary neopterin (CON) as well as the AUC of salivary neopterin by the AUC of cortisol (NOC). These various ratio computations are based on Ali and Pruessner's work on assessing sAA over cortisol ratio as a marker to assess deregulation of the stress system (Ali and Pruessner, 2012).

AUC of sAA, AUC of salivary cortisol, alpha amylase over cortisol (AOC), cortisol over alpha amylase (COA), alpha amylase over neopterin (AON), neopterin over alpha amylase (NOA), cortisol over neopterin (CON), and neopterin over cortisol (NOC) were then z-transformed to standardized measurements.

A Mann–Whitney test was applied to evaluate differences of AUC of sAA, AUC of salivary cortisol, and AUC of salivary neopterin between subjects with and without tinnitus. Spearman's Rho were computed between AUC of salivary cortisol and AUC of salivary neopterin and AUC of sAA and AUC of salivary cortisol.

A logistic regression including AUC of sAA, AUC of salivary cortisol and AUC of salivary neopterin as independent variables and group (subjects with tinnitus vs. subjects without tinnitus) as dependent variables was also conducted.

Spearman's correlations were conducted to examine the associations between the standardized AUC of sAA, AUC of salivary cortisol, α-amylase over cortisol, cortisol over α-amylase, α-amylase over neopterin, neopterin over α-amylase, cortisol over neopterin, and neopterin over cortisol with subjective indexes of stress. A 5% level of significance and a Spearman's Rho two-tailed analyses were adopted for all analyses. All statistical analyses were completed using the SPSS software package 22.

RESULTS

Descriptive Characteristics

Overall Subjects

Both subjects with tinnitus and subjects without tinnitus reported to have no serious health conditions, which required immediate or continuous medical attention. When given the choice to rate their overall health, 60% of subjects without tinnitus described their health as "excellent." The majority of subjects with tinnitus (80%) indicated their overall health as "good" or "excellent." Four subjects with tinnitus experienced one to three headaches per week in the month prior to experimentation; however, 80% reported these headaches not to be a significant problem. Exposure to noise was reported as one out of the two main causes of tinnitus. The remaining subjects reported exposure to stressful events as the primary cause of their tinnitus.

A Mann–Whitney test indicated that the PSQI scores were significantly greater for subjects with tinnitus ($M = 4.9$, $Sd = 2.18$, $Md = 5.50$) than subjects without tinnitus ($M = 2.70$, $Sd = 1.05$, $Md = 2$), $U = 20.50$, $p = 0.02$, $r = 0.51$. Similarly, the PSS score for subjects with tinnitus ($M = 20.30$, $Sd = 6.86$, $Md = 20$) were greater than subjects without tinnitus ($M = 10.10$, $Sd = 2.80$, $Md = 10$), $U = 6.50$, $p = 0.001$, $r = 0.73$. Pure tone audiometry results indicated that all subjects had normal hearing thresholds of 20 dB HL or better (with tinnitus, right ear $M = 16$, $Sd = 10.72$; without tinnitus, right ear $M = 19.66$, $Sd = 12.24$) and (with tinnitus, left ear $M = 22$, $Sd = 9.30$; without tinnitus, left ear $M = 14.50$, $Sd = 10.20$). A comparison between the pure tone averages revealed no significant effect between groups. No significant difference between groups was revealed for the pure tone averages.

Tinnitus Characteristics

Five tinnitus subjects reported to have a gradual onset of tinnitus, while five subjects reported to have a sudden onset. The average duration of tinnitus was 3.30 years ($Sd = 1.63$). Six subjects perceived their tinnitus bilaterally, while four perceived it unilaterally. The average pitch match for both the left and right ears were approximately 3 kHz (right ear $M = 3525$, $Sd = 2180$; left ear $M = 3050$, $Sd = 1978$), while average loudness match ranged from 13 to 58 dB HL. The range of loudness match varied from 13 to 44 dB HL in the right ear and 13 to 58 dB HL in the left ear (right ear $M = 30.50$, $Sd = 11.24$; left ear $M = 31.20$, $Sd = 13.33$).

According to the TSI scores ($M = 19.20$, $Sd = 6.90$), tinnitus was not considered to be a bothersome or debilitating problem for subjects with tinnitus. Pure tone ringing was the most common tinnitus sound described by the tinnitus subjects (70%), while hissing and music were the least described tinnitus sounds (20%); 10% reported their tinnitus to be a combination of different tones.

Baseline Measures

A Mann–Whitney test revealed significant difference for baseline sAA (μ/ml) which demonstrated lower score for subjects with tinnitus ($M = 42.84$, $Sd = 24.38$, $Md = 42.65$) than subjects without tinnitus ($M = 98.60$, $Sd = 61.51$, $Md = 65.45$), $U = 20$, $p = 0.023$, $r = -0.50$. Baseline concentrations of salivary cortisol (mg/dl) (subjects with tinnitus $M = 0.10$, $Sd = 0.09$, $Md = 0.07$; subjects without tinnitus $M = 0.09$, $Sd = 0.06$, $Md = 0.09$), $U = 49$, $p = 0.94$, $r = 0.01$, yielded no statistical significant difference. Similarly, salivary neopterin (ng/ml) yielded no significant difference (subjects with tinnitus $M = 2.35$, $Sd = 0.75$, $Md = 2.54$; subjects without tinnitus $M = 1.71$, $Sd = 0.99$, $Md = 1.79$), $U = 28$, $p = 0.09$, $r = 0.37$. See **Figures 1A–C**.

There was a significant correlation between scores the PSS and baseline measures of sAA (μ/ml) ($r_s = -0.49$ $p = 0.02$), indicating that higher stress rates corresponded to lower concentrations of sAA (see **Figure 2A**). The correlation between the related-stress psychometric scores of the PSS and baseline measures of salivary cortisol (mg/dl) ($r_s = -0.05$, $p = 0.81$) and salivary neopterin (ng/ml) ($r_s = 0.34$, $p = 0.14$) yielded no statistical significance. See **Figures 2B,C**.

Experiment

Stress Test

A Kruskal-Wallis test was conducted to determine whether baseline salivary stress-related measures of subjects with tinnitus and subjects without tinnitus varied from post-test measure. The test, which was corrected for tied ranks, showed that in regard to sAA (μ/ml) ($x^2 = 5.14$, $p = 0.02$) results yielded a significant effect from post-test measure. Specifically, baseline measures of sAA for subjects with tinnitus were significantly lower ($M = 42.84$, $Sd = 24.38$, $Md = 42.65$) than subjects without tinnitus ($M = 98.60$, $Sd = 61.51$, $Md = 65.45$), $U = 20$, $p = 0.02$, $r = -0.50$.

No statistical significant difference was found for salivary cortisol (mg/dl) at baseline ($x^2 = 0.006$, $p = 0.09$), and post-test measure ($x^2 = 0.07$, $p = 0.79$). Similarly, there was no statistical significance difference demonstrated for salivary

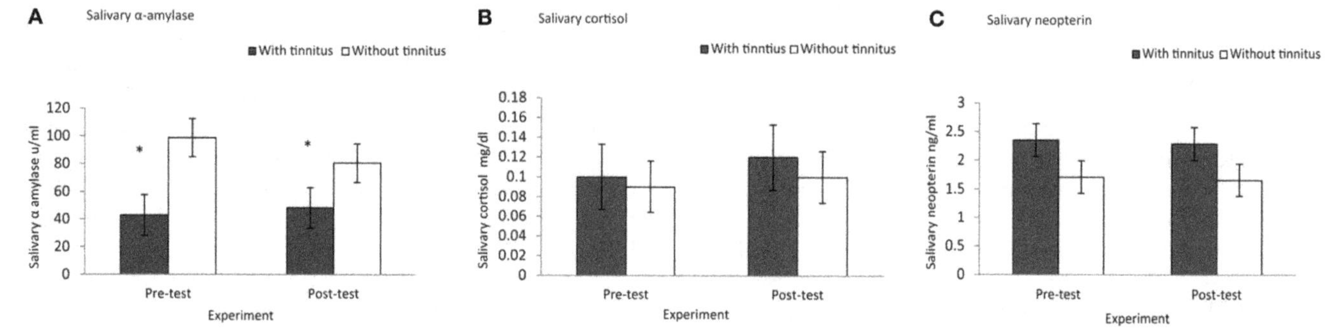

FIGURE 1 | Experimental effect of group differences at baseline vs.post-test for (A) salivary α amylase, (B) salivary cortisol, and (C) salivary neopterin. **(A)** Subjects with tinnitus ($M = 42.84$, $Sd = 24.38$) had lessened salivary α amylase scores than those without tinnitus ($M = 98.60$, $Sd = 61.51$). **(A)** *Indicates significant differences. **(B)** Salivary cortisol, and **(C)** salivary neopterin yielded no statistical significant differences between baseline and post-test measure.

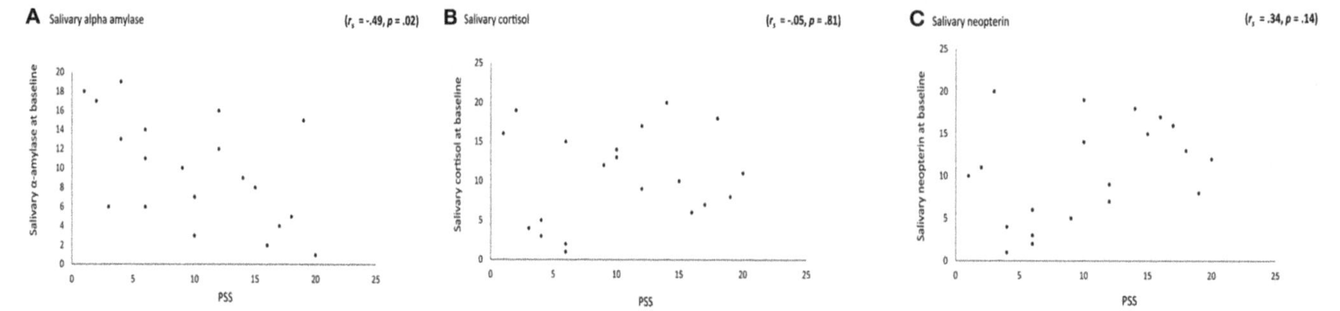

FIGURE 2 | Correlation between the perceived stress scale (PSS) and stress-related markers. **(A)** A significant negative correlation ($r_S = -0.49$ $p = 0.02$) between PSS and baseline measures of salivary α amylase, indicating the higher the stress the lower salivary α amylase concentrations. **(B)** No correlation between PSS scores and baseline measures of salivary cortisol was obtained ($r_S = -0.05$ $p = 0.81$). Similarly, **(C)** PSS with baseline measures of salivary neopterin ($r_S = 0.34$ $p = 0.14$), yielded no statistical significance.

neopterin (ng/ml) at baseline ($x^2 = 2.76, p = 0.09$), and post-test measure ($x^2 = 1.75, p = 0.18$).

Follow-Up

With regard to sAA (μ/ml) there was no statistical significant difference between post-test measure and 30 min fellow-up ($x^2 =$ 4.80, $p = 0.02$). However, a significant difference was obtained at 60 min follow-up ($x^2 = 7$, $p = 0.008$). Specifically, subjects with tinnitus ($M = 40.21$, $Sd = 30.06$, $Md = 22.95$) had lower measures of sAA than subjects without tinnitus ($M = 87.81$, $Sd = 48.04$, $Md = 80.20$), $U = 15$, $p = 0.008$, $r = -0.59$. See **Figure 3A**.

No statistical significant difference was demonstrated for salivary cortisol (mg/dl) at 30 min ($x^2 = 0.20$, $p = 0.65$), and 60 min ($x^2 = 14$, $p = 0.70$). Similarly, there was no significant difference demonstrated for salivary neopterin (ng/ml) at 30 min ($x^2 = 1.12, p = 0.29$), and 60 min follow up ($x^2 = 1.28, p = 0.25$). See **Figures 3B,C**.

Control of Flow Rate of Salivary α-Amylase

A Mann-Whitney test of sAA flow rate reveled no statistical significant difference of flow rate measures in (ml/min) at baseline (subjects with tinnitus $M = 1.85$, $Sd = 0.85$, $Md = 1.50$; subjects without tinnitus $M = 2.02$, $Sd = 1.20$, $Md = 1.75$), $U = 47, p = 0.81, r = -0.05$, at 5 min post-test measure (subjects with tinnitus $M = 2.21$, $Sd = 0.78$, $Md = 2$; subjects without tinnitus $M = 1.79$, $Sd = 0.88$, $Md = 1.62$), $U = 30.50$, $p = 0.13$, $r = -0.30$, at 30 min follow-up measure (subjects with tinnitus $M = 2.02$, $Sd = 0.45$, $Md = 2$; subjects without tinnitus $M =$ 1.79, $Sd = 0.84$, $Md = 1.50$), $U = 31$, $p = 0.13$, $r = -0.30$, as well as at 60 min follow-up measure (subjects with tinnitus $M =$ 1.77, $Sd = 0.40$, $Md = 2$; subjects without tinnitus $M = 1.59$, Sd $= 0.80$, $Md = 1.20$), $U = 34$, $p = 0.21$, $r = -0.27$. In addition, Spearman's Rho revealed no significant correlation between flow rate and sAA activity at baseline ($r_s = -0.21$, $p = 0.35$), 5 min ($r_s = 0.08$, $p = 0.73$), 30 min ($r_s = 0.22$, $p = 0.34$), and 60 min ($r_s = -0.07, p = 0.75$) post-test.

Experimental Validation (Baseline vs. 5 min Post-test)

A Kruskal–Wallis test was conducted for NRS at baseline and 5 min post-test, and revealed statistical difference at the edge of significance ($x^2 = 3.69, p = 0.05$), A Mann–Whitney test showed that subjects with tinnitus had a greater increase in NRS scores post-test ($M = 4.40, Sd = 2.50, Md = 4.50$) than subjects without tinnitus ($M = 2.80$, $Sd = 2.39$, $Md = 2.50$), $U = 25$, $p = 0.05$, $r = -0.42$. See **Figure 4**.

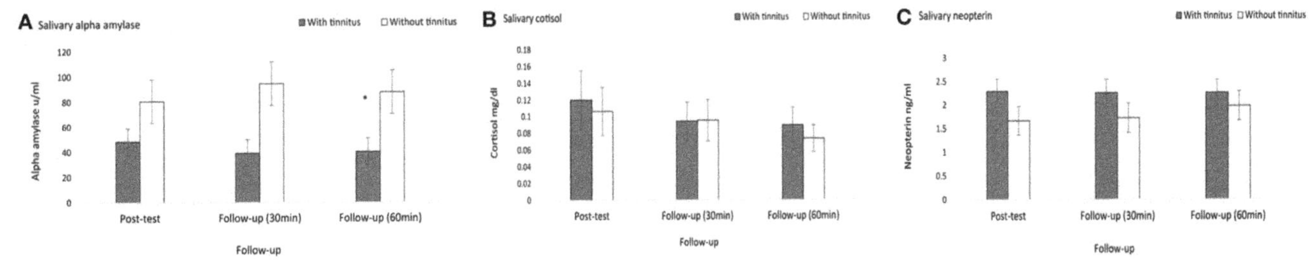

FIGURE 3 | Follow-up effect of group differences at 5, 30, and 60 min post-test measures. (A) Salivary α amylase yielded no statistical significant difference for 30 min post-test, however a significant difference was obtained for 60 min post-test Specifically, subjects with tinnitus ($M = 40.21$, $Sd = 30.06$) had lower measures of salivary α-amylase than subjects without tinnitus ($M = 87.81$, $Sd = 48.04$). **(B)** Salivary cortisol and **(C)** salivary neopterin yielded no statistical significant difference for the effect of time. *Indicates significant difference.

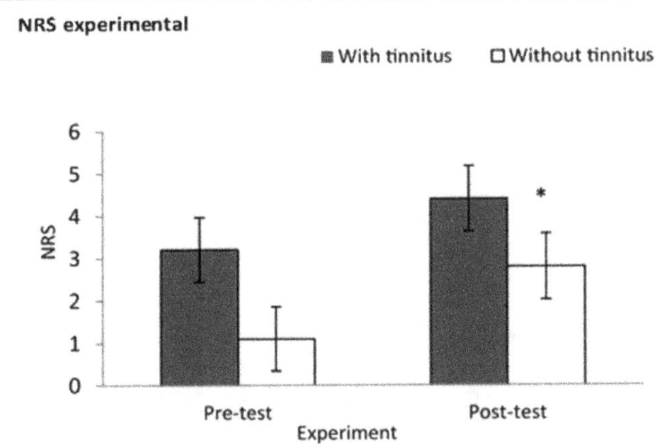

FIGURE 4 | Experimental validation using a numeric rating scale. Subjects had increases stress scores post-test in comparison to baseline; this was characterized by subjects with tinnitus ($M = 4.40$, $Sd = 2.50$) exhibiting higher stress scores than subjects without tinnitus ($M = 2.80$, $Sd = 2.39$). *Indicates significant difference.

Sensitivity Analysis

A Mann–Whitney test revealed a significant effect for AUC of sAA. Subjects with tinnitus ($M = 2510.20$, $Sd = 1566.34$, $Md = 2548.12$) had lower scores than subjects without tinnitus ($M = 5369.55$, $Sd = 2975.72$, $Md = 4317.75$), $U = 19$, $p = 0.01$, $r = -0.52$. No significant effects were obtained for AUC of salivary cortisol, AUC of salivary neopterin.

Significant correlations were obtained between AUC of salivary cortisol and AUC of salivary neopterin ($r_s = 0.53$, $p = 0.01$). Between AUC of sAA and respectively AUC of salivary cortisol ($r_s = 0.19$, $p = 0.40$) and AUC of salivary neopterin ($r_s = -0.22$, $p = 0.35$) no significant correlation could be obtained.

A logistic regression including AUC of sAA, AUC of salivary cortisol and AUC of salivary neopterin as independent variables and group (subjects with tinnitus vs. subjects without tinnitus) as dependent variable was conducted. This analysis revealed an overall effect, $c^2 = 11.87$, $p = 0.008$, Nagelkerke $R^2 = 0.62$. A closer look indicated that AUC of sAA was a good predictor ($W = 4.26$, $p = 0.04$, $\beta = -2.50$) indicating that 84.2% of the subjects could be correctly classified. The β-value further indicated that the lower the individual score is on AUC of sAA the higher the probability is that a subject has tinnitus. Neither AUC of salivary cortisol nor AUC of salivary neopterin reached significance. In addition, a Spearman's correlation revealed a significant effect between PSS and respectively, AUC of sAA ($r_s = -0.65$, $p = 0.002$), α-amylase over cortisol ($r_s = -0.68$, $p = 0.001$), cortisol over α-amylase ($r_s = 0.65$, $p = 0.002$), α-amylase over neopterin ($r_s = -0.62$, $p = 0.003$), neopterin over α-amylase ($r_s = 0.57$, $p = 0.008$), and cortisol over neopterin ($r_s = 0.62$, $p = 0.003$), but not neopterin over cortisol ($r_s = 0.22$, $p = 0.35$). The correlations suggest that the higher the stress score, the lower the individual score on AUC of sAA, α-amylase over cortisol, or α-amylase over neopterin, indicating a higher probability that a subject has stress and vice versa. The higher an individual score is on cortisol over α-amylase, neopterin over α-amylase, and cortisol over neopterin, the higher the likelihood is that a subject has chronic stress or vice versa (as suggested by the positive correlation). No significant correlations were obtained for AUC of salivary cortisol ($r_s = 0.11$, $p = 0.63$), and AUC of salivary neopterin ($r_s = 0.24$, $p = 0.29$). For an overview, see **Figure 5**.

DISCUSSION

This is a preliminary study to examine the feasibility of utilizing stress related markers in tinnitus. The data from this preliminary study will help us pursue a larger investigation on the feasibility of using salivary stress related responses in tinnitus. To our knowledge, this is the first study with regard to the examination of sAA, salivary cortisol, and salivary neopterin, simultaneously, in male subjects with tinnitus. The results of this preliminary study show that sAA levels were lower in the tinnitus group in comparison to subjects without tinnitus, suggesting impaired sympathetic activity in the tinnitus group. Furthermore, sAA remained stable throughout the stress experiment (i.e., acute stress); further confirming impaired sympathetic activity in the tinnitus group. The results of this preliminary study found no correlations between sAA and salivary cortisol and salivary neopterin, respectively, highlighting the distinctiveness of sAA as a stress-related marker. Furthermore, sAA ratio was found to be more strongly associated with measures of stress and depression

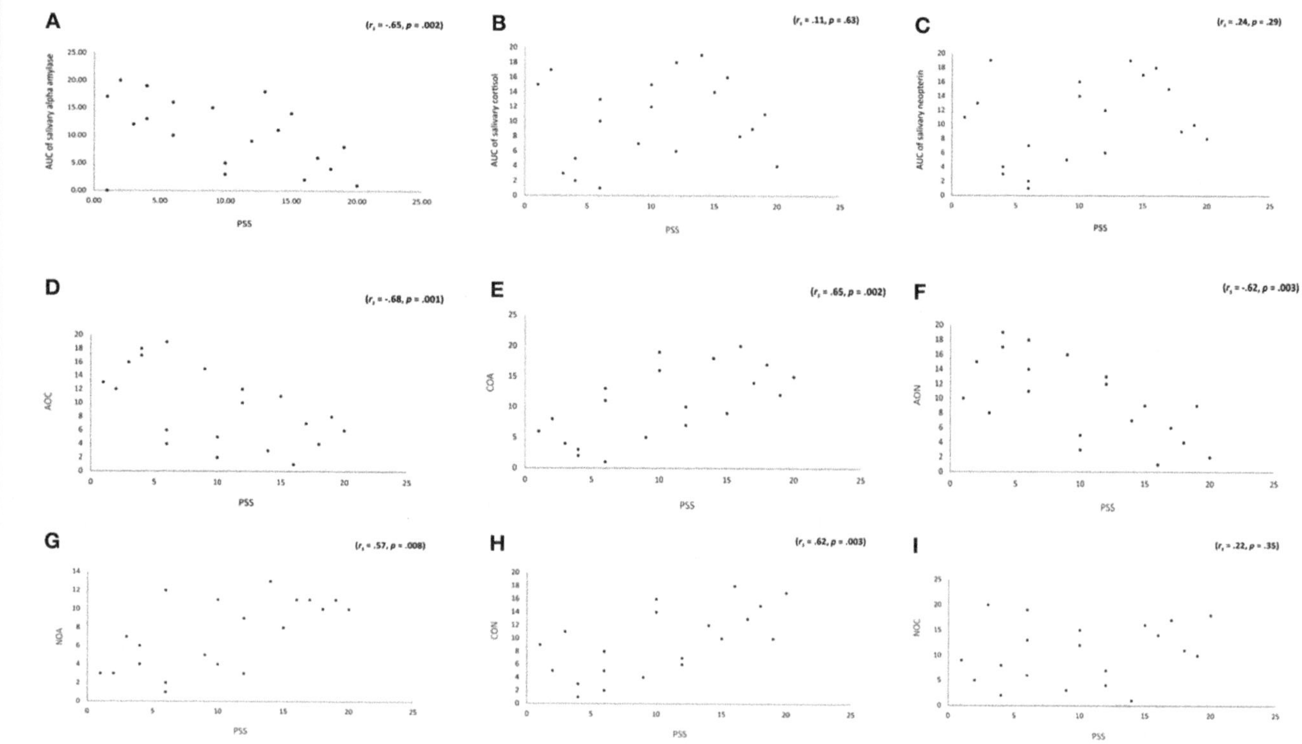

FIGURE 5 | (A) Significant correlations was obtained between AUC of salivary α-amylase, but not with **(B)** AUC salivary cortisol, or **(C)** AUC neopterin.Spearman's Rho were significant for **(D)** AOC, **(E)** COA, **(F)** AON, **(G)** NOA, and **(H)** CON, but not for **(I)** NOC. This suggests that the higher the scores of the PSS the lower the individual scores of AUC for salivary α-amylase, salivary cortisol, and salivary neopterin, and the higher the likelihood that subjects has chronic stress.

and is regarded as an index of deregulation in the stress system (Ali and Pruessner, 2012). In addition, this preliminary data found a strong effect observed for sAA in relation to baseline, stress test, follow-up and AUC, indicating that the expected value of sAA response decreases as stress increases, particularly for the tinnitus group.

Salivary α-amylase, Cortisol, and Neopterin

An increasing amount of research is supporting the proposal of a dynamic relationship between tinnitus and stress (Vanneste et al., 2010; De Ridder et al., 2011). Stress induces biological changes, such as alterations in stress-related markers. sAA was suggested as a valuable index for the assessment of pain (Shirasaki et al., 2007; Ahmadi-Motamayel et al., 2013; Ferrara et al., 2013; Liu et al., 2013), psychological stress (Chatterton et al., 1997) and physical stress (Chatterton et al., 1996). Thus, because of the symptomatic similarities between tinnitus, stress, and pain, it may be expected that a common pathophysiology may underlie these conditions. There are reports of lower sAA in chronically stressed patients with mood depressive disorders (Cubala and Landowski, 2014) and personality disorders (Nater et al., 2010). It is known that chronic activation of this stress system can lead to changes in functioning (i.e., allostatic load), leading to impaired or inadequate responses to subsequent challenges (Chrousos, 2009). This can be confirmed by our data. During a stress test, no changes could be obtained in the tinnitus group; in the healthy controls, immediate changes were observed. Previous research suggests that patients habituated to stress are indicated by a decrease or decline of sAA concentrations (Schumacher et al., 2013, 2014). Interestingly, previous research in tinnitus has revealed that highly distressed tinnitus patients show increased activity in specific brain areas (i.e., insula, dorsal, and subgenual anterior cingulate cortex; Vanneste et al., 2010, 2014) that are known to be mediated by the SNS (Vanneste and De Ridder, 2013).

With regard to salivary cortisol, no effect was found in relation to stress between the two groups at baseline. However, a significant positive relationship was obtained for salivary cortisol after correcting for salivary neopterin with stress independent of whether the subject had tinnitus or not. Our finding is in line with findings of a recent report showing no differences in responses of the HPA axis, as measured by salivary cortisol after exposure to stressful events (McKune et al., 2014). This could be indicative of the effect the type of stress (i.e., acute vs. chronic) has on the activation of the HPA axis. Taking into consideration that salivary cortisol is influenced by circadian rhythm (Lac, 2001), our finding can be considered a reflection of cortisol systematic influence by the circadian rhythm, with concentrations being higher during the day and lower in the evening.

A key characteristic of HPA functioning that has been frequently observed is the habituation after repeated exposure to an initially stressful event (i.e., tinnitus) (Wust et al., 2005).

Hebert and Lupien observed that basal levels of salivary cortisol are chronically changed in tinnitus patients (Hebert et al., 2004); however, they also report a blunted cortisol response to acute stress in patients who had experienced tinnitus for longer duration (Hebert and Lupien, 2007). Studies document that a habituation of adrenocortical responses does not necessarily occur (Al'Absi et al., 1997). It seems that characteristics of the stressor are important mediators determining the development of habituation, including intensity (Marti et al., 2001) and frequency (Ma and Lightman, 1998) of stress. Habituation to prolonged exposure to stressful events could possibly explain why tinnitus patients do not report any changes after the stress test. The lack of cortisol differences is in line with the findings of several other reports documenting no differences in endocrine responses to chronic stress (Hamilos et al., 1998; Scott and Dinan, 1998; Gaab et al., 2001).

In addition, while sAA levels were lower in the subjects with tinnitus, no changes could be obtained between subjects with tinnitus and healthy controls throughout the experiment for salivary cortisol. These findings further suggest dissociation between the two stress systems (endocrine vs. autonomic), and further point to a specific nature of the SNS-HPA axis relationship. Recent research already suggested an asymmetry between the HPA axis and SNS (Nater and Rohleder, 2009). The factors responsible for this asymmetry are largely unknown. One possible explanation could be that when it comes to habituation, these two systems operate at different rates. In support of this idea, evidence has been provided that in experimental animals, repeated stress exposure leads to a decreased response over time in the SNS with sustained HPA axis response (Britton et al., 1992). Whatever the causes, it has been suggested that asymmetry between these two biological systems may have unhealthy consequences (Bauer et al., 2002) and might contribute to pathogenesis development and/or maintenance (Monteleone et al., 2011).

Research has suggested that neopterin production might be linked with immune pathogenesis (Zhang et al., 2009; Chittiprol et al., 2010). It is known that neopterin is a significant and reliable indicator for the endogenous formation of IFN- γ (Fuchs et al., 2009). A prolonged elevation of IFN-γ was suggested to induce hyperexcitability neurons, which may lead to amplify pain perceptions, a process referred to as central sensitization (Vikman et al., 2007). Interestingly, tinnitus has also been considered a central sensitization phenomenon that results from an increase in responsivity to neural activity (Zenner, 2006; Zenner et al., 2006). Overall, numerous studies have shown an association between increase in immune system function due to infections (Fuchs et al., 1988, 1993b; Avanzas et al., 2004; Breinekova et al., 2007; Chittiprol et al., 2010; Euteneuer et al., 2012) and deregulation of endocrine and autonomic systems. However, we were unable to make such an assumption because in this study subjects were excluded if they had infectious or inflammatory diseases. On the other hand, our results do support variability in salivary neopterin that seems to be independent of fluctuation in sAA and salivary cortisol, suggesting that there also an asymmetry with neopterin. However, we are not aware of any former study that reports on the exact relationship between salivary measures of neopterin and respectively sAA or salivary cortisol; therefore, further examination of this assumption is necessary.

Feasibility of Using Salivary Stress-Related Biomarkers

sAA levels in this study showed statistically significant lower values in the subjects with tinnitus compared to subjects without tinnitus and sAA levels were correlated with stress. After correction for salivary cortisol and neopterin levels, the effects remained significant. As such, these results suggest a promising role of sAA as a possible biological stress marker in tinnitus. Given that in subjects without tinnitus, sAA was able to measure acute stress, it suggests that subjects with tinnitus had an impaired or inadequate functioning of the SNS.

LIMITATIONS

Although the present study has yielded significant findings in regard to the use of stress-related markers—specifically with regard to salivary α amylase—its design is not without limitations. Thus, a number of caveats need to be noted regarding the present work. First, this is a preliminary study, and thus it was primarily limited by its small sample size and statistical need to run multiple comparisons. Second, ideally including subjects of both sexes and increasing the collection range to longer time period would expand the sample size and further aid in generalizing the findings. Third, the small number of subjects may have led to an underestimation of the differences in salivary markers. Fourth, due to time constraints only a portion of the TSST test was administered, and although the portion administered is proven to induce stress, administering the entire TSST would have probably led to a larger increase in stress. Finally, although there was no significant rise in salivary cortisol secretions after the stressful event, subjective reports indicated that the stress-induced task used was effective enough to induce stress as measured by salivary α amylase.

CONCLUSION

Although stress can be a versatile event, reliable biological indicators of stress reactions have been shown to be valuable markers in both psycho physiological research and clinical practice. As such, alteration in the psychological state of a patient with tinnitus can alter biological indictors of stress reactions as measured by salivary stress related biomarkers. With this in mind, stress related markers have been emerged as potential non-invasive techniques with collection methods that can be administrated by health and non-health professionals. As a final point, it is important to note that even if salivary measures of stress do not map well due to their sensitivity, they may yet predictive of diseases and well-being. Future research relating the validity of using salivary stress related measures is needed to better determine their clinical relevance. Particularly, studies should further confirm whether sAA is a sensitive maker of stress and how it is associated with other mediators of the allostatic load network, such as pro- and anti-inflammatory cytokines (e.g., interleukin-6, tumor necrosis factor-alpha).

AUTHOR CONTRIBUTIONS

OA collected and analyzed the data, prepared and wrote the manuscript, as well as secured the funding. DT monitored data collection, advised on data analyses, advised on manuscript perpetration. SV data analyses, manuscript perpetration, and manuscript writing.

FUNDING

This work was supported by the American Tinnitus Association (ATA, funding #: 225352).

REFERENCES

Ahmadi-Motamayel, F., Shahriari, S., Goodarzi, M. T., Moghimbeigi, A., Jazaeri, M., and Babaei, P. (2013). The relationship between the level of salivary alpha amylase activity and pain severity in patients with symptomatic irreversible pulpitis. *Restor. Dent. Endod.* 38, 141–145. doi: 10.5395/rde.2013.38.3.141

Al'Absi, M., Bongard, S., Buchanan, T., Pincomb, G. A., Licinio, J., and Lovallo, W. R. (1997). Cardiovascular and neuroendocrine adjustment to public speaking and mental arithmetic stressors. *Psychophysiology* 34, 266–275. doi: 10.1111/j.1469-8986.1997.tb02397.x

Ali, N., and Pruessner, J. C. (2012). The salivary alpha amylase over cortisol ratio as a marker to assess dysregulations of the stress systems. *Physiol. Behav.* 106, 65–72. doi: 10.1016/j.physbeh.2011.10.003

Avanzas, P., Arroyo-Espliguero, R., Cosin-Sales, J., Quiles, J., Zouridakis, E., and Kaski, J. C. (2004). Prognostic value of neopterin levels in treated patients with hypertension and chest pain but without obstructive coronary artery disease. *Am. J. Cardiol.* 93, 627–629. doi: 10.1016/j.amjcard.2003.11.035

Bauer, A. M., Quas, J. A., and Boyce, W. T. (2002). Associations between physiological reactivity and children's behavior: advantages of a multisystem approach. *J. Dev. Behav. Pediatr.* 23, 102–113. doi: 10.1097/00004703-200204000-00007

Breinekova, K., Svoboda, M., Smutna, M., and Vorlova, L. (2007). Markers of acute stress in pigs. *Physiol. Res.* 56, 323–329.

Britton, K. T., Segal, D. S., Kuczenski, R., and Hauger, R. (1992). Dissociation between *in vivo* hippocampal norepinephrine response and behavioral/neuroendocrine responses to noise stress in rats. *Brain Res.* 574, 125–130. doi: 10.1016/0006-8993(92)90808-M

Carnuta, M., Crisan, L. G., Vulturar, R., Opre, A., and Miu, A. C. (2015). Emotional non-acceptance links early life stress and blunted cortisol reactivity to social threat. *Psychoneuroendocrinology* 51, 176–187. doi: 10.1016/j.psyneuen.2014.09.026

Chatterton, R. T. Jr., Vogelsong, K. M., Lu, Y. C., and Hudgens, G. A. (1997). Hormonal responses to psychological stress in men preparing for skydiving. *J. Clin. Endocrinol. Metab.* 82, 2503–2509. doi: 10.1210/jc.82.8.2503

Chatterton, R. T., Vogelsong, K. M., Lu, Y. C., Ellman, A. B., and Hudgens, G. A. (1996). Salivary alpha-amylase as a measure of endogenous adrenergic activity. *Clin. Physiol.* 16, 433–448. doi: 10.1111/j.1475-097X.1996.tb00731.x

Chittiprol, S., Venkatasubramanian, G., Neelakantachar, N., Babu, S. V., Reddy, N. A., Gangadhar, B. N., et al. (2010). Oxidative stress and neopterin abnormalities in schizophrenia: a longitudinal study. *J. Psychiatr. Res.* 44, 310–313. doi: 10.1016/j.jpsychires.2009.09.002

Chrousos, G. P. (2000). The role of stress and the hypothalamic-pituitary-adrenal axis in the pathogenesis of the metabolic syndrome: neuro-endocrine and target tissue-related causes. *Int. J. Obes. Relat. Metab. Disord.* 24(Suppl. 2), S50–S55. doi: 10.1038/sj.ijo.0801278

Chrousos, G. P. (2009). Stress and disorders of the stress system. *Nat. Rev. Endocrinol.* 5, 374–381. doi: 10.1038/nrendo.2009.106

Chrousos, G. P., and Gold, P. W. (1992). The concepts of stress and stress system disorders. Overview of physical and behavioral homeostasis. *JAMA* 267, 1244–1252. doi: 10.1001/jama.1992.03480090092034

Cohen, M., and Khalaila, R. (2014). Saliva pH as a biomarker of exam stress and a predictor of exam performance. *J. Psychosom. Res.* 77, 420–425. doi: 10.1016/j.jpsychores.2014.07.003

Cohen, S., Tyrrell, D. A., and Smith, A. P. (1991). Psychological stress and susceptibility to the common cold. *N. Engl. J. Med.* 325, 606–612. doi: 10.1056/NEJM199108293250903

Cubala, W. J., and Landowski, J. (2014). Low baseline salivary alpha-amylase in drug-naive patients with short-illness-duration first episode major depressive disorder. *J. Affect. Disord.* 157, 14–17. doi: 10.1016/j.jad.2013.12.043

De Ridder, D., Vanneste, S., and Congedo, M. (2011). The distressed brain: a group blind source separation analysis on tinnitus. *PLoS ONE* 6:e24273. doi: 10.1371/journal.pone.0024273

Euteneuer, F., Schwarz, M. J., Hennings, A., Riemer, S., Stapf, T., Rief, W., et al. (2012). Psychobiological aspects of somatization syndromes: contributions of inflammatory cytokines and neopterin. *Psychiatry Res.* 195, 60–65. doi: 10.1016/j.psychres.2011.07.032

Ferrara, P., Bottaro, G., Angeletti, S., Gatto, A., Vitelli, O., Battaglia, D., et al. (2013). Salivary alpha-amylase: a new non-invasive biomarker for assessment of pain perception in epileptic children. *Acta Neurol. Belg.* 113, 279–283. doi: 10.1007/s13760-013-0180-z

Folmer, R., and Griest, S. (2000). Tinnitus and insomnia. *Am. J. Otolaryngol.* 21, 287–293. doi: 10.1053/ajot.2000.9871

Folmer, R., Griest, S., Meikle, M., and Martin, W. (1999). Tunnitus severity, loudness, and depression. *Otolaryngol. Head Neck Surg.* 121, 48–51. doi: 10.1016/S0194-5998(99)70123-3

Fuchs, D., Avanzas, P., Arroyo-Espliguero, R., Jenny, M., Consuegra-Sanchez, L., and Kaski, J. C. (2009). The role of neopterin in atherogenesis and cardiovascular risk assessment. *Curr. Med. Chem.* 16, 4644–4653. doi: 10.2174/092986709789878247

Fuchs, D., Hausen, A., Reibnegger, G., Werner, E. R., Dierich, M. P., and Wachter, H. (1988). Neopterin as a marker in HIV infection. *Clin. Chem.* 34, 466–467.

Fuchs, D., Samsonov, M., Weiss, G., Reibnegger, G., Nasonov, E. L., and Wachter, H. (1993a). The clinical significance of neopterin in human diseases. *Ter. Arkh.* 65, 80–87.

Fuchs, D., Weiss, G., and Wachter, H. (1993b). Neopterin, biochemistry and clinical use as a marker for cellular immune reactions. *Int. Arch. Allergy Immunol.* 101, 1–6. doi: 10.1159/000236491

Gaab, J., Huester, D., Peisen, R., Engert, V., Schad, T., Schuermeyer, T., et al. (2001). Hypothalamus-pituitary-adrenal axis reactivity in chronic fatigue syndrome and health under psychological, physiological and pharmacological stimulation. *Psychosom. Med.* 63, 188–188.

Halford, J., and Anderson, S. (1991). Anxiety and depression in Tinnitus sufferers. *J. Psychosomatic Disord.* 35, 383–390. doi: 10.1016/0022-3999(91)90033-K

Hamilos, D. L., Nutter, D., Gershtenson, J., Redmond, D. P., Di Clementi, J. D., Jones, J. F., et al. (1998). Core body temperature is normal in chronic fatigue syndrome. *Biol. Psychiatry* 43, 293–302. doi: 10.1016/S0006-3223(97)83214-3

Hebert, S., and Lupien, S. J. (2007). The sound of stress: blunted cortisol reactivity to psychosocial stress in tinnitus sufferers. *Neurosci. Lett.* 411, 138–142. doi: 10.1016/j.neulet.2006.10.028

Hebert, S., Paiement, P., and Lupien, S. J. (2004). A physiological correlate for the intolerance to both internal and external sounds. *Hear. Res.* 190, 1–9. doi: 10.1016/S0378-5955(04)00021-8

Het, S., Vocks, S., Wolf, J. M., Hammelstein, P., Herpertz, S., and Wolf, O. T. (2015). Blunted neuroendocrine stress reactivity in young women with eating disorders. *J. Psychosom. Res.* 78, 260–267. doi: 10.1016/j.jpsychores.2014.11.001

Hinton, D. E., Chhean, D., Pich, V., Hofmann, S. G., and Barlow, D. H. (2006). Tinnitus among Cambodian refugees: relationship to PTSD severity. *J. Trauma. Stress* 19, 541–546. doi: 10.1002/jts.20138

Jastreboff, P. J., and Hazell, J. W. (1993). A neurophysiological approach to tinnitus: clinical implications. *Br. J. Audiol.* 27, 7–17. doi: 10.3109/03005369309077884

Kim, H. J., Lee, H. J., An, S. Y., Sim, S., Park, B. Choi, H. G., et al. (2015). Analysis of the prevalence and associated risk factors of tinnitus in adults. *PLoS ONE* 10:e0127578. doi: 10.1371/journal.pone.0127578

Kirschbaum, C., Pirke, K. M., and Hellhammer, D. H. (1993). The "Trier Social Stress Test"-a tool for investigating psychobiological stress responses in a laboratory setting. *Neuropsychobiology* 28, 76–81. doi: 10.1159/000119004

Kudielka, B. M., and Wust, S. (2010). Human models in acute and chronic stress: assessing determinants of individual hypothalamus-pituitary-adrenal axis activity and reactivity. *Stress* 13, 1–14. doi: 10.3109/10253890902874913

Lac, G. (2001). Saliva assays in clinical and research biology. *Pathol. Biol.* 49, 660–667. doi: 10.1016/S0369-8114(01)00228-0

Lindsay, A., Lewis, J., Scarrott, C., Draper, N., and Gieseg, S. P. (2015). Changes in acute biochemical markers of inflammatory and structural stress in rugby union. *J. Sports Sci.* 33, 882–891. doi: 10.1080/02640414.2014.971047

Liu, H., Dong, W. Y., Wang, J. B., Wang, T., Hu, P. Wei, S. F., et al. (2013). Association between salivary alpha-amylase activity and pain relief scale scores in cancer patients with bone metastases treated with radiotherapy. *Chin. Med. J.* 126, 4444–4447. doi: 10.3760/cma.j.issn.0366-6999.20130654

Lupis, S. B., Lerman, M., and Wolf, J. M. (2014). Anger responses to psychosocial stress predict heart rate and cortisol stress responses in men but not women. *Psychoneuroendocrinology* 49, 84–95. doi: 10.1016/j.psyneuen.2014.07.004

Ma, X. M., and Lightman, S. L. (1998). The arginine vasopressin and corticotrophin-releasing hormone gene transcription responses to varied frequencies of repeated stress in rats. *J. Physiol. 510(Pt* 2), 605–614. doi: 10.1111/j.1469-7793.1998.605bk.x

Marti, O., Garcia, A., Vellès, A., Harbuz, M. S., and Armario, A. (2001). Evidence that a single exposure to aversive stimuli triggers long-lasting effects in the hypothalamus-pituitary-adrenal axis that consolidate with time. *Eur. J. Neurosci.* 13, 129–136. doi: 10.1111/j.1460-9568.2001.01355.x

McKune, A. J., Bach, C. W., Semple, S. J., and Dyer, B. J. (2014). Salivary cortisol and alpha-amylase responses to repeated bouts of downhill running. *Am. J. Hum. Biol.* 26, 850–855. doi: 10.1002/ajhb.22605

Monteleone, P., Scognamiglio, P., Canestrelli, B., Serino, I., Monteleone, A. M., and Maj, M. (2011). Asymmetry of salivary cortisol and alpha-amylase responses to psychosocial stress in anorexia nervosa but not in bulimia nervosa. *Psychol. Med.* 41, 1963–1969. doi: 10.1017/S0033291711000092

Moynihan, J. A. (2003). Mechanisms of stress-induced modulation of immunity. *Brain Behav. Immun.* 17(Suppl. 1), S11–S16. doi: 10.1016/S0889-1591(02)00060-0

Nater, U. M., Bohus, M., Abbruzzese, E., Ditzen, B., Gaab, J., Kleindienst, N., et al. (2010). Increased psychological and attenuated cortisol and alpha-amylase responses to acute psychosocial stress in female patients with borderline personality disorder. *Psychoneuroendocrinology* 35, 1565–1572. doi: 10.1016/j.psyneuen.2010.06.002

Nater, U. M., and Rohleder, N. (2009). Salivary alpha-amylase as a non-invasive biomarker for the sympathetic nervous system: current state of research. *Psychoneuroendocrinology* 34, 486–496. doi: 10.1016/j.psyneuen.2009.01.014

Nondahl, D. M., Cruickshanks, K. J., Huang, G. H., Klein, B. E., Klein, R., Tweed, T. S., et al. (2011). Tinnitus and its risk factors in the Beaver Dam offspring study. *Int. J. Audiol.* 50, 313–320. doi: 10.3109/14992027.2010.551220

Pruessner, J. C., Kirschbaum, C., Meinlschmid, G., and Hellhammer, D. H. (2003). Two formulas for computation of the area under the curve represent measures of total hormone concentration versus time-dependent change. *Psychoneuroendocrinology* 28, 916–931. doi: 10.1016/S0306-4530(02)00108-7

Schumacher, S., Gaudlitz, K., Plag, J., Miller, R., Kirschbaum, C., Fehm, L., et al. (2014). Who is stressed? *A pilot study of salivary cortisol and alpha-amylase concentrations in agoraphobic patients and their novice therapists undergoing in vivo exposure. Psychoneuroendocrinology* 49, 280–289. doi: 10.1016/j.psyneuen.2014.07.016

Schumacher, S., Kirschbaum, C., Fydrich, T., and Strohle, A. (2013). Is salivary alpha-amylase an indicator of autonomic nervous system dysregulations in mental disorders?-a review of preliminary findings and the interactions with cortisol. *Psychoneuroendocrinology* 38, 729–743. doi: 10.1016/j.psyneuen.2013.02.003

Scott, L. V., and Dinan, T., G. (1998). Urinary free cortisol excretion in chronic fatigue syndrome, major depression and in healthy volunteers. *J. Affect. Disord.* 47, 49–54. doi: 10.1016/S0165-0327(97)00101-8

Shargorodsky, J., Curhan, G., and Farwell, W. (2010). Prevalence and characteristics of tinnitus among US adults. *Am. J. Med.* 123, 711–718. doi: 10.1016/j.amjmed.2010.02.015

Shirasaki, S., Fujii, H., Takahashi, M., Sato, T., Ebina, M., Noto, Y., et al. (2007). Correlation between salivary alpha-amylase activity and pain scale in patients with chronic pain. *Reg. Anesth. Pain Med.* 32, 120–123. doi: 10.1097/00115550-200703000-00005

Tsigos, C., and Chrousos, G. P. (2002). Hypothalamic-pituitary-adrenal axis, neuroendocrine factors and stress. *J. Psychosom. Res.* 53, 865–871. doi: 10.1016/S0022-3999(02)00429-4

van West, D., and Maes, M. (2001). Neuroendocrine and immune aspects of fibromyalgia. *Bio. Drugs* 15, 521–531. doi: 10.2165/00063030-200115080-00004

Vanneste, S., Congedo, M., and De Ridder, D. (2014). Pinpointing a highly specific pathological functional connection that turns phantom sound into distress. *Cereb. Cortex* 24, 2268–2282. doi: 10.1093/cercor/bht068

Vanneste, S., and De Ridder, D. (2013). Brain areas controlling heart rate variability in tinnitus and tinnitus-related distress. *PLoS ONE* 8:e59728. doi: 10.1371/journal.pone.0059728

Vanneste, S., Plazier, M., der Loo, E., de Heyning, P. V., Congedo, M., and De Ridder, D. (2010). The neural correlates of tinnitus-related distress. *Neuroimage* 52, 470–480. doi: 10.1016/j.neuroimage.2010.04.029

Vikman, K. S., Duggan, A. W., and Siddall, P. J. (2007). Interferon-gamma induced disruption of GABAergic inhibition in the spinal dorsal horn *in vivo*. *Pain* 133, 18–28. doi: 10.1016/j.pain.2007.02.010

Widner, B., Laich, A., Sperner-Unterweger, B., Ledochowski, M., and Fuchs, D. (2002). Neopterin production, tryptophan degradation, and mental depression–what is the link? *Brain Behav. Immun.* 16, 590–595. doi: 10.1016/S0889-1591(02)00006-5

Wust, S., Federenko, I. S., van Rossum, E. F., Koper, J. W., and Hellhammer, D. H. (2005). Habituation of cortisol responses to repeated psychosocial stress-further characterization and impact of genetic factors. *Psychoneuroendocrinology* 30, 199–211. doi: 10.1016/j.psyneuen.2004.07.002

Zenner, H. P. (2006). Tinnitus sensitization: a neurophysiological pathway of chronic complex tinnitus. *Otolaryngol. Pol.* 60, 485–489. doi: 10.1097/01.mao.0000231604.64079.77

Zenner, H. P., Pfister, M., and Birbaumer, N. (2006). Tinnitus sensitization: sensory and psychophysiological aspects of a new pathway of acquired centralization of chronic tinnitus. *Otol. Neurotol.* 27, 1054–1063. doi: 10.1097/01.mao.0000231604.64079.77

Zhang, X. Y., Zhou, D. F., Qi, L. Y., Chen, S., Cao, L. Y. C., Kosten, T. R., et al. (2009). Superoxide dismutase and cytokines in chronic patients with schizophrenia: association with psychopathology and response to antipsychotics. *Psychopharmacology* 204, 177–184. doi: 10.1007/s00213-008-1447-6

8

GLAST Deficiency in Mice Exacerbates Gap Detection Deficits in a Model of Salicylate-Induced Tinnitus

Hong Yu[1,2]*, Kim Vikhe Patil*[1]*, Chul Han*[3]*, Brian Fabella*[4]*, Barbara Canlon*[1]*, Shinichi Someya*[3] *and Christopher R. Cederroth*[1]*

[1] Laboratory of Experimental Audiology, Department of Physiology and Pharmacology, Karolinska Institutet, Stockholm, Sweden, [2] Department of Otolaryngology, Head and Neck Surgery, First Hospital of JiLin University, Changchun, China, [3] Department of Aging and Geriatric Research, University of Florida, Gainesville, FL, USA, [4] Howard Hughes Medical Institute and Laboratory of Sensory Neuroscience, The Rockefeller University, New York, NY, USA

***Correspondence:**
Christopher R. Cederroth
christopher.cederroth@ki.se

Gap detection or gap pre-pulse inhibition of the acoustic startle (GPIAS) has been successfully used in rat and guinea pig models of tinnitus, yet this system has been proven to have low efficacy in CBA mice, with low basal GPIAS and subtle tinnitus-like effects. Here, we tested five mouse strains (CBA, BalbC, CD-1, C57BL/6 and 129sv) for pre-pulse inhibition (PPI) and gap detection with varying interstimulus intervals (ISI) and found that mice from a CBA genetic background had the poorest capacities of suppressing the startle response in the presence of a pre-pulse or a gap. CD-1 mice displayed variable responses throughout all ISI. Interestingly, C57BL/6, 129sv and BalbC showed efficient suppression with either pre-pulses or gaps with shorter ISI. The glutamate aspartate transporter (GLAST) is expressed in support cells from the cochlea and buffers the excess of glutamate. We hypothesized that loss of GLAST function could sensitize the ear to tinnitus-inducing agents, such as salicylate. Using shorter ISI to obtain a greater dynamic range to assess tinnitus-like effects, we found that disruption of gap detection by salicylate was exacerbated across various intensities of a 32-kHz narrow band noise gap carrier in GLAST knockout (KO) mice when compared to their wild-type (WT) littermates. Auditory brainstem responses (ABR) and distortion-product otoacoustic emission (DPOAE) were performed to evaluate the effects on hearing functions. Salicylate caused greater auditory threshold shifts (near 15 dB) in GLAST KO mice than in WT mice across all tested frequencies, despite similarly reduced DPOAE. Despite these changes, inhibition using broad-band gap carriers and 32 kHz pre-pulses were not affected. Our study suggests that GLAST deficiency could become a useful experimental model to decipher the mechanisms underlying drug-induced tinnitus. Future studies addressing the neurological correlates of tinnitus in this model could provide additional insights into the mechanisms of tinnitus.

Keywords: hearing loss, salicylate, tinnitus, gap detection, pre-pulse inhibition, startle response, mouse, disease models

INTRODUCTION

Tinnitus remains an untreatable condition frequently associated with stress, anxiety or depression (Baguley et al., 2013), and affects 10–15% of the population. In spite of increasing attention towards the understanding and treatment of tinnitus, experimental efforts in the field remain relatively limited in comparison to the numerous clinical reports (Cederroth et al., 2013). Experimentally, the induction of tinnitus is achieved through noise overexposure or the administration of ototoxic drugs (e.g., salicylate, quinine or cisplatin; Stolzberg et al., 2012; von der Behrens, 2014).

Advances in the field of tinnitus have been made due to the development of behavioral methods to objectively assess the perception of non-existing sounds. Gap pre-pulse inhibition of the acoustic startle reflex (GPIAS), validated in a rat model of tinnitus using the operant conditioning paradigm (Turner et al., 2006; Turner and Parrish, 2008), resembles pre-pulse inhibition of the acoustic startle reflex (PPI or PPIAS), whereby a reduction in the response to an intense stimulus is observed when preceded by a subthreshold intensity pre-pulse (Ison et al., 1973; Graham, 1975). Animal models or humans with schizophrenia or bipolarity disorders have deficits in inhibiting the startle reflex with a pre-pulse as a consequence of a dysfunction in the sensorimotor gating mechanism (Braff et al., 1978; DelPezzo and Hoffman, 1980). In contrast to PPI, which uses a low-intensity pre-pulse to inhibit the startle reflex, GPIAS presents a silent gap embedded in a continuous carrier noise. Despite startle suppression being calculated similarly for both GPIAS and PPI, these use different neural pathways to regulate inhibition. Lesion studies have shown that the auditory cortex regulates GPIAS but not PPI (Bowen et al., 2003). When used in the context of tinnitus, as an animal's tinnitus closely matches the background noise, the startle reflex is less suppressed by the pre-pulse gap because tinnitus interferes with the optimal inhibition of the startle reflex mediated by the gap. As a consequence, affected animals display greater startle response (meaning less inhibited) than in the absence of tinnitus. The use of GPIAS for the assessment of tinnitus has been supported by additional neuronal correlates of tinnitus such as increased spontaneous firing rates in the dorsal cochlear nucleus (DCN; Li et al., 2013), hyperactivity in the inferior colliculus (Holt et al., 2010) and remapping of the auditory cortex (Engineer et al., 2011).

CBA mice have been conventionally used in auditory research for their excellent hearing abilities. In contrast, C57BL/6, in which mutant strains have been traditionally developed, display age-related hearing loss due to a point mutation on the *Cdh23* gene (Ohlemiller and Gagnon, 2004) and thus have been less accepted in the auditory field. However, in the absence of tinnitus, suppression of the startle response with the presence of a gap in narrow band carriers remains highly inefficient in CBA mice (10–50%; Middleton et al., 2011; Llano et al., 2012; Hickox and Liberman, 2014) when compared to that in rats (40–60%; Turner et al., 2006; Turner and Parrish, 2008; Engineer et al., 2011; Su et al., 2012; Yi et al., 2016), consequently offering a small dynamic range to distinguish tinnitus-like effects. Thus, improving the basal suppression of gap detection in mice would increase the confidence window for detecting tinnitus. Curiously, mice appear to be resistant to developing tinnitus, as only 20–50% of the mice that are exposed to noise display behavioral evidence of tinnitus (Middleton et al., 2011; Li et al., 2013), compared to 70–75% of that in rats (Wang et al., 2009; Zhang et al., 2011; Ruttiger et al., 2013). These observations are consistent with the notion that mice are more resilient than guinea pigs to drug-induced hearing loss by, for instance, aminoglycoside antibiotics or the anti-cancer drug cisplatin (Poirrier et al., 2010). Overall, a smaller number of mice display noise-induced changes in GPIAS than do rats, and this species appears more resistant to drug-induced hearing loss than are guinea pigs.

The glutamate aspartate transporter (GLAST) appears as a potential candidate to explain such differences. GLAST belongs to the family of glutamate transporters that stabilize the extracellular environment and maintain cell-to-cell communication. GLAST, but not GLT1, has been identified in the hearing organ, the cochlea (Jin et al., 2003). GLAST is present in the inner phalangeal cells (IPCs) that surround the sensory inner hair cells (IHCs) and afferent neuron synapse (Ruel et al., 2007), where it pumps back excessive glutamate released by sensory cells (Glowatzki et al., 2006) during noise exposure (Hakuba et al., 2000; Chen et al., 2010). As a consequence, mice lacking GLAST show greater hearing threshold shifts and synaptic damage than do wild-type (WT) mice after noise exposure (Hakuba et al., 2000; Chen et al., 2010). GLAST is hardly detectable in the cochlea of rats or guinea pigs and is abundant in the mouse cochlea (Jin et al., 2003). This is why we hypothesized that GLAST abundance in the murine cochlea could underlie the resilience of mice to inner ear insults by drugs, and potentially tinnitus.

Research on tinnitus would benefit from the use of mice, whose species offers facilitated genetic manipulations for understanding the mechanisms that are related to this auditory disorder. In the present study, we address the limitations of using mice by: (i) increasing the dynamic range of startle suppression in the presence of a gap; and (ii) identifying a protein whose disruption exacerbates gap detection deficits induced by salicylate. By combining these two advances, we propose a new mouse model for investigating tinnitus.

MATERIALS AND METHODS

Experimental Animals

Experimental procedures on animals performed at the Karolinska Institutet were in accordance with the guidelines and regulations set out by the University and *Stockholm's Norra Djurförsöksetiska Nämnd.* Experiments performed at the Rockefeller University were approved by the Institutional Animal Care and Use Committee of The Rockefeller University. GLAST knockout (KO) mice on a C57BL/6 background (Watase et al., 1998) and the other listed strains (from Charles Rivers) were maintained at 19–21°C in a 50%–50% light-dark cycle.

GLAST KO mice and their WT littermates were obtained from heterozygous crosses. We observed a non-mendelian distribution in the progeny of crosses between heterozygous KO mice ($n = 145$): 28% WT animals, 61% heterozygous KO animals, and only 10% homozygous KO animals. When crossing male homozygotes with female heterozygotes, we obtained 80% heterozygous and 20% homozygous KO animals among the progeny. In addition, homozygous females appeared highly anxious and displayed pup-killing behavior. Only male mice between 2 and 4 months of age were used in this study. Baseline auditory thresholds of GLAST KO mice measured by auditory brainstem responses (ABR) within this age range were similar to those of WT littermates (8 kHz = 35.71 ± 2; 16 kHz = 19.29 ± 0.7; 32 kHz = 29.64 ± 1.7; KO: 8 kHz = 38 ± 1.7; 16 kHz = 21 ± 1; 32 kHz = 32 ± 1.33; $p = 0.97$ by a 2-way ANOVA).

The animals had free access to water and food. They were injected daily with intraperitoneal (i.p.) sodium salicylate (Sigma, S3007) at 300 mg/kg diluted in 0.9% NaCl for three consecutive days. Hearing threshold measures and behavior tests were performed 2 h after the last injection, as previously described (Guitton et al., 2003).

Auditory Brainstem Responses

Mice were anesthetized with 80 mg/kg ketamine and 12 mg/kg xylazine for measurements of ABR. The positive needle electrode was inserted subdermally at the vertex, the negative electrode was placed beneath the pinna of the left ear, and the ground electrode was located near the tail. ABR were evoked by tone bursts of 8, 16 and 32 kHz, produced by a closed-field electrostatic speaker connected to a driver (EC-1 and ED-1, Tucker-Davis Technologies). The 5-ms signals were presented 33.3 times per second; their 0.5-ms onsets and offsets were tapered with a squared cosine function. The speaker's audio output was transmitted into the ear through a custom acoustic coupler. Sound pressure levels were measured with a calibrated microphone and preamplifier, connected to a conditioning amplifier (4939-A-011 and 2690-A-0S1, Brüel and Kjær). The response was amplified 10,000× and bandpass filtered at 0.3–3 kHz (P55, Natus Neurology Inc.). The amplified response was then digitally sampled at 10-μs intervals with a data acquisition device (USB-6210, National Instruments), controlled by custom software (LabVIEW 2010, National Instruments). The responses to 1000 bursts were averaged at each intensity level to determine the threshold; the threshold is defined as the lowest level at which a response peak is distinctly and reproducibly present. For each frequency, the sound pressure level was decreased from 100 dB SPL in 5 dB steps, until the threshold was reached and confirmed with one replicate measure. Threshold shifts were measured against individual's baseline values.

Distortion-Product Otoacoustic Emissions

Distortion-product otoacoustic emissions were elicited with an acoustic assembly, consisting of two electrostatic speakers (EC-1, Tucker-Davis Technologies), to generate primary tones and a miniature microphone (EK-23103, Knowles) to measure ear-canal sound pressure. The speakers and the microphone were both calibrated with the calibration microphone described above. The $2f_1 - f_2$ distortion product was measured with $f_1 = 6$–24 kHz, $f_2/f_1 = 1.25$ and the stimulus levels $L_1 = L_2 = 75$ dB SPL. The acoustic signal was amplified by a preamplifier (ER-10B+, Etymotic Research), and the sound pressure measured in the ear canal was digitally sampled at 10-μs intervals with the data acquisition system described above. Each frequency pair was presented for 1 s. After computing fast Fourier transforms and averaging them over 10 consecutive traces, we determined for each frequency pair the amplitudes of the $2f_1 - f_2$ distortion product and of the noise floor measured at ±100 Hz from $2f_1 - f_2$; this procedure required 17 s of data acquisition and processing.

Testing of the Interstimulus Interval

Interstimulus intervals (ISI) were tested using the SR-Lab startle response system from San Diego Instruments as previously described with minor modifications (Lowry et al., 2013). Animals were acclimated to the procedure on day 1, and were tested for PPI on day 2 and GPIAS on day 5. Background sound level (unfiltered white noise) was 65 dB SPL for PPI sessions, with pre-pulses of 75 dB SPL. For GPIAS, carrier level was 80 dB SPL and silent gaps (absence of stimulus) went down to the noise floor of the SR-Lab chamber. Startle pulses were presented at 115 dB SPL. Trials varied pseudo-randomly in their ISI by 10 ms, from 150 to 0 ms. Ten trials per ISI were tested. Inter-trial time interval varied randomly from 8 to 15 ms. Twenty startle-only trials were presented before the session, and five startle-only trials at the end in order to assess habituation. One whole session of PPI or GPIAS lasted 1 h.

Tinnitus Evaluation by the Gap Detection Method

To test frequency-specific gap detection deficits, we developed a custom-made set-up. Tests were performed in a sound-attenuating chamber (ENV-022S, Med Associates, Inc.). whose noise floor was 55 ± 0.5 dB SPL. In the case of PPI tests, which were used to verify the normal sensorimotor gating, white noise was generated by a function generator (DS340, Stanford Research Systems) and filtered (Wavetek 852 Dual HI/LO Variable Analog Filter, Butterworth filtered, 48 dB/octave roll-off) to 1 kHz-wide narrowband noise centered at a given frequency or broadband noise (BBN) and presented at a given sound intensity (60, 65, 70, 75, 80 dB SPL) in a silent environment for a duration of 50 ms through a speaker (NX-6, Power Acoustik) positioned in front of the animal. To startle an animal, a 20-ms white noise startle pulse of 115 dB SPL was delivered from a second speaker positioned above the animal, 70 ms after the pre-pulse. Calibration was done using the microphone, preamplifier and conditioning amplifier mentioned above.

For the gap detection tests that were used to evaluate tinnitus perception, the same set-up was used. The gap carrier was filtered as above into a broadband or 1 kHz-wide narrowband noise centered at a given frequency and presented at a given sound intensity (60, 65, 70, 75, 80 dB SPL). A relay switch was used to silence the noise for 50 ms, a gap with 0.1 ms rise and fall times (RT/FT), which was followed 15 ms later by a 20-ms white noise startle pulse of 115 dB SPL. The startle response was captured through an electromagnetic coil, bandpass filtered at 3–100 Hz and amplified 10× (P55, Natus Neurology Inc.). Gap detection or PPI was quantified as the percentage decrease in the peak amplitude of the startle response, when a warning gap or pre-pulse preceded the startling noise in comparison to the amplitude when no gap or pre-pulse was present [(1 − the ratio) × 100] (Engineer et al., 2011), using a similar representation as used in PPI studies (greater suppression of the startle reflex closer to 100%). The more tinnitus fills the gap, the less inhibition of the startle is observed. Only naïve animals were used in this study.

Experimental Procedure for the Screening of the Putative Tinnitus Frequency

This procedure was performed on a small group of animals ($n = 3$) to identify the putative tinnitus frequency at which a deeper analysis could be performed with a greater number of animals (see below). Here, PPI was not performed in order to avoid excessive habituation to the startle stimulus.

In order to acclimatize the animals to the testing procedure, a 30-min preliminary test was performed on day 1. On the following day (day 2), the experiment comprised a session of three consecutive blocks.

Block 1

The first block started with a 5-min acclimatization to silence, followed by 20 startle pulses; each of the pulses was 20 ms in duration and at 115 dB SPL. The time between each trial was random and varied between 8 and 12 s.

Block 2

The second block consisted in testing gap detection at various carrier frequencies (BBN, 8, 10, 12, 16, 20, 24, 32-kHz) of 80 dB SPL with 20 trials per frequency, with or without silent gaps (50 ms). Each frequency was tested sequentially with 20 trials. Each trial was performed with 20-ms startle pulses and an ISI of 15 ms.

Block 3

The final block comprised five trials only with startle pulses to be compared with those of the first block to assess habituation. A total of 185 trials was presented in approximately 40 min.

One day after the testing (day 3), animals were treated with salicylate daily for 2 days and tested on the third day of administration (day 5) with the same procedure.

Experimental Procedure for the Validation of the Putative Tinnitus Frequency

This procedure was performed to validate the findings from the frequency screening performed above. In order to acclimatize the animals to the testing procedure, a 30-min preliminary test was performed on day 1. On the following day (day 2), the experiment comprised a session of four consecutive blocks.

Block 1

The first block started with a 5-min acclimation to silence, followed by 20 startle pulses; each of the pulses was 20 ms in duration and at 115 dB SPL. The time between each trial was random and between 8 and 12 s.

Block 2

A second block of stimuli consisted in testing PPI with 20 trials with or without pre-pulses (50 ms), first consisting of a BBN of 75 dB SPL, and then consisting of a 32 kHz centered narrowband noise of successive intensities of 60, 65, 70, 75 and 80 dB SPL in a quiet background. Each trial was performed with 20-ms startle pulses and an ISI of 70 ms.

Block 3

The third block consisted in testing gap detection with 20 trials, with or without silent gaps (50 ms), first embedded in a broadband carrier noise at 75 dB SPL and then embedded in a 32-kHz centered narrowband noise of successive intensities of 60, 65, 70, 75 and 80 dB SPL. Each trial was performed with 20-ms startle pulses and an ISI of 15 ms.

Block 4

The final block comprised five trials only with startle pulses to be compared with those of the first block to assess habituation. A total of 265 trials were presented in approximately 55 min.

One day after the testing (day 3), animals were treated with salicylate daily for 2 days and tested on the third day of administration (day 5) with the same procedure.

Quantitative Real Time-PCR

SybrGreen qRT-PCR assays from cochlear extracts were performed as previously described (Meltser et al., 2014; Vikhe Patil et al., 2015). A mean quantity was calculated from triplicate PCR for each sample, and this quantity was normalized with the geometric mean of the three most stable genes out of six reference genes (tubulin β, Tubb; glyceraldehyde-3-phosphate dehydrogenase, G3pdh; transferring receptor 1, Trf1R; Tubulin α2, Tuba2; hypoxanthine phosphoribosyltransferase, HPRT; and Cyclophilin B) selected using the geNorm algorithm as described (Vandesompele et al., 2002). Normalized quantities were averaged for three technical replicates for each data point and represented as mean ± SD. The highest normalized relative quantity was arbitrarily designated 1.0. Fold changes were calculated from the quotient of means of these normalized quantities and reported as ± SEM. The primers for *eaat1* used are F: 5′-GGGAAGATGGGGATGCGAG-3′ and R: 5′-GCCGAAGCACATGGAGAAG-3′.

Statistical Analysis

Two-way ANOVA and a Bonferroni *post hoc* were used for statistical analysis (Prism version 4.0, GraphPad software). Differences were considered significant if $P < 0.05$. Animals that failed to respond to the startle (any peak-to-peak response above noise floor was considered a startle) or failed to inhibit the startle in the presence of a pre-pulse before salicylate treatment (any decrease in startle amplitude during pre-pulse trials vs. startle only trials) were excluded from the analysis (near 5%). When performing PPI tests using a pre-pulse of 80 dB SPL, nearly 10% of the pre-pulses elicited a startle, which then completely suppressed the startle response. The greater the intensity of the pre-pulse, more efficient was the inhibition of the startle response. As a consequence, trials in which the 80 dB pre-pulse induced a startle response before the startle pulse (10% of the 80 dB pre-pulse trials) were excluded from the analysis.

RESULTS

Shorter Interstimulus Interval Improves GPIAS in Specific Mouse Strains

When developing a custom-made gap detection set-up, we found that the ability of C57BL/6 mice to inhibit the startle response in the presence of a gap was almost null when using similar settings to those used for PPI (duration of the pre-pulse: 50 ms; ISI: 70 ms; startle duration: 20 ms; startle intensity: 115 dB). This particular paradigm only reduced the startle response by 20% (data not shown). We found that GPIAS was particularly sensitive to modifications of the ISI. We observed that in both C57BL/6 and 129sv mice, unlike for PPI, the shorter the ISI, the greater the inhibition of startle response, achieving up to 80% in C57BL/6 and 129sv mice (**Figures 1B,C**). Measures of the startle amplitude before and after each PPIAS or GPIAS session confirmed the lack of habituation during this test (data not shown). While this pattern was present in CBA mice, it did not exceed more than 50% at the lowest ISI, strongly suggesting that the inhibition of the startle reflex in this strain is not efficient (**Figure 1D**). This trend was not observed when using other genetic backgrounds such as CD-1 and Balb-C mice (**Figures 1E,F**). In Balb-C, PPI and GPIAS followed a similar course over varying ISIs, and CD-1 had highly variable responses, suggesting they would require additional acclimatization sessions (as typically performed with rats) to obtain a more robust reflex response. Overall, it is concluded that ISI is a critical parameter for improving gap detection in C57BL/6 and 129sv mice, and that shorter ISIs can be used to increase the basal level of suppression of the startle response in these strains in order to provide greater dynamic range to detect deficits in gap detection.

Salicylate Causes Severe Gap Detection Deficits in GLAST KO Mice

The basal level of startle suppression in the presence of a gap was further improved using Longenecker and Galazyuk (2012) recommendations by: (i) adjusting speaker non-linearity by calibrating the intensity output for each filtered narrowband noise; (ii) suppressing echo and reverberation by covering the interior walls with sound-insulating foam; and (iii) replacing the acrylic animal restrainer with a non-resonating perforated plastic pipette box. Because noise is effective in inducing tinnitus in nearly 50% of animals, we used salicylate, which is the most commonly used drug in animal models of tinnitus (Cazals, 2000; von der Behrens, 2014). Salicylate has an advantage over noise in that it has previously been used in humans to induce tinnitus

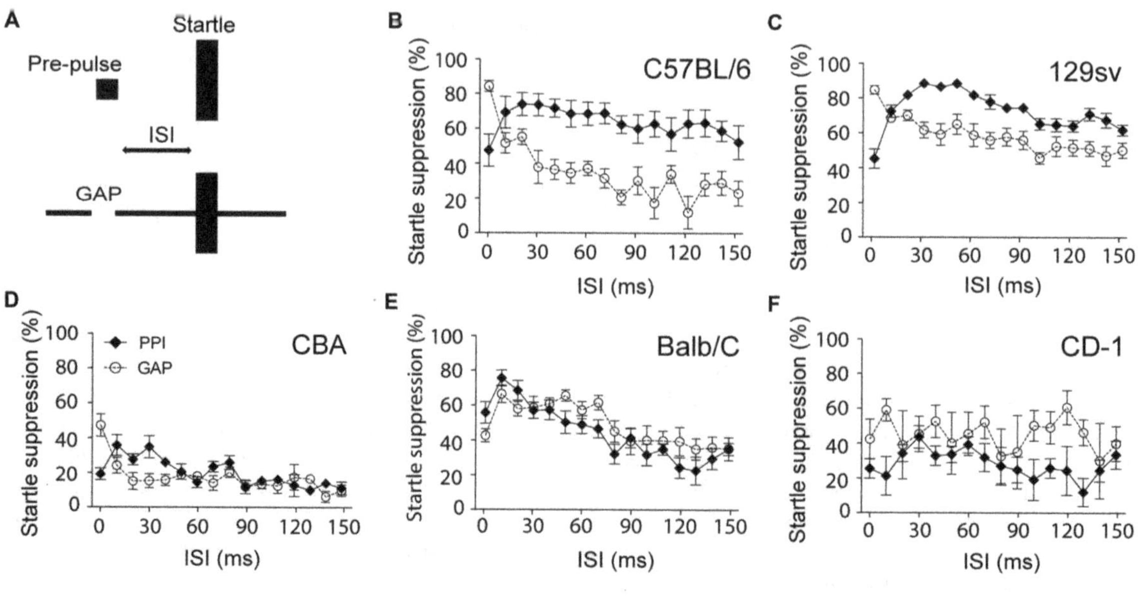

FIGURE 1 | Shorter interstimulus intervals (ISI) improves gap-mediated suppression of the startle response. (A) Schematic model of the experiment. Male C57BL/6 **(B)**, 129sv **(C)**, CBA **(D)**, Balb/C **(E)** and CD-1 **(F)** male mice (2–4 months old) were exposed to pre-pulse inhibition of the acoustic startle reflex (PPIAS) (black diamonds) and gap pre-pulse inhibition (PPI) of the acoustic startle (GPIAS; open circles) sequentially. ISI was modified by steps of 10 ms. Average startle amplitudes before and after each paradigm were not affected. Data represent means ± SEM ($n = 8$).

(3.9 g salicylate/day for 5 days; Mongan et al., 1973; McFadden et al., 1984).

We screened various 1-kHz narrowband frequencies (from 8 to 32 kHz) in a small group of animals ($n = 3$) to identify the putative tinnitus frequency, meaning the frequency at which GPIAS would be most affected by salicylate treatment according to a previous model (300 mg/kg/day for 3 days, Guitton et al., 2003). We used a carrier noise of high intensity (80 dB SPL) to maximize the inhibition of the startle by the gap and identify the frequencies with the greatest changes. This initial screening showed that both WT and KO mice treated with salicylate exhibit greater deficits in sensing the gap at 32 kHz (two-way ANOVA, Genotype and Treatment Factor: $F_{(7,64)} = 6.108$, $p < 0.0001$; Frequency Factor: $F_{(3,64)} = 11.44$, $p < 0.0001$, data not shown).

We next focused on the 32-kHz narrowband noise to perform both GPIAS, using different carrier intensities, and PPI, using increasing pre-pulse intensities. PPI was used as a control for normal temporal processing or sensory motor gating. Before salicylate administration, WT animals increasingly detected the gap with increasing intensities of a narrowband carrier noise centered at 32 kHz, inhibiting their startle reflexes up to 91% (**Figure 2A**). After 3 days of salicylate administration, the ability of WT mice to repress their startle reflexes decreased by 25% at all carrier intensities tested ($p < 0.0001$ by a two-way ANOVA with Bonferroni *post hoc* test, Treatment Factor, $F_{(1,110)} = 40.46$, $p < 0.0001$; Carrier Intensity Factor, $F_{(4,110)} = 35.36$, $p < 0.0001$; **Figure 2A**). Salicylate did not affect PPI with the exception of the lowest intensity of pre-pulse tested, suggestive of hyperacusis ($p = 0.03$ by a two-way ANOVA with Bonferroni *post hoc* test, Treatment Factor, $F_{(1,111)} = 4.64$, $p = 0.0333$; Pre-pulse Intensity Factor, $F_{(4,111)} = 25.40$, $p < 0.0001$; **Figure 2B**). The overall gap detection deficits, although significant, appeared to be relatively small.

Before salicylate treatment, GLAST KO mice displayed GPIAS as efficiently as WT mice (two-way ANOVA, Genotype Factor: $F_{(1,79)} = 0.4351$, $p = 0.5114$; Carrier Intensity Factor: $F_{(4,79)} = 57.0$, $p < 0.0001$). However, after salicylate treatment, the ability of GLAST KO mice to detect the gap was severely impaired throughout all carrier intensities tested (two-way ANOVA with Bonferroni *post hoc* test, Treatment Factor: $F_{(1,89)} = 117.5$, $p < 0.0001$; Carrier Intensity Factor: $F_{(4,89)} = 16.02$, $p < 0.0001$; **Figure 2C**). Although PPIAS at 32 kHz appeared to be lower in GLAST KO mice than in WT mice (two-way ANOVA, Genotype Factor: $F_{(1,105)} = 17.19$, $p < 0.0001$; Pre-pulse Intensity Factor: $F_{(4,105)} = 27.54$, $p < 0.0001$), it was not affected by salicylate administration (two-way ANOVA, Treatment Factor: $F_{(1,105)} = 0.2299$, $p = 0.6326$; Pre-pulse Intensity Factor: $F_{(4,105)} = 15.72$, $p < 0.0001$, **Figure 2D**), suggesting that the disruption of gap detection is more likely a tinnitus effect rather than a deficit in temporal processing or in auditory sensitivity (hyperacusis-like phenomenon).

To confirm the frequency-specific effects on GPIAS observed after the treatment with salicylate, we used a BBN Gap or pre-pulse (BBN PPI) at 75 dB SPL, and next verified whether inhibition of the startle response was affected before and after salicylate administration in both WT and GLAST KO mice. GPIAS in a BBN carrier was equally efficient before or after salicylate treatment in both genotypes (two-way ANOVA, Genotype Factor: $F_{(1,40)} = 0.7098$, $p = 0.4045$; Treatment Factor: $F_{(1,40)} = 0.2667$, $p = 0.6084$, **Figure 2E**). Similarly, the efficacy of BBN PPI, which is also used to assess normal temporal processing (Turner et al., 2006; Turner and Parrish, 2008; Middleton et al., 2011; Llano et al., 2012), was identical in WT and mutant animals both before and after the administration of salicylate (two-way ANOVA, Genotype Factor: $F_{(1,46)} = 0.4673$, $p = 0.4976$; Treatment Factor: $F_{(1,46)} = 0.009994$, $p = 0.9208$, **Figure 2F**). These control experiments confirmed that BBN PPIAS and GPIAS are not affected by salicylate in both WT and KO mice and support the notion that salicylate causes greater gap detection deficits at 32 kHz in GLAST KO than it does in WT mice.

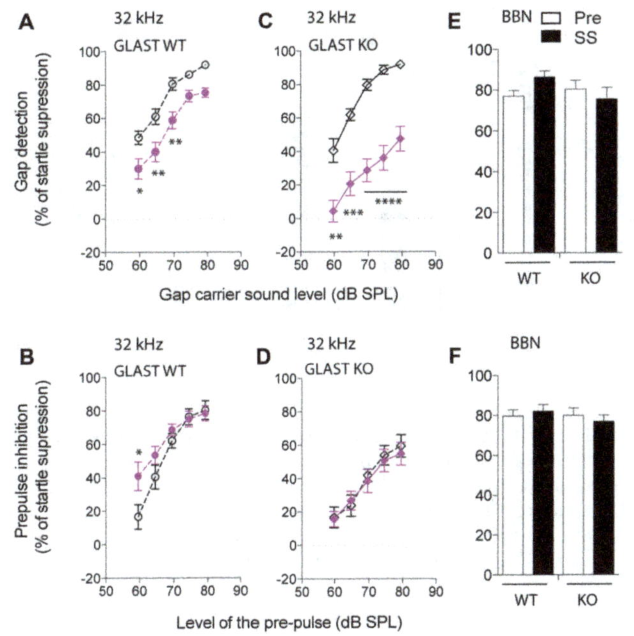

FIGURE 2 | Glutamate aspartate transporter (GLAST) deficiency facilitates the induction of tinnitus by salicylate. GPIAS in wild-type (WT) **(A)** and GLAST knockout (KO) **(C)** mice before (dark) and 2 h after the last salicylate (SS) administration (purple) using a 32-kHz narrowband carrier noise presented with a 5 dB step increase in intensity. PPIAS in WT **(B)** and GLAST KO **(D)** mice before (dark) and after (purple) salicylate treatment using a 32-kHz narrowband pre-pulse presented with a 5 dB step increase in intensity. Normal gap **(E)** and pre-pulse sensing **(F)** in WT and GLAST KO mice before (white) and after (black) the injection of SS using a broadband noise (BBN) at 75 dB SPL carrying a silent gap (GPIAS session) or a 75 dB SPL broadband pre-pulse presented in a silent environment (PPI session). Pre-treatment values are shown in dark, and SS values are shown in filled symbols in purple. WT mice are shown with circles and GLAST KO mice are shown with diamonds. Data represent means ± SEM (n = 8–14). *$P < 0.05$, **$P < 0.01$, ***$P < 0.001$ and ****$P < 0.0001$, by a two-way ANOVA with *post hoc* Bonferroni test.

We also assessed how basal startle amplitudes were affected in WT and GLAST KO mice by salicylate. Salicylate treatment increased the startle amplitude in response to startle pulses alone in KO mice (two-way ANOVA, Genotype Factor: $F_{(1,56)} = 37.90$, $p < 0.0001$; Treatment Factor: $F_{(1,56)} = 17.86$, $p < 0.0001$,

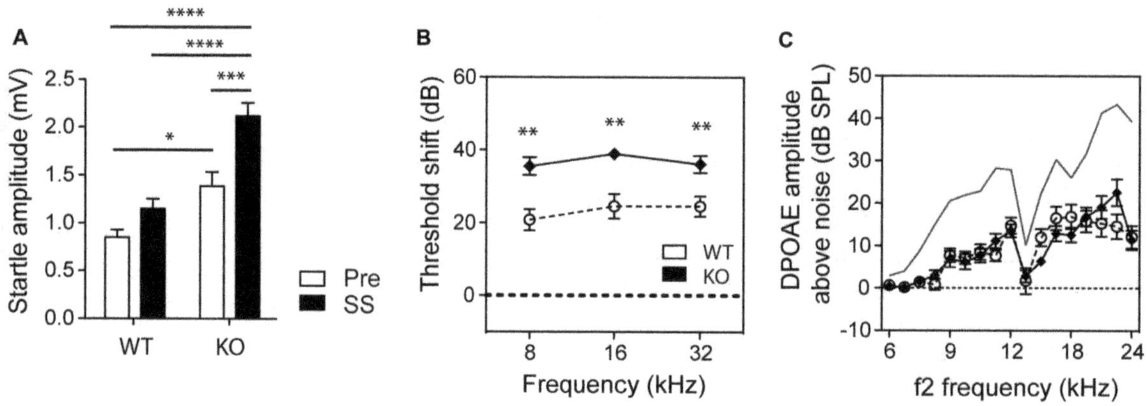

FIGURE 3 | GLAST deficiency sensitizes mice to salicylate-induced hearing loss but without affecting outer hair cell function. (A) GLAST KO mice subjected to startle pulses showed significantly larger startle responses than did WT mice. Salicylate (black, SS) enhanced the startle reflexes of GLAST KO mice. Pre-treatment values are shown in white. Data represent means ± SEM (n = 8–14). Auditory threshold shifts **(B)** and distortion-product otoacoustic emissions (DPOAEs **C)** of GLAST WT (white circles) and homozygous (black diamonds) mice with sodium salicylate at 300 mg/kg/day for 3 days, measured 2 h after the last injection. The uppermost curve (in gray) represents the mean for saline-treated WT control animals analyzed on the same day. Data of the auditory measures represent means ± SEM (n = 10–16). $^{*}P < 0.05$, $^{**}P < 0.01$, $^{***}P < 0.001$ and $^{****}P < 0.0001$, by a two-way ANOVA with *post hoc* Bonferroni test.

Figure 3A). Changes in hearing thresholds could account for differences in gap detection as well as in PPI. It is worth noting that salicylate caused a loss of hearing threshold by 20 dB across all frequencies (from 8 to 32 kHz) in WT mice and 35 dB in GLAST KO mice (two-way ANOVA, Genotype Factor, $F_{(1,57)} = 35.03, p < 0.0001$; Frequency Factor, $F_{(2,57)} = 0.8140$, $p = 0.4482$, n = 10–16, **Figure 3B**) with distortion-product otoacoustic emissions (DPOAEs) reduced by half, and in a similar way in WT and KO mice (Genotype Factor, $F_{(16,340)} = 19.05, p = 0.9188$; Frequency Factor, $F_{(16,340)} = 1.248$, $p < 0.0001$, **Figure 3C**). However, DPOAE measures were only performed at suprathreshold levels, and potential differences at threshold could have occurred. Still, the lack of differences in DPOAEs between WT and KO mice suggests that GLAST does not regulate outer hair cell function; rather GLAST could potentiate the effects of salicylate at the afferent synapse as suggested by the greater threshold shifts in GLAST KO mice. These findings are in agreement with previous work showing that salicylate potentiates glutamate-evoked responses in spiral ganglion neurons *ex vivo* (Ruel et al., 2008).

Such differences in salicylate-induced threshold shifts between WT and KO should have equally affected the perception of the pre-pulse or the perception of the gap and subsequent PPIAS and GPIAS. However, the findings indicate that this is not the case since PPI remained completely unaffected by salicylate treatment at 32 kHz where gap detection deficits were the greatest (**Figures 2B,D**). Second, we observed gap sensing deficits in GLAST WT and KO mice at 32 kHz but not when using a BBN as a carrier (**Figure 2E**), although similar hearing threshold shifts have been found across all frequencies tested (**Figure 3B**). Overall, our results suggest that the gap detection deficits observed here are reminiscent of tinnitus perception in the high-frequency area and are not due to hearing loss or defective temporal processing.

DISCUSSION

The present study shows that suppression of the startle response in the presence of a gap can be improved in C57BL/6 and 129sv mice by shortening the ISI and that constitutive loss of glutamate transporter function likely exacerbates the tinnitus-inducing effects of salicylate.

In some strains of mice, the efficacy of the startle suppression by the gap requires shorter ISI than with PPI. With a 15-ms ISI, gap detection suppressed the startle response by nearly 80% in C57BL/6 mice. Our findings contrast with those in the previous studies in rats by Ison and Bowen (2000), in which a biphasic response in the ability of the gap to suppress the startle was observed when varying the ISI . It is likely that these differences are related to species differences. Our results also underline the importance of the genetic background when performing GPIAS experiments. Previous studies have shown that PPI is highly influenced by genetic background and that the C57BL/6 strain displays rather efficient abilities to suppress the startle response in the presence of a pre-pulse (Willott et al., 2003). It would thus be interesting to evaluate how GPIAS is affected by varying ISIs in humans and how genetic background (e.g., different ethnicities) affects the efficacy of GPIAS.

In spite of the successful use of gap detection to identify physiological and molecular pathways involved in tinnitus (Engineer et al., 2011; Li et al., 2013, 2015; Kalappa et al., 2014, 2015), there has been a lot of debate regarding the use of gap detection for tinnitus evaluation (Campolo et al., 2013; Fournier and Hébert, 2013; Boyen et al., 2015; Galazyuk and Hébert, 2015). First, the low level of startle suppression in the presence of a gap reported in tinnitus studies that have used CBA mice leaves little margin to identify gap detection deficits and infer the presence of tinnitus (Longenecker and Galazyuk, 2011; Hickox and Liberman, 2014; Longenecker et al., 2014). Methods to discriminate between tinnitus and non-tinnitus animals have proven useful (Li et al., 2013, 2015) but an increase in the basal suppression level of the startle response offers a greater dynamic range for identifying tinnitus with greater confidence. Second, Hickox and Liberman (2014) performed a tinnitus study in which they adjusted the gap such that some of the trials were done with a gap closer to the startle stimulus (ISI = 0 ms) and some were done with a gap presented at greater lead times (ISI = 70 ms). Consistent with our findings (**Figure 1**), differences in gap detection between the two ISI conditions were found (being less efficient with greater lead times), however the authors interpreted that tinnitus "was not filling" the gap, since deficits in GPIAS were not observed at both ISIs (Hickox and Liberman, 2014). We believe the experimental conditions used were not optimal for inferring the presence of tinnitus as they used CBA mice, whose basal level of startle suppression in the presence of the gap was inefficient and even more variable with greater ISI. In addition, it has been shown that scopolamine, a muscarinic receptor blocker that disrupts cholinergic function in the brain, affects gap detection when the ISI is larger and not when the gap is closer to the startle stimulus (Ison and Bowen, 2000), meaning that different mechanisms operate GPIAS depending on the ISI. As a consequence, since GPIAS is a reflex response that relies on temporal processing and not on a conscious percept (meaning tinnitus does not fill the gap but interferes with the reflex response *per se*), gap detection deficits caused by tinnitus cannot be expected to be equally efficient at various lead times. The mechanism with which salicylate interferes solely with GPIAS and not PPI is not well understood, however it has been shown that gap detection operates in the auditory cortex, which is not the case of PPI (Bowen et al., 2003). Recent optogenetic studies in mice have shown that cortical inhibition is important in controlling perceptual gap detection (Weible et al., 2014). Since salicylate has been shown to alter the activity in the auditory cortex (Wang et al., 2006; Sun et al., 2009), we postulate that salicylate alters perceptual gap detection at the level of the auditory cortex. Additional behavioral methods in mice would be needed to confirm that the GPIAS deficits observed here correlate with a tinnitus percept.

Previous studies have shown that the ability to suppress the startle response in the presence of a gap improves with experience or with repeated pre-acclimatization sessions (Crofton et al., 1990; Ison and Bowen, 2000), and can reach 50% of startle suppression in CBA mice (Ison et al., 2002). The same applies to PPI (Plappert et al., 2006). We believe that the CBA strain, which is commonly used in the auditory field because of the well-preserved hearing, is not appropriate for PPIAS and GPIAS studies, unless longer acclimatization sessions are performed to achieve efficient gap processing. Instead, C57BL/6 or C57BL/6 × 129sv mixed mice (typical of most mouse mutant models available) would be most appropriate at an age when PPIAS/GPIAS responses are maximized and hearing deficits not yet detectable (between 3 and 4 months of age). Longenecker and Galazyuk (2012) also improved gap detection by decreasing the startle stimulus intensity to non-saturating levels (around 105 dB SPL), which has not been implemented in the current experiment. The differences we observe may also be due to differences in sound quality. With the exception of the initial study by Turner and Parrish (2008); Hickox and Liberman (2014), who describe a 48 dB/octave roll-off in their sound filtering like the one used in the present report, none of the other studies that used GPIAS describe the frequency filtering slope of their narrowband noises. Typically, when the shape of the filter is too narrow (e.g., when the slope of the filter is steep), perceptual artifacts are generated and could interfere with the ability of tinnitus to disrupt GPIAS. These artifacts decrease when using a 48 dB/octave roll-off, and could contribute to improved "detectability" of tinnitus. How the contour of the narrowband filtering affects the ability of tinnitus to interfere with GPIAS remains to be addressed. We believe that the appropriate selection of background strain, startle impulse level and ISI can provide robust PPI and gap detection responses when combined with adequate acclimatization sessions. Such parameters should be taken into account when testing gap detection for the assessment of tinnitus in humans.

The identification of GPIAS deficits in the 32-kHz frequency region when using salicylate in GLAST KO mice contrasts with previous research. A recent review article by Galazyuk and Hébert (2015) summarizes the results obtained with different tinnitus models using GPIAS. It appears that the generation of tinnitus by salicylate varies in terms of frequency depending on species and strains (i.e., Wistar rats get broader-range tinnitus, Brown Norways display tinnitus at 10, 12 and 24 kHz, and Sprague Dawleys at 16 kHz). The overall conclusion is that tinnitus does not seem to be focal and its frequency depends on the strain used. It is possible that we may have missed some frequencies in our screening that would have been otherwise revealed using lower carrier sound intensities and a greater number of animals throughout the procedure. Conversely, the protocols using GPIAS to assess tinnitus are very diverse and none of the salicylate studies (with the exception of the article by Turner and Parrish, 2008) have tested potential GPIAS deficits at 32 kHz (Galazyuk and Hébert, 2015). It is thus hard to determine whether our findings are specific to our model, or whether salicylate-induced tinnitus typically triggers high-frequency tinnitus, or simply whether the deficits in GPIAS are truly triggered by tinnitus *per se* and do not result from confounding effects of hearing loss. The control experiments we have performed rule out the potential bias of high-frequency hearing loss in the disrupted GPIAS observed in GLAST KO mice since: (i) auditory thresholds were equally affected by salicylate in WT and KO mice at all frequencies; (ii) salicylate did not affect GPIAS using a BBN carrier sound; (iii) basal auditory thresholds were normal and equivalent in both WT and KO mice at the time of the test; and (iv) salicylate treatment did not disrupt PPI in either WT or KO mice at 32 khZ, which otherwise would have been altered if hearing loss had contributed to the lower GPIAS at 32 kHz found in GLAST KO mice treated with salicylate. However, we do not rule out the possibility that in spite of the significant changes in GPIAS (in either genotype), the lack of changes in PPI upon salicylate administration could arise from salicylate-induced loudness recruitment, which may maintain suprathreshold PPI behavior.

Our study proposes the first gene potentially involved in tinnitus. GLASTs are mainly present in astrocytes in the central nervous system, buffering the excess of glutamate released at the synaptic cleft, converting it into glutamine, which is then transported back to pre-synaptic terminals to be recycled to glutamate. Two major glutamate transporters, namely GLAST (predominant in the cortex and hippocampus) and the glial GLutamate Transporter GLT1 (predominant in the cerebellum), are responsible for more than 80% of the glutamate uptake in the brain. Loss of glutamate transporters with subsequently uncontrolled extracellular glutamate levels has been associated with neurotoxic effects during seizures, amyotrophic lateral sclerosis, epilepsy and now, possibly, tinnitus. Although species comparison in gene expression levels is difficult to evaluate, given the broad changes in endogenous normalizing components (e.g., ubiquitously expressed genes), it appears likely that the resistance of mice to auditory insults could result, at least in part, from the higher expression of cochlear GLAST. On the other hand, a low abundance of cochlear GLAST would predict higher sensitivity to noise and drug-induced tinnitus. Consistent with this notion, we found that GLAST mRNA abundance was greater in CBA mouse cochleae than in those from CD-1 mice (CBA: 1.02 ± 0.06 relative expression level; CD-1: 0.76 ± 0.04; $p = 0.008$ by an unpaired two-tailed t-test, $n = 5$ per strain), which correlates with these strains' known auditory sensitivity and development of age-related hearing loss. In this regard, Shimizu et al. (2005) found that GLAST KO mice are more vulnerable to kanamycin ototoxicity. Ongoing data collection in our laboratory indicates that this is also the case for cisplatin (unpublished observations). In humans, whose susceptibility to ototoxic medications and noise varies from one individual to another, it remains unknown how cochlear GLAST levels correlate with tinnitus predisposition. A recent study failed to detect GLAST protein in support cells from the human cochlea (Ahmed et al., 2013), suggesting that the human cochlea expresses very low levels in GLAST at the afferent synapse. As a consequence, we predict that humans would show less glutamate-buffering capacity and thus greater vulnerability to noise and ototoxic medications. Genetic analyses of the human homolog of GLAST (*EAAT1*) in subjects with and without tinnitus could bring new knowledge about the mechanisms underlying the vulnerability and resilience to tinnitus.

It is rather widely accepted that peripherally generated tinnitus arises from a lack of cochlear output, rather than an increase in cochlear output. There are clear cochlear differences between salicylate and noise insults whereby spontaneous activity of the auditory nerve (AN) is increased after salicylate but decreased after noise (Eggermont and Roberts, 2004). However, most measures in noise-traumatized animals are performed after noise exposure and not *during* noise exposure. Thus, we would predict an early phase of increased AN activity during noise exposure (Searchfield et al., 2004) and a decrease in AN activity resulting from permanent synaptic damage. In contrast to noise, measures on salicylate-treated animals are performed shortly after the administration of salicylate—presumably when salicylate bioavailability peaks in the cochlea. Although there are to our knowledge no studies that report salicylate bioavailability in the cochlea after intraperitoneal injections, a peak is observed in other tissues after 30–60 min, with blood clearance after 8 h (Sturman et al., 1968). As salicylate potentiates glutamate-evoked responses in primary afferent neurons (Ruel et al., 2008), and lack of GLAST results in increased excess glutamate at the IHC-cochlear nerve synapse (Hakuba et al., 2000; Glowatzki et al., 2006), the overall cochlear output in GLAST KO mice would be expected to increase before salicylate is cleared out. Whether repeated administration of salicylate would cause permanent damage is unclear, but a recent rat model of chronic salicylate-administration leads tinnitus (Yi et al., 2016) and could prove useful to investigate whether more permanent damages would occur at the synapse, and reconcile salicylate-induced tinnitus with the decreased cochlear output theory.

The tinnitus effects observed here could also underlie central actions of salicylate and/or loss of GLAST function in the brain. Indeed, systemic administration of salicylate could activate non-auditory structures (Stolzberg et al., 2012; Chen et al., 2015) translating into broader central impacts than those happening after noise exposure (Holt et al., 2010). However, GLAST is predominant in the cortex and the hippocampus, and whether it is present in structures of the auditory pathway is unknown. The higher baseline startle amplitudes observed in GLAST KO mice could reflect hyperacusis. These findings are also consistent with the known higher anxiety levels in this model (Karlsson et al., 2009): increased locomotor activity in the open field, decreased sociability and social novelty preference, and poor nesting behavior. In addition, (Karlsson et al., 2009) found that pairwise discrimination learning is also affected in GLAST KO mice. The startle responses we obtain are however inconsistent with Karlsson et al.'s (2009) findings, which were not controlled—as we did with ABR—for hearing levels (as acknowledged by the authors), known to be affected at 6 months of age in GLAST KO mice (Hakuba et al., 2000). Importantly, unlike the auditory field, which uses startle response as an indicator of hearing abilities, all biological psychiatry textbooks mention the use of the startle response as a gauge of fear or anxiety. For instance, people with post-traumatic stress disorder have greater startle responses (Grillon et al., 1998). After an animal has learned to associate a specific stimulus with fear, such as light being paired with shocks, greater startle response is observed after presenting a fear signal just before the startle stimulus. Conversely, signals associated with pleasure decrease the startle amplitude response (Schmid et al., 1995). Fear or pleasure signals fail to modulate the startle response in amygdala-lesioned animals, showing that the amygdala is involved in the startle response system (Hitchcock and Davis, 1991). We thus believe that the increased startle response seen in GLAST KO mice in the presence of salicylate is an indicator of amygdala-mediated effects. The recent evidence linking tinnitus with the amygdala suggests that central-GLAST deficiency in the amygdala could contribute to the increased tinnitus severity observed in GLAST KO mice. Nonetheless, Karlsson et al. (2009) also found that PPI was not affected in GLAST KO mice and hence reasoned that these mice display *some* of the multiple and complex symptoms belonging to schizophrenia (e.g., GLAST KO mice would belong to a subgroup of schizophrenia of lesser severity). Salicylate, which is known to be anxiogenic in high doses (Puel and Guitton, 2007; Guitton, 2009), exacerbated this anxiety effect by increasing startle amplitude responses in KO animals (**Figure 3A**), something that we were able to qualitatively observe when handling the animals. It is thus possible that the higher basal anxiety levels of GLAST KO mice facilitated the tinnitus-inducing effects of salicylate, thereby increasing tinnitus intensity. Specific deletion of GLAST either in the brain or in the ear should enable discrimination of the contribution of all of these factors.

CONCLUSION

Our results suggest a potential role for GLAST in the vulnerability to salicylate-induced tinnitus. Given the magnitude of the disruption in gap detection observed in GLAST KO mice treated with salicylate, we propose that GLAST deficiency may serve as a useful model to distinguish more subtle, yet unidentified mechanisms on how tinnitus is triggered and maintained. Finally, optimizing parameters in gap detection in humans may uncover a potential use of this technology in the objective diagnosis of tinnitus (Galazyuk and Hébert, 2015).

AUTHOR CONTRIBUTIONS

HY, KVP, CH, BF and CRC carried out the experiments; HY, KVP and CRC analyzed the results; CRC designed and directed the research; BC, SS and CRC discussed the results and wrote the manuscript; all authors reviewed the manuscript.

FUNDING

CRC was a recipient of postdoctoral fellowships from the Swiss National Science Foundation (SNF; n° PBGEP3-125837), the Schweizerischen Stiftung für medizinisch-biologische Stipendien (SSMBS; n° PASMP3-136979), the Nicholson Fund and the Wenner Gren Foundation, and has received funding from Vetenskapsrådet, Lars Hiertas Minne, Magnus Bergvalls Stiftelserna, Loo och Hans Ostermans, Tysta Skolan, Karolinska Institutet and an independent research program funded under the Biomedicine and Molecular Biosciences European Cooperation in Science and Technology (COST) Action framework (TINNET BM1306). BC received funding from Karolinska Institutet, Vetenskapsrådet, Tysta Skola, Hörselskadades Riksförbund, FORTE and AFA Försäkring. SS is funded by the American Federation for Aging Research, by National Institutes of Health grant DC011840, and by a Claude D. Pepper Older Americans Independence Center Junior Scholar Award.

ACKNOWLEDGMENTS

We would like to thank the Hudspeth laboratory for their continuous and generous support, Y. Castellanos for technical assistance, S. Rasmussen for dedicated veterinary advice and J. Dyrhfjeld-Johnsen for his insightful comments on the manuscript. With the approval of K. Tanaka, V. P. Sarthy kindly provided the GLAST KO mice. We are grateful to J. G. Turner and T. Tzounopoulos for advice concerning the gap detection method; M. Ravitch, I. J. Stefanov-Wagner and M. C. Liberman for suggestions about the apparatus for recording ABR and distortion-product otoacoustic emissions, and for providing an acoustic coupler and calibration software.

REFERENCES

Ahmed, S., Vorasubin, N., Lopez, I. A., Hosokawa, S., Ishiyama, G., and Ishiyama, A. (2013). The expression of glutamate aspartate transporter (GLAST) within the human cochlea and its distribution in various patient populations. *Brain Res.* 1529, 134–142. doi: 10.1016/j.brainres.2013.06.040

Baguley, D., McFerran, D., and Hall, D. (2013). Tinnitus. *Lancet* 382, 1600–1607. doi: 10.1016/S0140-6736(13)60142-7

Bowen, G. P., Lin, D., Taylor, M. K., and Ison, J. R. (2003). Auditory cortex lesions in the rat impair both temporal acuity and noise increment thresholds, revealing a common neural substrate. *Cereb. Cortex* 13, 815–822. doi: 10.1093/cercor/13.8.815

Boyen, K., Başkent, D., and van Dijk, P. (2015). The gap detection test: can it be used to diagnose tinnitus? *Ear Hear.* 36, e138–e145. doi: 10.1097/aud.0000000000000156

Braff, D., Stone, C., Callaway, E., Geyer, M., Glick, I., and Bali, L. (1978). Prestimulus effects on human startle reflex in normals and schizophrenics. *Psychophysiology* 15, 339–343. doi: 10.1111/j.1469-8986.1978.tb01390.x

Campolo, J., Lobarinas, E., and Salvi, R. (2013). Does tinnitus "fill in" the silent gaps? *Noise Health* 15, 398–405. doi: 10.4103/1463-1741.121232

Cazals, Y. (2000). Auditory sensori-neural alterations induced by salicylate. *Prog. Neurobiol.* 62, 583–631. doi: 10.1016/s0301-0082(00)00027-7

Cederroth, C. R., Canlon, B., and Langguth, B. (2013). Hearing loss and tinnitus-are funders and industry listening? *Nat. Biotechnol.* 31, 972–974. doi: 10.1038/nbt.2736

Chen, Z., Kujawa, S. G., and Sewell, W. F. (2010). Functional roles of high-affinity glutamate transporters in cochlear afferent synaptic transmission in the mouse. *J. Neurophysiol.* 103, 2581–2586. doi: 10.1152/jn.00018.2010

Chen, Y. C., Li, X., Liu, L., Wang, J., Lu, C. Q., Yang, M., et al. (2015). Tinnitus and hyperacusis involve hyperactivity and enhanced connectivity in auditory-limbic-arousal-cerebellar network. *Elife* 4:e06576. doi: 10.7554/elife.06576

Crofton, K. M., Dean, K. F., Sheets, L. P., and Peele, D. B. (1990). Evidence for an involvement of associative conditioning in reflex modification of the acoustic startle response with gaps in background noise. *Psychobiology* 18, 467–474.

DelPezzo, E. M., and Hoffman, H. S. (1980). Attentional factors in the inhibition of a reflex by a visual stimulus. *Science* 210, 673–674. doi: 10.1126/science.7433993

Eggermont, J. J., and Roberts, L. E. (2004). The neuroscience of tinnitus. *Trends Neurosci.* 27, 676–682. doi: 10.1016/j.tins.2004.08.010

Engineer, N. D., Riley, J. R., Seale, J. D., Vrana, W. A., Shetake, J. A., Sudanagunta, S. P., et al. (2011). Reversing pathological neural activity using targeted plasticity. *Nature* 470, 101–104. doi: 10.1038/nature09656

Fournier, P., and Hébert, S. (2013). Gap detection deficits in humans with tinnitus as assessed with the acoustic startle paradigm: does tinnitus fill in the gap? *Hear. Res.* 295, 16–23. doi: 10.1016/j.heares.2012.05.011

Galazyuk, A., and Hébert, S. (2015). Gap-Prepulse Inhibition of the Acoustic Startle Reflex (GPIAS) for tinnitus assessment: current status and future directions. *Front. Neurol.* 6:88. doi: 10.3389/fneur.2015.00088

Glowatzki, E., Cheng, N., Hiel, H., Yi, E., Tanaka, K., Ellis-Davies, G. C., et al. (2006). The glutamate-aspartate transporter GLAST mediates glutamate uptake at inner hair cell afferent synapses in the mammalian cochlea. *J. Neurosci.* 26, 7659–7664. doi: 10.1523/JNEUROSCI.1545-06.2006

Graham, F. K. (1975). Presidential Address, 1974. The more or less startling effects of weak prestimulation. *Psychophysiology* 12, 238–248. doi: 10.1111/j.1469-8986.1975.tb01284.x

Grillon, C., Morgan, C. A. III, Davis, M., and Southwick, S. M. (1998). Effects of experimental context and explicit threat cues on acoustic startle in Vietnam veterans with posttraumatic stress disorder. *Biol. Psychiatry* 44, 1027–1036. doi: 10.1016/s0006-3223(98)00034-1

Guitton, M. J. (2009). Tinnitus-provoking salicylate treatment triggers social impairments in mice. *J. Psychosom. Res.* 67, 273–276. doi: 10.1016/j.jpsychores.2008.10.017

Guitton, M. J., Caston, J., Ruel, J., Johnson, R. M., Pujol, R., and Puel, J. L. (2003). Salicylate induces tinnitus through activation of cochlear NMDA receptors. *J. Neurosci.* 23, 3944–3952.

Hakuba, N., Koga, K., Gyo, K., Usami, S. I., and Tanaka, K. (2000). Exacerbation of noise-induced hearing loss in mice lacking the glutamate transporter GLAST. *J. Neurosci.* 20, 8750–8753.

Hickox, A. E., and Liberman, M. C. (2014). Is noise-induced cochlear neuropathy key to the generation of hyperacusis or tinnitus? *J. Neurophysiol.* 111, 552–564. doi: 10.1152/jn.00184.2013

Hitchcock, J. M., and Davis, M. (1991). Efferent pathway of the amygdala involved in conditioned fear as measured with the fear-potentiated startle paradigm. *Behav. Neurosci.* 105, 826–842. doi: 10.1037/0735-7044.105.6.826

Holt, A. G., Bissig, D., Mirza, N., Rajah, G., and Berkowitz, B. (2010). Evidence of key tinnitus-related brain regions documented by a unique combination of manganese-enhanced MRI and acoustic startle reflex testing. *PLoS One* 5:e14260. doi: 10.1371/journal.pone.0014260

Ison, J. R., and Bowen, G. P. (2000). Scopolamine reduces sensitivity to auditory gaps in the rat, suggesting a cholinergic contribution to temporal acuity. *Hear. Res.* 145, 169–176. doi: 10.1016/s0378-5955(00)00088-5

Ison, J. R., Castro, J., Allen, P., Virag, T. M., and Walton, J. P. (2002). The relative detectability for mice of gaps having different ramp durations at their onset and offset boundaries. *J. Acoust. Soc. Am.* 112, 740–747. doi: 10.1121/1.1490352

Ison, J. R., McAdam, D. W., and Hammond, G. R. (1973). Latency and amplitude changes in the acoustic startle reflex of the rat produced by variation in auditory prestimulation. *Physiol. Behav.* 10, 1035–1039. doi: 10.1016/0031-9384(73)90185-6

Jin, Z. H., Kikuchi, T., Tanaka, K., and Kobayashi, T. (2003). Expression of glutamate transporter GLAST in the developing mouse cochlea. *Tohoku J. Exp. Med.* 200, 137–144. doi: 10.1620/tjem.200.137

Kalappa, B. I., Brozoski, T. J., Turner, J. G., and Caspary, D. M. (2014). Single unit hyperactivity and bursting in the auditory thalamus of awake rats directly correlates with behavioural evidence of tinnitus. *J. Physiol.* 592, 5065–5078. doi: 10.1113/jphysiol.2014.278572

Kalappa, B. I., Soh, H., Duignan, K. M., Furuya, T., Edwards, S., Tzingounis, A. V., et al. (2015). Potent KCNQ2/3-specific channel activator suppresses *in vivo* epileptic activity and prevents the development of tinnitus. *J. Neurosci.* 35, 8829–8842. doi: 10.1523/JNEUROSCI.5176-14.2015

Karlsson, R. M., Tanaka, K., Saksida, L. M., Bussey, T. J., Heilig, M., and Holmes, A. (2009). Assessment of glutamate transporter GLAST (EAAT1)-deficient mice for phenotypes relevant to the negative and executive/cognitive symptoms of schizophrenia. *Neuropsychopharmacology* 34, 1578–1589. doi: 10.1038/npp.2008.215

Li, S., Choi, V., and Tzounopoulos, T. (2013). Pathogenic plasticity of Kv7.2/3 channel activity is essential for the induction of tinnitus. *Proc. Natl. Acad. Sci. U S A* 110, 9980–9985. doi: 10.1073/pnas.1302770110

Li, S., Kalappa, B. I., and Tzounopoulos, T. (2015). Noise-induced plasticity of KCNQ2/3 and HCN channels underlies vulnerability and resilience to tinnitus. *Elife* 4:e07242. doi: 10.7554/eLife.07242

Llano, D. A., Turner, J., and Caspary, D. M. (2012). Diminished cortical inhibition in an aging mouse model of chronic tinnitus. *J. Neurosci.* 32, 16141–16148. doi: 10.1523/JNEUROSCI.2499-12.2012

Longenecker, R. J., and Galazyuk, A. V. (2011). Development of tinnitus in CBA/CaJ mice following sound exposure. *J. Assoc. Res. Otolaryngol.* 12, 647–658. doi: 10.1007/s10162-011-0276-1

Longenecker, R. J., and Galazyuk, A. V. (2012). Methodological optimization of tinnitus assessment using prepulse inhibition of the acoustic startle reflex. *Brain Res.* 1485, 54–62. doi: 10.1016/j.brainres.2012.02.067

Longenecker, R. J., Chonko, K. T., Maricich, S. M., and Galazyuk, A. V. (2014). Age effects on tinnitus and hearing loss in CBA/CaJ mice following sound exposure. *Springerplus* 3:542. doi: 10.1186/2193-1801-3-542

Lowry, E. R., Kruyer, A., Norris, E. H., Cederroth, C. R., and Strickland, S. (2013). The GluK4 kainate receptor subunit regulates memory, mood and excitotoxic neurodegeneration. *Neuroscience* 235, 215–225. doi: 10.1016/j.neuroscience.2013.01.029

McFadden, D., Plattsmier, H. S., and Pasanen, E. G. (1984). Aspirin-induced hearing loss as a model of sensorineural hearing loss. *Hear. Res.* 16, 251–260. doi: 10.1016/0378-5955(84)90114-x

Meltser, I., Cederroth, C. R., Basinou, V., Savelyev, S., Lundkvist, G. S., and Canlon, B. (2014). TrkB-mediated protection against circadian sensitivity to noise trauma in the murine cochlea. *Curr. Biol.* 24, 658–663. doi: 10.1016/j.cub.2014.01.047

Middleton, J. W., Kiritani, T., Pedersen, C., Turner, J. G., Shepherd, G. M., and Tzounopoulos, T. (2011). Mice with behavioral evidence of tinnitus exhibit dorsal cochlear nucleus hyperactivity because of decreased GABAergic inhibition. *Proc. Natl. Acad. Sci. U S A* 108, 7601–7606. doi: 10.1073/pnas.1100223108

Mongan, E., Kelly, P., Nies, K., Porter, W. W., and Paulus, H. E. (1973). Tinnitus as an indication of therapeutic serum salicylate levels. *JAMA* 226, 142–145. doi: 10.1001/jama.1973.03230020014004

Ohlemiller, K. K., and Gagnon, P. M. (2004). Apical-to-basal gradients in age-related cochlear degeneration and their relationship to "primary" loss of cochlear neurons. *J Comp Neurol* 479, 103–116. doi: 10.1002/cne.20326

Plappert, C. F., Kuhn, S., Schnitzler, H. U., and Pilz, P. K. (2006). Experience increases the prepulse inhibition of the acoustic startle response in mice. *Behav. Neurosci.* 120, 16–23. doi: 10.1037/0735-7044.120.1.16

Poirrier, A. L., Van den Ackerveken, P., Kim, T. S., Vandenbosch, R., Nguyen, L., Lefebvre, P. P., et al. (2010). Ototoxic drugs: difference in sensitivity between mice and guinea pigs. *Toxicol. Lett.* 193, 41–49. doi: 10.1016/j.toxlet.2009.12.003

Puel, J. L., and Guitton, M. J. (2007). Salicylate-induced tinnitus: molecular mechanisms and modulation by anxiety. *Prog. Brain Res.* 166, 141–146. doi: 10.1016/s0079-6123(07)66012-9

Ruel, J., Chabbert, C., Nouvian, R., Bendris, R., Eybalin, M., Leger, C. L., et al. (2008). Salicylate enables cochlear arachidonic-acid-sensitive NMDA receptor responses. *J. Neurosci.* 28, 7313–7323. doi: 10.1523/JNEUROSCI.5335-07.2008

Ruel, J., Wang, J., Rebillard, G., Eybalin, M., Lloyd, R., Pujol, R., et al. (2007). Physiology, pharmacology and plasticity at the inner hair cell synaptic complex. *Hear. Res.* 227, 19–27. doi: 10.1016/j.heares.2006.08.017

Ruttiger, L., Singer, W., Panford-Walsh, R., Matsumoto, M., Lee, S. C., Zuccotti, A., et al. (2013). The reduced cochlear output and the failure to adapt the central auditory response causes tinnitus in noise exposed rats. *PLoS One* 8:e57247. doi: 10.1371/journal.pone.0057247

Schmid, A., Koch, M., and Schnitzler, H. U. (1995). Conditioned pleasure attenuates the startle response in rats. *Neurobiol. Learn. Mem.* 64, 1–3. doi: 10.1006/nlme.1995.1037

Searchfield, G. D., Munoz, D. J., and Thorne, P. R. (2004). Ensemble spontaneous activity in the guinea-pig cochlear nerve. *Hear. Res.* 192, 23–35. doi: 10.1016/j.heares.2004.02.006

Shimizu, Y., Hakuba, N., Hyodo, J., Taniguchi, M., and Gyo, K. (2005). Kanamycin ototoxicity in glutamate transporter knockout mice. *Neurosci. Lett.* 380, 243–246. doi: 10.1016/j.neulet.2005.01.066

Stolzberg, D., Salvi, R. J., and Allman, B. L. (2012). Salicylate toxicity model of tinnitus. *Front. Syst. Neurosci.* 6:28. doi: 10.3389/fnsys.2012.00028

Sturman, J. A., Dawkins, P. D., McArthur, N., and Smith, M. J. (1968). The distribution of salicylate in mouse tissues after intraperitoneal injection. *J. Pharm. Pharmacol.* 20, 58–63. doi: 10.1111/j.2042-7158.1968.tb09619.x

Su, Y. Y., Luo, B., Jin, Y., Wu, S. H., Lobarinas, E., Salvi, R. J., et al. (2012). Altered neuronal intrinsic properties and reduced synaptic transmission of the rat's medial geniculate body in salicylate-induced tinnitus. *PLoS One* 7:e46969. doi: 10.1371/journal.pone.0046969

Sun, W., Lu, J., Stolzberg, D., Gray, L., Deng, A., Lobarinas, E., et al. (2009). Salicylate increases the gain of the central auditory system. *Neuroscience* 159, 325–334. doi: 10.1016/j.neuroscience.2008.12.024

Turner, J. G., Brozoski, T. J., Bauer, C. A., Parrish, J. L., Myers, K., Hughes, L. F., et al. (2006). Gap detection deficits in rats with tinnitus: a potential novel screening tool. *Behav. Neurosci.* 120, 188–195. doi: 10.1037/0735-7044.120.1.188

Turner, J. G., and Parrish, J. (2008). Gap detection methods for assessing salicylate-induced tinnitus and hyperacusis in rats. *Am. J. Audiol.* 17, S185–S192. doi: 10.1044/1059-0889(2008/08-0006)

Vandesompele, J., De Preter, K., Pattyn, F., Poppe, B., Van Roy, N., De Paepe, A., et al. (2002). Accurate normalization of real-time quantitative RT-PCR data by geometric averaging of multiple internal control genes. *Genome Biol.* 3:RESEARCH0034. doi: 10.1186/gb-2002-3-7-research0034

Vikhe Patil, K., Canlon, B., and Cederroth, C. R. (2015). High quality RNA extraction of the mammalian cochlea for qRT-PCR and transcriptome analyses. *Hear. Res.* 325, 42–48. doi: 10.1016/j.heares.2015.03.008

von der Behrens, W. (2014). Animal models of subjective tinnitus. *Neural Plast.* 2014:741452. doi: 10.1155/2014/741452

Wang, H. T., Luo, B., Zhou, K. Q., Xu, T. L., and Chen, L. (2006). Sodium salicylate reduces inhibitory postsynaptic currents in neurons of rat auditory cortex. *Hear. Res.* 215, 77–83. doi: 10.1016/j.heares.2006.03.004

Wang, H., Brozoski, T. J., Turner, J. G., Ling, L., Parrish, J. L., Hughes, L. F., et al. (2009). Plasticity at glycinergic synapses in dorsal cochlear nucleus of rats with behavioral evidence of tinnitus. *Neuroscience* 164, 747–759. doi: 10.1016/j.neuroscience.2009.08.026

Watase, K., Hashimoto, K., Kano, M., Yamada, K., Watanabe, M., Inoue, Y., et al. (1998). Motor discoordination and increased susceptibility to cerebellar injury in GLAST mutant mice. *Eur. J. Neurosci.* 10, 976–988. doi: 10.1046/j.1460-9568.1998.00108.x

Weible, A. P., Moore, A. K., Liu, C., DeBlander, L., Wu, H., Kentros, C., et al. (2014). Perceptual gap detection is mediated by gap termination responses in auditory cortex. *Curr. Biol.* 24, 1447–1455. doi: 10.1016/j.cub.2014.05.031

Willott, J. F., Tanner, L., O'Steen, J., Johnson, K. R., Bogue, M. A., and Gagnon, L. (2003). Acoustic startle and prepulse inhibition in 40 inbred strains of mice. *Behav. Neurosci.* 117, 716–727. doi: 10.1037/0735-7044.117.4.716

Yi, B., Hu, S., Zuo, C., Jiao, F., Lv, J., Chen, D., et al. (2016). Effects of long-term salicylate administration on synaptic ultrastructure and metabolic activity in the rat CNS. *Sci. Rep.* 6:24428. doi: 10.1038/srep24428

Zhang, J., Zhang, Y., and Zhang, X. (2011). Auditory cortex electrical stimulation suppresses tinnitus in rats. *J. Assoc. Res. Otolaryngol.* 12, 185–201. doi: 10.1007/s10162-010-0246-z

9

Genetics of Tinnitus: Time to Biobank Phantom Sounds

Christopher R. Cederroth[1]*, Anna K. Kähler[2], Patrick F. Sullivan[2,3,4] and Jose A. Lopez-Escamez[5,6]*

[1] Experimental Audiology, Department of Physiology and Pharmacology, Karolinska Institutet, Stockholm, Sweden, [2] Department of Molecular Epidemiology and Biostatistics, Karolinska Institutet, Stockholm, Sweden, [3] Department of Genetics, University of North Carolina, Chapel Hill, NC, United States, [4] Department of Psychiatry, University of North Carolina, Chapel Hill, NC, United States, [5] Otology & Neurotology Group, Department of Genomic Medicine, Pfizer-Universidad de Granada-Junta de Andalucía Centre for Genomics and Oncology Research (GENyO), Granada, Spain, [6] Department of Otolaryngology, Instituto de Investigación Biosanitaria ibs.GRANADA, Hospital Virgen de las Nieves, Universidad de Granada, Granada, Spain

***Correspondence:**
Christopher R. Cederroth
christopher.cederroth@ki.se
Jose A. Lopez-Escamez
antonio.lopezescamez@genyo.es

Tinnitus is a common phantom sensation resulting most often from sensory deprivation, and for which little knowledge on the molecular mechanisms exists. While the existing evidence for a genetic influence on the condition has been until now sparse and underpowered, recent data suggest that specific forms of tinnitus have a strong genetic component revealing that not all tinnitus percepts are alike, at least in how they are genetically driven. These new findings pave the way for a better understanding on how phantom sensations are molecularly driven and call for international biobanking efforts.

Keywords: tinnitus, genetics, heritability, subtype, neuropsychiatry, GWAS (genome-wide association study), whole exome sequencing

PERSPECTIVE

For decades, tinnitus was considered a consequence of environmental factors, with low genetic contribution. The numerous etiologies, such as aging (presbycusis), noise exposure, stress, hypertension, diabetes, ototoxic medications, temporomandibular joint disorders, traumatic or ischemic damage, vascular problems, middle-ear problems, and the complex pathophysiology involving peripheral and central auditory and non-auditory structures, have led to the belief that tinnitus is a consequence of some other disease.

The knowledge on the genetic basis of tinnitus was recently reviewed (Vona et al., 2017) and phenotyping strategies have been proposed based on the assumption that tinnitus should be considered as an ensemble of sub-entities called subtypes (Lopez-Escamez et al., 2016). A small familial aggregation study ($n = 198$ families) found no obvious heritability (Hendrickx et al., 2007), and the first large population-based family study ($n = 52{,}045$) made an estimate of heritability of 0.11 (Kvestad et al., 2010). But a recent twin study revealed a higher heritability of 0.4, indicating that a larger fraction of the variance can be due to genetic variants than previously reported (Bogo et al., 2016). Such discrepancies may originate from differences in the design and formulation of the questionnaires, which have been found to vary greatly in prevalence studies on tinnitus (McCormack et al., 2016).

The tinnitus phenotype could also be grounds for diverging heritability values, but what defines a tinnitus phenotype is highly debated. We indeed consider that a more precise definition of a homogeneous phenotype will be essential in the design of genetic studies. A larger twin study performed by members of the TINNET[1] consortium recently

[1] http://tinnet.tinnitusresearch.net/

considered the laterality of tinnitus as a potential genetic subtype (Maas et al., 2017). A key finding was that bilateral tinnitus had higher heritability than unilateral tinnitus. The study was based on self-reported data from the Swedish Twin Registry, one of the largest twin registries in the world (Lichtenstein et al., 2002, 2006; Pedersen et al., 2002; van Dongen et al., 2012). Of a total of 70,186 twins that answered questions related to tinnitus, 15% of them experienced tinnitus. 10,464 concordant or discordant pairs for tinnitus were identified, in which 6,990 subjects had tinnitus. When considering tinnitus as a whole, a moderate genetic contribution (near 40%) was found (Bogo et al., 2016). However, when twins were stratified - based on tinnitus experienced in one ear (unilateral) or in both ears (bilateral) as well as on gender - bilateral tinnitus reached a heritability of 0.68 in men (Maas et al., 2017). Such values are close to the levels of heritability for schizophrenia and attention deficit hyperactive disorder (ADHD), two well known heritable conditions (**Table 1**). Although more work is required for establishing the contribution of hearing loss in such high heritability values (e.g., by including exhaustive auditory data), these findings open the possibility of specific forms of tinnitus being more genetically driven than others and pave the way for future genetic studies considering subtypes. These findings, however, need to be replicated in other twin cohorts as well as familial studies.

In line with genetic association studies of other complex traits, published studies to find genetic markers for chronic tinnitus patients in candidate genes have been underpowered (n = 95–288) and failed to identify robustly associated genetic variants (Sand et al., 2010, 2011, 2012a,b; Gallant et al., 2013). In spite of a lowly powered tinnitus group (N = 167) and no significant associations found, a recent genome-wide association study (GWAS) identified some pathways (e.g., oxidative stress, endoplasmatic reticulum stress, and serotonin reception mediated signaling) potentially involved in tinnitus (Gilles et al., 2017). Supporting the need of better characterizing the tinnitus cases, Pawelczyk and colleagues investigated 99 single nucleotide polymorphisms targeting 10 genes involved in the potassium recycling pathway in the inner ear (128 tinnitus cases and 498 controls both exposed to occupational noise) (Pawelczyk et al., 2012). However, two of the identified SNPs were not subjected to multiple testing and were thus considered nominally significant. An important lesson from GWAS on other complex traits, such as schizophrenia and major depressive disorder (Sullivan et al., in press), is that far larger sample sizes are needed in order to identify genome-wide significant genetic variants. Therefore, an important next step in the search for genetic variants associated with tinnitus will be to perform joint GWAS analysis of thousands of tinnitus patients and healthy controls.

Since familial tinnitus is a rare condition, the selection of multiplex tinnitus families, in addition to unrelated cases and controls, for exome sequencing, is another potential strategy to be used for the discovery of genes involved in tinnitus. This strategy has been successful in the identification of *DTNA*, *PRKCB*, *SEMA3D* and *DPT* in autosomal dominant Meniere disease (Requena et al., 2015; Martin-Sierra et al., 2016, 2017).

With tinnitus being a condition with highly unmet clinical needs (Cederroth et al., 2013), the recent identification of a high heritability opens door to exciting research. Since it is more than likely that tinnitus is a polygenic trait and it will require the study of several thousand samples, audiologists and ENT doctors should optimize their phenotyping strategies for instance by using high frequency audiometry and multivariate questionnaire data (Muller et al., 2016; Schlee et al., 2017), initiate incentives to allocate a specific ICD-code for bilateral tinnitus, and start biobanking samples (Lopez-Escamez et al., 2016). Regarding the latter, since it is not custom for an ENT clinic to collect samples for DNA biobanking, guidelines should emerge to promote good practice (Fuller et al., 2017) and enable the creation of a large consortium to join efforts to decipher the genetic basis of tinnitus.

TABLE 1 | Classification of tinnitus heritability against other disorders.

Trait	Heritability	Number of Twin pairs
Diabetes, type 1	0.88	22 650
Schizophrenia	0.81	Meta-analysis
ADHD	0.76	Review
Autism	0.71	11 535
Bilateral tinnitus (men)	0.68	10 464
Diabetes, type 2	0.64	13 888
Coronary heart disease	0.57	10 483
Alzheimer's disease	0.48	662
Any tinnitus	0.43	10 464
Prostate cancer	0.42	21 000
Systolic blood pressure	0.42	1 617
Bilateral tinnitus (women)	0.41	10 464
Colorectal cancer	0.35	44 788
Parkinson's disease	0.34	46 436
Breast cancer	0.27	23 788
Unilateral tinnitus	0.27	10 464
MS	0.25	Review

Modified from van Dongen et al. (2012) with permission from the Nature Publishing Group. Tinnitus values are marked in red.

AUTHOR CONTRIBUTIONS

CC conceived the paper and prepared the table. CC co-wrote the paper with JL-E. AK and PS helped to develop the scientific arguments. All authors played a role in writing the manuscript and approved the final version.

FUNDING

CC has received funding from Tysta Skolan, Karolinska Institutet, Lars Hiertas Minne, Magnus Bergvalls Stiftelserna, Hörselforskningsfonden, and Loo och Hans Ostermans. The work was supported by an independent research program funded under the Biomedicine and Molecular Biosciences European Cooperation in Science and Technology (COST) Action framework (TINNET BM1306).

REFERENCES

Bogo, R., Farah, A., Karlsson, K. K., Pedersen, N. L., Svartengren, M., and Skjonsberg, A. (2016). Prevalence, incidence proportion, and heritability for tinnitus: a longitudinal twin study. *Ear Hear.* 38, 292–300. doi: 10.1097/AUD.0000000000000397

Cederroth, C. R., Canlon, B., and Langguth, B. (2013). Hearing loss and tinnitus–are funders and industry listening? *Nat. Biotechnol.* 31, 972–974. doi: 10.1038/nbt.2736

Fuller, T. E., Haider, H. F., Kikidis, D., Lapira, A., Mazurek, B., Norena, A., et al. (2017). Different teams, same conclusions? A systematic review of existing clinical guidelines for the assessment and treatment of tinnitus in adults. *Front. Psychol.* 8:206. doi: 10.3389/fpsyg.2017.00206

Gallant, E., Francey, L., Fetting, H., Kaur, M., Hakonarson, H., Clark, D., et al. (2013). Novel COCH mutation in a family with autosomal dominant late onset sensorineural hearing impairment and tinnitus. *Am. J. Otolaryngol.* 34, 230–235. doi: 10.1016/j.amjoto.2012.11.002

Gilles, A., Van Camp, G., Van de Heyning, P., and Fransen, E. (2017). A pilot genome-wide association study identifies potential metabolic pathways involved in tinnitus. *Front. Neurosci.* 11:71. doi: 10.3389/fnins.2017.00071

Hendrickx, J. J., Huyghe, J. R., Demeester, K., Topsakal, V., Van Eyken, E., Fransen, E., et al. (2007). Familial aggregation of tinnitus: a European multicentre study. *B-ENT* 3(Suppl. 7), 51–60.

Kvestad, E., Czajkowski, N., Engdahl, B., Hoffman, H. J., and Tambs, K. (2010). Low heritability of tinnitus: results from the second Nord-Trondelag health study. *Arch. Otolaryngol. Head Neck Surg.* 136, 178–182. doi: 10.1001/archoto.2009.220

Lichtenstein, P., De Faire, U., Floderus, B., Svartengren, M., Svedberg, P., and Pedersen, N. L. (2002). The Swedish Twin Registry: a unique resource for clinical, epidemiological and genetic studies. *J. Intern. Med.* 252, 184–205. doi: 10.1046/j.1365-2796.2002.01032.x

Lichtenstein, P., Sullivan, P. F., Cnattingius, S., Gatz, M., Johansson, S., Carlstrom, E., et al. (2006). The Swedish Twin Registry in the third millennium: an update. *Twin Res. Hum. Genet.* 9, 875–882. doi: 10.1375/183242706779462444

Lopez-Escamez, J. A., Bibas, T., Cima, R. F., Van de Heyning, P., Knipper, M., Mazurek, B., et al. (2016). Genetics of tinnitus: an emerging area for molecular diagnosis and drug development. *Front. Neurosci.* 10:377. doi: 10.3389/fnins.2016.00377

Maas, I. L., Bruggemann, P., Requena, T., Bulla, J., Edvall, N. K., Hjelmborg, J. V., et al. (2017). Genetic susceptibility to bilateral tinnitus in a Swedish twin cohort. *Genet Med.* doi: 10.1038/gim.2017.4 [Epub ahead of print].

Martin-Sierra, C., Gallego-Martinez, A., Requena, T., Frejo, L., Batuecas-Caletrio, A., and Lopez-Escamez, J. A. (2017). Variable expressivity and genetic heterogeneity involving DPT and SEMA3D genes in autosomal dominant familial Meniere's disease. *Eur. J. Hum. Genet.* 25, 200–207. doi: 10.1038/ejhg.2016.154

Martin-Sierra, C., Requena, T., Frejo, L., Price, S. D., Gallego-Martinez, A., Batuecas-Caletrio, A., et al. (2016). A novel missense variant in PRKCB segregates low-frequency hearing loss in an autosomal dominant family with Meniere's disease. *Hum. Mol. Genet.* 25, 3407–3415. doi: 10.1093/hmg/ddw183

McCormack, A., Edmondson-Jones, M., Somerset, S., and Hall, D. (2016). A systematic review of the reporting of tinnitus prevalence and severity. *Hear. Res.* 337, 70–79. doi: 10.1016/j.heares.2016.05.009

Muller, K., Edvall, N. K., Idrizbegovic, E., Huhn, R., Cima, R., Persson, V., et al. (2016). Validation of online versions of tinnitus questionnaires translated into Swedish. *Front. Aging Neurosci.* 8:272. doi: 10.3389/fnagi.2016.00272

Pawelczyk, M., Rajkowska, E., Kotylo, P., Dudarewicz, A., Van Camp, G., and Sliwinska-Kowalska, M. (2012). Analysis of inner ear potassium recycling genes as potential factors associated with tinnitus. *Int. J. Occup. Med. Environ. Health* 25, 356–364. doi: 10.2478/S13382-012-0061-3

Pedersen, N. L., Lichtenstein, P., and Svedberg, P. (2002). The Swedish Twin Registry in the third millennium. *Twin Res.* 5, 427–432. doi: 10.1375/136905202320906219

Requena, T., Cabrera, S., Martin-Sierra, C., Price, S. D., Lysakowski, A., and Lopez-Escamez, J. A. (2015). Identification of two novel mutations in FAM136A and DTNA genes in autosomal-dominant familial Meniere's disease. *Hum. Mol. Genet.* 24, 1119–1126. doi: 10.1093/hmg/ddu524

Sand, P. G., Langguth, B., Itzhacki, J., Bauer, A., Geis, S., Cardenas-Conejo, Z. E., et al. (2012a). Resequencing of the auxiliary GABA(B) receptor subunit gene KCTD12 in chronic tinnitus. *Front. Syst. Neurosci.* 6:41. doi: 10.3389/fnsys.2012.00041

Sand, P. G., Langguth, B., and Kleinjung, T. (2011). Deep resequencing of the voltage-gated potassium channel subunit KCNE3 gene in chronic tinnitus. *Behav. Brain Funct.* 7:39. doi: 10.1186/1744-9081-7-39

Sand, P. G., Langguth, B., Schecklmann, M., and Kleinjung, T. (2012b). GDNF and BDNF gene interplay in chronic tinnitus. *Int. J. Mol. Epidemiol. Genet.* 3, 245–251.

Sand, P. G., Luettich, A., Kleinjung, T., Hajak, G., and Langguth, B. (2010). An examination of KCNE1 mutations and common variants in chronic tinnitus. *Genes* 1, 23–37. doi: 10.3390/genes1010023

Schlee, W., Hall, D., Edvall, N. K., Langguth, B., Canlon, B., and Cederroth, C. R. (2017). Visualization of global disease burden for the optimization of patient management and treatment. *Front. Med.* 4:86. doi: 10.3389/fmed.2017.00086

Sullivan, P. F., Agrawal, A., Bulik, C. M., Andreassen, O. A., Børglum, A. D., Breen, G., et al. (in press). Psychiatric genomics: an update and an agenda. *Am. J. Psychiatry.*

van Dongen, J., Slagboom, P. E., Draisma, H. H., Martin, N. G., and Boomsma, D. I. (2012). The continuing value of twin studies in the omics era. *Nat. Rev. Genet.* 13, 640–653. doi: 10.1038/nrg3243

Vona, B., Nanda, I., Shehata-Dieler, W., and Haaf, T. (2017). Genetics of tinnitus: still in its infancy. *Front. Neurosci.* 11:236. doi: 10.3389/fnins.2017.00236

10

Impairments of Speech Comprehension in Patients with Tinnitus

Daniela Ivansic, Orlando Guntinas-Lichius, Boris Müller, Gerd F. Volk, Gerlind Schneider and Christian Dobel *

Tinnitus-Centre, Department of Otorhinolaryngology, Jena University Hospital, Jena, Germany

*Correspondence:
Christian Dobel
christian.dobel@med.uni-jena.de

Tinnitus describes the subjective perception of a sound despite the absence of external stimulation. Being a sensory symptom the majority of studies focusses on the auditory pathway. In the recent years, a series of studies suggested a crucial involvement of the limbic system in the manifestation and development of chronic tinnitus. Regarding cognitive symptoms, several reviews addressed the presence of cognitive impairments in tinnitus as well and concluded that attention and memory processes are affected. Despite the importance for social communication and the reliance on a highly functional auditory system, speech comprehension remains a largely neglected field in tinnitus research. This is why we review here the existing literature on speech and language functions in tinnitus patients. Reviewed studies suggest that speech comprehension is impaired in patients with tinnitus, especially in the presence of competing noise. This is even the case in tinnitus patients with normal hearing thresholds. Additionally, speech comprehension measures seem independent of other measures such as tinnitus severity and perceived tinnitus loudness. According to the majority of authors, the speech comprehension difficulties arise as a result of central processes or dysfunctional neuroplasticity.

Keywords: tinnitus, speech comprehension, speech processing, cognition, review, aging

INTRODUCTION

Impairment of General Cognitive Functions in Tinnitus

Tinnitus describes the perception of a sound in the absence of physical stimulation and is also called a phantom percept. As tinnitus is characterized as a sensory and auditory phenomenon, most studies addressed dysfunctions of the auditory pathways. Several studies suggested that not only peripheral, but also central auditory systems and dysfunctional neuroplastic processes as a consequence of deafferentation contribute to the development of the impairment (Møller, 2007). Consequently, therapeutic approaches focused on the auditory system (e.g., Jastreboff et al., 1996; Eysel-Gosepath et al., 2004; Stein et al., 2016). However, research provided evidence that not only auditory pathways are affected, but also the limbic system which is involved in affective processing (see e.g., Husain, 2016). The support for this was not only provided by imaging studies, but was also gained from clinical reports stressing the high comorbidity of tinnitus with psychiatric disorders (Andersson, 2002).

Reviews on Cognitive Functions

Due to neuroplasticity and the strong linkage of auditory pathways, the limbic system and central processes, it is not surprising that a range of cognitive processes are impaired in tinnitus patients. To date, there are three reviews with each having a slightly different focus (Andersson and McKenna, 2006; Mohamad et al., 2016; Tegg-Quinn et al., 2016).

In their review, Andersson and McKenna (2006) grouped studies in three areas: (1) neuropsychological measures evidenced that control of attention is impaired under conditions when attentional demands are neither high nor low, but average; (2) regarding cognitive biases, selective attention bias was described as an emphasis on disorder-related information (e.g., found in patients suffering from anxiety disorders), while memory bias has been found among depressive patients, who tend to remember negative information better than positive. Such biases were present in tinnitus patients as well, but there may be two subgroups of tinnitus patients with one exhibiting a focus on tinnitus related information (similar to anxiety disorders) and the other displaying memory distortions as seen in depression; and (3) finally, Andersson and McKenna (2006) report the literature on the conscious appraisal of tinnitus (i.e., in terms of remembering and reporting the intrusiveness of tinnitus) and they stress the prominent role of complaints, worries and anxious thoughts.

In a systematic literature search on tinnitus and cognition with a focus on attention and memory, Mohamad et al. (2016) reviewed nine studies. While there is mixed evidence for the notion that working memory and selective attention are affected in tinnitus patients, a clearer picture evolved for executive attention. This function encompasses the engagement and disengagement to a specific stimulus, as well as the switch to a different stimulus to reach a specific goal. These processes enhance processing of relevant stimuli and in turn achieve a better representation of information in working memory. For instance, tinnitus patients were generally slower than controls in Stroop tasks (Andersson et al., 2000; Jackson et al., 2014) and also exhibited a deficit in an "attention network test" which is used as an index measure for executive control (Heeren et al., 2014). Additionally, self-reported tinnitus symptoms correlated with behavioral measures for executive control (Heeren et al., 2014; Jackson et al., 2014). Reviewing this evidence, Mohamad et al. (2016) concluded that there is at least preliminary evidence that tinnitus interferes with executive attention.

Recently Tegg-Quinn et al. (2016) performed a similar systematic review, however, with a broader search criterion and a focus on clinical management of invasive tinnitus. They report 18 studies employing a variety of measures on cognitive functions in tinnitus. Based on nine studies reporting attentional impairments, the authors state that executive control of attention is impaired and impacts on cognitive function in tinnitus patients.

Apart from these reviews, Roberts et al. (2015) also stress the crucial involvement of attentional processes in the generation of chronic tinnitus and provide a model for these dysfunctional processes. In normal hearing persons, neural patterns from actual inputs are compared to predicted representations generated from long-term memory. If the factual and the predicted inputs match, the comparison leads to a cancellation and no mismatch signal is generated. In tinnitus patients, cochlear damage and/or subsequent neuroplastic processes lead to a mismatch between the two inputs and the comparison process draws attention towards the auditory input to generate a better representation of the acoustic environment.

Taken together, several reviews agree that tinnitus is accompanied by cognitive impairments particularly affecting attentional executive functions. Given the reliance of speech comprehension on detailed and stable representations of the acoustic environment, it seems surprising that speech is not a more dominant topic regarding cognitive impairments. This is even more so, when considering the tight connections between attention and language. We will briefly describe these processes before we review the studies on speech, language and tinnitus.

Language Comprehension, Production, Working Memory and Attention

There is a strong link between language and attention at several levels and a comprehensive overview would go far beyond the scope of the current review. The best example for this link is the role of joint attention during language acquisition when infants want that their communication partners devote their attention to the same object in space as they do (Moore and Dunham, 1995). Similarly, speakers generally look at objects before they name them and so the order of naming becomes evident from the order of looking (e.g., Meyer and Dobel, 2004; Dobel et al., 2011) and listeners look at objects that are mentioned by a speaker (e.g., Henderson et al., 2003). Besides this overt behavior, there are earlier states of processing when attention plays an important role. The connection between language comprehension, working memory capacity (WMC) and attention is possibly best captured by the *Ease of Language Understanding* (ELU) model (for a recent overview of the model see Rönnberg et al., 2013). With regard to early encoding of auditory stimuli, the interplay of attention and WMC ensures a fine-tuning of processing even under adverse conditions. Several neurophysiological studies suggest that attentional processes interact with WMC already at subcortical levels (Zouridakis et al., 1998; Sörqvist et al., 2012; Tsuchida et al., 2012). Next to these early effects, the interplay of attention with WMC and their influence on short-term retention was evidenced by studies on persons wearing hearing aids, where short-term memory performance correlated with the degree of hearing impairment under conditions of divided attention (Tun et al., 2009; Rönnberg et al., 2011). Thus, on one hand, hearing aids reduce attentional costs when persons listen to speech in noise and can improve speech comprehension (Rönnberg et al., 2013). On the other hand, tinnitus is likely to put strong demands on speech processing in everyday listening situations, or more explicitly: "signal distortion will tax WMC during speech understanding" (Rönnberg et al., 2013; p. 10).

On this background, i.e., the presence of cognitive and particularly attentional deficits in tinnitus patients and the strong link between attention and speech, we predict that speech comprehension impairments might be a prominent symptom in patients with chronic tinnitus, especially under difficult listening conditions. Here, we want to substantiate this claim by a systematic review. Second, we want to find out if this impairment is caused by peripheral cochlear damage and is as such a rather trivial phenomenon. Finally, we would like to give some recommendations for future research based on our findings.

METHODS

Search Strategy

A literature search with no date restriction using the search terms (((tinnitus) AND ("speech perception" OR "speech recognition")) NOT (implant* OR transplant*) NOT review NOT Schwannoma NOT cancer NOT sudden NOT Menière) was undertaken in the PubMed and PsycINFO databases as well as the Cochrane Library in September 2016. Additional articles were obtained through the references of studies identified during the initial search (see **Figure 1**). The search resulted in $N = 13$ publications reported below and summarized in **Table 1**.

RESULTS

With regard to our hypothesis, we will briefly outline the overall results (for an overview see **Table 1**). From the 13 studies reported here, 12 evidenced impairments of speech perception in patients suffering from chronic tinnitus. Across studies a variety of tests was used with and without competing noise. Patients were native speakers of rather different languages. As the only exception, Tugumia et al. (2016) did not report impaired speech perception in tinnitus patients. Six studies contrasted speech comprehension under easy (e.g., no competing noise) and difficult conditions. Five of those reported stronger impairments under difficult conditions. In 8 of the 13 studies, the authors interpreted their results in terms of central contributions to the generation of speech comprehension impairments. In the remaining studies, the authors did not comment on this. In the following we will present the reviewed studies in more detail and focus on the hypotheses outlined in the "Introduction" Section.

Newman et al. (1994) investigated the relationship between psychoacoustic measures and speech perception abilities in patients with hearing loss and tinnitus (THL group) compared to patients with hearing loss only (HL group; $N = 23$ in each group). Even though peripheral hearing loss was similar in both groups, the THL group performed worse than the HL group in speech-in-noise tasks, particularly for difficult items. There was no correlation between speech perception abilities and perceived handicap. The authors suggested that tinnitus should be considered as a symptom which may also have central causes rather than only peripheral damage. Hearing loss does not even have to be present for the occurrence of impairment in speech perception as reported by Soalheiro et al. (2012). This study evidenced impaired speech perception measured without competing noise in 81% of almost 300 workers exposed to occupational stress.

Goldstein and Shulman (1999) investigated 25 individuals with severely disturbing tinnitus. About half of these participants (52%) displayed low scores in at least one of the central auditory speech tests. More specifically, in the low-pass filtered speech test and the competing sentence test, patients complaining about interference of tinnitus with daily communication displayed low performance. Similar to Newman et al. (1994), Goldstein and Shulman stressed the contribution of central processes to the generation of chronic tinnitus. Huang et al. (2007) investigated speech perception in 20 chronic tinnitus patients speaking Mandarin. Compared to controls, tinnitus patients displayed generally lower scores in perceiving sentences in noise and, as it appears (though it was not analyzed), this was more so when sentences were hard to predict, i.e., with low contextual cues. As above, these measures did not correlate with tinnitus loudness or disability, again arguing for a contribution of central processes to the symptomatology. A corroborating result for the influence of hearing condition was obtained with 19 Portuguese patients suffering from tinnitus and hyperacusis (Hennig et al., 2011). Compared to normal hearing controls they demonstrated lower abilities to comprehend sentences in noise, but performed normally without noise. Using the Korean version of the hearing in noise test, Ryu et al. (2012) showed that tinnitus patients with normal pure tone audiometry ($N = 20$), thus arguing for no peripheral impairment, performed worse than normal hearing controls, both when sentences were displayed in silence and with competing noise, i.e., there was no influence of hearing condition. Similar findings were reported on 15 Dutch speakers wearing cochlear implants suffering from one-sided tinnitus (Mertens et al., 2013). Importantly, this study evidenced impaired speech-in-noise comprehension in the unaffected ear which argues again for impairment with strong contributions from central processes (note that publications studying patients with hearing aids were excluded from this review; this study was included, however, because the unaffected ear was tested). Similarly arguing for an involvement of central processes, Cuny et al. (2004) reported left hemispheric dominance (i.e., a right ear advantage) in controls employing a word dichotic listening and lateralized decision task. In contrast, tinnitus patients did not show such a hemispheric asymmetry for language processing. Importantly, tinnitus was simulated in normal hearing participants by a tinnitus-like noise and thus the difference between groups could not be attributed to the tinnitus noise *per se* (note that the inclusion of white band noise worsens speech intelligibility even in normal hearing participants, Paglialonga et al., 2011). Consequently, the authors argued for functional reorganization as a consequence of the peripheral damage. The same conclusion was reached by Moon et al. (2015) who measured the speech recognition threshold in noise in 21 patients suffering from tinnitus. Patients performed worse than a control group in this test, but not in a variety on tests on auditory spectral and temporal resolution. This dissociation argues again against the hypothesis that tinnitus depends on damage to outer hair cells, but rather on plastic changes in the central auditory pathways after damage to the cochlea.

To further investigate the dissociation between inconspicuous pure tone audiograms and speech perception, Jain and Sahoo (2014) tested 20 patients suffering from mild to moderate tinnitus in comparison to a control group. Tests

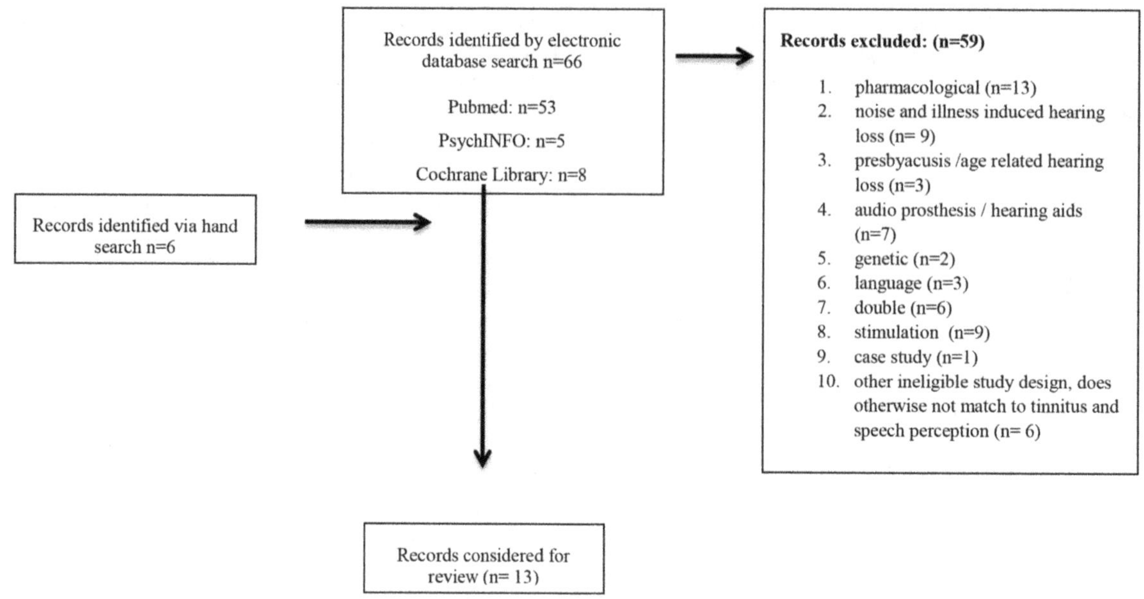

FIGURE 1 | Flow chart for the identification of studies included in the review.

included speech perception in noise, frequency discrimination, differential limen of intensity and frequency, gap detection and modulation detection thresholds. The results demonstrated that tinnitus patients were impaired in various aspects of auditory perception such as frequency discrimination, temporal resolution and speech recognition in noise, i.e., aspects that are not reflected in a pure tone audiogram. Corroborating results were presented from 19 young adults exposed to leisure noise who developed noise-induced tinnitus (Gilles et al., 2016). While these participants did not show differences to a control group with regard to hearing thresholds, otoacoustic emissions and ABR, participants with noise induced tinnitus displayed worse abilities for sentence comprehension in noise. Thus, even if measures indicating peripheral damage are inconspicuous, speech perception tests argue for impairment.

DISCUSSION AND CONCLUSION

Given the small but recently increasing literature on problems with speech perception in tinnitus, it appears that these functions are impaired in tinnitus patients across a wide variety of languages. Despite the small number of studies, the reported evidence for tinnitus-related impairments of speech perception goes far beyond just a few cases. From an experimental viewpoint, in most studies the investigated group sizes allowed to make robust conclusions (all $N > 14$). The only study that did not find evidence for speech comprehension impairments is by Tugumia et al. (2016). They used a Portuguese version of a speech-in-Noise test (Pereira and Schochat, 2011) as a validation of an auditory training procedure. Speech comprehension did not improve due to training and was already in the normal range before training. Reasons for this divergence to other studies might be the rather mild condition of the studied patients as well as their young age.

As a particularly important finding in several studies, speech measures were impaired even if audiological measures were inconspicuous (e.g., Ryu et al., 2012; Mertens et al., 2013; Gilles et al., 2016). Thus, a speech impairment was even demonstrated when no peripheral damage was evidenced. We take this as an argument that reduced speech comprehension is a phenomenon *per se* and not only attributable to impaired hearing. Consequently, it is not a trivial problem as one might have quite understandably suggested.

Nevertheless, the underlying mechanism is far from understood. Despite the strong link between attention and speech comprehension as well as language in general, it is not yet clear what the nature of their relation is. Are the impairments in speech processing a direct consequence of attentional impairments or are they both the consequence of underlying common functions? The majority of authors agree that for the development of chronic tinnitus peripheral damage is accompanied by neuroplastic processes of central functions (e.g., Newman et al., 1994; Cuny et al., 2004; Paglialonga et al., 2011; Mertens et al., 2013). If attentional functions and/or working memory and/or language processing are *per se* affected, then this should become obvious independent from the domain of input. This assumption is to some degree supported by the very high percentage of tinnitus patients reporting difficulties with concentration (Watts et al., 2016) and by evidence for poorer reading performance in these patients (Sanchez and Stephens, 1997). As a working hypothesis, we propose that difficulties in speech comprehension arise via a central mechanism. The phantom noise attracts attention and as a consequence these resources are not available for

TABLE 1 | Overview of reviewed studies: basic participant characteristics, employed speech comprehension tests, main results and conclusions regarding our hypothesis language.

	Methods			Results		Conclusion
Study	**Participants**	**Speech comprehension (SC) test(s)**	**Language**	**Impairment in SC for T**	**Impact of hearing condition**	**Involvement of central processes**
Newman et al. (1994)	*N* = 23: UT + BHL *N* = 23: BHL	Harvard Psychoacoustic Laboratory word test, synthetic sentence identification test, speech perception in noise test, dichotic sentence identification test	English	yes	yes	yes
Goldstein and Shulman (1999)	*N* = 25: severe T + NH	Monaural low-pass filtered speech, binaural fusion test, rapid alternating speech test, competing sentence test, staggered spondaic word test	English	yes	yes	yes
Cuny et al. (2004)	*N* = 20: UT *N* = 10: BT *N* = 30: healthy controls	Dichotic listening, lateralized lexical decision	French	yes	n.a.	yes
Huang et al. (2007)	*N* = 20: T + NH	Mandarin speech perception in noise test	Mandarin	yes	yes	yes
Hennig et al. (2011)	*N* = 19: T + NH + hyperacusis *N* = 23: controls	Sentences recognition threshold in silence and in noise	Portuguese	yes	yes	n.s.
Paglialonga et al. (2011)	*N* = 10: NH	Speech in noise test with three-alternative, forced-choice paradigm	Italian	yes	yes	n.s.
Ryu et al. (2012)	*N* = 20: T + NH *N* = 20: healthy controls	Korean version of hearing in noise test	Korean	yes	no	n.s.
Soalheiro et al. (2012)	*N* = 495: T	Logoaudiometric thresholds without competing noise	Portuguese	yes	n.a.	n.s.
Mertens et al. (2013)	*N* = 15: UHL and ipsilateral T	Speech reception threshold using the Leuven intelligibility sentences test	Dutch	yes	n.a.	yes
Jain and Sahoo (2014)	*N* = 10: mild T *N* = 10: moderate T *N* = 20: controls	Speech perception in noise based on sentences from the Kannada quick speech in noise test	Canarese	yes	n.a.	yes
Moon et al. (2015)	*N* = 9: UT + NH *N* = 12: UT + HL *N* = 9: BT + HL *N* = 15: healthy controls	Speech recognition in noise	Korean	yes	n.a.	yes
Gilles et al. (2016)	*N* = 19: T *N* = 68: controls	Speech-in-noise testing with continuous and modulated noise based on the Leuven intelligibility sentence test	Dutch	yes	n.a.	yes
Tugumia et al. (2016)	*N* = 12: UT + BT	Speech-in-noise test (not specified)	Portuguese	no	n.a.	n.s.

U, unilateral; B, bilateral; T, Tinnitus; HL, hearing loss; NH, normal hearing; SC, speech comprehension; n.a., not applicable; n.s, not stated.

other processes. This becomes expressed as deficits of divided or selective attention. As described in the introduction and emphasized by the ELU model, language processing depends on all levels on attentional capacities and is consequently impaired. We outline below some possibilities to investigate this on a detailed functional level. As an alternative hypothesis, this mechanism could be mediated via stress responses to the tinnitus. Such a possibility seems plausible regarding the recent evidence for the involvement of the limbic system (e.g., Husain, 2016).

Outlook

We propose that future research should aim at disentangling the various factors that contribute to impaired speech perception in tinnitus as well as the causal relationships between attention and speech comprehension. By comparing complex sentences (with e.g., relative clauses) to simpler sentences, the interaction with working memory can be tested. The use of text passages requiring frequent or rare shifts of attention could evidence the interplay of speech processing with attentional requirements. Eye-tracking proved as a useful technique to measure shifts and the locus of attention and could therefore be applied in tinnitus-research to investigate the interplay of speech processing and attentional focus (e.g., Andersson et al., 2011). Moreover, keeping in mind that different phonemes are plotted on different frequency areas in an audiogram, it would be interesting to investigate which phonemes are harder to understand than others. As an example on the single word level, it is highly plausible that words with fricatives are particularly hard to process, especially with competing white noise. While these are only a few suggestions, they necessitate the development of systematic, standardized test batteries employing speech stimuli involving not only tinnitus-researchers but linguists, phoneticians and neuroscientists alike. The multitude and variability of symptoms demand that tinnitus research becomes even more interdisciplinary than it already is.

AUTHOR CONTRIBUTIONS

DI, BM and CD: literature search, conception of review; wrote the manuscript. OG-L, GFV and GS: conception of review; wrote the manuscript.

ACKNOWLEDGMENTS

We thank Dr. Romi Zäske, MD Christina Lauer and Dr. Susanne Duncker for reading and commenting earlier versions of the manuscript.

REFERENCES

Andersson, G. (2002). Psychological aspects of tinnitus and the application of cognitive-behavioral therapy. *Clin. Psychol. Rev.* 22, 977–990. doi: 10.1016/s0272-7358(01)00124-6

Andersson, G., Eriksson, J., Lundh, L. G., and Lyttkens, L. (2000). Tinnitus and cognitive interference: a stroop paradigm study. *J. Speech Lang. Hear. Res.* 43, 1168–1173. doi: 10.1044/jslhr.4305.1168

Andersson, G., and McKenna, L. (2006). The role of cognition in tinnitus. *Acta Otolaryngol. Suppl.* 126, 39–43. doi: 10.1080/03655230600895226

Andersson, R., Ferreira, F., and Henderson, J. M. (2011). I see what you're saying: the integration of complex speech and scenes during language comprehension. *Acta Psychol.* 137, 208–216, doi: 10.1016/j.actpsy.2011.01.007

Cuny, C., Chéry-Croze, S., Bougeant, J. C., and Koenig, O. (2004). Investigation of functional hemispheric asymmetry of language in tinnitus sufferers. *Neuropsychology* 18, 384–392. doi: 10.1037/0894-4105.18.2.384

Dobel, C., Glanemann, R., Kreysa, H., Zwitserlood, P., and Eisenbeiss, S. (2011). "Visual encoding of meaningful and meaningless scenes," in *Event Representation in Language and Cognition*, eds E. Pedersen, and J. Bohnemeyer (Cambridge: Cambridge University Press), 189–215.

Eysel-Gosepath, K., Gerhards, F., Schicketanz, K.-H., Teichmann, K., and Benthien, M. (2004). Aufmerksamkeitslenkung in der Tinnitustherapie. Vergleich von Effekten unterschiedlicher Behandlungsmethoden. *HNO* 52, 431–439. doi: 10.1007/s00106-003-0929-4

Gilles, A., Schlee, W., Rabau, S., Wouters, K., Fransen, E., and Van de Heyning, P. (2016). Decreased speech-in-noise understanding in young adults with tinnitus. *Front. Neurosci.* 10:288. doi: 10.3389/fnins.2016.00288

Goldstein, B., and Shulman, A. (1999). Central auditory speech test findings in individuals with subjective idiopathic tinnitus. *Int. Tinnitus J.* 5, 16–19.

Heeren, A., Maurage, P., Perrot, H., De Volder, A., Renier, L., Araneda, R., et al. (2014). Tinnitus specifically alters the top-down executive control sub-component of attention: evidence from the attention network task. *Behav. Brain Res.* 269, 147–154. doi: 10.1016/j.bbr.2014.04.043

Henderson, J. M., Williams, C. C., Castelhano, M. S., and Falk, R. J. (2003). Eye movements and picture processing during recognition. *Percept. Psychophys.* 65, 725–734. doi: 10.3758/bf03194809

Hennig, T. R., Costa, M. J., Urnau, D., Becker, K. T., and Schuster, L. C. (2011). Recognition of speech of normal-hearing individuals with tinnitus and hyperacusis. *Int. Arch. Otorhinolaryngol.* 15, 21–28. doi: 10.1590/S1809-48722011000100003

Huang, C. Y., Lee, H. H., Chung, K. C., Chen, H. C., Shen, Y. J., and Wu, J. L. (2007). Relationships among speech perception, self-rated tinnitus loudness and disability in tinnitus patients with normal pure-tone threshold s of hearing. *ORL* 69, 25–29. doi: 10.1159/000096713

Husain, F. T. (2016). Neural networks of tinnitus in humans: elucidating severity and habituation. *Hear Res.* 334, 37–48. doi: 10.1016/j.heares.2015.09.010

Jackson, J. G., Coyne, I. J., and Clough, P. J. (2014). A preliminary investigation of potential cognitive performance decrements in non-help-seeking tinnitus sufferers. *Int. J. Audiol.* 53, 88–93. doi: 10.3109/14992027.2013.846481

Jain, C., and Sahoo, J. P. (2014). The effect of tinnitus on some psychoacoustical abilities in individuals with normal hearing sensitivity. *Int. Tinnitus J.* 19, 28–35. doi: 10.5935/0946-5448.20140004

Jastreboff, P. J., Gray, W. C., and Gold, S. L. (1996). Neurophysiological approach to tinnitus patients. *Am. J. Otol.* 17, 236–240.

Mertens, G., Kleine Punte, A., De Ridder, D., and Van de Heyning, P. (2013). Tinnitus in a single-sided deaf ear reduces speech reception in the nontinnitus ear. *Otol. Neurotol.* 34, 662–666. doi: 10.1097/MAO.0b013e31828779f0

Meyer, A. S., and Dobel, C. (2004). "Application of eye tracking in speech production research," in *The Mind's Eye: Cognitive and Applied Aspects of Eye Movement Research*, eds J. Hyöna, J. R. Radach, and H. Deubel (Oxford: Elsevier Science), 253–272.

Mohamad, N., Hoare, D. J., and Hall, D. A. (2016). The consequences of tinnitus and tinnitus severity on cognition: A review of the behavioural evidence. *Hear. Res.* 332, 199–209. doi: 10.1016/j.heares.2015.10.001

Møller, A. R. (2007). The role of neural plasticity in tinnitus. *Prog. Brain Res.* 166, 37–45. doi: 10.1016/S0079-6123(07)66003-8

Moon, I. J., Won, J. H., Kang, H. W., Kim, D. H., An, Y. H., and Shim, H. J. (2015). Influence of tinnitus on auditory spectral and temporal resolution and speech perception in tinnitus patients. *J. Neurosci.* 35, 14260–14269. doi: 10.1523/JNEUROSCI.5091-14.2015

Moore, C., and Dunham, P. J. (1995). *Joint Attention: Its Origins and Role in Development*. Hillsdale, NJ: Lawrence Erlbaum Associates.

Newman, C. W., Wharton, J. A., Shivapuja, B. G., and Jacobson, G. P. (1994). Relationships among psychoacoustic judgments, speech understanding ability and self-perceived handicap in tinnitus subjects. *Audiology* 33, 47–60. doi: 10.3109/00206099409072954

Paglialonga, A., Fiocchi, S., Del Bo, L., Ravazzani, P., and Tognola, G. (2011). Quantitative analysis of cochlear active mechanisms in tinnitus subjects with normal hearing sensitivity: time-frequency analysis of transient evoked otoacoustic emissions and contralateral suppression. *Auris Nasus Larynx* 38, 33–40. doi: 10.1016/j.anl.2010.04.006

Pereira, L. D., and Schochat, E. (2011). *Testes Auditivos e Comportamentais para Avaliação do Processamento Auditivo Central.* São Paulo: Pró Fono.

Roberts, L. E., Bosnyak, D. J., Bruce, I. C., Gander, P. E., and Paul, B. T. (2015). Evidence for differential modulation of primary and nonprimary auditory cortex by forward masking in tinnitus. *Hear. Res.* 327, 9–27. doi: 10.1016/j.heares.2015.04.011

Rönnberg, J., Danielsson, H., Rudner, M., Arlinger, S., Sternäng, O., Wahlin, A., et al. (2011). Hearing loss is negatively related to episodic and semantic long-term memory but not to short-term memory. *J. Speech Lang. Hear. Res.* 54, 705–726. doi: 10.1044/1092-4388(2010/09-0088)

Rönnberg, J., Lunner, T., Zekveld, A., Sörqvist, P., Danielsson, H., Lyxell, B., et al. (2013). The ease of language understanding (ELU) model: theoretical, empirical and clinical advances. *Front. Syst. Neurosci.* 7:31. doi: 10.3389/fnsys.2013.00031

Ryu, I. S., Ahn, J. H., Lim, H. W., Joo, K. Y., and Chung, J. W. (2012). Evaluation of masking effects on speech perception in patients with unilateral chronic tinnitus using the hearing in noise test. *Otol. Neurotol.* 33, 1472–1476. doi: 10.1097/MAO.0b013e31826dbcc4

Sanchez, L., and Stephens, D. (1997). A tinnitus problem questionnaire in a clinic population. *Ear Hear.* 18, 210–217.doi: 10.1097/00003446-199706000-00004

Soalheiro, M., Rocha, L., do Vale, D. F., Fontes, V., Valente, D., and Teixeira, L. R. (2012). Speech recognition index of workers with tinnitus exposed to environmental or occupational noise: a comparative study. *J. Occup. Med. Toxicol.* 22:6. doi: 10.1186/1745-6673-7-26

Sörqvist, P., Stenfelt, S., and Rönnberg, J. (2012). Working memory capacity and visual-verbal cognitive load modulate auditory-sensory gating in the brainstem: toward a unified view of attention. *J. Cogn. Neurosci.* 24, 2147–2154. doi: 10.1162/jocn_a_00275

Stein, A., Wunderlich, R., Lau, P., Engell, A., Wollbrink, A., Shaykevich, A., et al. (2016). Clinical trial on tonal tinnitus with tailor-made notched music training. *BMC Neurol.* 16:38. doi: 10.1186/s12883-016-0558-7

Tegg-Quinn, S., Bennett, R. J., Eikelboom, R. H., and Baguley, D. M. (2016). The impact of tinnitus upon cognition in adults: A systematic review. *Int. J. Audiol.* 55, 533–540. doi: 10.1080/14992027.2016.1185168

Tsuchida, Y., Katayama, J., and Murohashi, H. (2012). Working memory capacity affects the interference control of distractors at auditory gating. *Neurosci. Lett.* 516, 62–66. doi: 10.1016/j.neulet.2012.03.057

Tugumia, D., Samelli, A. G., Matas, C. G., Magliaro, F. C., and Rabelo, C. M. (2016). Auditory training program in subjects with tinnitus. *Codas* 28, 27–33. doi: 10.1590/2317-1782/20162015113

Tun, P. A., McCoy, S., and Wingfield, A. (2009). Aging, hearing acuity and the attentional costs of effortful listening. *Psychol. Aging* 24, 761–766. doi: 10.1037/a0014802

Watts, E., Fackrell, K., Smith, S., Sheldrake, J., and Hoare, D. (2016). "Why is tinnitus a problem? A qualitative analysis of problems reported by tinnitus patients," in *Poster presented at 10th International Tinnitus Research Initiative Conference and 1st EU Cost Action (TINNET) Conference, 16th–18th March 2016* (Nottingham).

Zouridakis, G., Simos, P. G., and Papanicolaou, A. C. (1998). Multiple bilaterally asymmetric cortical sources account for the auditory N1m component. *Brain Topogr.* 10, 183–189.

11

Tinnitus in Normal-Hearing Participants after Exposure to Intense Low-Frequency Sound and in Ménière's Disease Patients

Margarete Anna Ueberfuhr[1,2], *Lutz Wiegrebe*[2,3], *Eike Krause*[1,4], *Robert Gürkov*[1,4] *and Markus Drexl*[1]*

[1]*German Center for Vertigo and Balance Disorders, University Hospital Munich, Ludwig-Maximilians Universität München, Munich, Germany,* [2]*Graduate School of Systemic Neurosciences, Ludwig-Maximilians-Universität München, Martinsried, Germany,* [3]*Division of Neurobiology, Department Biology II, Ludwig-Maximilians-Universität München, Martinsried, Germany,* [4]*Department of Otorhinolaryngology, Head and Neck Surgery, Grosshadern Medical Centre, Ludwig-Maximilians Universität München, Munich, Germany*

Correspondence:
Markus Drexl
markus.drexl@med.uni-muenchen.de

Tinnitus is one of the three classical symptoms of Ménière's disease (MD), an inner ear disease that is often accompanied by endolymphatic hydrops. Previous studies indicate that tinnitus in MD patients is dominated by low frequencies, whereas tinnitus in non-hydropic pathologies is typically higher in frequency. Tinnitus of rather low-frequency (LF) quality was also reported to occur for about 90 s in normal-hearing participants after presentation of intense, LF sound (120 dB SPL, 30 Hz, 90 s). LF sound has been demonstrated to also cause temporary endolymphatic hydrops in animal models. Here, we quantify tinnitus in two study groups with chronic (MD patients) and presumably transient endolymphatic hydrops (normal-hearing participants after LF exposure) with a psychophysical procedure. Participants matched their tinnitus either with a pure tone of adjustable frequency and level or with a noise of adjustable spectral shape and level. Sensation levels of matching stimuli were lower for MD patients (mean: 8 dB SL) than for normal-hearing participants (mean: 15 dB SL). Transient tinnitus after LF-exposure occurred in all normal-hearing participants (N = 28). About half of the normal-hearing participants matched noise to their tinnitus, the other half chose a pure tone with frequencies below 2 kHz. MD patients matched their tinnitus with either high-frequency pure tones, mainly above 3 kHz, or with a noise. Despite a significant proportion of MD patients matching low-pass (roaring) noises to their tinnitus, the range of matched stimuli was more heterogeneous than previous data suggested. We propose that in those participants with noise-like tinnitus, the percept is probably generated by increased spontaneous activity of auditory nerve fibers with a broad range of characteristic frequencies, due to an impaired ion balance in the cochlea. For tonal tinnitus, additional mechanisms are conceivable: focal hair cell loss can result in decreased auditory nerve firing and a central auditory overcompensation. Also, normal-hearing participants after LF-exposure experience alterations in spontaneous otoacoustic emissions, which may contribute to a transient tonal tinnitus.

Keywords: tinnitus, low-frequency, Ménière's disease, bounce phenomenon, endolymphatic hydrops

---

Abbreviations: BP, bounce phenomenon; DPOAE, distortion product otoacoustic emission; ICC, intra-class correlation coefficients; IHCs, inner hair cells; LF, low-frequency; MD, Ménière's disease; NH, normal-hearing; OAE, otoacoustic emission; OHCs, outer hair cells; SOAE, spontaneous otoacoustic emission.

INTRODUCTION

Tinnitus is defined as the perception of sound in the absence of external acoustic stimulation and can take various forms from pure tones to more atonal percepts (1, 2).

Tinnitus can be distinguished into two main classes: objective tinnitus and subjective tinnitus. Objective tinnitus is caused by sounds originating from internal sources, e.g., from the patient's inner ear such as prominent spontaneous otoacoustic emissions (SOAEs) (3, 4). Subjective tinnitus is characterized by an abnormal spontaneous activity within the auditory periphery or the central auditory pathway in the absence of any acoustic stimulation, which is interpreted by the brain as sound (5, 6). A psychophysical characterization of tinnitus serves to quantify loudness and pitch/timbre, which can, in the second step, contribute to the understanding of the underlying pathology (7). For the sake of simplicity, in the following, the term pitch will be applied to pure tones and noises, although the term pitch refers to pure tones only and the equivalent for noises would be timbre. Pitch and loudness of a tinnitus sensation are typically characterized by matching a synthesized sound to the tinnitus percept [see Ref. (8, 9) for an overview]. Pitch matches of tinnitus patients are usually in the rather high-frequency region above 3 kHz and only rarely below 1 kHz (10).

However, patients with Ménière's disease (MD) seem to be an exception regarding tinnitus pitch. MD is classically characterized by a triad of symptoms: fluctuating hearing loss, episodes of vertigo, and tinnitus (11). In early stages of the disease, tinnitus seems to be related to episodes of vertigo, being more intense before and during attacks. With progression of the disease, which is typically associated with increasing hearing loss and ceasing of vertigo, tinnitus stays and its intensity increases (12–14). Descriptions of tinnitus in MD patients range from roaring over buzzing to ringing (13, 15); except for few MD patients presumably in later stages of the disease, who describe their tinnitus as tonal and containing high-pitched components (12, 13). Overall, studies concluded that tinnitus in the majority of MD patients was confined to lower-frequency ranges below 1 kHz and in particular between 125 and 250 Hz (16–21).

An excess of endolymph volume, termed endolymphatic hydrops, is often suggested to cause MD and specifically symptoms such as tinnitus. A transient endolymphatic hydrops was experimentally induced in rodents by an intense low-frequency (LF) sound (22).

In human participants, transient endolymphatic hydrops induced by an intense LF sound has not been shown directly. However, a post-LF-exposure phenomenon called "Bounce Phenomenon" (BP), lasting only a few minutes, was found in humans. The BP includes a transient tinnitus percept, fluctuating hearing thresholds with transient improvement and subsequent worsening (23–26), and biphasic amplitude level changes in otoacoustic emissions (OAEs) (27–31). As OAEs are sounds emitted by the cochlea due to active amplification processes by outer hair cells (OHCs) (32), the origin of the BP is thought to be cochlear (33). Increased endocochlear potentials in the cochlea have been recorded after presentation of LF sound (22) and were suggested to lead to an increase in the spontaneous firing rate of auditory nerve fibers, resulting in a "rate tinnitus" (34), presumably in the absence of any structural cochlear impairment.

In BP studies, human participants reported a transient "roaring" tinnitus immediately after LF sound exposure (23, 26, 27). The time course and relative loudness of the transient tinnitus percept were characterized with psychophysical studies (26, 30), but tinnitus pitch has not been systematically described with psychophysical measures yet. This study employed a tinnitus-matching procedure to quantify and compare tinnitus percepts in MD patients and normal-hearing (NH) participants after exposure to intense LF sound. Both study groups presumably presented with impaired cochlear ion balance that might manifest in endolymphatic hydrops in MD patients and shows indirectly as BP after LF sound in NH participants.

MATERIALS AND METHODS

Subjects

The study population consisted of two groups: a group of NH participants and a group of patients with MD. In the following, members of both groups will be referred to as participants. NH participants comprised 18 females and 10 males (age range 20–29, mean age 23.7) with no reported hearing problems, no ear surgery, no recent ear infections, and no tinnitus. All NH participants had hearing thresholds of less than 25 dB HL between 0.25 and 8 kHz, tested with a Matlab-based automated procedure [Automatic Pure Tone Audiometry APTA-HF 2012 V2.28 (HörTech, Oldenburg, Germany)]. One ear was pseudo-randomly chosen (14 left ears, 14 right ears) and exposed to a LF sound. The transient tinnitus was lateralized and perceived on the exposed side only.

The group of MD patients consisted of nine females and nine males (age range 26–74, mean age 53.1) diagnosed with definite MD according to the criteria recently formulated by the Bárány Society joint with several national and international organizations (14). Additionally, endolymphatic hydrops had been detected with magnetic resonance imaging after intra-tympanic gadolinium injection (35) before study participation in 15 of 18 patients.

Ménière's disease patients were included when they were unilaterally affected only (10 left ears, 8 right ears) and when they reported tinnitus localized to the affected ear.

Patients with middle ear disorders, pathologies of the auditory nerve or recent ear infections were excluded from the study. Patients with obvious noise-related hearing damage (i.e., notched audiograms) as well as patients with a history of noise exposure were not eligible either. All MD patients were required to be in a stage of the disease with fluctuating symptoms, with at least one vertigo attack during the 6 months preceding the experiment. In the contralateral, non-affected ear patients were required to have hearing thresholds better than 40 dB HL below 2 kHz, and better than 70 dB HL at higher frequencies.

This study was approved by the ethics committee of the University Hospital of the Ludwig-Maximilians-Universität Munich, Germany, in agreement with the Code of Ethics of the World Medical Association for experiments involving humans

(Declaration of Helsinki) and all participants (MD and NH) gave their written informed consent.

Experiments with NH participants were conducted in a double-walled, sound-attenuated booth at the Department of Biology, Ludwig-Maximilians-Universität Munich, Martinsried. Experiments with MD patients were carried out in a sound-attenuated booth at the ENT Department at the University Hospital of the Ludwig-Maximilians-Universität Munich, Germany.

Signal Generation and Data Acquisition

Signal generation and data acquisition was implemented with scripts written in MATLAB 7.5 (MathWorks, Natick, MA, USA). Sound generation and acquisition was done with an RME Fireface UC 24-bit external sound card (RME, Audio AG, Haimhausen, Germany). The sampling rate was 44.1 kHz. For sound stimulation, SoundMexPro (HörTech GmbH, Oldenburg, Germany) was employed, which enables low-latency multi-channel Audio Stream Input/Output and interactive changes of stimuli properties within the MATLAB environment.

SOAEs Recording

In NH participants, SOAEs were recorded with the ER-10C distortion product otoacoustic emission (DPOAE) probe microphone (Etymotic Research Inc., Elk Grove Village, IL, USA). The recorded signal was amplified 30 dB by the preamplifier of the external sound card. Level and frequency of SOAEs were recorded in the control trial for 120 s (measured in 21 of 28 NH participants) and after LF stimulation for 240 s (measured in 15 of 28 NH participants). In an artificial ear (B&K 4157, Brüel & Kjaer Sound and Vibration Measurement A/S, Denmark), no artifacts exceeding the noise floor of the system could be detected during recording. A probe-fit-check procedure preceded and concluded each measurement by presenting a band-stop noise consisting of a low- and a high-frequency band and analyzing the ear response using a Fourier transform analysis. If the probe-fit-check procedure at the end of a trial indicated that the probe position had changed, the trial was rejected and repeated.

Tinnitus-Matching Procedure

In experiments with MD patients, the output of the sound card was sent to HDA 200 headphones (Sennheiser, Wedemark-Wennebostel, Germany). In NH participants, two different sound systems were used for the two ears: an ER4 insert ear phone (Etymotic Research Inc., Elk Grove Village, IL, USA) was used to present the matching stimuli to one ear. An ER-10C DPOAE probe system with an additional tube coupled to an external transducer was used to present LF sounds (30 Hz sine wave, 120 dB SPL, 90 s, including 0.1 s raised-cosine ramps) to the other ear in order to elicit a tinnitus sensation.

The external transducer was a small broadband unit (NSW1-205-8A, Aura Sound Inc., Santa Fe Springs, CA, USA) driven by a RB-960BX power amplifier (Rotel, Worthing, UK). This transducer was connected to a 50-cm long polyethylene tube (inner diameter 1 mm), the tip of which was fed through the foam ear tip of the ER-10C DPOAE probe. The ER-10C includes a microphone for recording sound pressure in the ear canal enabling the examiners to calibrate the LF sound. The amplitude response of the DPOAE probe microphone was compared with the amplitude response in an artificial ear (B&K 4157, Brüel & Kjaer Sound and Vibration Measurement A/S, Denmark) and corrected for deviations. The level of the first harmonic of the LF sound was at least 50 dB lower than the level of the desired LF frequency.

Participants (NH and MD) were given standardized, written and illustrated instructions for the tinnitus-matching procedure. In NH participants, each trial was started with LF-sound exposure to one ear, thereby inducing a transient tinnitus percept in the exposed ear (see **Figure 1A**). Since the transient tinnitus lasted only for about 90 s after LF exposure (30), NH participants were allowed to restart the LF stimulus playback if necessary. As tinnitus was a unilateral symptom in both groups, matching stimuli were presented to the contralateral, unaffected ear (see **Figures 1A,B**). Participants were able to interactively adjust matching stimuli regarding loudness and pitch with a gamepad (Bigben Interactive GmbH, Bergheim, Germany). Matching stimuli were continuous and generated in real time by a SoundMexPro plug-in.

The matching procedure was split into two stages. The first stage served to determine whether the participants' tinnitus was matched best either with a pure tone or with a noise. Therefore, 10 different synthesized stimuli were presented. The stimuli comprised pure tones of five different frequencies, equally spaced on a logarithmic frequency axis between 0.25 and 8 kHz (0.25, 0.595, 1.414, 3.364, and 8.0 kHz) and five noises derived from Gaussian noise with different filter slopes (see **Figure 1C**). In the following, those slopes are referred to as spectral tilts with units of decibel per octave. They ranged from negative values with dominant LF components (−12 and −6 dB/octave) over white Gaussian noise (0 dB/octave) to positive values with dominant high-frequency components (+6 and +12 dB/octave). Stimuli were filtered such that linear phase and frequency distortions of the transducers (NH participants: ER4, Etymotic Research; MD patients: HDA 200, Sennheiser) were exactly compensated for. Participants started the playback of the individual stimuli successively by choosing from a graphical representation of the stimuli on a user interface. No information regarding the physical properties of the stimuli was available from the graphical representation. The 10 stimuli were identical but reordered on the user interface for each trial.

After having listened to all stimuli, participants were asked to select the stimulus best matching their tinnitus. After stimulus selection, participants had to adjust the stimulus level, such that the selected tone matched their tinnitus as well as possible. Selecting 1 out of the 10 stimuli and adjusting its loudness was counted as one trial in the first stage of the matching procedure. In NH participants, trials were repeated until the same stimulus class was selected in two successive trials. In MD patients, due to time constraints, only two trials were carried out regardless of whether participants selected the same stimulus or different stimuli in those two trials.

In the second stage, participants carried out fine adjustments of level and pitch of either a pure tone or a noise. Matching stimuli were presented with a starting frequency or starting spectral tilt corresponding to the selected stimulus of the first stage, respectively. In MD patients selecting two different stimuli in the first stage, the matching stimulus was chosen based on the patient's statement of which of the two selected stimuli was the better fit.

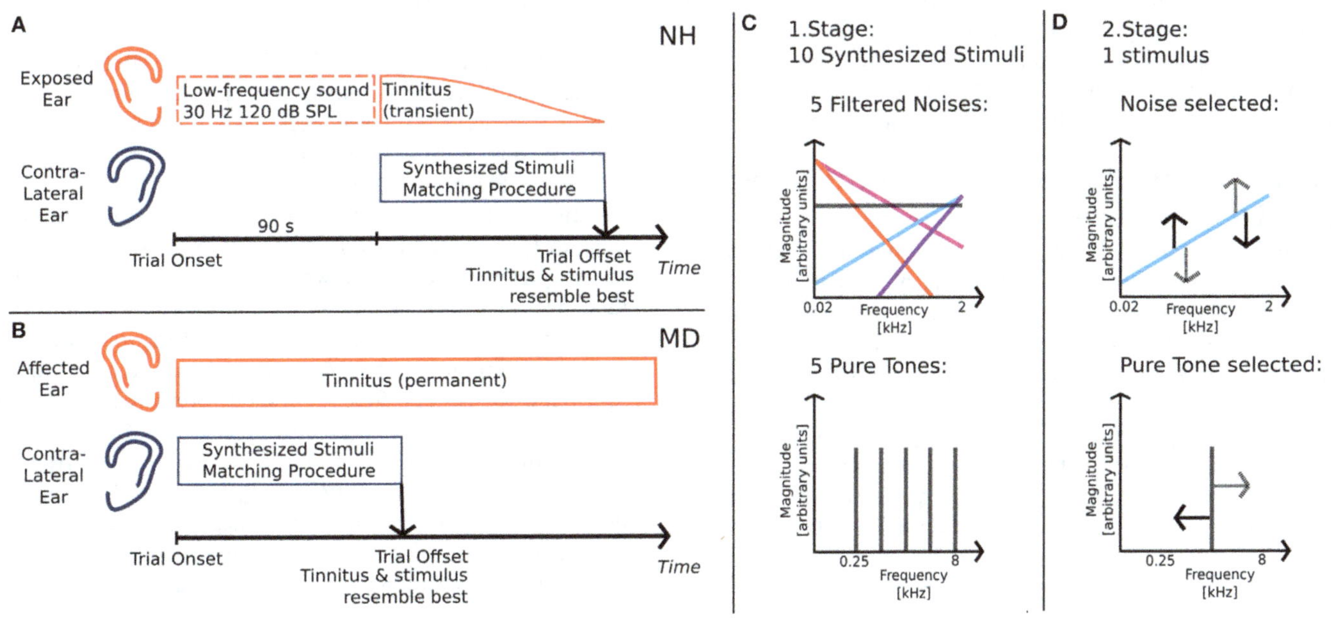

FIGURE 1 | Tinnitus-matching procedure. **(A)** Matching procedure for normal-hearing participants with intense low-frequency sound exposure prior to matching; **(B)** matching procedure for Ménière's disease patients with unilateral disease; **(C)** first stage of matching procedure: determining stimulus class of tinnitus percept; **(D)** second stage of matching procedure: adjusting stimulus regarding pitch/timbre and loudness of tinnitus.

The starting sound level was the mean sound level derived from the last two trials of the first stage.

During presentation of the matching stimulus, participants could continuously adjust loudness and frequency or spectral tilt (see **Figure 1D**). When participants found an adjustment for the matching stimulus that resembled their tinnitus, they stopped the adjustment procedure. Subsequently, the adjusted matching stimulus was again presented continuously and participants were required to adjust its sound level such that it was just audible. Similar to a Békésy tracking procedure, participants decreased the level of their adjusted matching stimulus until they did not perceive it anymore and then increased its intensity until they heard the stimulus again. This was done to estimate the sensation level of the matching stimulus. Adjusting the matching stimulus pitch and level and tracking the corresponding hearing threshold was considered as one trial in the second stage of the matching procedure.

In this second matching stage, NH participants always ran five trials and MD patients two to five trials depending on how many they were capable of doing due to time constraints and cognitive load.

After each trial, NH participants and MD patients were asked to describe their transient tinnitus in their own words. In NH participants, measurements were taken on two to four different days and lasted between 25 and 60 min each. In MD patients, testing was embedded in their clinical routine and carried out on 1 or 2 days. Measurements lasted 40–60 min.

All data analysis and statistics were carried out with scripts written in MATLAB 7.5 (MathWorks, Natick, MA, USA). Visualizations were done either with MATLAB 7.5 or Inkscape 0.91 (The Inkscape Team, http://www.inkscape.org).

RESULTS

Estimates of Level and Pitch of Tinnitus in NH Participants after LF Sound Exposure

All 28 NH participants exposed to the LF sound experienced a transient tinnitus percept and were able to match its pitch and level with a matching stimulus presented to the contralateral ear. Matching stimuli were adjusted after offset of the LF exposure, on average within 68.7 ± 32.5 s (mean ± SD, $N = 28$). This suggests that most NH participants concluded the matching while still hearing the transient tinnitus, which lasts about 90 s on average (30).

Conclusions drawn from questioning the NH participants after the software-based adjustment procedure are summarized as follows: 7 of the 28 NH participants described their tinnitus as tonal, 8 NH participants as a noise. The remaining 13 NH participants reported a hybrid percept consisting of noise and one or more tones. During the matching procedure, 8 out of those 13 NH participants experiencing a hybrid percept selected a matching tone and only 5 selected a matching noise. Altogether, 15 NH participants selected and adjusted a tone and 13 NH participants selected a noise (**Figure 2A**). Subjective descriptions of tinnitus perceived by NH participants after LF exposure are summarized in **Table 1**.

The loudness of the transient tinnitus percept was reported to be faint up to clearly audible with the tinnitus starting to fade out after a minute. Some participants also described qualitative changes in their tinnitus percept over time. Most of those participants reported a hybrid percept of pure tone(s) and noise. In those cases, the relative contribution of noise and tones to the tinnitus percept shifted over time. The tonal components seemed to fade out over time, while the noise serving as a background noise at the beginning of the BP got more prominent at later time points. Participants did not complain about the percept and its loudness. At most participants stated the tinnitus to be irritating, especially in combination with a feeling of aural fullness.

Tonal Tinnitus Percepts in NH Participants after LF Exposure

Fifteen NH participants selected pure tones to characterize their tonal tinnitus. The pure tone frequency was determined by averaging all adjustments per subject. The selected matching tone frequencies (see **Figures 3A,B**) show an accumulation between 0.1 and 2 kHz, where 14 out of 15 participants selected matching tones below 2 kHz.

The mean frequency of the 15 averaged pure tones chosen was 0.96 ± 0.89 kHz (mean ± SD, $N = 15$). As the SD across adjustments in hertz is only of limited value, frequency deviations were also expressed logarithmically as fraction of an octave in cent, where 100 cents equal a semitone, so that 1,200 cents correspond to an octave.

In 13 of 15 NH participants, SDs for single participants comprised less than 1,200 cents, and for some participants, the SD was as low as 30 cents. The inter-subject mean of the sound pressure level of the adjusted matching tone was around 49.5 ± 15.9 dB SPL (mean ± SD, $N = 15$).

Sound levels for matching tones decreased with increasing frequency from 90 dB SPL at 70 Hz to 30–35 dB SPL at 2–4 kHz. Matched pure tone levels followed equal-loudness contours for human hearing within a loudness level range of 25–60 phons (see **Figure 3A**). Thus, for NH participants, matching tones at lower frequencies were not generally perceived louder than at higher frequencies, despite the difference in sound pressure levels. For an interpretation of how loud participants (NH and MD) perceived their tinnitus, sensation levels were calculated (see **Figure 4A**). The sensation level is the difference (in decibel) between the presented sound level and the absolute hearing threshold for the same sound. The mean sensation level for tonal tinnitus matches of NH participants was 15.2 ± 6.7 dB SL (mean ± SD, $N = 15$).

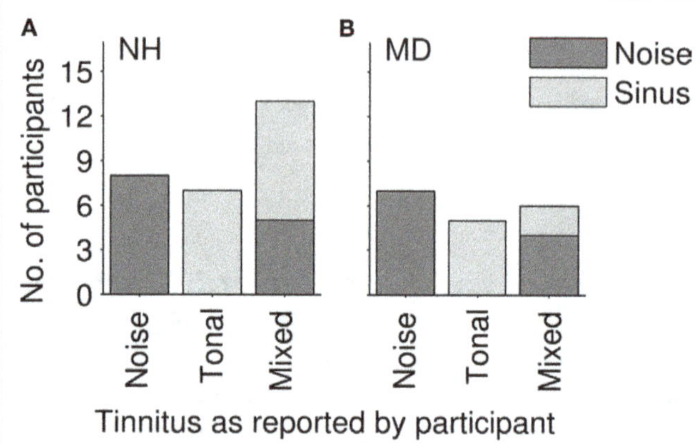

FIGURE 2 | Distribution of reported tinnitus quality. (A) Normal-hearing participants ($N = 28$). **(B)** Ménière's disease patients ($N = 18$); gray tones code for the stimulus class that participants selected in the tinnitus-matching procedure (light gray—pure tone; dark gray—noise).

TABLE 1 | Qualitative description of transient tinnitus after intense low-frequency sound exposure (30 Hz, 120 dB SPL, 90 s) by normal-hearing participants ($N = 28$).

	N
Noise-like tinnitus	**8**
Noise—exactly like matching noise	5
Low-Pitched Noise (Roaring like a fan)	2
Noise but tonal character	1
Tonal tinnitus	**7**
Pure Tone—exactly like matching tone	2
Two Tones—alternating/simultaneously (1 tone faint + 1 tone more intense) (Ringing like church bell, Chinese meditation balls)	5
Hybrid tinnitus percept	**13**
Low-Pitched Noise (Roaring) + tone	5
High-Frequency Tone(s) + machine-like sound (Rattling, jackhammer, sewing machine)	5
Other: noise with low-frequency (LF) modulation LF tone with tinny ring Sound of pressure valve	3

Noise-Like Tinnitus Percepts in NH Participants after LF Exposure

Thirteen NH participants chose noises to match their LF-induced transient tinnitus. Adjusted spectral tilts showed a bimodal distribution slightly shifted toward negative tilts with an average adjusted spectral tilt of −1.8 ± 7.9 dB/octave (mean ± SD, $N = 13$) (see **Figures 5A,B**). Except for one participant choosing white noise (mean tilt: ~0 dB/octave) to match the tinnitus percept, all NH participants selected either noises with a clearly positive tilt (mean ± SD = 6.7 ± 3.3 dB/octave, $n = 5$) or with a clearly negative tilt (mean ± SD = −8.1 ± 3.1 dB/octave, $n = 7$).

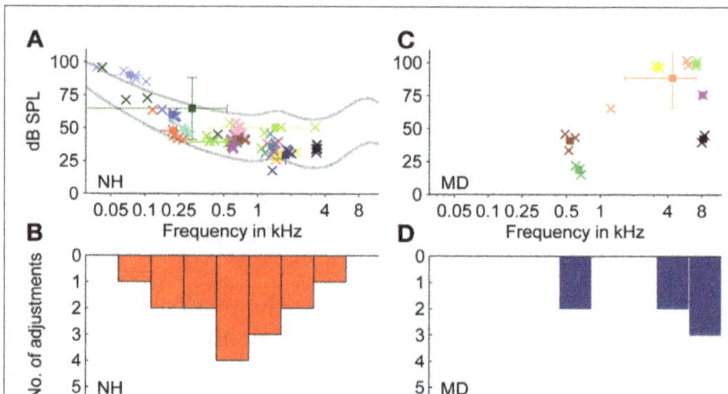

FIGURE 3 | Adjustments of level and frequency of externally presented pure tones to match a tonal tinnitus percept. (A,B) Normal-hearing participants ($N = 15$). **(C,D)** Ménière's disease patients ($N = 7$). **(A,C)** Plots show adjusted pure tones of individual participants. Data from individual participants are represented by different colors. Square symbols represent the mean of the two to five individual adjustments of one participant (indicated by cross symbols). Error bars represent the SD regarding sound pressure level (dB SPL) (vertically) and frequency (Hz) (horizontally). Lines in **(A)** represent equal-loudness contours for loudness levels at 25 and 60 phons. **(B,D)** Distribution of the selected matching tone frequencies of data shown in **(A,C)**, respectively (bin width = 1,249 cents).

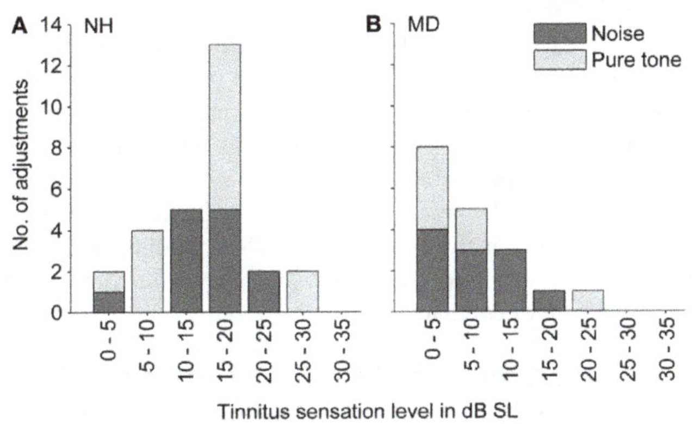

FIGURE 4 | Distribution of tinnitus loudness (expressed as sensation level). (A) Normal-hearing participants (N = 28). **(B)** Ménière's disease patients (N = 18). Colors code for the stimulus class that participants selected in the tinnitus-matching procedure (light gray – pure tone; dark gray – noise).

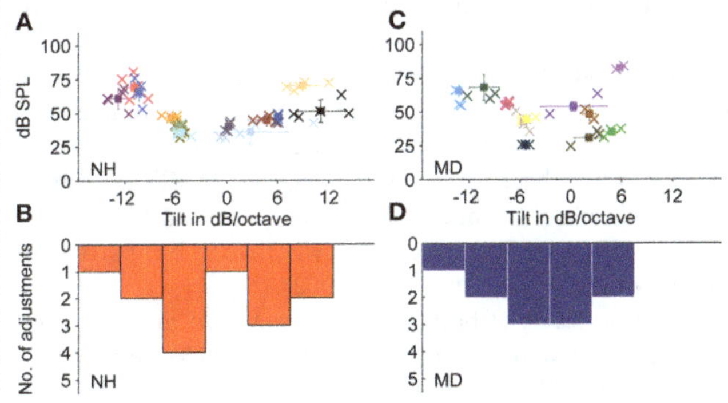

FIGURE 5 | Adjustments of level and frequency content of externally presented noises to match a noise-like tinnitus percept. (A,B) Normal-hearing participants (N = 13). **(C,D)** Ménière's disease patients (N = 11). **(A,C)** Plots show adjusted noises of individual participants. Error bars represent the SD regarding sound pressure level (dB SPL) (vertically) and frequency content (dB/octave) (horizontally). **(B,D)** Distribution of the matching noise tilts of the data shown in **(A,C)**, respectively, within the range of −17.5 to +17.5 dB/octave (bin width = 5 dB/octave). Color coding and symbols as in **Figure 3**.

Within-participant variability between adjustments was quite small (SD between 0.02 and 4.4 dB/octave).

Sound levels of the matching noises were within the range of 36–70 dB SPL with a mean of around 49.5 ± 12.9 dB SPL (mean ± SD, N = 13). Matching noises with highest sound pressure levels were noises with the steepest spectral tilts, either negative or positive. The mean sensation levels of matching noises were 15.3 ± 5.6 dB SL (mean ± SD, N = 13).

Sensation levels of both selected matching tones and matching noises in NH participants were summarized (see **Figure 4A**), and the mean was calculated as 15.2 ± 6.1 dB SL (mean ± SD, N = 28).

Estimates of Level and Pitch of Tinnitus in MD Patients

In all 18 MD patients, the tinnitus was a permanent sensation, sometimes varying in loudness over time. In eight patients, the loudness of the tinnitus was apparently correlated to the vertigo attacks increasing right before and/or during an attack. Three patients reported not only a loudness change correlated to the attacks but also an increase of tinnitus pitch. In this case, patients were asked to match their current tinnitus percept. Seven patients reported their tinnitus to be a noise, and five patients reported it to be a pure tone. The other six patients reported to hear a hybrid percept of pure tone(s) and noise. In the tinnitus-matching procedure, two of those patients perceiving a hybrid tinnitus matched their tinnitus with a pure tone and four of them with a noise (see **Figure 2B**). Qualitative tinnitus descriptions by the patients are summarized in **Table 2**. Descriptions included low-pitched noise, modulated noise, and high-frequency whistling.

Tonal Tinnitus in MD Patients

Seven MD patients selected pure tones in the matching procedure. Thereby, data did not show the previously suggested correlation that older patients or patients in later stages of the disease were more likely to experience tonal tinnitus of high-frequency quality instead of noise-like tinnitus (linear correlation coefficients, age: $r = -0.12$, p-value = 0.64, stage of disease $r = 0.08$, p-value = 0.76).

TABLE 2 | Qualitative description of tinnitus by Ménière's disease patients (N = 18) with unilateral disease and one-sided, permanent tinnitus.

	N
Noise-like tinnitus	**7**
Low-pitched noise (roaring, buzzing)	4
Noise with modulation/pulsatile (rushing blood)	2
Other: humming	1
Tonal tinnitus	**5**
Pure Tone—exactly like matching tone	2
High-frequency whistling, swishing	3
Hybrid tinnitus percept	**6**
High-frequency tone(s) + low-pitched noise (angle sander, whistling, and dull roaring)	4
Other: rushing blood Swarm of bees	2

Selected matching tone frequencies showed a bimodal distribution with peaks around 500 Hz and around 5 kHz (see **Figures 3C,D**). The mean frequency was 4.6 ± 3.3 kHz (mean ± SD, N = 13).

Matched sound levels increased with increasing frequency from 20 dB SPL at 0.6 kHz to 80–100 dB SPL at 7–8 kHz. Sensation levels of matching tones, however, were small (mean ± SD = 7.0 ± 7.8 dB SL, N = 7).

Noise-Like Tinnitus Percepts in MD Patients

Eleven of 18 MD patients selected noises to describe their tinnitus percept. The matching noise properties were averaged across the two to three trials for each patient.

Across patients, the average spectral tilt of matched noises was −2.9 ± 6.3 dB/octave (mean ± SD, N = 11). Matching noises showed adjusted tilts between −13 and +4 dB/octave and resulted in an almost normal distribution with a shift toward negative tilts (see **Figures 5C,D**).

On average, the noise level adjusted by MD patients was 50.4 ± 17.3 dB SPL (mean ± SD, N = 11), which was comparable to noise levels of noises matched by NH participants with transient tinnitus. Due to hearing loss in the majority of MD patients, the sensation levels of the matching tones were with 8.5 ± 4.9 dB SL (mean ± SD, N = 11) significantly lower than in NH participants (Mann–Whitney test, p-value = 0.0002).

Sensation levels of both matched tones and matched noises in MD patients were summarized (see **Figure 4B**), and the mean was 7.9 ± 6.0 dB SL (mean ± SD, N = 18).

Comparison of Tinnitus Percepts in MD Patients and in NH Participants after LF-Sound Exposure

Tonal Tinnitus Percepts

Pure tones matched by MD patients and matched by NH participants differed in their distribution (see **Figure 3**) (two-sample Kolmogorov–Smirnov test, p-value = 0.019). While the majority of MD patients chose pure tones above 3 kHz, which is comparable to most tinnitus percepts of tinnitus patients (10, 16), the majority of NH participants selected pure tones below 2 kHz.

Noise-Like Tinnitus Percepts

Comparing the two subgroups of MD patients selecting noises and NH participants with BP-induced tinnitus selecting noises did not show pronounced differences. Although the distribution appeared bimodal for NH participants and rather normally distributed in MD patients, the null hypothesis stating that the two subgroups were from equal distributions could not be rejected (two-sample Kolmogorov–Smirnov test; p-value = 0.86). Both subgroups had a tendency to select noises with a negative spectral tilt, which corresponds to previous reports from the literature (16–18, 23, 30).

Test–Retest Reliability

In general, the pitch and loudness matches obtained with the current two-stage procedure showed good test–retest reliability. Intra-class correlation coefficients (ICC) were calculated for the five trials of fine matching run in one to three different sessions in NH participants (pitch matching: ICC = 0.92; loudness matching: ICC = 0.85). In MD patients, data were usually collected in one session only, but for the two to three different adjustments ICC indicated very strong test–retest reliability, too (pitch matching: ICC = 0.93; loudness matching: ICC = 0.92).

SOAE Measurements in NH Participants

In 15 of the 28 NH participants, SOAEs were measured in the same ear that was exposed to the LF sound. The first measurement was run before LF exposure to find SOAEs. The second SOAE measurement was carried out immediately after LF exposure during the BP, while NH participants perceived the corresponding transient tinnitus. During the BP, "new" SOAEs could develop and existing SOAEs increased in level. Occasionally, those SOAEs exceeded the hearing threshold determined for the same ear by audiometric testing at the beginning of the experiments. In 10 NH participants, SOAEs could be found. In all of those participants, SOAEs were slightly altered when recorded during the BP compared to baseline before LF exposure. In eight NH participants, SOAE levels exceeded the individual hearing threshold at the SOAE characteristic frequency during the BP. From these eight participants, five matched their tinnitus with a pure tone, three with a noise. **Figure 6** shows SOAEs, hearing threshold and selected tinnitus-matching tones from three participants with "audible" SOAEs. These data suggest that some NH participants might possibly have matched their tinnitus to a transiently audible SOAE.

DISCUSSION

The current study, by applying a comprehensive tinnitus-matching procedure, compared tinnitus in two groups with

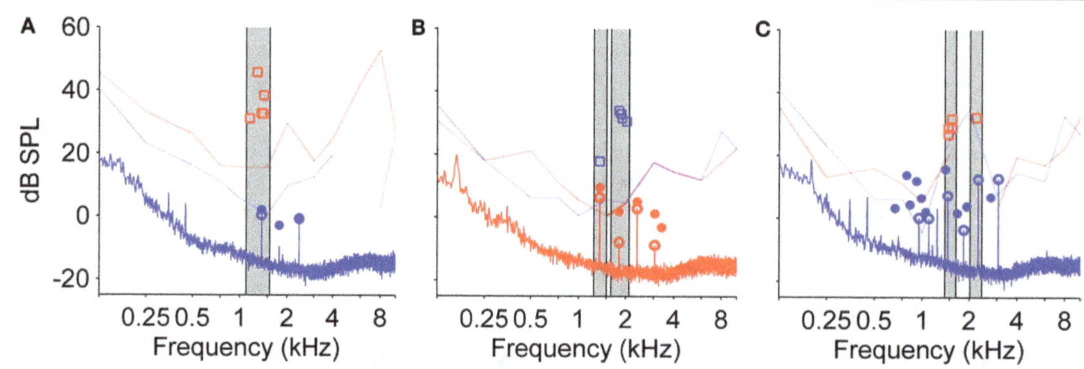

FIGURE 6 | Audiograms from both ears, spontaneous otoacoustic emissions (SOAEs), and level and frequency estimates of the tinnitus percept after low-frequency (LF) sound exposure for three different normal-hearing participants (A–C). SOAEs were recorded in ipsilateral ears before and immediately after exposure to a 30 Hz tone at 120 dB SPL for 90 s. In all three measures, red color refers to the right ear, blue color refers to the left ear. Light lines indicate audiogram thresholds (gaps within light lines are due to lack of valid data points of audiometric testing), open squares represent five adjustments of level and frequency of the matching tone presented to the contralateral ear. Solid lines represent the spectrum of the SOAE recording. Open circles represent SOAEs before LF sound exposure, filled circles represent SOAEs after LF sound exposure. Gray patches highlight SOAEs and corresponding matching tone adjustments.

chronic (MD patients) and transiently (NH participants after LF exposure) challenged cochlear homeostasis presumably resulting in hydropic conditions.

Our results show that sensation levels of tinnitus percepts were on average between 8 dB SL (MD patients) and 15 dB SL (NH participants after LF sound). Tinnitus pitch varied substantially both within and across MD patients and NH participants. While MD patients matched their tinnitus mainly with either high-pitched pure tones or noises with a tendency to low-pitched (roaring) noises, NH participants perceiving a transient tinnitus after LF-exposure matched that tinnitus with high- or low-pitched noises or low-pitched pure tones. In the few studies available in the literature, MD patients were found to perceive mainly LF tinnitus (16–21), albeit reports on MD patients with high-frequency tinnitus exist (12, 13, 36). Tinnitus percepts of MD patients in the current study were more diverse, and this is probably due to the following reasons: first, the matching procedures employed in the available literature differed from our advanced matching paradigm, in that participants could adjust matching stimuli on their own without any interference or bias caused by the examiner. Furthermore, participants could choose between two matching stimulus classes (pure tones and noises). Second, participating MD patients were heterogeneous regarding age (26–74 years). As the onset of MD symptoms generally occurs around 30–50 years (37, 38), younger MD patients without age-related hearing loss are underrepresented in our patient population. Nevertheless, contralateral, unaffected ears of all participating patients were within the normal hearing range when considering the age-corrected pure-tone average at 2, 3, and 4 kHz. This is important as the matching stimulus was delivered to the unaffected ear. All patients, despite their age, were in a stage of the disease with fluctuating symptoms.

In the following, we will dissect tinnitus percepts into tonal and noise-like tinnitus and discuss tinnitus loudness for both kinds of percepts in the end. Underlying mechanisms possibly generating the tinnitus percepts in both MD patients and NH participants after LF exposure will be proposed for tonal and noise-like tinnitus separately.

Tonal Tinnitus Generation

MD patients mainly chose high-frequency matching tones when their tinnitus was predominantly tonal. This is comparable to the tinnitus quality typically related to inner hair cell (IHC) and OHC damage (39). Here, it was suggested that the tinnitus frequency roughly corresponds to characteristic frequency of the impaired hair cells or to the frequency at the boundary between intact and impaired hair cells (40, 41). This tinnitus mechanism might generate the tonal tinnitus percepts MD patients perceive. Audiograms of MD patients often show LF hearing loss but high-frequency hearing loss also occurs, mostly in later stages of the disease (12, 13). The majority of MD patients in this study showed greatly reduced DPOAE levels as judged from measurements acquired during the clinical routine. This indicates some degree of OHC function impairment, but it is unclear if this is age-related or due to the presence of endolymphatic hydrops. OHC loss might not suffice to induce tinnitus. Therefore, damage to IHCs or the auditory nerve, which cannot be detected with DPOAE measurements, might also be required. Given the presence of both IHC and OHC dysfunction, tonal tinnitus could also be the result of endolymphatic hydrops (or its underlying pathology) combined with the pre-existing hair cell dysfunction.

Tonal tinnitus in NH participants after LF exposure showing frequencies below 2 kHz is presumably triggered by transiently challenged cochlear homeostasis. Intense, LF sound causes broad excitation patterns peaking at the apical part of the cochlea. Thus, effects on cochlear homeostasis are not restricted to the characteristic frequency region of LF sound and higher-frequency regions can be affected as well.

Temporary tinnitus in humans is generally thought to be caused by temporary decrease of OHC amplification, which results in increased firing in the central auditory system and tinnitus generation (42). Although this generation mechanism cannot be ruled out, especially for participants showing temporary worsening of hearing threshold after LF exposure, it seems to be unlikely because of concurrent, increasing OAE levels typically following LF exposure due to enhanced OHC amplification (30). Temporary enhanced amplification and increased OAE levels might contribute to a different generation mechanism.

In three participants, it could be shown that frequencies of the selected matching tones roughly corresponded to the recorded SOAE frequencies. Besides the fact that permanent tinnitus percepts originating from an SOAE are rare [between 2 and 4.5% (4, 43)], SOAEs seem to be a plausible explanation in the case of transient tonal tinnitus after LF sound exposure for the following reasons:

Tinnitus frequencies selected by NH participants in the present study correspond to typical SOAE frequencies. SOAEs in human adults are usually in the range between 0.9 and 4 kHz with distribution maxima near 1.5 and 3 kHz (44, 45).

Under normal conditions, SOAEs are relatively stable in both frequency and level (46). After intense LF exposure, however, frequency and level of SOAEs slowly cycle for a time period of about 2 min in a stereotypic manner with a level maximum typically occurring about 50 s after LF sound offset (27, 31). SOAEs presumably buried in the noise floor become detectable during that period. Typically, SOAEs are not perceived by their owner (47). It has been shown, however, that induced frequency or level changes of SOAEs can result in SOAEs becoming transiently audible (47–49), as the inhibition of SOAE perception at higher stages of auditory processing (45) might not be active anymore. Not all NH participants perceiving tonal tinnitus had SOAEs with frequencies similar to the chosen matching tone frequency. NH participants with recordable SOAEs often showed more than one SOAE, which would have resulted in a percept difficult to match with a single pure tone.

In NH participants without recordable SOAEs, SOAE levels might be significantly underestimated by external recordings after OAE back-propagation, compared to sound pressure level of OAEs within the cochlea (47). This is strongly supported by the comparison of DPOAE sound levels measured in the gerbil meatus and the electrophysiological response to the same DPOAE in the gerbil cochlear nucleus (50). Thus, for SOAEs to be perceived by their owner, it might not be necessary that SOAE levels, as measured in the meatus, exceed the individual hearing thresholds at the SOAE characteristic frequency.

Noise-Like Tinnitus Generation

In both subject groups, a major proportion of tinnitus matches indicated a noise-like tinnitus. In experimental animals, it has been shown that the endocochlear potential increases temporarily with intense LF exposure (22, 51), resulting in a depolarization of IHCs and consequently in an increased spontaneous activity of the auditory nerve (34).

While direct recordings of the endolymphatic potential in MD patients are not feasible, a similar mechanism is nonetheless conceivable. Increased spontaneous activity of the auditory nerve could lead to the perception of a tinnitus, for which Patuzzi (34) coined the term "rate tinnitus." If a large expanse of the cochlea was affected by the above mechanism, a noise-like percept would result.

MD patients perceiving noise-like tinnitus percepts chose mainly noises with negative tilts (low pitches). This is in line with reports that MD patients typically show LF hearing loss at frequencies below 3 kHz (14), suggesting that, for hitherto unknown reasons, the apical part of the cochlea is most affected, resulting in a LF rate tinnitus. But, presumably depending on the duration of the disease, audiograms of MD patients reveal a broad range of affected frequencies (15), which is also reflected in our study population. This might explain why MD patients selected matching noises not necessarily limited to the LF range.

During intense LF stimulation, cochlear excitation is not restricted to the characteristic frequency, but the whole cochlea is excited and individual differences in cochlear excitation patterns might exist. LF stimulation affects the apical end of the cochlea strongest and LF components should be more prominent in noise-like tinnitus after intense LF exposure in NH participants (corresponding to selected noises with negative tilt). Those NH participants that chose high-pitched noises to match their LF-induced tinnitus may have done so as a compromise to represent hybrid tinnitus percepts consisting of both noise and tonal components or cochlear locations other than the apex dominate the tinnitus percept.

Tinnitus Sensation Levels

Sensation levels of tinnitus percepts were estimated with previously selected matching stimuli. In MD patients, hearing thresholds even on the contralateral, unaffected ear were slightly elevated at higher frequencies due to age-related hearing loss. Therefore, for MD patients choosing a high-pitched pure tone to match their tinnitus, loudness matches might have resulted in lower values than loudness matches using frequencies at which hearing was normal (8, 52). Loudness recruitment could also contribute: for participants suffering from cochlear hearing loss, low to moderate sensation levels may be much louder than for NH participants because the lack of cochlear compression decreases the overall dynamic range of loudness perception dramatically (52, 53). Furthermore, low sensation levels of matching tones in MD patients can be due to tinnitus loudness fluctuations. Patients were measured between vertigo attacks when tinnitus loudness was typically lower than immediately before or during attacks.

On the other hand, high loudness values in NH participants could be explained with a shift of attention toward the suddenly occurring tinnitus percept. Tinnitus sensation levels after LF exposure were on average higher than tinnitus sensation levels in MD patients and higher than tinnitus sensation levels in most patients with pathologies other than MD. Studies showed that tinnitus loudness was generally matched with stimuli below 10 dB SL, even in participants referring to their tinnitus as loud (8, 10, 54).

Procedural Limitations

Participants were presented with a limited range of sounds from which they had to select. Although this limited range of sounds was chosen to facilitate the matching procedure, participants complained about not being able to adjust amplitude modulations or about being restricted to one stimulus class when hearing hybrid percepts with both pure tones and noises. Furthermore, for both MD patients and NH participants with an LF-induced transient tinnitus, tinnitus loudness, and sometimes even tinnitus pitch were varying over time. In case of MD patients, these variations can take place over days or weeks depending on vertigo attacks or the current stage of the disease (12, 13). In NH participants, fluctuations appear within the 1–2 min of tinnitus duration. This is inherent to the transient percept after LF exposure. To guarantee consistency, NH participants were able to retrigger the tinnitus percept by turning on the LF stimulation again.

In either case, tinnitus-matching results can only represent approximations of actual tinnitus percepts, constrained by both choice of offered stimuli and experimental procedures.

CONCLUSION

Estimates of tinnitus pitch reported in the literature are heterogeneous and depend heavily on the methods used. Here, we implemented a tinnitus-matching procedure with fewer constraints than in previous, comparable studies, including noises with adjustable spectral shapes. As a consequence, our results revealed a relatively large proportion of participants with noise-like tinnitus, which might have not been detected in previous studies mostly employing sinusoidal matching tones. Contrary to reports in the literature, tinnitus pitch in NH participants after LF sound exposure and in MD patients is not exclusively LF, and hybrid percepts with noise-like and tonal components can occur.

Noise-like tinnitus cannot easily be explained with localized damage to cochlear regions. Rather, a mechanism affecting a broad frequency range is needed. An increase of spontaneous activity of the auditory nerve was suggested to cause the noise-like tinnitus observed here. However, further experiments are now required to identify unusual patterns in auditory nerve spontaneous activity as a potential tinnitus generator in chronic and induced hydropic conditions.

AUTHOR CONTRIBUTIONS

MU contributed to study design, performed data acquisition, statistical analysis and interpretation of results, drafting of the manuscript, revised the manuscript, and approved the final manuscript. LW contributed to study design and data acquisition, critically reviewed and approved the final manuscript. EK contributed to data acquisition, revised and approved the final manuscript. RG contributed to data acquisition, revised and approved the final manuscript. MD conceptualized and designed the study, contributed to data acquisition, interpretation of results, drafting of the manuscript, critically reviewed and approved the final manuscript. All authors are agreeable to be accountable for the content of the work, integrity, and accuracy of the data.

ACKNOWLEDGMENTS

The authors wish to thank Benedikt Grothe for his valuable support of the study and Kathrin Kugler for critically reading earlier versions of the manuscript. Parts of this work have been presented at the 39th MidWinter Meeting of the Association for Research in Otolaryngology in San Diego, CA, USA.

FUNDING

This work was funded by a grant (01EO1401) from the German Ministry of Education and Research (BMBF) to the German Center for Vertigo and Balance Disorders (DSGZ) (project TRFII-6).

REFERENCES

Meikle MB, Vernon J, Johnson RM. The perceived severity of tinnitus. Some observationsconcerningalargepopulationoftinnitusclinicpatients.*Otolaryngol Head Neck Surg* (1984) 92(6):689–96. doi:10.1177/019459988409200617

Baguley DM. Mechanisms of tinnitus. *Br Med Bull* (2002) 63:195–212. doi:10.1093/bmb/63.1.195

Penner MJ. An estimate of the prevalence of tinnitus caused by spontaneous otoacoustic emissions. *Arch Otolaryngol Head Neck Surg* (1990) 116(4):418–23. doi:10.1001/archotol.1990.01870040040010

Baskill JB, Coles RRA. Current studies of tinnitus caused by spontaneous otoacoustic emissions. In: Aran JM, Dauman R, editors. *Fourth International Tinnitus Seminar*. Amsterdam: Kugler (1992). p. 79–83.

Bento RF, Sanchez TG, Miniti A, Tedesco-Marchesi AJ. Continuous, high-frequency objective tinnitus caused by middle ear myoclonus. *Ear Nose Throat J* (1998) 77(10):814–8.

Jastreboff PJ. Phantom auditory perception (tinnitus): mechanisms of generation and perception. *Neurosci Res* (1990) 8(4):221–54. doi:10.1016/0168-0102(90)90031-9

Norena A, Micheyl C, Chery-Croze S, Collet L. Psychoacoustic characterization of the tinnitus spectrum: implications for the underlying mechanisms of tinnitus. *Audiol Neurootol* (2002) 7(6):358–69.

Henry JA, Meikle MB. Psychoacoustic measures of tinnitus. *J Am Acad Audiol* (2000) 11(3):138–55. Available from: http://www.audiology.org/ publications-resources/journal-american-academy-audiology/jaaa-archives/ jaaa-archives-2000

Moore BC. *The Psychophysics of Tinnitus. Tinnitus*. New York: Springer (2012). p. 187–216.

Meikle M, Taylor-Walsh E. Characteristics of tinnitus and related observations in over 1800 tinnitus clinic patients. *J Laryngol Otol Suppl* (1984) 9:17–21. doi:10.1017/S1755146300090053

Ménière P. Sur une forme de surdité grave dépendant d'une lésion de l'oreille interne. *Gaz Méd de Paris* (1861) 16:29.

Paolino M, Ghulyan-Bedikian V. *Ménière's Disease and Tinnitus. Textbook of Tinnitus*. New York: Springer (2011). p. 477–86.

Ying Y-LM, Arriaga MA. *Tinnitus and Ménière's Disease. Textbook of Tinnitus*. New York: Springer (2011). p. 311–6.

Lopez-Escamez JA, Carey J, Chung WH, Goebel JA, Magnusson M, Mandala M, et al. Diagnostic criteria for Meniere's disease. Consensus document of the Barany Society, the Japan Society for Equilibrium Research, the European Academy of Otology and Neurotology (EAONO), the American Academy of Otolaryngology-Head and Neck Surgery (AAO-HNS) and the Korean Balance Society. *Acta Otorrinolaringol Esp* (2015) 67(1):1–7. doi:10.3233/ VES-150549

Havia M, Kentala E, Pyykko I. Hearing loss and tinnitus in Meniere's disease. *Auris Nasus Larynx* (2002) 29(2):115–9. doi:10.1016/S0385-8146(01)00142-0

Reed GF. An audiometric study of two hundred cases of subjective tinnitus. *AMA Arch Otolaryngol* (1960) 71(1):84–94. doi:10.1001/ archotol.1960.03770010088009

Graham JT, Newby HA. Acoustical characteristics of tinnitus. An analysis. *Arch Otolaryngol* (1962) 75:162–7. doi:10.1001/archotol.1962. 00740040168015

Douek E, Reid J. The diagnostic value of tinnitus pitch. *J Laryngol Otol* (1968) 82(11):1039–42. doi:10.1017/S0022215100069838

Nodar RH, Graham JT. An investigation of frequency characteristics of tinnitus associated with Meniere's disease. *Arch Otolaryngol* (1965) 82(1):28–31. doi:10.1001/archotol.1965.00760010030007

Caparosa RJ. Medical treatment for Meniere's disease. *Laryngoscope* (1963) 73(6):666–72. doi:10.1288/00005537-196306000-00003

Day KM. Twenty-five years' experience with Meniere's disease. *Laryngoscope* (1963) 73(6):693–8. doi:10.1288/00005537-196306000-00006

Salt AN. Acute endolymphatic hydrops generated by exposure of the ear to nontraumatic low-frequency tones. *J Assoc Res Otolaryngol* (2004) 5(2):203–14. doi:10.1007/s10162-003-4032-z

Hirsh I, Ward W. Recovery of the auditory threshold after strong acoustic stimulation. *J Acoust Soc Am* (1952) 24:131. doi:10.1121/1.1906867

Hughes JR. Auditory sensitization. *J Acoust Soc Am* (1954) 26(6):1064–70. doi:10.1121/1.1907450

Zwicker E, Hesse A. Temporary threshold shifts after onset and offset of moderately loud low-frequency maskers. *J Acoust Soc Am* (1984) 75(2):545–9. doi:10.1121/1.390488

Patuzzi R, Wareing N. Generation of transient tinnitus in humans using low-frequency tones and its mechanism. In: Patuzzi R, editor. *Proceedings of the Seventh International Tinnitus Seminar*. Crawley: The University of Western Australia (2002). p. 16–24.

Kemp DT. Otoacoustic emissions, travelling waves and cochlear mechanisms. *Hear Res* (1986) 22:95–104. doi:10.1016/0378-5955(86)90087-0

Kemp DT, Brill OJ. Slow oscillatory cochlear adaptation to brief overstimulation: cochlear homeostasis dynamics. In: Cooper NP, Kemp DT, editors. *Concepts and Challenges in the Biophysics of Hearing*. Singapore: World Scientific Publ Co Pte Ltd (2009). p. 168–74.

Kevanishvili Z, Hofmann G, Burdzgla I, Pietsch M, Gamgebeli Z, Yarin Y, et al. Behavior of evoked otoacoustic emission under low-frequency tone exposure: objective study of the bounce phenomenon in humans. *Hear Res* (2006) 222(1–2):62–9. doi:10.1016/j.heares.2006.05.014

Drexl M, Uberfuhr M, Weddell TD, Lukashkin AN, Wiegrebe L, Krause E, et al. Multiple indices of the 'bounce' phenomenon obtained from the same human ears. *J Assoc Res Otolaryngol* (2014) 15(1):57–72. doi:10.1007/ s10162-013-0424-x

Kugler K, Wiegrebe L, Grothe B, Kössl M, Gürkov R, Krause E, et al. Low-frequency sound affects active micromechanics in the human inner ear. *R Soc Open Sci* (2014) 1(2). doi:10.1098/rsos.140166

Kemp DT. Stimulated acoustic emissions from within the human auditory system. *J Acoust Soc Am* (1978) 64(5):1386–91. doi:10.1121/1.382104

Kirk DL, Patuzzi RB. Transient changes in cochlear potentials and DPOAEs after low-frequency tones: the 'two-minute bounce' revisited. *Hear Res* (1997) 112(1–2):49–68. doi:10.1016/S0378-5955(97)00105-6

Patuzzi R, editor. Outer hair cells, EP regulation and tinnitus. *Proceedings of the Seventh International Tinnitus Seminar*. Crawley: The University of Western Australia (2002).

Nakashima T, Naganawa S, Sugiura M, Teranishi M, Sone M, Hayashi H, et al. Visualization of endolymphatic hydrops in patients with Meniere's disease. *Laryngoscope* (2007) 117(3):415–20. doi:10.1097/MLG.0b013e31802c300c

Herraiz C, Tapia MC, Plaza G. Tinnitus and Ménière's disease: characteristics and prognosis in a tinnitus clinic sample. *Eur Arch Otorhinolaryngol* (2006) 263(6):504–9. doi:10.1007/s00405-006-0019-9

Watanabe Y, Mizukoshi K, Shojaku H, Watanabe I, Hinoki M, Kitahara M. Epidemiological and clinical characteristics of Meniere's disease in Japan. *Acta Otolaryngol Suppl* (1995) 519:206–10. doi:10.3109/00016489509121906

Gates GA. Meniere's disease review 2005. *J Am Acad Audiol* (2006) 17(1):16–26. doi:10.3766/jaaa.17.1.3

Jastreboff PJ, Hazell JW. A neurophysiological approach to tinnitus: clinical implications. *Br J Audiol* (1993) 27(1):7–17. doi:10.3109/03005369309077884

Robertson D, Irvine DR. Plasticity of frequency organization in auditory cortex of guinea pigs with partial unilateral deafness. *J Comp Neurol* (1989) 282(3):456–71. doi:10.1002/cne.902820311

Eggermont J. Cortical tonotopic map reorganization and its implications for treatment of tinnitus. *Acta Otolaryngol* (2006) 126(sup 556):9–12. doi:10.1080/03655230600895259

Nuttall AL, Meikle MB, Trune DR. Peripheral processes involved in tinnitus. In: Snow JB, editor. *Tinnitus: Theory and Management*. Shelton: PMPH-USA (2004). p. 52–68.

Penner M. Spontaneous otoacoustic emissions and tinnitus. In: Tyler RS, editor. *Tinnitus Handbook*. San Diego: Singular (2000). p. 203–20.

Yongbing S, Martin W. Spontaneous otoacoustic emissions in tinnitus patients. *J Otol* (2006) 1(1):35–9. doi:10.1016/S1672-2930(06)50006-6

Braun M. A retrospective study of the spectral probability of spontaneous otoacoustic emissions: rise of octave shifted second mode after infancy. *Hear Res* (2006) 215(1–2):39–46. doi:10.1016/j.heares.2006.03.008

Burns EM. Long-term stability of spontaneous otoacoustic emissions. *J Acoust Soc Am* (2009) 125(5):3166–76. doi:10.1121/1.3097768

Long G. Perceptual consequences of the interactions between spontaneous otoacoustic emissions and external tones. I. Monaural diplacusis and after- tones. *Hear Res* (1998) 119(1–2):49–60. doi:10.1016/S0378-5955(98)00032-X

Long GR, Tubis A. Modification of spontaneous and evoked otoacoustic emis- sions and associated psychoacoustic microstructure by aspirin consumption. *J Acoust Soc Am* (1988) 84(4):1343–53. doi:10.1121/1.396633

Long GR, Tubis A. Investigations into the nature of the association between threshold microstructure and otoacoustic emissions. *Hear Res* (1988) 36(2–3):125–38. doi:10.1016/0378-5955(88)90055-X

Faulstich M, Kossl M. Neuronal response to cochlear distortion products in the anteroventral cochlear nucleus of the gerbil. *J Acoust Soc Am* (1999) 105(1):491–502. doi:10.1121/1.424586

Salt AN, Lichtenhan JT, Gill RM, Hartsock JJ. Large endolymphatic potentials from low-frequency and infrasonic tones in the guinea pig. *J Acoust Soc Am* (2013) 133(3):1561–71. doi:10.1121/1.4789005

Goodwin PE, Johnson RM. The loudness of tinnitus. *Acta Otolaryngol* (1980) 90(5–6):353–9. doi:10.3109/00016488009131736

Buus S, Florentine M. Growth of loudness in listeners with cochlear hearing losses: recruitment reconsidered. *J Assoc Res Otolaryngol* (2002) 3(2):120–39. doi:10.1007/s101620010084

Fowler EP. The "illusion of loudness" of tinnitus – its etiology and treatment. *Laryngoscope* (1942) 52(4):275–85.

12

Cognitive Mechanisms in Chronic Tinnitus: Psychological Markers of a Failure to Switch Attention

Krysta J. Trevis, Neil M. McLachlan and Sarah J. Wilson*

Psychological Sciences, The University of Melbourne, Melbourne, VIC, Australia

***Correspondence:**
Krysta J. Trevis
kjtrevis@gmail.com

The cognitive mechanisms underpinning chronic tinnitus (CT; phantom auditory perceptions) are underexplored but may reflect a failure to switch attention away from a tinnitus sound. Here, we investigated a range of components that influence the ability to switch attention, including cognitive control, inhibition, working memory and mood, on the presence and severity of CT. Our participants with tinnitus showed significant impairments in cognitive control and inhibition as well as lower levels of emotional well-being, compared to healthy-hearing participants. Moreover, the subjective cognitive complaints of tinnitus participants correlated with their emotional well-being whereas complaints in healthy participants correlated with objective cognitive functioning. Combined, cognitive control and depressive symptoms correctly classified 67% of participants. These results demonstrate the core role of cognition in CT. They also provide the foundations for a neurocognitive account of the maintenance of tinnitus, involving impaired interactions between the neurocognitive networks underpinning attention-switching and mood.

Keywords: tinnitus, cognition, attention, depression, salience, neurocognitive networks

INTRODUCTION

Chronic tinnitus (CT), commonly described as 'ringing in the ears,' can have a broad impact on an individual, affecting cognition, mood, social functioning, and general well-being. The overall prevalence of tinnitus varies across studies, ranging from 5 to 43% depending on the definition and criteria used (McCormack et al., 2016), with CT typically occurring in 10–15% of the general population (Henry et al., 2005). Despite its significant impact, there remains no cure or agreement on the mechanisms underpinning the maintenance of CT.

Tinnitus is often conceptualized as the result of a failure in the process of habituation (Hallam et al., 1984). Habituation is the ability to suppress information that is not primary to our goals, or indicative of a threat to our well-being. This process is important for facilitating our ability to control our cognitive resources and switch toward information that is of primary concern at a given moment in time. Since our cognitive capacity is limited, cognitive control of attention plays an important role in prioritizing access to relevant resources (Engle and Kane, 2004; Unsworth et al., 2014). This is achieved by modulating or 'switching' attention toward more salient or relevant stimuli and inhibiting stimuli less salient or relevant to task goals (Gazzaley and Nobre, 2012).

A Neurocognitive Account of Attention-Switching

Cognitive control of attention is a core aspect of our executive functions, and is thought to involve three neural networks: the cognitive control network (CCN), the salience network (SN), and the affective network (AN; **Table 1**). Cognitive control of attention can be conceptualized as arising from the flexible balance of interactions between self-directed (the CCN) and sensory-directed (the SN) neural networks to determine the information that crosses an individual's awareness threshold for further processing (Corbetta and Shulman, 2002; Menon and Uddin, 2010; Cocchi et al., 2013). This may be modulated by the emotional associations of a given stimulus (AN), resulting in increased monitoring of emotional information through increased SN–AN connectivity, or reduced top–down regulation from the CCN (Ochsner and Gross, 2005). In other words, the emotions associated with stimuli are important to consider, particularly with regard to engagement of the SN due to its high connectivity with the CCN and limbic system structures and proposed role in facilitating network de/activation (Seeley et al., 2007; Craig, 2009; Bonnelle et al., 2012).

The ability to switch our attention may be influenced by (1) our ability to control our cognitive resources, drawing on processes of inhibitory control and working memory to support flexible cognitive processing of incoming stimuli, and (2) our ability to down regulate our emotions in response to these stimuli. Specifically, proficient cognitive control enables effective attention-switching by utilizing working memory resources to maintain awareness of relevant information, and inhibitory control to resist distraction from irrelevant stimuli or thoughts (Diamond, 2013). Proficient emotion regulation influences our ability to switch attention by limiting the potential intrusion of goal-irrelevant emotionally salient information via top–down modulation of the emotions associated with a given stimulus (Ochsner and Gross, 2005; Buhle et al., 2014). In the case of tinnitus, a failure to switch attention resulting from impaired cognitive control and poor emotional down regulation may lead to ongoing engagement with the tinnitus sound, thus maintaining awareness of the sound (**Figure 1**).

TABLE 1 | Neural networks proposed to underpin attention-switching.

Network	Function	Core structures
CCN	Goal directed orientation of cognitive, attention, and memory resources	Prefrontal cortex, intraparietal sulcus[1]
SN	Identification of relevant sensory inputs and facilitation of further processing	Dorsal anterior cingulate cortex, insula[2]
AN	Regulates the experience of emotions	Cingulate cortex, prefrontal cortex, amygdala, nucleus accumbens[3]

CCN, cognitive control network; SN, salience network; AN, affective network; [1]Corbetta and Shulman (2002), [2]Menon and Uddin (2010), [3]Ochsner and Gross (2005).

Cognitive Functioning in Chronic Tinnitus

The literature on unipolar depression has identified CCN dysfunction, notably hypoactivation, as potentially underpinning symptoms of rumination, poor attention-switching, and emotion dysregulation (Rayner et al., 2016). Behavioral indicators of these symptoms include (1) biased information processing and poor disengagement from negative stimuli, and (2) difficulties with cognitive flexibility that can be detected when assessing attention, working memory, and inhibitory control (Gotlib and Joormann, 2010). People with CT have shown impaired performance on tasks assessing these behavioral markers of CCN dysfunction when compared to people without CT (Andersson et al., 2007; Stevens et al., 2007; Pierce et al., 2012).

In particular, highly distressed individuals with tinnitus have reported greater personal salience of emotive tinnitus sentences than low-distressed and tinnitus-free individuals, which was associated with increased activation of hubs of the CCN and SN, including the insula, prefrontal cortex, and cingulate cortex (Golm et al., 2013). In addition, research investigating the cognitive functioning of people with and without tinnitus in groups matched for emotional well-being (anxiety and depressive symptoms) show impaired performance of the tinnitus group on tasks relying on cognitive control processes (Heeren et al., 2014; Jackson et al., 2014). Such findings suggest CT is associated with cognitive deficits, independent of any emotional effects that may impair cognitive function.

A recent systematic review of nine studies of working memory and attention abilities in people with tinnitus investigated subcomponents of attention, such as sustained, alerting, selective and executive attention. This showed preliminary evidence for impaired executive attention, including inhibition and switching, whereas, findings for other subcomponents were mixed (Mohamad et al., 2016). Supporting this, people with CT subjectively report a greater number of attention and memory failures in everyday life compared to hearing impaired and healthy-hearing individuals (Hallam et al., 2004; Alam et al., 2012).

These results support the hypothesis that there may be an overarching failure of cognitive control processes in people with CT, reflected in a reduced ability to switch attention away from the tinnitus sound to achieve efficient cognitive performance. This, in part, may be due to the heightened salience of the tinnitus, and its association with negative emotions, particularly anxiety (Pattyn et al., 2016) and depression (Langguth et al., 2011). Stated another way, an imbalance in the regulation of the interactions between the CCN, SN, and AN may contribute to the maintenance of tinnitus by continued assignment of attentional resources and emotional salience to the tinnitus sound (**Figure 1**). As such, furthering our understanding of cognitive control, and how this relates to the emotional well-being and subjective cognitive experiences of individuals with CT represents an important next step in understanding the role of cognition in the maintenance of CT.

The aim of the current study was to investigate cognitive markers of the ability to switch attention in people with CT to determine the role of impaired cognitive control and emotional down regulation in the maintenance of tinnitus. We

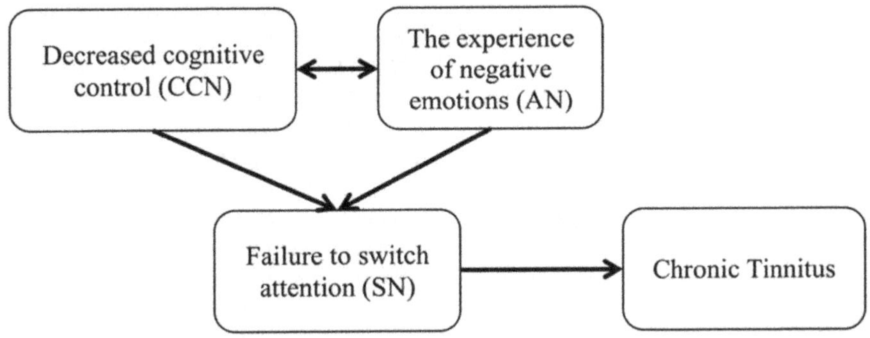

FIGURE 1 | Flow diagram of the proposed relationship between attention-switching and chronic tinnitus (CT), resulting from decreased cognitive control and emotional down regulation.

hypothesized that (1) participants with CT would have slower reaction times on a cognitive control task compared to healthy-hearing participants, reflecting less efficient CCN functioning; (2) participants with CT would report poorer emotional well-being than healthy-hearing participants, reflecting the emotional impact and salience of the tinnitus; (3) both poor cognitive control and emotional well-being would predict the experience of tinnitus, reflecting their dual contribution to the maintenance of CT; and (4) subjective report of cognitive difficulties would be associated with objective cognitive task performance.

MATERIALS AND METHODS

Participants

We recruited 26 people with self-identified CT who formed the CT group, and 29 healthy-hearing controls (HC) between 18 and 60 years using advertisements in local online newsletters and on noticeboards. Using G*Power (v3.1.9.2), a minimum total sample size of 42 was estimated to detect a moderate effect size (f = 0.39, derived from Heeren et al., 2014) in a repeated measures ANOVA, with power of 0.80 and $\alpha = 0.05$. Inclusion criteria for the CT group were (1) the experience of tinnitus for $\geq$3 months, and (2) experiencing the tinnitus as constantly (always) present (Hoffman and Reed, 2004). For the HC group, individuals were screened for tinnitus symptoms and hearing impairments, resulting in the exclusion of three individuals. The study was approved by the Human Research Ethics Committee at The University of Melbourne, and all participants gave written informed consent in accordance with the Declaration of Helsinki. There were no significant differences between the two groups for age, gender or education level (all $p > 0.10$). Demographic characteristics of the two groups are summarized in **Table 2**.

We used the World Health Organisation's definition of hearing impairment to determine the degree of hearing health for all participants for whom an audiogram was available (CT $n = 25$, HC $n = 26$; **Figure 2**; Concha-Barrientos et al., 2004). For each participant we calculated average hearing thresholds (dB) across four main frequencies (500, 1000, 2000, 4000 Hz) for each ear. The resulting average hearing threshold for the better ear was

TABLE 2 | Participant characteristics.

	Chronic tinnitus group (n = 26)	Healthy control group (n = 26)
Mean age, years (*SD*)	40.31 (14.67)	34.15 (11.55)
Gender	42% female	54% female
Education level	77% tertiary	92% tertiary

then classified using the World Health Organisation's hearing impairment grading system to classify the potential impact of hearing loss on daily life. This scale ranges from no impairment ($\leq$25 dB) to profound impairment ($\geq$81 dB; Concha-Barrientos et al., 2004). We found no significant difference between the two groups with regard to hearing impairment [$\chi^2(2, n = 51)$, 3.32, $p = 0.19$] and the average hearing threshold for each frequency was <25 dB in both groups, suggesting normal hearing ability at the group-level at each frequency. However, Mann–Whitney U-test comparing the groups at each frequency indicated that hearing thresholds in the CT group were significantly lower than the HC group at 2000 Hz (U = 212.50, p = 0.03) and 4000 Hz (U = 155.50, p < 0.001). Thus, we examined the data individually and found that all HC participants had normal hearing, while three participants in the CT group (12%) had impaired hearing (one slight impairment, two moderate impairment). Since removal of these three participants from the main analyses of the study did not change the significance of the results, all participants were retained for sample completeness and to reflect the heterogeneity of the presentation of CT. The tinnitus characteristics of the CT group are summarized in **Table 3**.

Cognitive Tasks

The cognitive control and inhibition tasks were programmed using Presentation software (Neurobehavioral Systems Inc, 2014) and delivered on a 13″ laptop screen, with responses made using a wireless mouse. The stimuli were capital letters in white Tahoma 24 point font on a black background, presented centrally on the screen. Participants were tested in a sound proof booth, and sat at a desk at a comfortable viewing distance and angle from the screen.

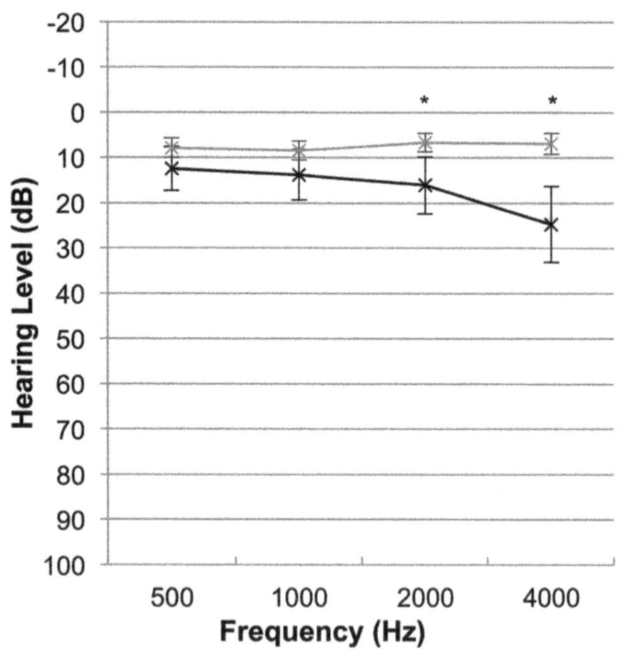

FIGURE 2 | Mean audiograms for the chronic tinnitus (CT; black line) and healthy control (HC; gray line) groups (*p < 0.05). 25 dB is considered the impairment threshold.

TABLE 3 | Tinnitus characteristics (n = 26).

Mean years with tinnitus (SD)	13.50 (14.08)
Mean tinnitus awareness, range 0–100 (SD)	39.35 (26.45)
Mean tinnitus annoyance, range 0–100 (SD)	17.17 (21.57)
Mean tinnitus loudness, range 0–100 (SD)	41.92 (22.18)
Tinnitus laterality	
Left ear	2 (8%)
Both ears, worse in left	2 (8%)
Both ears/inside the head	14 (53%)
Both ears, worse in right	5 (19%)
Right ear	3 (12%)
Onset	
Sudden	7 (27%)
Gradual	18 (69%)
Unknown	1 (4%)
Believed cause	
Known[a]	17 (65%)
Unknown	9 (35%)

[a]65% of individuals reported known causes of their tinnitus including stress (25%), music (25%), medical causes (20%), loud sound blast (10%), prolonged noise exposure (10%), head injury (5%), and hearing changes (5%).

Cognitive Control

We utilized an established cognitive control task also known to activate the CCN in neuroimaging work; the 'n-back' task (Owen et al., 2005; Niendam et al., 2012). We measured cognitive control in conditions of low and high cognitive load as reaction times on this task are sensitive to manipulations of cognitive load (Braver et al., 1997; Jaeggi et al., 2007). One of eight capital letters ("C", "G", "H", "K", "P", "Q", "T", or "W") was shown on the laptop screen in a pseudorandom order for 500 ms, followed by a blank screen for 2500 ms. Participants were asked to respond by clicking the mouse whenever a target letter was shown. In the low cognitive load condition (0-back), the target was a specific letter that participants were instructed to respond to at the start of each block (e.g., "C"). In the high cognitive load condition (2-back), participants were instructed to respond to the target which occurred when a letter was the same as the one seen two previously. Each block lasted approximately 1 min and comprised 20 letters, of which 30% were targets. Each participant completed one run of the task, comprising three blocks of the 0-back and three blocks of the 2-back, presented in random order. Before each block, participants were reminded of the instructions, and could take a break if required. We also used a short 10-letter practice block to train participants on the task, for which 60% of targets had to be correctly identified in both the 0-back and 2-back conditions prior to commencing the experimental run.

Inhibitory Control

We used the gold-standard Stop-Signal Task to assess the inhibitory control of attention given this contributes to performance on the n-back task (Logan et al., 1997; Avila and Parcet, 2001). Participants were required to respond as quickly as possible to the letters 'A' and 'Z' when they appeared on the laptop screen using the left ('A') and right ('Z') mouse buttons respectively. The letters were preceded by a fixation cross (500 ms) and displayed for 1000 ms. Participants were instructed to inhibit their response if a letter 'X' was also shown on the screen (the 'stop signal'). The 'stop signal' was presented in red font for 150 ms, with a delay between the onset of the primary letter ('A' or 'Z') and the stop signal of 250 ms. This delay varied by ±50 ms based on the participant's stopping accuracy (with a minimum delay of 50 ms and a maximum of 500 ms). There was a 1000 ms break between each trial, with 25% stop trials randomly presented over a total of 160 trials (80 for each letter), presented in random order. A rest break was provided half-way through the task. Before completing the task, participants were required to achieve a minimum of 50% correct responses on the practice trials, with a minimum of 10 practice trials shown.

Working Memory

We used the digit-span subtest of the Wechsler Adult Intelligence Scale – Fourth edition (Wechsler, 2008) to assess working memory given its contribution to cognitive control task performance. For this test, participants were asked to repeat back strings of numbers that gradually increased in length. All three subtests of the digit-span test were administered according to the test manual. In the first subtest, Digit Span Forward, participants repeated the numbers in the same order. In the second subtest, Digit Span Backward, participants were asked to recall the numbers in the backward order. Finally in the third subtest, Digit Span Sequencing, participants recalled the numbers in ascending order (from low to high). Each correct response is awarded one point, with a maximum of 16 points for each subtest. The total score for the three subtests formed the overall digit-span score. All raw scores on this test were converted to age-scaled scores, estimated using the norms in the WAIS-IV manual (Wechsler, 2008).

Emotional Well-being Measures

We used established questionnaires with well-documented psychometric properties as indicated by their internal consistency scores (α) to assess anxiety-proneness and depressive symptoms. The trait subscale of the State Trait Anxiety Inventory (STAI; Spielberger et al., 1983) was used to assess anxiety-proneness ($\alpha = 0.91$) and depressive symptoms were assessed using the Beck Depression Inventory (BDI-II, $\alpha = 0.93$; Beck et al., 1996).

Procedure

After providing informed consent, participants underwent a hearing test and provided sociodemographic information. The CT group also provided a history of their tinnitus experiences using the Tinnitus Case Sample History Questionnaire (Langguth et al., 2007), and we assessed the subjective impact of their tinnitus on daily life using the Tinnitus Handicap Inventory (THI; Newman et al., 1996). All participants also completed the Cognitive Failures Questionnaire (CFQ) to assess the subjective experience of memory and attention failures (Broadbent et al., 1982). Participants then completed the working memory and inhibition tasks, presented in counter-balanced order, after which they completed the cognitive control task in conditions of silence and in the presence of a repetitive background noise (control condition), with the order counterbalanced. Participants finished with the emotional well-being questionnaires.

Data Analysis

The Statistical Package for the Social Sciences Version 22 (SPSS) was used for all analyses. We tested the data for assumptions of parametric testing and identified extreme outliers, for which we applied a 90% winsorisation (<1% of data; Field, 2008). Where the assumptions of parametric tests were not upheld, more conservative non-parametric tests and log transformations for reaction time data were used to confirm the results. As no differences between parametric and non-parametric test outcomes were observed, the results of parametric tests on the raw data are reported here. We calculated effect size estimates for all statistical tests using eta squared (η^2) for analysis of variance models (ANOVA) and Cohen's (*d*) for independent sample *t*-test (Fritz et al., 2012).

To test hypothesis 1, that the CT group would have slower mean reaction times on the cognitive control task compared to the HC group, we performed an ANOVA on the reaction time data, with group as the between-subjects factor and cognitive load (0-back, 2-back) as the within-subjects factor. For the inhibitory control task, individual performance was first estimated using the integration method to calculate each participant's mean stop signal reaction time (SSRT; Verbruggen et al., 2013). We then compared the average performance of the CT and HC groups using an independent samples *t*-test. For the working memory task, we compared the Digit Span scaled scores for the CT and HC groups using independent samples *t*-test for the total test score and for each subtest. As inhibitory control and working memory are component skills of the n-back task, we performed secondary level analyses to adjust for these on the cognitive control task using analysis of covariance (ANCOVA) models.

To test hypothesis 2, that the CT group would report poorer emotional well-being than the HC group, we performed independent samples *t*-test on the group mean scores of the BDI-II and STAI-T measures. As mood and anxiety can influence cognitive performance, we also performed secondary level analyses to adjust for these on the cognitive control task, again using ANCOVA models.

To test hypothesis 3, that poor cognitive control and emotional well-being would independently predict the experience of tinnitus (i.e., group membership) we conducted a stepwise discriminant function analysis (DFA) with $\alpha = 0.05$ as the criterion for variables entering the analysis. We identified relevant cognitive and emotional well-being variables from those showing significant group differences in the analyses described above, and then examined their effectiveness in differentiating people with and without CT.

Finally, to test hypothesis 4, that subjective report of cognitive difficulties would be associated with objective cognitive task performance, we used one-tailed Pearson correlations (*r*) to determine if measures of objective cognitive ability and emotional well-being were significantly correlated with participant scores on the CFQ.

RESULTS

Decreased Cognitive Control in Chronic Tinnitus

In support of our first hypothesis there was a significant main effect of group, indicating that individuals with tinnitus responded more slowly on the 2-back and 0-back conditions of the cognitive control task compared to the HC group in silence [$F(1,50) = 7.23$, $p = 0.010$, $\eta^2 = 0.13$; see **Figure 3**]. As expected, there was also a main effect of cognitive load [$F(1,50) = 92.33$, $p < 0.001$, $\eta^2 = 0.64$], with faster reaction times in the 0-back condition ($M = 440.12$, $SE = 8.79$, 95%CI 422.46, 457.77) compared to the 2-back condition ($M = 602.53$, $SE = 19.21$, 95%CI 563.95, 641.11). There was no interaction between cognitive load and group [$F(1,50) = 1.95$, $p = 0.169$, $\eta^2 = 0.01$].

In addition to group differences on the cognitive control task, the CT group were also significantly slower on the inhibitory control task ($M = 242.01$, $SD = 47.25$) than the HC group [$M = 217.31$, $SD = 35.80$, $t(50) = 2.13$, $p = 0.039$, $d = 0.59$]. In contrast, there were no significant working memory differences between the CT ($M = 11.23$, $SD = 3.14$) and HC groups [$M = 11.65$, $SD = 3.17$, $t(50) = -0.48$, $p > 0.250$, $d = 0.13$] on the Digit Span total or subtest scores (all $p > 0.250$).

When we adjusted cognitive control scores for performance on the inhibitory control task by entering SSRT as a covariate, the main effect for group remained, although exhibited a smaller effect size and marginal significance [$F(1,49) = 3.96$, $p = 0.052$, $\eta^2 = 0.07$]. This suggests cognitive control task performance partially reflects inhibitory control performance. When we adjusted scores for working memory ability by entering

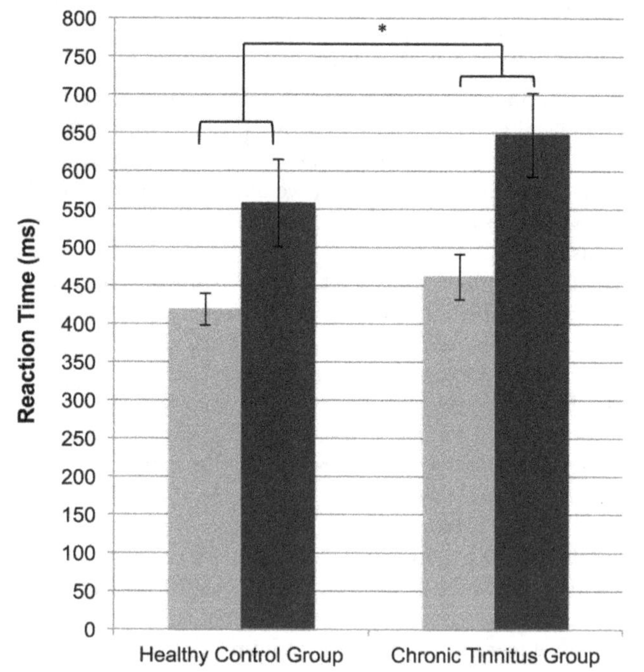

FIGURE 3 | Mean reaction times for the chronic tinnitus (CT) and healthy control (HC) groups on the 0-back (light gray) and 2-back (dark gray) versions of the cognitive control task (*$p < 0.05$).

whether these results were due to the presence of the tinnitus sound *per se* or a failure to switch attention away from the sound in the CT group, we compared the CT group's task performance in silence (tinnitus sound present) to the HC group's performance in the presence of the repetitive background sound. Here, we found a larger interaction effect [$F(1,50) = 5.74$, $p = 0.020$, $\eta^2 = 0.10$] indicating that when a noise source is present (tinnitus or background sound), there is a greater performance cost for the CT group as cognitive load increases (**Figure 4**). Consistent with the earlier analyses, we also observed main effects for group [$F(1,50) = 13.38$, $p = 0.001$, $\eta^2 = 0.21$] and cognitive load [$F(1,50) = 85.27$, $p < 0.001$, $\eta^2 = 0.63$].

Poor Emotional Well-being in Chronic Tinnitus

In support of our second hypothesis, the CT group reported significantly more symptoms of depression ($M = 11.79$, $SD = 10.03$) than the HC group ($M = 6.38$, $SD = 5.78$); $t(39.96) = 2.38$, $p = 0.022$, $d = 0.68$. In the CT group, 43% of people reported depressive symptoms in the mild-severe range (23% mild, 12% moderate, 8% severe) compared to 12% of the HC group (8% mild, 4% moderate, 0% severe). One tinnitus participant had a current diagnosis of clinical depression and was identified as a statistical outlier, however, removal of this participant did not change the significance of any of the described effects, and hence she was retained for sample

the Digit Span total test score as a covariate, the main effect for group remained significant and showed a similar effect size [$F(1,49) = 6.85$, $p = 0.012$, $\eta^2 = 0.12$]. While the groups did not differ significantly for demographic or hearing abilities, these factors could influence cognitive control and as such we assessed each factor as a potential covariate to determine the robustness of our findings. In support of our results, the main effect of group remained significant after accounting for age [$F(1,49) = 4.33$, $p = 0.043$, $\eta^2 = 0.07$], hearing ability [$F(1,48) = 7.32$, $p = 0.009$, $\eta^2 = 0.13$], gender [$F(1,49) = 6.64$, $p = 0.013$, $\eta^2 = 0.12$], and education [$F(1,49) = 6.26$, $p = 0.016$, $\eta^2 = 0.12$].

We also assessed if reduced cognitive control was associated with CT factors, including (a) the subjective loudness of the tinnitus sound, (b) the perceived impact of tinnitus on daily life, and (c) any perceived worsening of the tinnitus during task performance. Spearman correlations indicated that neither subjective loudness nor tinnitus handicap were associated with performance of any of the cognitive tasks (all $p > 0.10$). Similarly, independent t-test showed no significant differences for participants who experienced a worsening of their tinnitus ($n = 12$) compared to no change ($n = 14$) whilst performing the tasks (all $p > 0.10$).

Finally, we assessed whether our main effects could be replicated in the presence of background sound and found a significant main effect for group [$F(1,50) = 6.51$, $p = 0.014$, $\eta^2 = 0.12$] and cognitive load [$F(1,50) = 83.74$, $p < 0.001$, $\eta^2 = 0.63$], as well as an interaction effect where reaction times increased more for the CT group between the 0- and 2-back conditions [$F(1,50) = 4.23$, $p = 0.045$, $\eta^2 = 0.08$]. To distinguish

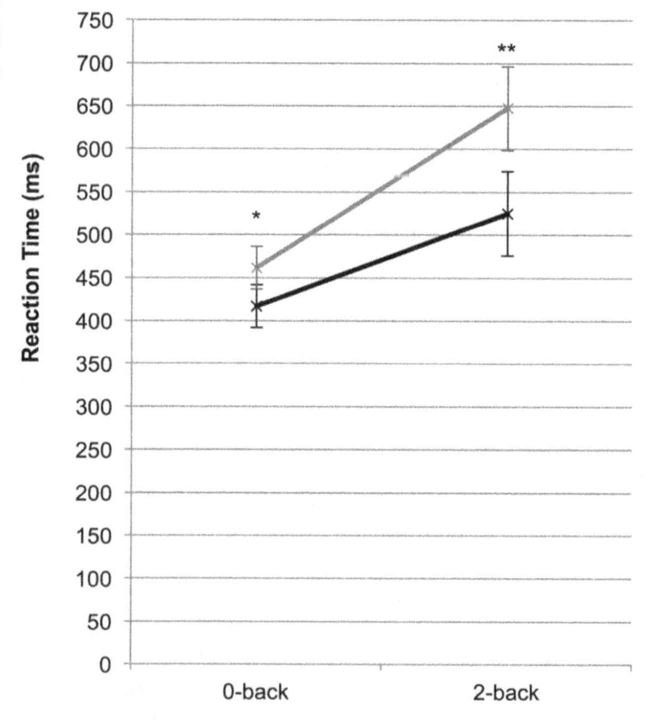

FIGURE 4 | Mean reaction time for the chronic tinnitus group (CT; gray line) in silence (i.e., tinnitus sound present) and the healthy control group (HC; black line) in the presence of a repetitive background sound while performing the cognitive control task (*$p < 0.05$, **$p < 0.001$).

completeness. No differences were observed between groups for the trait of anxiety-proneness $t(50) = 1.35$, $p = 0.182$, $d = 0.37$. We also assessed the influence of emotional well-being on performance of the cognitive control task, first by entering BDI-II scores as a covariate in the analysis. This indicated that the main effect of group remained significant with a similar effect size [$F(1,49) = 7.54$, $p = 0.008$, $\eta^2 = 0.13$]. Similarly, when we entered anxiety-proneness as a covariate the groups remained significantly different, again with similar effect size [$F(1,49) = 8.50, p = 0.005, \eta^2 = 0.14$].

Predictors of Chronic Tinnitus

For factors that showed group differences (cognitive control, inhibitory control, and depressive symptoms), we conducted a DFA to identify those factors that were most significant in discriminating between people with CT and healthy controls. Assumption checks for the stepwise DFA showed moderately strong correlations between the 0-back and 2-back conditions of the cognitive control task for both groups [$r_s(CT) = 0.40$, $p = 0.022$; $r_s(HC) = 0.40$, $p = 0.025$]. As such, to address the assumption of multicollinearity we removed the 0-back condition from the DFA in favor of the more cognitively demanding 2-back task. In this model, 2-back performance was identified as the core discriminating factor of people with and without CT, Wilk's $\lambda = 0.90$, $F(1,50) = 5.47$, $p = 0.023$, with the addition of depressive symptoms in the second step further improving the model, Wilk's $\lambda = 0.81$, $\chi^2(2) = 10.12$, $p = 0.006$. Combined, these two factors correctly classified 67% of cases and showed good sensitivity for participants with CT (65%), indicating that poor cognitive control and greater depressive symptoms were predictive of CT group membership. There was also good specificity (69%) for the HC group, suggesting low depressive symptoms and more effective cognitive control were consistent features of this group. Inhibitory control did not significantly contribute to the model.

To explore the data for effects relating to tinnitus severity, we conducted Spearman correlation (r_s) analyses between severity of tinnitus impact, cognitive control performance, and depressive symptoms. Since severity of the impact is considered a separate factor from the constant presence of the sound in the 'vicious cycle' of CT (Jastreboff et al., 1996), this analysis aimed to identify if either factor relating to its presence, also related to its perceived severity. We found that the degree of tinnitus impact was selectively associated with depressive symptoms ($r_s = 0.42, p = 0.033$), but not with cognitive control ($r_s = -0.32$, $p = 0.112$) despite both factors playing a role in correctly classifying people with and without CT. Combined these findings suggest ongoing awareness of the tinnitus sound may relate to reduced cognitive control, whereas depressive symptoms may determine the severity of its impact on an individual's daily life.

Correlates of Subjective Cognitive Complaints

The CT group reported significantly more subjective cognitive complaints ($M = 43.07$, $SD = 12.00$) than the HC group ($M = 34.35$, $SD = 14.51$); $t(50) = 2.36$, $p = 0.022$, $d = 0.66$, consistent with their objective performance on the cognitive control and inhibition tasks. Interestingly, we found differences in the pattern of associations between the CT and HC groups. The HC group showed an association between objective cognitive performance and subjective cognitive complaints, with significant correlations between scores on the CFQ and 2-back performance ($r = 0.38, p = 0.028$), between CFQ and SSRT scores ($r = 0.57$, $p = 0.001$), but no significant associations between CFQ scores and depressive symptoms or anxiety-proneness. In contrast, the CT group showed no significant associations between objective cognitive performance and subjective cognitive complaints. Rather, CFQ scores were associated with anxiety-proneness ($r = 0.69$, $p < 0.001$) and with depressive symptoms ($r = 0.55, p = 0.002$).

DISCUSSION

The present study addresses the role of attention-switching in CT by investigating two key aspects of attention-switching hypothesized to show impairments in this population, namely cognitive control and the experience of negative emotions. Consistent with our first hypothesis, we demonstrated slower reaction times in cognitive and inhibitory control in people with CT, whereas working memory function was similar to healthy controls. Consistent with our second hypothesis, we also found poorer emotional well-being in people with CT reflected by elevated depressive symptoms, whereas trait anxiety (anxiety-proneness) was similar to healthy controls. Third, we demonstrated a core role of reduced cognitive control in accurately classifying people with CT, while depressive symptoms were associated with its perceived severity. Taken together, these findings suggest that reduced control of the ability to switch attention may constitute a cognitive mechanism that maintains the awareness and severity of the tinnitus sound.

Cognitive Control and Tinnitus Awareness

Our results indicate that people with CT are less proficient at performing a cognitive control task compared to people with healthy-hearing, an effect which remained after adjusting for (1) performance on tasks assessing the component skills of inhibitory control and working memory, and (2) emotional well-being, including depressive symptoms and anxiety-proneness. Importantly, all participants were able to accurately perform and execute the cognitive tasks (n-back, stop-signal, and digit-span) and the groups were similar in age and hearing ability, two factors thought to influence cognitive abilities (Baltes and Lindenberger, 1997). Therefore, given the similarities in demographic variables between the groups, and the robustness of the effect after accounting for other cognitive, emotional and behavioral factors that could influence the results, it appears likely that the observed impairment in cognitive control is primarily related to the presence of CT.

An additional investigation of task performance in the presence of repetitive background sound provided further support for a failure to switch attention underpinning the observed impairment in cognitive control. In particular, replication of poorer performance of the CT group on the cognitive control task compared to the HC group in the presence of background noise suggests that the results were not due to the presence of the constant tinnitus sound itself, but rather a failure in attention-switching in people with CT. Specifically, there was a greater performance cost for people with CT as cognitive load increased when both groups were exposed to potential auditory distractors, suggesting that impaired top–down regulation of less relevant sensory information may underpin maintained awareness of the tinnitus sound. Consistent with this interpretation, we found no evidence that cognitive performance was influenced by factors relating to the tinnitus sound itself, including its volume, impact, or perceived worsening during task performance.

Since we found no overall differences in hearing ability between the groups, nor any influence of hearing ability on cognitive performance, and our main findings did not change with removal of participants with hearing impairment in the CT group, we feel it is unlikely that hearing ability accounts for the present results. However, given previous research has shown an association between uncorrected hearing impairment and cognitive functioning, particularly in older adults (Wayne and Johnsrude, 2015), the inclusion of individuals with hearing impairments may represent a limitation of our study. Future research directly investigating the relationships between cognition, age, and hearing ability may help to clarify the potential influence of these factors on the experience of CT, including the point at which hearing loss may pose a significant risk to cognition.

The similarity between groups for working memory may reflect this task's reliance on performance accuracy over processing speed, the latter being crucial to the performance of the cognitive control and inhibition tasks. This suggests that tasks relying on information processing speed may provide more sensitive measures of attention-switching in people with CT than measures of accuracy alone, potentially accounting for discrepant findings in previous research (Mohamad et al., 2016).

Psychological Salience and Tinnitus Severity

We have shown that there is a subjective emotional cost associated with the severity of tinnitus. Depressive symptoms not only predicted the presence of tinnitus but were also correlated with its severity, suggesting they play a specific role in determining the psychosocial impact of CT. This is consistent with recent findings of a core role of depressive symptoms in maintaining the awareness and impact of CT (Trevis et al., 2016). Depressive symptoms were also correlated with perceived cognitive difficulties in everyday life in the CT group, which may reflect the presence of a negative cognitive bias, which is a characteristic feature of depression (Rayner et al., 2016). These findings emphasize the importance of considering the psychological well-being of people with CT with regard to both effective treatment, and furthering our understanding of how cognition and emotion regulation, particularly with regard to low mood, can interact to maintain tinnitus awareness and severity. In addition, assessing the cognitive functioning of people with CT with or without depression would help delineate the contributions of mood and cognitive control to the presence and severity of CT.

Chronic Tinnitus and Attention-Switching

The present results indicate that both cognitive control and emotional regulation, two processes proposed to influence the ability to switch attention, are impaired in people with CT. Importantly, our results also suggest these processes serve different functions that are consistent with research on chronic pain, a condition considered to have similar underlying mechanisms to CT (Moller, 2007). In particular, our results suggest that depressive symptoms, cognitive control, and to some degree inhibitory control, may relate to the ongoing perception of the tinnitus sound, while emotion regulation, specifically of depressive symptoms, may relate to the perceived severity of its impact. Of note, symptoms of depression appear to be involved in maintaining both the awareness and severity of CT, which may reflect distinct roles for the cognitive and affective features of depression in specific aspects of tinnitus maintenance. For example, cognitive depressive symptoms (associated with CCN dysfunction) may be involved in the ongoing awareness of the sound while affective or somatic depressive symptoms (associated with AMN/AN dysfunction) may increase the severity and psychological salience of the tinnitus sound. In the chronic pain literature, research suggests that attention factors selectively modulate the awareness of pain, while mood selectively modulates the unpleasantness of the pain (Bushnell et al., 2013). Impaired cognitive control has also been implicated in anxiety (Derryberry and Reed, 2002) and depression (Fales et al., 2008), with both psychological conditions having a high incidence rate in CT populations (Zirke et al., 2013). As such, we propose that the ongoing awareness and severity of CT is underpinned by a failure of top–down cognitive resources, specifically cognitive and emotional control, resulting in a reduced ability to switch attention away from the tinnitus sound.

A Neurocognitive Approach to Chronic Tinnitus

A strength of our study involved the use of the *n*-back task, which is well-established in the cognitive neuroimaging literature to activate the CCN. In light of this, our findings suggest that people with CT may show hypoactivation of the CCN, decreasing top–down inhibition of the tinnitus sound. This, in turn, would increase the psychological salience of the sound (SN), which, in combination with reduced top–down inhibition of the AN by the CCN, may facilitate negative thinking about the sound (e.g., rumination) and emotion dysregulation (e.g., low mood).

In addition, the CCN is antithetical to the autobiographical memory network (AMN), also known as the 'resting state' or 'default mode' network, which is associated with introspection and rumination (Sheline et al., 2009; Rayner et al., 2016). To engage with the outside world through goal-directed behaviors we need to reduce self-focused thinking by suppressing the AMN, allowing the CCN to direct our cognitive resources and actions (Rayner et al., 2016). In CT, hypoactivation of the CCN may be related to a hyperactive, internally focused AMN, as suggested by resting-state connectivity data showing a highly connected auditory-limbic resting state network in people with tinnitus compared to people without tinnitus (Maudoux et al., 2012).

As illustrated in **Figure 5**, this neurocognitive account conceives tinnitus as a functional imbalance in the interaction of neurocognitive networks. Importantly, it distinguishes the neural networks associated with maintained awareness of the tinnitus sound, underpinned by a hypoactive CCN and hyperactive AMN, which facilitates ongoing attention toward a salient tinnitus sound. It also distinguishes the severity of the impact of tinnitus, underpinned by dysfunction of the AN, AMN, and SN, facilitating negative, internally focused processing of the sound. Considered this way, CT may reflect a fundamental failure of the CCN to inhibit the tinnitus percept when it is emotionally salient to an individual.

In support of the neurocognitive model, auditory processing of aversive sounds has shown reliable activation in the affective and SNs, particularly in the amygdala which is a core AN hub with strong connections to auditory processing (Zald and Pardo, 2002; Kumar et al., 2012). In addition, rapid habituation of the amygdala to aversive auditory stimuli has been proposed to be mediated by the SN (Büchel et al., 1998). There is also evidence of top–down control of auditory processing and associated neuroplasticity of auditory regions via CCN and SN hubs, including pre-frontal and parietal cortices, insula and the anterior cingulate cortex (Tzourio et al., 1997; Westerhausen et al., 2010). As such, there are established links between the functioning and plasticity of auditory pathways and the neurocognitive networks associated with cognitive control, emotion regulation and the salience of incoming sensory information (Westerhausen et al., 2010; Moore, 2013; Moreno and Bidelman, 2014). In light of this, the application of neuroimaging techniques to assess the integrity of these networks in people with and without CT would be beneficial to further assess the potential role of neurocognitive mechanisms in CT.

These network interactions are exemplified in a pilot real-time fMRI auditory control training study which found that conscious suppression of auditory cortex activation was associated with greater activation of the CCN and deactivation of the antithetical AMN, supporting the proposed role for these large-scale neurocognitive networks in the maintenance of CT (Haller et al., 2009). Consistent with this, a range of auditory-based activities have been shown to be protective of the psychological impact of CT, including auditory training therapies, real-time fMRI training of auditory control, and music training (Flor et al., 2004; Haller et al., 2009; Schneider et al., 2009). In particular, music training may be effective in alleviating tinnitus symptoms due to its effectiveness in improving (1) emotion regulation through its effect on the AN (Moore, 2013), and (2) cognitive functions via 'far transfer' effects on attention and working memory processes, which are mediated by CCN functions (Strait et al., 2010; Argstatter et al., 2012; Moreno and Bidelman, 2014). Investigating the possibility of training attention abilities through music or auditory control tasks may be a potential mechanism to attenuate the awareness and severity of CT worthy of further research.

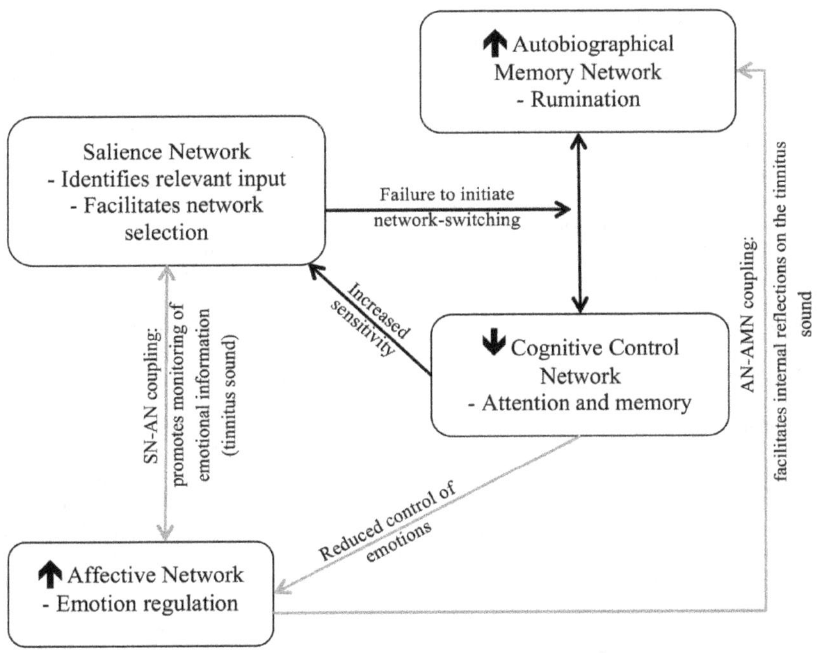

FIGURE 5 | Neurocognitive networks proposed to maintain tinnitus awareness (black arrows) and tinnitus severity (gray arrows).

Furthermore, psychological treatments aimed at strengthening goal-directed attentional control, such as mindfulness and cognitive behavior therapy (CBT) may benefit people with CT by increasing the proficiency of the CCN and improving its regulation of associated networks (SN, AN). Both CBT and mindfulness have been shown to be effective in lessening the impact of CT and improving psychosocial well-being (Philippot et al., 2011; Cima et al., 2012, 2014; Kreuzer et al., 2012). Specifically, evidence of neuroplasticity in regions of the neurocognitive networks proposed to underpin the impact and presence of CT have been found following CBT or mindfulness interventions (Frewen et al., 2008; Chiesa and Serretti, 2009; Brewer et al., 2011). In addition, the functioning of core hubs in these networks, including the dorsal anterior cingulate cortex and regions of the prefrontal cortex have been found to predict the effectiveness of CBT. This suggests that examining the functioning of the CCN and SN as part of 'treatment readiness' prior to commencing CBT may help to improve prognosis, engagement, and potential treatment benefits (Klumpp et al., 2014).

CONCLUSION

Our findings suggest that people with CT are less proficient in switching attention away from the tinnitus sound compared to people with healthy hearing. This highlights a core role of cognition, particularly cognitive control, in maintaining awareness of the tinnitus, as well as reduced emotional down regulation, with depressive symptoms associated with the severity of the tinnitus. Importantly, cognitive control and depressive symptoms provide targets for future treatment studies aimed at reducing awareness of the tinnitus sound and improving the well-being of people with CT. Finally, our results provide a foundation for establishing a new neurocognitive account of CT. This account suggests that a functional imbalance of specific large-scale neural networks associated with processes of attention-switching and emotion regulation may underpin chronic awareness of the tinnitus sound and the severity of its impact.

AUTHOR CONTRIBUTIONS

All authors contributed to the study concept. KT collected the data and completed the data analysis and interpretation under the supervision of SW. KT and SW wrote the manuscript, and NM provided critical revisions. All authors approved the final version of the manuscript for submission.

FUNDING

This work was supported by the National Health and Medical Research Council (grant number 1032042), awarded by the Australian Government. KT was supported by an Australian Postgraduate Award.

REFERENCES

Alam, N., Katarkar, A., Shah, P., Jalvi, R., Jain, A., and Shah, M. (2012). Audiological, psychological and cognitive characteristics of tinnitus sufferers. *Indian J. Otol.* 18, 20–25. doi: 10.4103/0971-7749.98288

Andersson, G., Kyrre Svalastog, O., Kaldo, V., and Sarkohi, A. (2007). Future thinking in tinnitus patients. *J. Psychosom. Res.* 63, 191–194. doi: 10.1016/j.jpsychores.2007.02.012

Argstatter, H., Grapp, M., Hutter, E., Plinkert, P., and Bolay, H. V. (2012). Long-term effects of the äúheidelberg model of music therapy äù in patients with chronic tinnitus. *Int. J. Clin. Exp. Med.* 5, 273–288.

Avila, C., and Parcet, M. A. (2001). Personality and inhibitory deficits in the stop-signal task: the mediating role of Gray's anxiety and impulsivity. *Pers. Individ. Dif.* 31, 975–986. doi: 10.1016/S0191-8869(00)00199-9

Baltes, P. B., and Lindenberger, U. (1997). Emergence of a powerful connection between sensory and cognitive functions across the adult life span: a new window to the study of cognitive aging? *Psychol. Aging* 12, 12–21. doi: 10.1037/0882-7974.12.1.12

Beck, A. T., Steer, R. A., and Brown, G. K. (1996). *Beck Depression Inventory-II.* San Antonio, TX: The Psychological Corporation.

Bonnelle, V., Ham, T. E., Leech, R., Kinnunen, K. M., Mehta, M. A., Greenwood, R. J., et al. (2012). Salience network integrity predicts default mode network function after traumatic brain injury. *Proc. Natl. Acad. Sci. U. S. A.* 109, 4690–4695. doi: 10.1073/pnas.1113455109

Braver, T. S., Cohen, J. D., Nystrom, L. E., Jonides, J., Smith, E. E., and Noll, D. C. (1997). A parametric study of prefrontal cortex involvement in human working memory. *NeuroImage* 5, 49–62. doi: 10.1006/nimg.1996.0247

Brewer, J. A., Worhunsky, P. D., Gray, J. R., Tang, Y.-Y., Weber, J., and Kober, H. (2011). Meditation experience is associated with differences in default mode network activity and connectivity. *Proc. Natl. Acad. Sci. U. S. A.* 108, 20254–20259. doi: 10.1073/pnas.1112029108/-/DCSupplemental

Broadbent, D. E., Cooper, P. F., FitzGerald, P., and Parkes, K. R. (1982). The cognitive failures questionnaire (CFQ) and its correlates. *Br. J. Clin. Psychol.* 21, 1–16. doi: 10.1111/j.2044-8260.1982.tb01421.x

Büchel, C., Morris, J., Dolan, R. J., and Friston, K. J. (1998). Brain systems mediating aversive conditioning: an event related fMRI study. *Neuron* 20, 947–957. doi: 10.1016/S0896-6273(00)80476-6

Buhle, J. T., Silvers, J. A., Wager, T. D., Lopez, R., Onyemekwu, C., Kober, H., et al. (2014). Cognitive reappraisal of emotion: a meta-analysis of human neuroimaging studies. *Cereb. Cortex* 24, 2981–2990. doi: 10.1093/cercor/bht154

Bushnell, M. C., Čeko, M., and Low, L. A. (2013). Cognitive and emotional control of pain and its disruption in chronic pain. *Nat. Rev. Neurosci.* 14, 502–511. doi: 10.1038/nrn3516

Chiesa, A., and Serretti, A. (2009). A systematic review of neurobiological and clinical features of mindfulness meditations. *Psychol. Med.* 40, 1239–1252. doi: 10.1017/S0033291709991747

Cima, R. F., Maes, I. H., Joore, M. A., Scheyen, D. J., Ei Refaie, A., Baguley, D. M., et al. (2012). Specialised treatment based on cognitive behaviour therapy versus usual care for tinnitus: a randomised controlled trial. *Lancet* 379, 1951–1959. doi: 10.1016/S0140-6736(12)60469-3

Cima, R. F. F., Andersson, G., Schmidt, C. J., and Henry, J. A. (2014). Cognitive-behavioral treatments for tinnitus: a review of the literature. *J. Am. Acad. Audiol.* 25, 29–61. doi: 10.3766/jaaa.25.1.4

Cocchi, L., Zalesky, A., Fornito, A., and Mattingley, J. B. (2013). Dynamic cooperation and competition between brain systems during cognitive control. *Trends Cogn. Sci.* 17, 493–501. doi: 10.1016/j.tics.2013.08.006

Concha-Barrientos, M., Campbell-Lendrum, D., and Steenland, K. (2004). *Occupational Noise: Assessing the Burden of Bisease from Work-related Hearing Impairment at National and Local Levels. WHO. Environmental Burden of Disease Series, No. 9.* Geneva: World Health Organization.

Corbetta, M., and Shulman, G. L. (2002). Control of goal-directed and stimulus-driven attention in the brain. *Nat. Rev. Neurosci.* 3, 215–229. doi: 10.1038/nrn755

Craig, A. D. (2009). How do you feel—now? the anterior insula and human awareness. *Nat. Rev. Neurosci* 10, 59–70.

Derryberry, D., and Reed, M. A. (2002). Anxiety-related attentional biases and their regulation by attentional control. *J. Abnorm. Psychol.* 111, 225–236. doi: 10.1037//0021-843X.111.2.225

Diamond, A. (2013). Executive Functions. *Annu. Rev. Psychol.* 64, 135–168. doi: 10.1146/annurev-psych-113011-143750

Engle, R. W., and Kane, M. J. (2004). Executive attention, working memory capacity, and a two-factor theory of cognitive control. *Psychol. Learn. Motiv.* 44, 145–199. doi: 10.1016/S0079-7421(03)44005-X

Fales, C. L., Barch, D. M., Rundle, M. M., Mintun, M. A., Snyder, A. Z., Cohen, J. D., et al. (2008). Altered emotional interference processing in affective and cognitive-control brain circuitry in major depression. *Biol. Psychiatry* 63, 377–384. doi: 10.1016/j.biopsych.2007.06.012

Field, A. (2008). *Discovering Statistics Using SPSS*. Thousand Oaks, CA: SAGE Publications.

Flor, H., Hoffmann, D., Struve, M., and Diesch, E. (2004). Auditory discrimination training for the treatment of tinnitus. *Appl. psychophysiol. Biofeedback* 29, 113–120.

Frewen, P. A., Dozios, D. J. A., and Lanius, R. (2008). Neuroimaging studies of psychological interventions for mood and anxiety disorders: empirical and methodological review. *Clin. Psychol. Rev.* 28, 228–246. doi: 10.1016/j.cpr.2007.05.002

Fritz, C. O., Morris, P. E., and Richler, J. J. (2012). Effect size estimates: current use, calculations, and interpretation. *J. Exp. Psychol. Gen.* 141, 2–18. doi: 10.1037/a0024338

Gazzaley, A., and Nobre, A. C. (2012). Top-down modulation: bridging selective attention and working memory. *Trends Cogn. Sci.* 16, 128–134. doi: 10.1016/j.tics.2011.11.014

Golm, D., Schmidt-Samoa, C., Dechent, P., and Kröner-Herwig, B. (2013). Neural correlates of tinnitus related distress: an fMRI-study. *Hear. Res.* 295, 87–99. doi: 10.1016/j.heares.2012.03.003

Gotlib, I. H., and Joormann, J. (2010). Cognition and depression: current status and future directions. *Annu. Rev. Clin. Psychol.* 6, 285–312. doi: 10.1146/annurev.clinpsy.121208.131305

Hallam, R. S., McKenna, L., and Shurlock, L. (2004). Tinnitus impairs cognitive efficiency. *Int. J. Audiol.* 43, 218–226. doi: 10.1080/14992020400050030

Hallam, R. S., Rachman, S., and Hinchcliffe, R. (1984). "Psychological aspects of tinnitus," in *Contributions to Medical Psychology* Vol. 3, ed. S. Rachman, (Oxford: Pergamon Press), 31–53.

Haller, S., Birbaumer, N., and Veit, R. (2009). Real-time fMRI feedback training may improve chronic tinnitus. *Eur. Radiol.* 20, 696–703. doi: 10.1007/s00330-009-1595-z

Heeren, A., Maurage, P., Perrot, H., De Volder, A., Renier, L., Araneda, R., et al. (2014). Tinnitus specifically alters the top-down executive control sub-component of attention: evidence from the attention network task. *Behav. Brain Res.* 269, 147–154. doi: 10.1016/j.bbr.2014.04.043

Henry, J. A., Dennis, K. C., and Schechter, M. A. (2005). General review of tinnitus: prevalence, mechanisms, effects, and management. *J. Speech Lang. Hear. Res.* 48, 1204–1235. doi: 10.1044/1092-4388(2005/084)

Hoffman, H. J., and Reed, G. W. (2004). "Epidemiology of tinnitus," in *Tinnitus Theory and Management*, ed. J. B. Snow Jr. (Lewiston, ME: BC Decker Inc.), 16–41.

Jackson, J. G., Coyne, I. J., and Clough, P. J. (2014). A preliminary investigation of potential cognitive performance decrements in non-help-seeking tinnitus sufferers. *Int. J. Audiol.* 53, 88–93. doi: 10.3109/14992027.2013.846481

Jaeggi, S. M., Buschkuehl, M., Etienne, A., Ozdoba, C., Perrig, W. J., and Nirkko, A. C. (2007). On how high performers keep cool brains in situations of cognitive overload. *Cogn. Affect. Behav. Neurosci.* 7, 75–89. doi: 10.3758/CABN.7.2.75

Jastreboff, P. J., Gray, W. C., and Gold, S. L. (1996). Neurophysiological approach to tinnitus patients. *Am. J. Otol.* 17, 236–240.

Klumpp, H., Fitzgerald, D. A., Angstadt, M., Post, D., and Phan, K. L. (2014). Neural response during attentional control and emotion processing predicts improvement after cognitive behavioral therapy in generalized social anxiety disorder. *Psychol. Med.* 44, 3109–3121. doi: 10.1017/S0033291714000567

Kreuzer, P. M., Goetz, M., Holl, M., Schecklmann, M., Landgrebe, M., Staudinger, S., et al. (2012). Mindfulness-and body-psychotherapy-based group treatment of chronic tinnitus: a randomized controlled pilot study. *BMC Complement. Altern. Med.* 12:235. doi: 10.1186/1472-6882-12-235

Kumar, S., Kriegsteinvon, K., Friston, K., and Griffiths, T. D. (2012). Features versus feelings: dissociable representations of the acoustic features and valence of aversive sounds. *J. Neurosci.* 32, 14184–14192. doi: 10.1523/JNEUROSCI.1759-12.2012

Langguth, B., Goodey, R., Azevedo, A., Bjorne, A., Cacace, A., Crocetti, A., et al. (2007). "Consensus for tinnitus patient assessment and treatment outcome measurement: Tinnitus research initiative meeting, regensburg, july 2006," in *Progress in Brain Research Progress in Brain Research*, eds B. Langguth, G. Hajak, T. Kleinjung, A. Cacace, and A. R. Moller (Amsterdam: Elsevier), 525–536. doi: 10.1016/S0079-6123(07)66050-6

Langguth, B., Landgrebe, M., Kleinjung, T., Sand, G. P., and Hajak, G. (2011). Tinnitus and depression. *World J. Biol. Psychiatry* 12, 489–500. doi: 10.3109/15622975.2011.575178

Logan, G. D., Schachar, R. J., and Tannock, R. (1997). Impulsivity and inhibitory control. *Psychol. Sci.* 8, 60–64. doi: 10.1111/j.1467-9280.1997.tb00545.x

Maudoux, A., Lefebvre, P., Cabay, J.-E., Demertzi, A., Vanhaudenhuyse, A., Laureys, S., et al. (2012). Auditory resting-state network connectivity in tinnitus: a functional mri study. *PLoS ONE* 7:e36222. doi: 10.1371/journal.pone.0036222.t004

McCormack, A., Edmondson-Jones, M., Somerset, S., and Hall, D. (2016). A systematic review of the reporting of tinnitus prevalence and severity. *Hear. Res.* 337, 70–79. doi: 10.1016/j.heares.2016.05.009

Menon, V., and Uddin, L. Q. (2010). Saliency, switching, attention and control: a network model of insula function. *Brain Struct. Funct.* 214, 655–667. doi: 10.1007/s00429-010-0262-0

Mohamad, N., Hoare, D. J., and Hall, D. A. (2016). The consequences of tinnitus and tinnitus severity on cognition: a review of the behavioural evidence. *Hear. Res.* 332, 199–209. doi: 10.1016/j.heares.2015.10.001

Moller, A. R. (2007). Tinnitus and pain. *Prog. Brain Res.* 166, 47–53. doi: 10.1016/S0079-6123(07)66004-X

Moore, K. S. (2013). A systematic review on the neural effects of music on emotion regulation: implications for music therapy practice. *J. Music Ther.* 50, 198–242. doi: 10.1093/jmt/50.3.198

Moreno, S., and Bidelman, G. M. (2014). Examining neural plasticity and cognitive benefit through the unique lens of musical training. *Hear. Res.* 308, 84–97. doi: 10.1016/j.heares.2013.09.012

Neurobehavioral Systems Inc (2014). Presentation®, Version 17. Berkeley, CA. Available at: www.neurobs.com

Newman, C. W., Jacobson, G. P., and Spitzer, J. B. (1996). Development of the tinnitus handicap inventory. *Arch. Otolaryngol. Head Neck Surg.* 122, 143–148. doi: 10.1001/archotol.1996.01890140029007

Niendam, T. A., Laird, A. R., Ray, K. L., Dean, Y. M., Glahn, D. C., and Carter, C. S. (2012). Meta-analytic evidence for a superordinate cognitive control network subserving diverse executive functions. *Cogn. Affec. Behav. Neurosci.* 12, 241–268. doi: 10.3758/s13415-011-0083-5

Ochsner, K. N., and Gross, J. J. (2005). The cognitive control of emotion. *Trends Cogn. Sci.* 9, 242–249. doi: 10.1016/j.tics.2005.03.010

Owen, A. M., McMillan, K. M., Laird, A. R., and Bullmore, E. (2005). N-back working memory paradigm: a meta-analysis of normative functional neuroimaging studies. *Hum. Brain Mapp.* 25, 46–59. doi: 10.1002/hbm.20131

Pattyn, T., Van Den Eede, F., Vanneste, S., Cassiers, L., Veltman, D. J., Van de Heyning, P., et al. (2016). Tinnitus and anxiety disorders: a review. *Hear. Res.* 333, 255–265. doi: 10.1016/j.heares.2015.08.014

Philippot, P., Nef, F., Clauw, L., Romrée, M., and Segal, Z. (2011). A randomized controlled trial of mindfulness-based cognitive therapy for treating tinnitus. *Clin. Psychol. Psychother.* 19, 411–419. doi: 10.1002/cpp.756

Pierce, K. J., Kallogjeri, D., Piccirillo, J. F., Garcia, K. S., Nicklaus, J. E., and Burton, H. (2012). Effects of severe bothersome tinnitus on cognitive function measured with standardized tests. *J. Clin. Exp. Neuropsychol.* 34, 126–134. doi: 10.1080/13803395.2011.623120

Rayner, G., Jackson, G., and Wilson, S. (2016). Cognition-related brain networks underpin the symptoms of unipolar depression: evidence from a systematic review. *Neurosci. Biobehav. Rev.* 61, 53–65. doi: 10.1016/j.neubiorev.2015.09.022

Schneider, P., Andermann, M., Wengenroth, M., Goebel, R., Flor, H., Rupp, A., et al. (2009). Reduced volume of Heschl's gyrus in tinnitus. *NeuroImage* 45, 927–939. doi: 10.1016/j.neuroimage.2008.12.045

Seeley, W. W., Menon, V., Schatzberg, A. F., Keller, J., Glover, G. H., Kenna, H., et al. (2007). Dissociable intrinsic connectivity networks for salience processing and executive control. *J. Neurosci.* 27, 2349–2356. doi: 10.1523/JNEUROSCI.5587-06.2007

Sheline, Y. I., Barch, D. M., Price, J. L., Rundle, M. M., Vaishnavi, S. N., Snyder, A. Z., et al. (2009). The default mode network and self-referential processes in depression. *Proc. Natl. Acad. Sci. U. S. A.* 106, 1942–1947.

Spielberger, C. D., Gorsuch, R., Lushene, R. E., Vagg, P. R., and Jacobs, G. A. (1983). *Manual for the State-Trait Anxiety Inventory*. Palo Alto, CA: Consulting Psychologists Press.

Stevens, C., Walker, G., Boyer, M., and Gallagher, M. (2007). Severe tinnitus and its effect on selective and divided attention. *Int. J. Audiol.* 46, 208–216. doi: 10.1080/14992020601102329

Strait, D. L., Kraus, N., Parbery-Clark, A., and Ashley, R. (2010). Musical experience shapes top-down auditory mechanisms: evidence from masking and auditory attention performance. *Hear. Res.* 261, 22–29. doi: 10.1016/j.heares.2009.12.021

Trevis, K. J., McLachlan, N. M., and Wilson, S. J. (2016). Psychological mediators of chronic tinnitus: the critical role of depression. *J. Affect. Disord.* 204, 234–240. doi: 10.1016/j.jad.2016.06.055

Tzourio, N., Massioui, El, F., Crivello, F., Joliot, M., Renault, B., et al. (1997). Functional anatomy of human auditory attention studied with PET. *NeuroImage* 5, 63–77. doi: 10.1006/nimg.1996.0252

Unsworth, N., Fukuda, K., Awh, E., and Vogel, E. K. (2014). Working memory and fluid intelligence: capacity, attention control, and secondary memory retrieval. *Cognit. Psychol.* 71, 1–26. doi: 10.1016/j.cogpsych.2014.01.003

Verbruggen, F., Chambers, C. D., and Logan, G. D. (2013). Fictitious inhibitory differences how skewness and slowing distort the estimation of stopping latencies. *Psychol. Sci.* 24, 352–362. doi: 10.1177/0956797612457390

Wayne, R. V., and Johnsrude, I. S. (2015). A review of causal mechanisms underlying the link between age-related hearing loss and cognitive decline. *Ageing Res. Rev.* 23, 154–166. doi: 10.1016/j.arr.2015.06.002

Wechsler, D. (2008). *Wechsler Adult Intelligence Scale, 4th Edn.* San Antonio, TX: Psychological Corporation.

Westerhausen, R., Moosmann, M., Alho, K., Belsby, S. O., Hämäläinen, H., Medvedev, S., et al. (2010). Identification of attention and cognitive control networks in a parametric auditory fMRI study. *Neuropsychologia* 48, 2075–2081. doi: 10.1016/j.neuropsychologia.2010.03.028

Zald, D. H., and Pardo, J. V. (2002). The neural correlates of aversive auditory stimulation. *NeuroImage* 16, 746–753. doi: 10.1006/nimg.2002.1115

Zirke, N., Seydel, C., Arsoy, D., Klapp, B. F., Haupt, H., Szczepek, A. J., et al. (2013). Analysis of mental disorders in tinnitus patients performed with composite international diagnostic interview. *Qual. Life Res.* 22, 2095–2104. doi: 10.1007/s11136-012-0338-9

13

Decreased Speech-in-Noise Understanding in Young Adults with Tinnitus

Annick Gilles[1, 2, 3], Winny Schlee[4], Sarah Rabau[1, 2], Kristien Wouters[2, 5], Erik Fransen[6] and Paul Van de Heyning[1, 2]*

[1] University Department of Otorhinolaryngology and Head and Neck Surgery, Antwerp University Hospital, Edegem, Belgium, [2] Department of Translational Neurosciences, Faculty of Medicine and Health Sciences, University of Antwerp, Wilrijk, Belgium, [3] Department of Human and Social Welfare, University College Ghent, Ghent, Belgium, [4] University Department of Psychology, University of Konstanz, Konstanz, Germany, [5] University Department of Scientific Coordination and Biostatistics, Antwerp University Hospital, Edegem, Belgium, [6] Department of Medical Genetics, Faculty of Medicine and Health Sciences, University of Antwerp, Wilrijk, Belgium

***Correspondence:**
Annick Gilles
annick.gilles@uza.be

Objectives: Young people are often exposed to high music levels which make them more at risk to develop noise-induced symptoms such as hearing loss, hyperacusis, and tinnitus of which the latter is the symptom perceived the most by young adults. Although, subclinical neural damage was demonstrated in animal experiments, the human correlate remains under debate. Controversy exists on the underlying condition of young adults with normal hearing thresholds and noise-induced tinnitus (NIT) due to leisure noise. The present study aimed to assess differences in audiological characteristics between noise-exposed adolescents with and without NIT.

Methods: A group of 87 young adults with a history of recreational noise exposure was investigated by use of the following tests: otoscopy, impedance measurements, pure-tone audiometry including high-frequencies, transient and distortion product otoacoustic emissions, speech-in-noise testing with continuous and modulated noise (amplitude-modulated by 15 Hz), auditory brainstem responses (ABR) and questionnaires.Nineteen students reported NIT due to recreational noise exposure, and their measures were compared to the non-tinnitus subjects.

Results: No significant differences between tinnitus and non-tinnitus subjects could be found for hearing thresholds, otoacoustic emissions, and ABR results.Tinnitus subjects had significantly worse speech reception in noise compared to non-tinnitus subjects for sentences embedded in steady-state noise (mean speech reception threshold (SRT) scores, respectively −5.77 and −6.90 dB SNR; $p = 0.025$) as well as for sentences embedded in 15 Hz AM-noise (mean SRT scores, respectively −13.04 and −15.17 dB SNR; $p = 0.013$). In both groups speech reception was significantly improved during AM-15 Hz noise compared to the steady-state noise condition ($p < 0.001$). However, the modulation masking release was not affected by the presence of NIT.

Conclusions: Young adults with and without NIT did not differ regarding audiometry, OAE, and ABR.However, tinnitus patients showed decreased speech-in-noise reception. The results are discussed in the light of previous findings suggestion NIT may occur in the absence of measurable peripheral damage as reflected in speech-in-noise deficits in tinnitus subjects.

Keywords: noise-induced tinnitus, homeostatic plasticity, young adults, recreational noise exposure, ABR, speech-in-noise testing, otoacoustic emissions, speech-in-noise understanding

INTRODUCTION

Due to the large amount of social activities in which adolescents are exposed to high music levels such as concerts, night clubs, sports events, pubs, bars, etc., the younger population is at risk to develop noise-induced symptoms such as hearing loss, hyperacusis, and tinnitus (Smith et al., 2000; Serra et al., 2005; Beach et al., 2013) of which noise-induced tinnitus (NIT) is the symptom most frequently reported by adolescents (Widen and Erlandsson, 2004; Gilles A. et al., 2013). Tinnitus is often perceived temporarily after noise exposure, usually disappearing within a few hours. Prevalence numbers of temporary tinnitus vary from 45 to 85% depending on the definition of temporary tinnitus used by the authors (Mercier and Hohmann, 2002; Chung et al., 2005; Quintanilla-Dieck et al., 2009; Gilles A. et al., 2013). However, a significant amount of young people perceive permanent NIT for which prevalence numbers range from 3 to 15% (Widen and Erlandsson, 2004; Gilles A. et al., 2013). Several studies suggest that the amount of young people suffering from noise-induced symptoms has increased over the years (Niskar et al., 1998, 2001; Henderson et al., 2011).

Often, tinnitus is perceived in the absence of measurable hearing loss (Schaette and McAlpine, 2011). Spiral ganglion neurons are the first neural structures of the auditory system. The ganglion is almost entirely (95%) composed of type I neurons which receive synaptic input from a single inner hair cell. On the other hand, each inner hair cell forms synapses with 10–30 type I neurons (Davis and Liu, 2011). Previous research has shown that the characteristics of the sensory receptors largely determine the fundamental parameters but that the intrinsic properties of primary afferent neurons also contribute (Scroggs and Fox, 1992). Spiral ganglion neurons possess tonotopic specializations due to the tonotopically varying soma and axon diameter of putative type I neurons with the largest neurons situated toward the basal regions (Liberman and Oliver, 1984). As such, frequency coding and intensity coding is modulated by the spiral ganglion neurons by respectively gradation of the spiral ganglion neuron soma along the cochlear axis and spiral ganglion axon diameter variations around the inner hair cell circumference (Davis and Liu, 2011). Kujawa and Liberman presented an animal model showing that noise exposure caused suprathreshold response decrements (measured by auditory brainstem responses) while auditory threshold sensitivity recovered. In addition, degeneration of both the pre- and post-synaptic elements of the inner hair cell occurred throughout the basal part of the cochlea despite normal hair cell populations. It was shown that the loss of peripheral terminals of the cochlear neurons occurs almost instantly after noise exposure but that cell death and disappearance of the somata were extremely slow with a decrease of spiral ganglion cells of around 50% over a time period of 2 years (Kujawa and Liberman, 2009).

Pure-tone audiometry and otoacoustic emissions (OAEs) are well-known audiological measurements used in the daily clinical practice investigating the presence of hearing damage. Sometimes, auditory brainstem responses (ABR) are also measured in order to provide more information. However, the sensitivity of these tests in an early stage of noise damage is still under debate as it is suggested that OAEs and ABR thresholds are sensitive metrics of hair cell damage, they are insensitive to neuronal degeneration in cases loss of cochlear neurons occur in the absence of hair cell loss (Kujawa et al., 1995). Lately the focus has been on the use of speech tests for this purpose. The sensitivity of speech tests in quiet and in noise might have a higher sensitivity for subtle changes in hearing function (Jansen et al., 2013). Some studies reported that subjects with sensorineural hearing loss have worse speech reception compared to normal-hearing people during speech-in-noise testing using a steady state noise (Bacon et al., 1998; Lorenzi et al., 2006a). The use of amplitude-modulated noise during speech-in-noise testing might add important information concerning the underlying pathology in subclinical noise-induced damage. Many mechanisms are involved in the phenomenon of the so-called "masking release effect" but it is well known that "dip listening" plays an important role (Fullgrabe et al., 2006). Dip listening or "valley listening" comprises the ability to take advantage of relatively short temporal minima in the fluctuating background noise to detect important speech cues and normal hearing subjects benefit from it to a greater extent than hearing impaired persons (Festen and Plomp, 1990; Gustafsson and Arlinger, 1994; Dubno et al., 2002; Fullgrabe et al., 2006). It was suggested that this loss of ability may be attributed to an impaired temporal resolution in the hearing function of the patient group. However, studies have shown that the reduction of masking release is rather caused by impaired suprathreshold processing of the temporal and spectral domain such as abnormal coding of temporal fine-structure information and degraded frequency selectivity, rather than less-than-normal audibility (Gustafsson and Arlinger, 1994; Fullgrabe et al., 2006; Lorenzi et al., 2006a,b). Furthermore, some studies focused on the effects of tinnitus on speech reception in noise. Newman et al. showed that a group of hearing impaired tinnitus patients had significantly worse speech reception abilities compared to a control group with similar hearing impairment (Newman et al., 1994). In addition, the presence of tinnitus in the deaf ear of patients with single-sided deafness and tinnitus in the deaf ear, also affects speech reception in the non-tinnitus ear (Mertens et al., 2013). It is however still unclear whether subjects with NIT (even with normal hearing thresholds) also show decreased masking release during speech-in-noise testing. To our knowledge, amplitude-modulated noise has not yet been used in the assessment of early noise-induced hearing damage.

To date, little is known about the early signs of noise damage and it is unclear which audiological tests can detect and localize early noise-induced damage in adolescents caused by recreational noise exposure. Therefore, an extensive test protocol on a group of students was performed comprising: otoscopy, reflex measurements, tympanometry, pure-tone audiometry including high-frequency audiometry, otoacoustic emissions, speech-in-noise testing (with two types of noise masker: continuous and amplitude modulated), auditory brainstem responses, and tinnitus analysis and questionnaires in cases tinnitus was present (see **Table 1**). The present study aimed to reveal early signs of recreational noise damage in noise-exposed young adults by use of audiological tests available in clinical settings. It is hypothesized that young adults with tinnitus show more peripheral deficit of the auditory system compared to non-tinnitus subjects which might be expressed by poorer auditory thresholds, decreased or absent otoacoustic emissions and/or deviating ABR results. Furthermore, it might be the case that tinnitus subjects perform worse compared to the control group at a suprathreshold level reflected in poorer masking release during speech-in-modulated-noise testing.

METHODS

A test protocol was developed in order to detect early-stage noise-induced damage in a young population in an early stage. The test protocol comprised the following audiological measurements: otoscopy, impedance and reflex measurements, pure-tone audiometry (including high-frequency audiometry), tinnitus analysis (in cases where tinnitus was present), otoacoustic emissions, speech-in-noise testing, auditory brainstem responses and questionnaires concerning hyperacusis and tinnitus (when present). This study was approved by the ethics committee of the University Hospital Antwerp (identification: 11/12/108). Written informed consent was obtained of all subjects. The original informed consents were archived and added to the personal medical document of the patients.

TABLE 1 | Demographic information concerning the study subjects.

	Mean age (years)	Total of subjects (N)	Tinnitus (N)	No tinnitus (N)
Male	23.1 ± 3.9	23	11	12
Female	23.5 ± 1.9	64	8	56

Subjects

Subjects were recruited by sending an email for participation to all Medicine students of the University Antwerp (N = 650) of which 91 students replied for participation. Exclusion criteria were: the presence of pulsatile tinnitus, middle ear pathology, known neurologic diseases, history of depression, and asymmetric sensorineural hearing loss. Students had to be below the age of 30 years old and should attend parties, concerts or festivals on a weekly basis. It was however stated that students could not attend such events 2 days prior to the testing date in order to control for temporary symptoms at the time of testing. A brief and limited questionnaire concerning tinnitus presence, tinnitus etiology, and noise exposure was answered by all subjects. Nineteen students perceived permanent tinnitus defined as tinnitus present for more than 3 months at the time of testing. All tinnitus subjects indicated recreational noise exposure as the most likely causal factor of their tinnitus (next to other possibilities: occupational noise exposure, head trauma, recurrent middle ear infections, other). Students were only included when going to a party/concert for at least once a week and/or when they used personal listening devices (PLDs) several times a week at a volume level of 70% or more of the maximum capacity of the device.

In total, four students were excluded from the study due to middle ear pathology. **Table 1** shows the demographic data on the test population. The following paragraphs elucidate on the methodology of the various audiological tests performed in the current protocol. ABR testing and speech-in-amplitude-modulated-noise (AM noise) was added to the test protocol in a later phase. As such, after initial testing, all participants were invited a second time for additional testing. Fifty two percent of the participants returned for the second testing moment. **Table 2** provides information on the amount of subjects who underwent the various audiological measurements. In all cases the ear of each participant with the worst PTA was included for statistical analysis. In the control group (non-tinnitus group) 43 subjects showed the worst PTA score on the right side and 25 on the left side. In the tinnitus group 8 subjects showed the worst PTA score on the right side and 11 on the left side. In the latter group, the included ears also corresponded with the ear in which the tinnitus was (most loudly) perceived.

Pure Tone Audiometry

Pure tone audiometry was measured in all participating subjects according to the clinical standards (ISO 8253-1, 1989) using a two-channel Interacoustics AC-40 audiometer in a soundproof booth. Air conduction thresholds were measured at 125 Hz, 250 Hz, 500 Hz, 1 kHz, 2 kHz, 3 kHz, 4 kHz, 6 kHz, and 8 kHz. In addition, extended HFA was performed including 9, 10, 11.2, 12.5, 14, and 16 kHz. Bone conduction thresholds were measured between 250 Hz and 4 kHz.

The auditory thresholds of tinnitus and non-tinnitus subjects were compared by use of Mann–Whitney U-tests. A $p \leq 0.05$ was considered as significant. Bonferroni–Holm was applied in order to correct for multiple testing. In addition, to test whether the tinnitus group contained a significantly larger number of clinically relevant outliers, the phenotype was recoded into

TABLE 2 | Overview of the audiological test protocol performed in subjects with and without NIT.

Audiological measurement		Number of subjects included	
		Tinnitus	No Tinnitus
Otoscopy		19	68
Impedance and reflex measurement		19	68
Tinnitus analysis		19	n.a.
Pure tone audiometry	Classical	19	68
	High-frequency	19	68
Otoacoustic emissions	TEOAEs	19	68
	DPOAEs	19	68
Speech-in-noise testing	Steady-state noise	19	68
	AM-noise	19	23
Auditory brainstem responses		19	23
Questionnaires	Hyperacusis questionnaire	18	50
	Tinnitus questionnaire	19	n.a.
	Visual analogue scale for tinnitus loudness	19	n.a.

HQ, hyperacusis questionnaire; TQ, Tinnitus Questionnaire and VAS-L; n.a., not applicable.

two groups: normal (<25 dB HL) and hearing loss (≥25 dB HL), and this recoded variable was tested for association with the presence/absence of tinnitus using a Chi Square test or a Fisher's exact test (in cases where the conditions did not fit the requirements for the Chi Square test).

Tinnitus Analysis and Questionnaires

To rate the personal tinnitus disturbance two instruments were used: the Tinnitus Questionnaire (TQ) for annoyance grading and a Visual Analogue Scale (VAS) for loudness grading. The TQ is an instrument which differentiates between emotional and cognitive distress, auditory perceptual difficulties, and self-experienced intrusiveness caused by the tinnitus (Goebel and Hiller, 1994). Looking at the total score going from 0 to 84, subjects are assigned to a distress category: slight (score = 0–30, grade 1), moderate (score = 31–46, grade 2), severe (score = 47–59, grade 3), and very severe (score = 60–84, grade 4). In the present study, a Dutch validated version of the TQ was used (41). In addition, tinnitus loudness was also assessed by a VAS (VAS-L) going from 0 to 10 (0 = tinnitus is not heard at all, 10 = an extremely loud tinnitus).

The type of tinnitus was evaluated by asking whether one perceived a pulsatile or non-pulsatile tinnitus, whether the tinnitus was perceived constantly or not, unilaterally or bilaterally, and whether the tinnitus sound was a pure-tone (ringing), a noise (hissing) or a mixture of different sounds (polyphonic). Tinnitus duration was questioned during the tinnitus analysis by asking the participants for how long they have had experienced constant tinnitus.

The presence of hyperacusis was evaluated by a Flemish validated version of Khalfa's Hyperacusis Questionnaire (HQ; Khalfa et al., 2002). According to Khalfa's HQ one is diagnosed with hyperacusis when the score on the HQ is 28 or more. While validating the Dutch version of the HQ, Meeus also compared the HQ scores with other hyperacusis measurements and found one can already speak of clinically relevant hyperacusis with a score of 22 on the Flemish HQ (Meeus et al., 2010). Therefore, the score of 22 was applied as a cut-off score for the presence of hyperacusis in the present study.

Otoacoustic Emissions

Transient evoked otoacoustic emissions (TEOAEs) as well as distortion product otoacoustic emissions (DPOAEs) were measured in all subjects. TEOAEs were elicited using biphasic click sounds of 80 μs presented at an intensity level of 80 dB SPL and recorded over a frequency range of 500–4000 Hz.

DPOAEs were elicited by use of a pair of two pure tone frequencies (f1 and f2) closely spaced and presented simultaneously at a level of 55 dB SPL for f1 and 65 dB SPL for f2 (frequency ratio f2/f1 = 1.22). The largest and most robust distortion product is 2f1–f2 and can be detected in almost all normal ears.

Non-parametric tests (Mann–Whitney U) were applied to assess possible differences between tinnitus subjects and non-tinnitus subjects for TEOAEs as well as DPOAEs. A $p \leq 0.05$ was considered as significant and the Bonferroni–Holm method was used to correct for multiple testing. In addition, to test whether the tinnitus group contained a significantly larger number of clinically relevant TEOAE and DPOAE outliers (SNR <3 dB and SNR <6 dB, respectively), the phenotype was recoded into two groups. For TEOAE analysis OAEs were considered as present when the SNR exceeded 3 dB and were considered as absent when the SNR was below 2.99 dB. For DPOAE analysis OAE were considered present when the SNR ≥6 dB. The presence/absence of TEOAEs/DPOAEs were tested for association with the presence/absence of tinnitus using a Pearson Chi Square test or a Fisher's exact test (in cases where the conditions did not fit the requirements for the Chi Square test).

Speech-in-Noise Testing

The Leuven Intelligibility Sentence Test (LIST; Van Wieringen and Wouters, 2008), a Dutch sentence test, was applied. The LIST consists of 35 lists of 10 sentences that are a reflection of daily communication and are of equivalent difficulty. An adaptive procedure is used with the noise at a fixed level of 65 dB SPL. The procedure starts at a signal-to-noise ratio (SNR) of 0 dB meaning that speech and noise are presented equally loud (65 dB SPL). Subsequently, the intensity level within a list of sentences is varied in steps of 2 dB adaptively in a 1-down (when the keywords in the sentence are correctly repeated), 1-up (when the keywords in the sentence are incorrectly repeated) procedure to determine the 50% correct identification point which is called the speech reception threshold (SRT), expressed in dB SNR. Before starting the actual procedure, one list was performed as a training list. Speech reception was calculated as the mean SNR obtained by the subject. For example, a score of −5 dB SNR means that the speech could be 5 dB quieter than the noise which is fixed at 65 dB SPL.

During the presentation of the sentences two kinds of noise masker were applied. A first noise masker was a steady-state noise spectrally matched with the long-term average speech spectrum so that the SNR would be, on average, approximately equal at all frequencies (Van Wieringen and Wouters, 2008). For the other masker used during the second testing moment, the stationary noise was amplitude-modulated by 15 Hz with a modulation depth of 100%, from now on referred to as AM noise.

Subjects were seated in a quiet room and the sentences were presented monaurally through headphones. The sentences were played directly from a computer using software interface TigerSpeech Technology (2012) and passed through an audiometer. Sentence levels were adjusted by the software during adaptive testing depending whether the keywords in the sentences were repeated correctly or incorrectly. Also the noise was played from the same software passing through the audiometer and was presented to the ipsilateral ear at a fixed level of 65 dB SPL. The levels of speech and noise were calibrated by a licensed company prior to the commencement of the experiment.

In order to test for normal distributions of the components, Shapiro–Wilk test of normality was applied and Q-Q plots were visually inspected. All variables were normally distributed ($p > 0.05$ for Shapiro–Wilk) in both groups. Consequently, parametric tests (student-t) were performed in order to find differences between speech reception in tinnitus and non-tinnitus subjects for steady-state noise as well as AM noise. In addition, parametric tests were performed to reveal possible differences in performance between speech reception during stationary noise and during AM noise for tinnitus as well as non-tinnitus subjects separately. Bonferroni–Holm correction was applied to correct for multiple testing.

In addition, a repeated measures ANOVA analysis was performed in order to see whether there was a different masking release effect of AM-noise for tinnitus subjects and non-tinnitus subjects when compared to the steady-state noise condition.

Auditory Brainstem Responses

Auditory brainstem responses (ABR) were recorded in a subset of tinnitus and non-tinnitus patients with the Bio-Logic Auditory Evoked Potentials system (version 6.2.1.1) and a Bio-Logic Navigator Pro® interface. The skin was prepared by use of a Nuprep gel in order to lower the skin impedance which had to be below 5 kOhm and inter-electrode impedance had to be below 2 kOhm. Electrodes were placed on both mastoids and on the high forehead with the common electrode on the lower forehead. Subjects laid down on a comfortable bed and the light was subdued. Subjects were also instructed to keep the eyes closed during the measurements and to minimize all muscle activity as much as possible.

100 μs-duration clicks were presented with alternating polarity through ER-3A earphones at a rate of 31.0 stimuli/s and a level of 80 dBnHL (= dB normalized hearing level). Contralateral white noise masking was applied with an intensity of 55 dBnHL. The signal was high pass filtered from 100 Hz and low pass filtered from 3000 Hz. Artifact rejection was set at 23.8 μV and a maximum of 2000 averages was recorded. In order to obtain the best possible outcome of the ABR testing, all recordings were repeated 3 times to ensure reproducibility.

ABR component amplitudes (baseline-to-peak) and latencies were determined by visual inspection of the waveforms I–V. Wave V is the most robust waveform in an adult population. Other waveforms may not always occur or be accurately identified by the clinician. In addition, latency ratios I–III, I–V, and III–V were calculated as well as the interpeak ratios I–III, I–V, and III–V.

Previous research has shown that the exact matching for pure-tone audiometry thresholds (with maximum differences of 5 dB HL) of groups is a prerequisite in order to be able to correctly analyze ABR data (Gu et al., 2012). As such, two separate analyses were performed. The first analysis was based on the data matched at a group level. Subsequently, a more precise matching was performed where every tinnitus subject was age- and gender-matched as well as matched until the level of 5 dB HL for pure-tone thresholds from 1 to 4 kHz (as this is the maximum frequency spectrum tested by the ABR). Therefore, in the second analysis, less participants were included to ensure the exact matching and only 10 pairs of perfectly matched subjects were obtained. The latter analysis was performed in addition to the group analysis in order to obtain reliable results. If Shapiro–Wilk test for normality showed normal data distributions, parametric testing was used.

RESULTS

Nineteen subjects had permanent tinnitus, corresponding with 22% of the sample. Noise exposure was briefly evaluated by a short questionnaire. All students with tinnitus attributed their tinnitus to recreational noise exposure. Party/concert attendance of students was approximately once a week. Sixty four percent of the control group and 52% of the tinnitus group attended a musical venue more than once a week.

Details on the tinnitus type, side and severity are shown in **Tables 3, 4**. Most young adults perceived a bilateral, pure-tone tinnitus with only limited tinnitus distress (on average a grade 1 on the TQ). The mean tinnitus duration was 2 years ($SD = 1.2$ years) and none of the tinnitus subjects reported tinnitus from childhood. The HQ was filled out by most subjects showing a clear difference between non-tinnitus and tinnitus subjects. Tinnitus subjects scored significantly higher on the HQ (mean = 15.39; $SD = 6.65$) compared to non-tinnitus subjects (mean = 7.71; $SD = 7.96$; $p = 0.001$). Only few subjects were diagnosed with hyperacusis though this symptom was relatively more prevalent in the tinnitus group. In the non-tinnitus group ($N = 68$) three subjects had a score >22 on the HQ while already four subjects of the tinnitus group ($N = 19$) had scores above 22. The sample of students with hyperacusis was too small to perform further statistical analysis.

Figures 1, 2 illustrate the median and the variability for the conventional audiometry and the HFA respectively as well as the differences between the tinnitus and non-tinnitus subjects.

TABLE 3 | Distribution of tinnitus type and tinnitus side characteristics assessed in the tinnitus group.

Tinnitus characteristic		*N* subjects
Type	Pure-tone	13
	Noise	6
	Polyphonic	0
Side	Unilateral	2
	Bilateral	16
	Central	1

TABLE 4 | Mean scores for the TQ and VAS-L, including standard deviations for the tinnitus subjects.

Tinnitus questionnaires	Mean	*SD*
TQ score	27.72	15.23
VAS-L score	5.44	2.46

No significant differences in hearing thresholds between tinnitus subjects and non-tinnitus subjects were apparent (see **Table 5**). Some outliers could be noted where the hearing thresholds exceeded 25 dB HL which no longer could be considered as normal hearing. It was investigated whether such outliers were more prevalent in the tinnitus group compared to the controls by use of a Fisher's exact test. Within the power of the current study, there is no indication that the tinnitus group contained a significantly larger fraction of outliers compared to the control group. More insight into the audiometric data is provided in the Supplementary Materials section.

TEOAE and DPOAE were compared between tinnitus and non-tinnitus subjects for each frequency band. **Tables 6, 7** summarize the otoacoustic emissions data which is also plotted in **Figures 3, 4**. No significant differences in OAE strength were found between groups for the measured TEOAE as well as DPOAE frequency bands. By the use Mann–Whitney *U*-tests to compare OAEs between the tinnitus and the control group it is likely to miss crucial differences between the two groups. In particular, clinically relevant outliers in the case group may be missed, since nonparametric tests transform the observed values into ranks. Therefore, additional dichotomizing was performed where TEOAEs were considered as present when the SNR was equal to or exceeded 3 dB SNR and DPOAEs were considered as present when ≥6 dB SNR. Chi square tests and Fisher's exact tests did not show—within the power of the current study—significant differences in the prevalence of present/absent OAEs in both groups. More insight into the latter analyses is provided in the Supplementary Material section.

Concerning the speech-in-noise testing, tinnitus subjects had significantly worse SRT scores compared to non-tinnitus subjects for sentences embedded in steady-state noise (mean SRT scores, respectively −5.77 and −6.90 dB SNR; $p = 0.025$) as well as for sentences embedded in 15 Hz AM-noise (mean SRT scores, respectively −13.04 and −15.17 dB SNR; $p = 0.013$) as illustrated in **Figure 5**. In the repeated measures ANOVA the between subject effect was "group" and the within subject effect was "noise type." In addition, the interaction between noise type and group was investigated. Significant effects were shown for group and speech-in-noise ($p < 0.001$) but no interaction effect was apparent ($p = 0.162$) meaning that the increase of masking release when going from steady-state noise to AM noise were quite similar for both groups with the difference that tinnitus subjects had a worse starting point. Also, a logistic regression was performed in order to explain the variance provided by speech-in-noise testing in NIT subjects. By use of this analysis it was confirmed that speech-in-noise testing by use of steady-state noise was worse in NIT subjects ($p = 0.018$) as well as in AM-15 Hz noise ($p = 0.011$). In addition, it was found that speech-in-noise testing explains 40% of the variance (Nagelkerke $R^2 = 0.403$).

Visual inspection of the ABR waveforms were performed. Wave V is the most robust wave in an adult population. Other waves may not always occur or be accurately identified by the clinician by use of visual inspection. Independent student's *t*-tests were performed in order to reveal differences between the tinnitus and control group for the latency and/or amplitude of the different ABR waveforms. **Table 8** provides an overview of the mean latencies, amplitudes, interpeak latencies/amplitudes, standard deviations, and the outcome of the independent student's *t*-test between tinnitus subjects and controls. After correction for multiple testing by Bonferroni–Holm, no statistical differences could be shown between tinnitus subjects and controls within the power of the current study.

For the second analysis, for which a very thorough matching was applied (see ABR description in the Methods Section), paired student's *t*-tests were performed but again did not show any statistical different ABR results between tinnitus and non-tinnitus subjects concluding the ABR data did not differ between groups in the present dataset.

DISCUSSION AND CONCLUSIONS

Audiological Tests Assessing the Peripheral Pathway

The current study examined a group of 87 recreationally noise-exposed university students. In total 19 students, corresponding to 22% of the study population, experienced NIT which was present for more than 3 months at the time of testing. Earlier epidemiological studies on noise-induced symptoms in Belgian adolescents has shown a high prevalence of NIT in this population in line with the current findings (Gilles et al., 2012; Gilles A. et al., 2013; Degeest et al., 2014). The present study compared test results of various audiological tests between the students with and without tinnitus. The testing consisted of pure-tone audiometry (including high frequencies), otoacoustic emissions, ABR, and speech-in-noise testing (with steady-state noise and amplitude-modulated noise). No significant differences in audiometric thresholds between tinnitus and control subjects could be observed. Most had normal hearing thresholds and the prevalence of outliers (thresholds >25 dB HL) was equal in both groups.

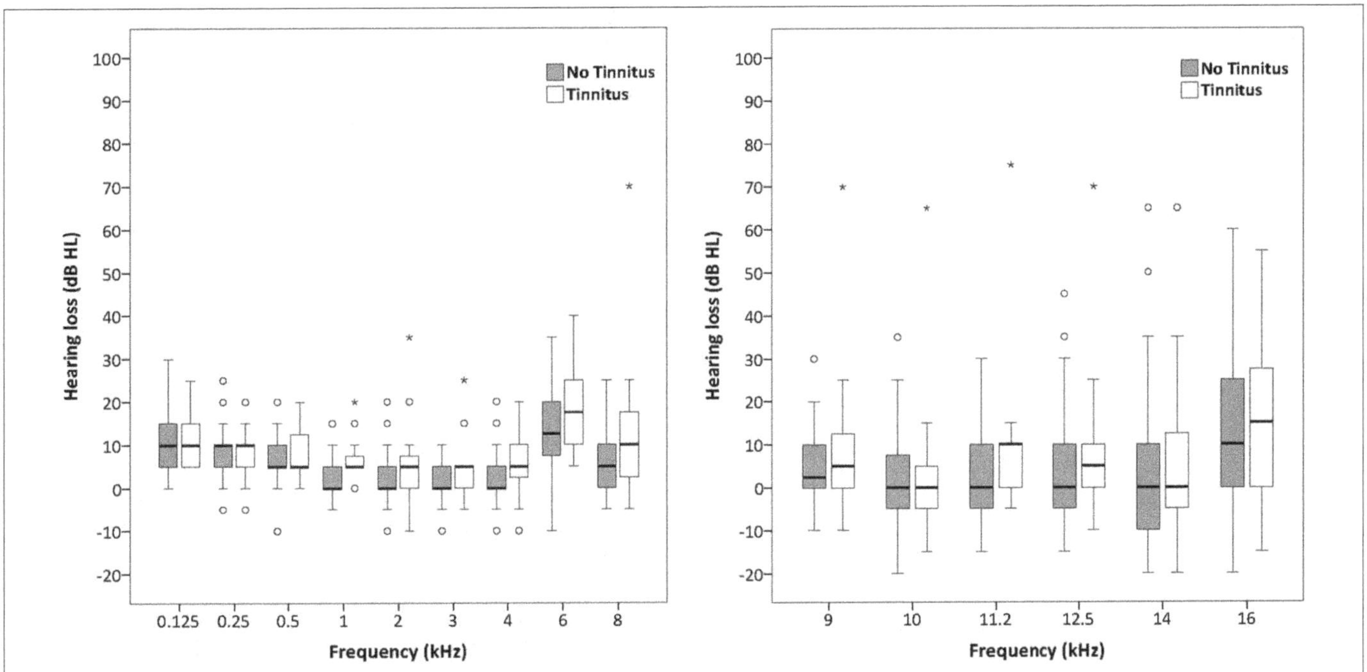

FIGURES 1, 2 | Boxplots representing pure tone audiometry for conventional frequencies (125–8 kHz) and high frequencies (9–16 kHz) for tinnitus subjects and non-tinnitus subjects. The box length is the interquartile range (IQR). A circle represents outliers with values between 1.5 and 3 box lengths from the upper or lower edge of the box. Asterisks represent extreme outliers (more than 3 times the IQR).

Furthermore, TEOAEs, DPOAEs, and ABRs did not show significant differences between the groups. However, speech-in-noise reception was significantly decreased in tinnitus subjects. The following paragraphs discuss these findings in the light of previous findings suggesting the presence of (noise-induced) tinnitus may occur in the absence of measurable peripheral damage and might cause more central plasticity than expected.

It has been suggested that extended high frequency audiometry (HFA) testing might reveal cochlear damage at higher frequencies than investigated by a conventional audiogram (Yildirim et al., 2010; Mehrparvar et al., 2011). Concerning the application of HFA in young people exposed to recreational noise, only limited research has been performed so far. However, it has been shown that, when no signs of noise-induced hearing damage can be detected on the conventional audiometry (125 Hz to 8 kHz), hearing thresholds at the higher frequencies (9–16 kHz) can be significantly increased (Sulaiman et al., 2013). However, the current study shows that adolescents with NIT do not necessarily have decreased hearing thresholds on conventional nor high-frequency audiometry. Also, audiometric outliers (>25 dB HL) were not more prevalent in the tinnitus group compared to controls indicating that there were no significant differences in hearing thresholds between the groups. This fact raises questions concerning the applicability of pure-tone audiometry as an assessment tool for the evaluation of early noise-induced damage. Besides HFA, evidence for the clinical use of OAEs in the early detection of noise-induced damage is growing (Sliwinska-Kowalska and Kotylo, 1997; Prasher and Sulkowski, 1999). It has been suggested that OAEs might reveal outer hair cell damage before it is reflected in the audiogram (Sliwinska-Kowalska and Kotylo, 1997, 2001). Sulaiman et al. showed increased high-frequency thresholds and decreased DPOAE amplitudes in a group of PLD users in the absence of measurable hearing loss between 125 Hz and 8 kHz (Sulaiman et al., 2013). Also McKee and Stephens showed decreased OAEs in tinnitus subjects with normal hearing (McKee and Stephens, 1992). In the current study, TEOAEs as well as DPOAEs were performed in all students but no significant differences between tinnitus and non-tinnitus subjects could be observed. Similar results were obtained in a younger population in a recent study by Sanchez et al. assessing 168 adolescents by use of pure-tone audiometry (250 Hz to 16 kHz), TEOAEs and DPOAEs. 28.6% of the sample experienced permanent tinnitus, 28% sporadic tinnitus and the remaining 43.4% did not have tinnitus. No significant differences were observed between the groups regarding audiometric thresholds and TEOAEs/DPOAEs (Sanchez et al., 2015). Considering the present results as well as findings from previous studies, the use of OAEs in noise-exposed subjects is still under debate. Possibly OAEs might render more information in cases of acute acoustic trauma with temporary threshold shift in order to more precisely investigate specific frequency regions such as the 3–6 kHz region (Buchler et al., 2012). However, as a tool for early noise-induced hearing damage screening, the overall results of studies are rather inconclusive at this point (Shupak et al., 2007), suggesting that the addition of OAE measurements to the golden standard of audiometry, is not

TABLE 5 | Audiometric differences between the tinnitus and the non-tinnitus group for all measured frequencies.

Audiometric frequency	*p*-value (uncorrected)	*p*-value (corrected)
125 Hz	0.52	1.00
250 Hz	0.75	1.00
500 Hz	0.52	1.00
1 kHz	<0.01	0.06
2 kHz	0.24	1.00
3 kHz	0.34	1.00
4 kHz	0.02	0.25
6 kHz	0.07	0.86
8 kHz	0.19	1.00
9 kHz	0.76	1.00
10 kHz	0.95	0.95
11.2 kHz	0.16	1.00
12.5 kHz	0.33	1.00
14 kHz	0.26	1.00
16 kHz	0.64	1.00

Bonferroni-Holm correction was applied for multiple testing correction but uncorrected values are provided as well.

TABLE 6 | Differences in TEOAE band-frequency strength [signal-to-noise ratio (SNR)] between tinnitus and non-tinnitus subjects.

TEOAE band-frequency (kHz)	Median TEOAE strength (dB SNR)		*p*-value (uncorrected)	*p*-value (corrected)
	Tinnitus	No tinnitus		
1	3.90	1.95	0.83	1.0
1.4	6.90	7.50	0.98	0.98
2	7.90	5.20	0.86	1.0
2.8	5.30	5.90	0.63	1.0
4	2.60	3.85	0.25	1.0

Uncorrected p-values are given and were corrected for multiple testing by use of Bonferroni–Holm.

sufficient in detecting early-staged noise-induced hearing damage.

The current study did not find any differences in ABR results between tinnitus subjects and controls. This is in line with the study by Barnea et al. who performed HFA and ABR testing on a tinnitus group with normal hearing sensitivity in the range of 125 Hz to 8 kHz compared to an age- and gender-matched control group. Similar to the present study, high-frequency and ABR audiometric data did not differ between the considered groups (Barnea et al., 1990). Although not found in the present study, an I–V amplitude ratio alteration was previously reported. Schaette and McAlpine found reduced wave I potentials in normal-hearing female tinnitus subjects but normal amplitude of the more centrally generated wave V. The authors concluded that the deviation of wave I, which is generated by the primary auditory nerve fibers, provides direct evidence for "hidden hearing loss" that manifests as reduced neural output coming from the cochlea followed by renormalization of neural response

TABLE 7 | Differences in DPOAE band-frequency strength between tinnitus and control subjects.

DPOAE band-frequency (kHz)	Median DPOAE strength (dB SNR)		*p*-value (uncorrected)	*p*-value
	Tinnitus	No tinnitus		
1	6.10	9.10	0.80	0.80
1.4	15.00	12.40	0.15	0.45
2	13.00	10.60	0.28	0.57
2.8	10.40	7.40	0.01	0.07
4	14.20	10.45	0.10	0.41

Uncorrected p-values are given and were corrected for multiple testing by use of Bonferroni–Holm.

magnitude within the brainstem reflected by normal wave V amplitudes (Schaette and McAlpine, 2011). Similar results were obtained for male subjects in another study where tinnitus subjects also showed reduced wave I amplitudes but, in addition, enhanced wave V reflecting elevated input to the inferior colliculi. Also elevated I–III and I/V amplitude ratios were apparent implicating disproportionally high activity in spherical bush cells in the ventral cochlear nucleus (Gu et al., 2012). Intergender differences exist in auditory brainstem response amplitudes and latencies (Durrant et al., 1990). Therefore, the current study also investigated possible differences in ABR results within male and female subjects for tinnitus subjects vs. controls (see also Supplementary Material). No gender differences were apparent in the current data set. However, it has to be pointed out that the control group contained more female subjects than males and therefore these results should be interpreted with caution.

Peripheral vs. Central Deficits

The deteriorating effects of hearing loss on speech reception in noise have been thoroughly investigated in previous research (Festen and Plomp, 1990; Bacon et al., 1998; Peters et al., 1998; Bernstein and Grant, 2009; Rhebergen et al., 2010). The decreased release of masking that occurs in hearing impaired subjects could only be partly explained by reduced audibility (Bacon et al., 1998). The ability to correctly detect the temporal fine structure of speech (Fullgrabe et al., 2006; Lorenzi et al., 2006a) and to process spectral details (Nelson et al., 2003; Nelson and Jin, 2004), seems critical for dip-listening. As loss of ability to use temporal and spectral cues in speech is highly associated with sensorineural hearing loss (Bacon et al., 1998) the question arises why speech reception in noise is also sometimes decreased in normal hearing subjects in the absence of hearing loss (Middelweerd et al., 1990). In the present study, tinnitus subjects had significantly worse speech reception in steady-state noise as well as in AM noise. Ryu et al. also found decreased speech perception ability (in quiet as well as in noise) in normal-hearing tinnitus subjects compared to controls (Ryu et al., 2012) in line with earlier findings by Huang et al. (2007). A recent study including tinnitus subjects with and without hearing loss and a control group, measured spectral and temporal

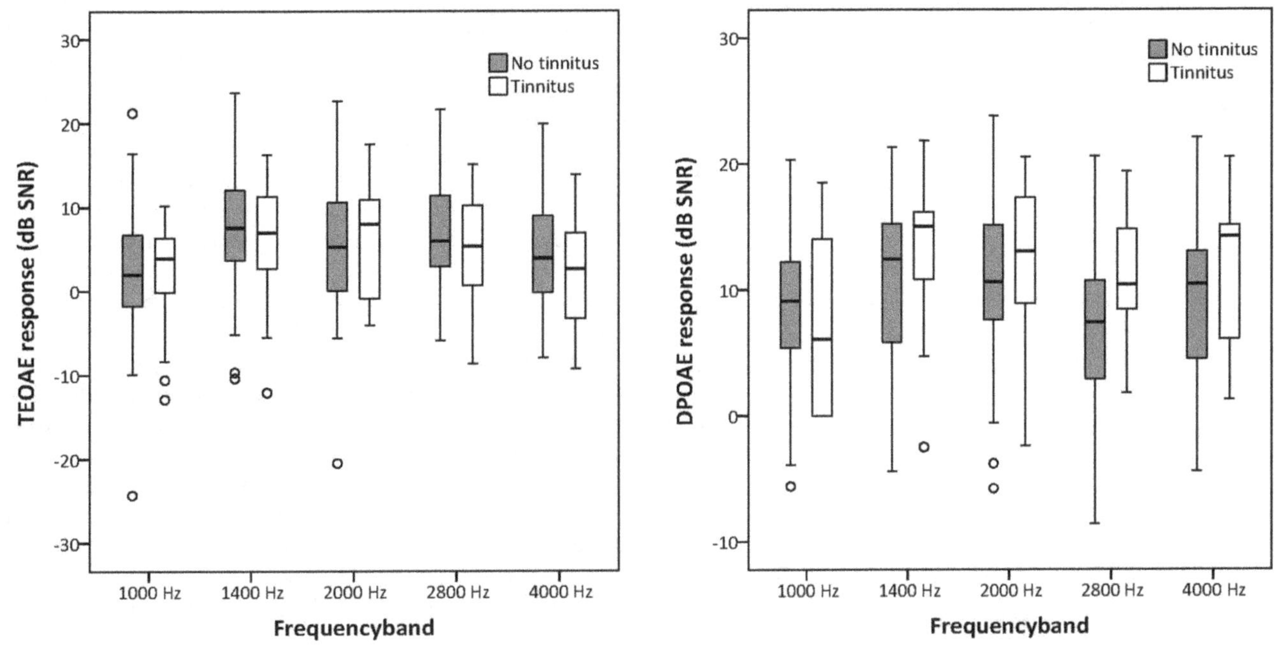

FIGURES 3, 4 | Boxplots representing TEOAE and DPOAE data for tinnitus subjects and controls. The box length is the interquartile range (IQR). A circle represents outliers with values between 1.5 and 3 box lengths from the upper or lower edge of the box.

resolution as well as speech-in-noise reception. No significant differences between tinnitus subjects and controls were found concerning spectral and temporal abilities. However, SRT scores were significantly worse in tinnitus subjects (Moon et al., 2015). It is discussed that normal temporal and spectral resolution in tinnitus subjects reflect the undisturbed functionality of OHCs in the cochlea. In case of cochlear damage, the basilar membrane response would be more linear and broadly tuned resulting in reduced compression and broadening of the auditory filters which would negatively affect both frequency selectivity and temporal resolution (Moore and Glasberg, 1986; Oxenham and Bacon, 2003). The findings of decreased SRT scores in the absence of temporal/spectral resolution deficits imply that tinnitus can occur without OHC damage and might depend more on plastic changes in the central auditory system (Moon et al., 2015). The present results confirm the latter findings as no differences in peripheral functioning, tested by pure-tone audiometry, and OAEs, could be observed. In this study however, spectral and temporal resolution was not specifically tested but speech-in-amplitude-modulated noise testing gives a robust idea of temporal encoding when listening in the gaps. Speech reception in AM noise was significantly worse in tinnitus patients compared to controls but to the same extent as speech reception in steady-state noise. Hence, no additional temporal deficits are apparent in the tinnitus group. It can be suggested that speech reception testing in AM noise does not add useful information to the classical speech reception test in steady-state noise. However, in line with previous findings by Moon et al. the suggestion can be made that the decreased speech reception in subjects with NIT, in the absence of measurable cochlear lesions, might be due to a more central deficit.

The presence of tinnitus in the absence of measurable cochlear hearing loss, as is the case in the present study, forms a serious challenge to the model of cortical hyperactivity. However, Kujawa and Liberman earlier reported that in an animal experiment 50–60% of the auditory nerve fibers in the high-frequency region of the cochlea were deafferented after mild acoustic trauma without any permanent auditory threshold elevation suggesting that normal hearing thresholds do not necessarily exclude the possibility of cochlear damage (Kujawa and Liberman, 2009). It is posited that acoustic overexposure can produce a rapid and irreversible loss of cochlear nerve peripheral terminals on IHCs and a slow degeneration of spiral ganglion cells, despite full recovery of cochlear thresholds and no loss of IHCs or OHCs (Kujawa and Liberman, 2009; Lin et al., 2011). The phenomenon of noise-induced cochlear neuronal degeneration in mice independent of auditory threshold changes, described by Kujawa and Liberman is recently described as "cochlear synaptopathy" (Liberman et al., 2015). Recently, it has been shown that a deficiency in pejvakin protein can cause exceptional vulnerability to sound as pejvakin deficient cochleae exhibit features of marked oxidative stress and impaired antioxidant defenses (Delmaghani et al., 2015). Although aforementioned studies are animal studies, a study by Weisz et al. supported the presence of deafferentiation in the absence of audiometrically detectable hearing loss in humans with tinnitus by use of the Threshold Equalizing Noise test (TEN test; Weisz et al., 2006). However, these results were not confirmed in one of our

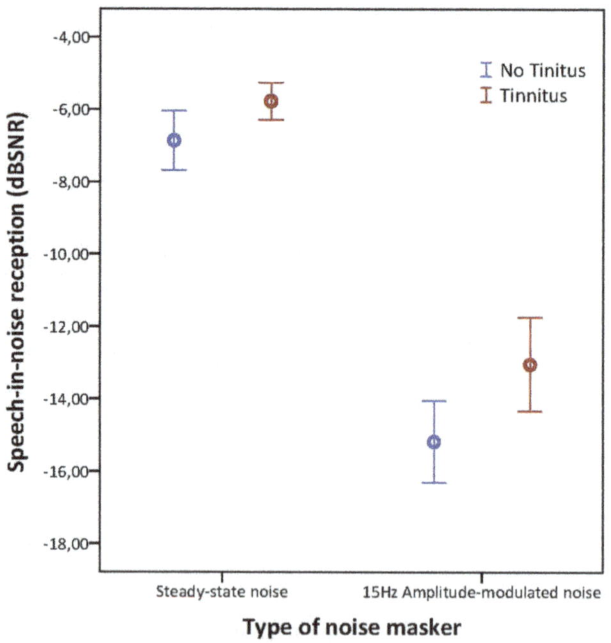

FIGURE 5 | Error barchart illustrating speech-in-noise reception in steady state noise and AM-15 Hz noise of tinnitus and non-tinnitus subjects. The bars represents the 95% confidence interval and the standard error is depicted by the whiskers.

previous studies (Gilles A. D. et al., 2013). The authors believe that in case of presence of cochlear synaptopathy or pejvakin deficiency in the tinnitus subjects, ABR data of the tinnitus subjects would have shown amplitude and latency decrements which were not apparent in the present study. Not-withstanding, the results of the current study does not exclude the possible interference of (currently unmeasurable) peripheral damage in NIT.

However, it can also be argued that when all audiometric findings show normal results in NIT subjects, retrocochlear deficits are present which result into the tinnitus percept on one hand but may also influence performance on a broader scale. The neural correlates of tinnitus have been described as auditory as well as non-auditory (Langers and Melcher, 2011; Langguth et al., 2012; Vanneste and De Ridder, 2012) suggesting that speech performance may also be altered as a consequence of cortical reorganization. It was shown by a previous study that brainstem responses evoked by speech in subjects with speech message decoding difficulties, may reveal miscoding in subcortical structures as an origin (Kraus and Nicol, 2005). In addition, deficiencies in higher-order cortical networks have been found in tinnitus subjects with normal hearing thresholds (Melcher et al., 2009).

CONCLUSIONS AND FUTURE RESEARCH

The current study examined a group of 87 recreationally noise-exposed university students. The argument can be made that, ideally, also a group of non-exposed students should be included in order to investigate their audiological characteristics and compare them to the subject groups with occasional recreational noise exposure. However, as recreational noise exposure is an undeniable part of the current society, it is rather impossible to find young subjects who did not have any kind of noise exposure during their lifespan. Therefore, the decision was made to only include young adults with a certain amount of noise exposure. Noise exposure was evaluated by use of a very limited questionnaire broadly evaluating the current frequency of social events with high music levels as well as noise exposure caused by PLDs. However, noise exposure during the lifespan was not assessed meaning that, inevitably, there were possibly (small to large) differences in the total amount of noise exposure. As such, it cannot be ruled out by the current analysis that tinnitus subjects did not have more noise exposure. Nevertheless, the scope of the present study was not to investigate nor calculate noise exposure in adolescents but the focus was on the effects of recreational noise on the audiological characteristics. As some students experienced NIT, which can be considered as a symptom of noise damage, this symptom was used to make a comparison in audiological characteristics between tinnitus and non-tinnitus subjects.

No peripheral lesions could be observed in the current study evaluated by pure-tone audiometry, OAEs, and ABR. Speech-in-noise testing however was significantly decreased in tinnitus subjects possibly suggesting more centrally located deficits in tinnitus subjects. In addition, it can be said that cortical reorganization may occur due to frequent exposure to recreational noise exposure in the absence of any measurable peripheral hearing loss. The present article underlines the need for further testing besides the conventional audiometry. The sensitivity of pure-tone audiometry as well as OAE measurements might be insufficient to detect peripheral noise-induced damage at an early stage and one must interpret normal outcome results with this technique with caution. The authors like to mention the theory of "homeostatic plasticity" described by Gourévitch et al. (2014). These authors showed that reversible noise-induced threshold shifts may mask progressive underlying neuropathology that likely has profound long-term consequences on auditory processing. A normal audiogram is considered as the "golden standard." However, although the peripheral parts of the auditory system seem to be functioning normal (expressed by normal audiogram and OAE measurements in the present study), substantial changes may occur in the auditory brain post noise exposure. The mechanism of "central gain" at the level of the auditory brainstem, or more cortically located, causes initially a decrease in synaptic efficacy in central parts of the auditory system in the noise-exposed frequency region. Long-lasting changes in synaptic efficacy after prolonged noise exposure could affect the expression of inhibition (Gourévitch et al., 2014). Gourevitch et al. provided evidence that the peripheral auditory system can be harmed without decreased auditory thresholds and that long-lasting disturbance of the excitation-inhibition balance in the central auditory system may eventually lead to cortical reorganization as a result of homeostatic plasticity (Gourévitch et al., 2014). Homeostatic plasticity mechanisms may regulate

TABLE 8 | overview of the detectability of each wave (= N), mean values for wave latency (in ms) and amplitude (in μV) and standard deviations.

Variable	Group	N	Mean	*SD*	*p*-value for independent *t*-test (uncorrected)	*p*-value for independent *t*-test (corrected)
LATENCY						
Wave I	Controls	23	1.57	0.11	0.63	1.00
	Tinnitus	19	1.60	0.17		
Wave II	Controls	17	2.74	0.17	0.57	1.00
	Tinnitus	7	2.78	0.11		
Wave III	Controls	23	3.75	0.24	0.17	1.00
	Tinnitus	19	3.67	0.18		
Wave IV	Controls	9	5.01	0.16	0.07	0.98
	Tinnitus	5	4.81	0.19		
Wave V	Controls	23	5.51	0.23	0.88	1.00
	Tinnitus	19	5.53	0.33		
INTERPEAK LATENCY						
Wave I–III	Controls	23	2.18	0.17	0.16	1.00
	Tinnitus	19	2.06	0.28		
Wave III–V	Controls	23	1.78	0.12	0.05	0.75
	Tinnitus	19	1.91	0.31		
Wave I–V	Controls	23	3.94	0.18	0.54	1.00
	Tinnitus	19	3.98	0.22		
AMPLITUDE						
Wave I	Controls	23	0.10	0.08	0.12	1.00
	Tinnitus	19	0.14	0.08		
Wave II	Controls	17	0.06	0.06	0.09	1.00
	Tinnitus	7	0.11	0.07		
Wave III	Controls	23	0.20	0.10	0.18	1.00
	Tinnitus	19	0.26	0.15		
Wave IV	Controls	10	0.10	0.06	0.38	1.00
	Tinnitus	5	0.07	0.05		
Wave V	Controls	23	0.23	0.13	0.14	1.00
	Tinnitus	19	0.18	0.07		
INTERPEAK AMPLITUDE						
Wave I–III	Controls	23	0.10	0.15	0.77	1.00
	Tinnitus	19	0.12	0.15		
Wave III–V	Controls	23	0.02	0.14	0.04	0.64
	Tinnitus	19	0.08	0.17		
Wave I–V	Controls	23	0.13	0.19	0.08	1.00
	Tinnitus	19	0.04	0.12		

Corrected and uncorrected p-values are shown for the independent samples t-test.

a central gain mechanism, and tinnitus might be a side-effect of these changes (Norena and Farley, 2013; Brotherton et al., 2015). In addition, it has to be noted that hyperacusis was more prevalent in the tinnitus sample than in the controls. Psychoacoustic measurements in the tinnitus subjects might have rendered additional, important information and it can be considered as a limitation of the study that these measurements were not performed. Further research is required in order to investigate the role of homeostatic plasticity in recreational noise exposure.

In conclusion, speech-in-noise testing forms a reliable and clinically feasible technique to assess noise-induced damage in patients with normal peripheral function but with complaints of NIT. The present study shows promising results concerning the use of speech-in-noise testing in detection of noise-induced damage in adolescents. The use of amplitude-modulated noise however, requires more research in order to further investigate the mechanism of homeostatic plasticity in recreational noise exposure as well as the peripheral involvement. Furthermore, late-auditory evoked potentials might provide additional information on higher-order cortical processing of (speech) sounds (Joos et al., 2014) and might therefore also render useful information in normal-hearing tinnitus subjects.

AUTHOR CONTRIBUTIONS

AG: This author has substantially contributed to the design of the study, the acquisition, analysis, and interpretation of the data, is the main author for drafting the manuscript. WS: This author has substantially contributed to the interpretation of the study and the writing of the manuscript. He agrees to be accountable for all aspects of the work. SR: This author has substantially contributed to the collection of the data and the final version of the manuscript. KW: This author has substantially contributed to the analysis of the data and reviewed the final draft very carefully. EF: This author has substantially contributed to the analysis of the data and reviewed the final draft very carefully. PV: This author was involved in the design, analysis and interpretation of the study and has contributed to the writing of the manuscript. All authors gave final approval of this version to be published as such and agrees to be accountable for all aspects of the work in ensuring that questions related to the accuracy or integrity of any part of the work are appropriately investigated and resolved.

FUNDING

The main author is an employee of the University Hospital Antwerp and as such, this research is funded by the hospital. No external funding bodies were involved in the current study.

ACKNOWLEDGMENTS

The authors thank David Landberger for his help with the installation and protocol of the TigerSpeech software for the speech-in-noise-testing. This study was financially supported by a TOP-BOF grant of the University of Antwerp.

REFERENCES

Bacon, S. P., Opie, J. M., and Montoya, D. Y. (1998). The effects of hearing loss and noise masking on the masking release for speech in temporally complex backgrounds. *J. Speech Lang. Hear. Res.* 41, 549–563. doi: 10.1044/jslhr.4103.549

Barnea, G., Attias, J., Gold, S., and Shahar, A. (1990). Tinnitus with normal hearing sensitivity: extended high-frequency audiometry and auditory-nerve brain-stem-evoked responses. *Audiology* 29, 36–45. doi: 10.3109/00206099009081644

Beach, E., Williams, W., and Gilliver, M. (2013). Estimating young Australian adults' risk of hearing damage from selected leisure activities. *Ear Hear.* 34, 75–82. doi: 10.1097/AUD.0b013e318262ac6c

Bernstein, J. G., and Grant, K. W. (2009). Auditory and auditory-visual intelligibility of speech in fluctuating maskers for normal-hearing and hearing-impaired listeners. *J. Acoust. Soc. Am.* 125, 3358–3372. doi: 10.1121/1.3110132

Brotherton, H., Plack, C. J., Maslin, M., Schaette, R., and Munro, K. J. (2015). Pump up the volume: could excessive neural gain explain tinnitus and hyperacusis? *Audiol. Neurootol.* 20, 273–282. doi: 10.1159/000430459

Büchler, M., Kompis, M., and Hotz, M. A. (2012). Extended frequency range hearing thresholds and otoacoustic emissions in acute acoustic trauma. *Otol. Neurotol.* 33, 1322. doi: 10.1097/MAO.0b013e318263d598

Chung, J. H., Des Roches, C. M., Meunier, J., and Eavey, R. D. (2005). Evaluation of noise-induced hearing loss in young people using a web-based survey technique. *Pediatrics* 115, 861–867. doi: 10.1542/peds.2004-0173

Davis, R. L., and Liu, Q. (2011). Complex primary afferents: what the distribution of electrophysiologically-relevant phenotypes within the spiral ganglion tells us about peripheral neural coding. *Hear. Res.* 276, 34–43. doi: 10.1016/j.heares.2011.01.014

Degeest, S., Corthals, P., Vinck, B., and Keppler, H. (2014). Prevalence and characteristics of tinnitus after leisure noise exposure in young adults. *Noise Health* 16, 26–33. doi: 10.4103/1463-1741.127850

Delmaghani, S., Defourny, J., Aghaie, A., Beurg, M., Dulon, D., Thelen, N., et al. (2015). Hypervulnerability to sound exposure through impaired adaptive proliferation of peroxisomes. *Cell* 163, 894–906. doi: 10.1016/j.cell.2015.10.023

Dubno, J. R., Horwitz, A. R., and Ahlstrom, J. B. (2002). Benefit of modulated maskers for speech recognition by younger and older adults with normal hearing. *J. Acoust. Soc. Am.* 111, 2897–2907. doi: 10.1121/1.1480421

Durrant, J. D., Sabo, D. L., and Hyre, R. J. (1990). Gender, head size, and ABRs examined in large clinical sample. *Ear Hear.* 11, 210–214. doi: 10.1097/00003446-199006000-00008

Festen, J. M., and Plomp, R. (1990). Effects of fluctuating noise and interfering speech on the speech-reception threshold for impaired and normal hearing. *J. Acoust. Soc. Am.* 88, 1725–1736. doi: 10.1121/1.400247

Füllgrabe, C., Berthommier, F., and Lorenzi, C. (2006). Masking release for consonant features in temporally fluctuating background noise. *Hear. Res.* 211, 74–84. doi: 10.1016/j.heares.2005.09.001

Gilles, A., De Ridder, D., Van Hal, G., Wouters, K., Kleine Punte, A., and Van de Heyning, P. (2012). Prevalence of leisure noise-induced tinnitus and the attitude toward noise in university students. *Otol. Neurotol.* 33, 899–906. doi: 10.1097/mao.0b013e31825d640a

Gilles, A., Van Hal, G., De Ridder, D., Wouters, K., and Van de Heyning, P. (2013). Epidemiology of noise-induced tinnitus and the attitudes and beliefs towards noise and hearing protection in adolescents. *PLoS ONE.* 8:e70297. doi: 10.1371/journal.pone.0070297

Gilles, A. D., Ridder, D., and Van de Heyning, P. (2013). No cochlear dead regions detected in non-pulsatile tinnitus patients: an assessment with the threshold equalizing noise (sound pressure level) test. *Noise Health 15*, 129–133. doi: 10.4103/1463-1741.110297

Goebel, G., and Hiller, W. (1994). The tinnitus questionnaire. A standard instrument for grading the degree of tinnitus. Results of a multicenter study with the tinnitus questionnaire. *HNO* 42, 166–172.

Gourevitch, B., Edeline, J. M., Occelli, F., and Eggermont, J. J. (2014). Is the din really harmless? *Long-term effects of non-traumatic noise on the adult auditory system. Nat. Rev. Neurosci.* 15, 483–491. doi: 10.1038/nrn3744

Gu, J. W., Herrmann, B. S., Levine, R. A., and Melcher, J. R. (2012). Brainstem auditory evoked potentials suggest a role for the ventral cochlear nucleus in tinnitus. *J. Assoc. Res. Otolaryngol.* 13, 819–833. doi: 10.1007/s10162-012-0344-1

Gustafsson, H. A., and Arlinger, S. D. (1994). Masking of speech by amplitude-modulated noise. *J. Acoust. Soc. Am.* 95, 518–529. doi: 10.1121/1.408346

Henderson, E., Testa, M. A., and Hartnick, C. (2011). Prevalence of noise-induced hearing-threshold shifts and hearing loss among US youths. *Pediatrics* 127, e39–e46. doi: 10.1542/peds.2010-0926

Huang, C. Y., Lee, H. H., Chung, K. C., Chen, H. C., Shen, Y. J., and Wu, J. L. (2007). Relationships among speech perception, self-rated tinnitus loudness and disability in tinnitus patients with normal pure-tone thresholds of hearing. *ORL J. Otorhinolaryngol. Relat. Spec.* 69, 25–29. doi: 10.1159/000096713

Jansen, S., Luts, H., Dejonckere, P., van Wieringen, A., and Wouters, J. (2013). Efficient hearing screening in noise-exposed listeners using the digit triplet test. *Ear Hear. 34*, 773–778. doi: 10.1097/AUD.0b013e318297920b

Joos, K., Gilles, A., Van de Heyning, P., De, R. D., and Vanneste, S. (2014). From sensation to percept: the neural signature of auditory event-related potentials. *Neurosci. Biobehav. Rev.* 42C, 148–156. doi: 10.1016/j.neubiorev.2014.02.009

Khalfa, S., Dubal, S., Veuillet, E., Perez-Diaz, F., Jouvent, R., and Collet, L. (2002). Psychometric normalization of a hyperacusis questionnaire. *ORL J. Otorhinolaryngol. Relat. Spec.* 64, 436–442. doi: 10.1159/000067570

Kraus, N., and Nicol, T. (2005). Brainstem origins for cortical 'what' and 'where' pathways in the auditory system. *Trends Neurosci.* 28, 176–181. doi: 10.1016/j.tins.2005.02.003

Kujawa, S. G., Fallon, M., and Bobbin, R. P. (1995). Time-varying alterations in the f2-f1 DPOAE response to continuous primary stimulation. *I: response characterization and contribution of the olivocochlear efferents. Hear. Res.* 85, 142–154. doi: 10.1016/0378-5955(95)00041-2

Kujawa, S. G., and Liberman, M. C. (2009). Adding insult to injury: cochlear nerve degeneration after "temporary" noise-induced hearing loss. *J. Neurosci.* 29, 14077–14085. doi: 10.1523/JNEUROSCI.2845-09.2009

Langers, D. R., and Melcher, J. R. (2011). Hearing without listening: functional connectivity reveals the engagement of multiple nonauditory networks during basic sound processing. *Brain Connect.* 1, 233–244. doi: 10.1089/brain.2011.0023

Langguth, B., Schecklmann, M., Lehner, A., Landgrebe, M., Poeppl, T. B., Kreuzer, P. M., et al. (2012). Neuroimaging and neuromodulation: complementary approaches for identifying the neuronal correlates of tinnitus. *Front. Syst. Neurosci.* 6:15. doi: 10.3389/fnsys.2012.00015

Liberman, L. D., Suzuki, J., and Liberman, M. C. (2015). Dynamics of cochlear synaptopathy after acoustic overexposure. *J. Assoc. Res. Otolaryngol.* 16, 205–219. doi: 10.1007/s10162-015-0510-3

Liberman, M. C., and Oliver, M. E. (1984). Morphometry of intracellularly labeled neurons of the auditory nerve: correlations with functional properties. *J. Comp. Neurol.* 223, 163–176. doi: 10.1002/cne.902230203

Lin, H. W., Furman, A. C., Kujawa, S. G., and Liberman, M. C. (2011). Primary neural degeneration in the Guinea pig cochlea after reversible noise-induced threshold shift. *J. Assoc. Res. Otolaryngol.* 12, 605–616. doi: 10.1007/s10162-011-0277-0

Lorenzi, C., Gilbert, G., Carn, H., Garnier, S., and Moore, B. C. (2006a). Speech perception problems of the hearing impaired reflect inability to use temporal fine structure. *Proc. Natl. Acad. Sci. U.S.A.* 103, 18866–18869. doi: 10.1073/pnas.0607364103

Lorenzi, C., Husson, M., Ardoint, M., and Debruille, X. (2006b). Speech masking release in listeners with flat hearing loss: effects of masker fluctuation rate on identification scores and phonetic feature reception. *Int. J. Audiol.* 45, 487–495. doi: 10.1080/14992020600753213

McKee, G. J., and Stephens, S. D. (1992). An investigation of normally hearing subjects with tinnitus. *Audiology* 31, 313–317. doi: 10.3109/00206099209072919

Meeus, O. M., Spaepen, M., Ridder, D. D., and Heyning, P. H. (2010). Correlation between hyperacusis measurements in daily ENT practice. *Int. J. Audiol.* 49, 7–13. doi: 10.3109/14992020903160868

Mehrparvar, A. H., Mirmohammadi, S. J., Ghoreyshi, A., Mollasadeghi, A., and Loukzadeh, Z. (2011). High-frequency audiometry: a means for early diagnosis of noise-induced hearing loss. *Noise Health* 13, 402–406. doi: 10.4103/1463-1741.90295

Melcher, J. R., Levine, R. A., Bergevin, C., and Norris, B. (2009). The auditory midbrain of people with tinnitus: abnormal sound-evoked activity revisited. *Hear. Res.* 257, 63–74. doi: 10.1016/j.heares.2009.08.005

Mercier, V., and Hohmann, B. W. (2002). Is electronically amplified music too loud? what do young people think? *Noise Health* 4, 47–55.

Mertens, G., Punte, A. K., De Ridder, D., and Van de Heyning, P. (2013). Tinnitus in a single-sided deaf ear reduces speech reception in the nontinnitus ear. *Otol. Neurotol.* 34, 662–666. doi: 10.1097/mao.0b013e31828779f0

Middelweerd, M. J., Festen, J. M., and Plomp, R. (1990). Difficulties with speech intelligibility in noise in spite of a normal pure-tone audiogram. *Audiology* 29, 1–7. doi: 10.3109/00206099009081640

Moon, I. J., Won, J. H., Kang, H. W., Kim, D. H., An, Y. H., and Shim, H. J. (2015). Influence of tinnitus on auditory spectral and temporal resolution and speech perception in tinnitus patients. *J. Neurosci.* 35, 14260–14269. doi: 10.1523/JNEUROSCI.5091-14.2015

Moore, B. C., and Glasberg, B. R. (1986). Comparisons of frequency selectivity in simultaneous and forward masking for subjects with unilateral cochlear impairments. *J. Acoust. Soc. Am.* 80, 93–107. doi: 10.1121/1.394087

Nelson, P. B., and Jin, S. H. (2004). Factors affecting speech understanding in gated interference: cochlear implant users and normal-hearing listeners. *J. Acoust. Soc. Am.* 115, 2286–2294. doi: 10.1121/1.1703538

Nelson, P. B., Jin, S. H., Carney, A. E., and Nelson, D. A. (2003). Understanding speech in modulated interference: cochlear implant users and normal-hearing listeners. *J. Acoust. Soc. Am.* 113, 961–968. doi: 10.1121/1.1531983

Newman, C. W., Wharton, J. A., Shivapuja, B. G., and Jacobson, G. P. (1994). Relationships among psychoacoustic judgments, speech understanding ability and self-perceived handicap in tinnitus subjects. *Audiology* 33, 47–60. doi: 10.3109/00206099409072954

Niskar, A. S., Kieszak, S. M., Holmes, A., Esteban, E., Rubin, C., and Brody, D. J. (1998). Prevalence of hearing loss among children 6 to 19 years of age: the Third National Health and Nutrition Examination Survey. *JAMA* 279, 1071–1075. doi: 10.1001/jama.279.14.1071

Niskar, A. S., Kieszak, S. M., Holmes, A. E., Esteban, E., Rubin, C., and Brody, D. J. (2001). Estimated prevalence of noise-induced hearing threshold shifts among children 6 to 19 years of age: the Third National Health and Nutrition Examination Survey, 1988-1994, United States. *Pediatrics* 108, 40–43. doi: 10.1542/peds.108.1.40

Noreña, A. J., and Farley, B. J. (2013). Tinnitus-related neural activity: theories of generation, propagation, and centralization. *Hear. Res.* 295, 161–171. doi: 10.1016/j.heares.2012.09.010

Oxenham, A. J., and Bacon, S. P. (2003). Cochlear compression: perceptual measures and implications for normal and impaired hearing. *Ear Hear.* 24, 352–366. doi: 10.1097/01.AUD.0000090470.73934.78

Peters, R. W., Moore, B. C., and Baer, T. (1998). Speech reception thresholds in noise with and without spectral and temporal dips for hearing-impaired and normally hearing people. *J. Acoust. Soc. Am.* 103, 577–587. doi: 10.1121/1.421128

Prasher, D., and Sulkowski, W. (1999). The role of otoacoustic emissions in screening and evaluation of noise damage. *Int. J. Occup. Med. Environ. Health* 12, 183–192.

Quintanilla-Dieck, M. L., Artunduaga, M. A., and Eavey, R. D. (2009). Intentional exposure to loud music: the second MTV.com survey reveals an opportunity to educate. *J. Pediatr.* 155, 550–555. doi: 10.1016/j.jpeds.2009.04.053

Rhebergen, K. S., Versfeld, N. J., de Laat, J. A., and Dreschler, W. A. (2010). Modelling the speech reception threshold in non-stationary noise in hearing-impaired listeners as a function of level. *Int. J. Audiol.* 49, 856–865. doi: 10.3109/14992027.2010.498446

Ryu, I. S., Ahn, J. H., Lim, H. W., Joo, K. Y., and Chung, J. W. (2012). Evaluation of masking effects on speech perception in patients with unilateral chronic tinnitus using the hearing in noise test. *Otol. Neurotol.* 33, 1472–1476. doi: 10.1097/mao.0b013e31826dbcc4

Sanchez, T. G., Oliveira, J. C., Kii, M. A., Freire, K., Cota, J., and Moraes, F. V. (2015). Tinnitus in adolescents: the start of the vulnerability of the auditory pathways. *Codas* 27, 5–12. doi: 10.1590/2317-1782/20152013045

Schaette, R., and McAlpine, D. (2011). Tinnitus with a normal audiogram: physiological evidence for hidden hearing loss and computational model. *J. Neurosci.* 31, 13452–13457. doi: 10.1523/JNEUROSCI.2156-11.2011

Scroggs, R. S., and Fox, A. P. (1992). Multiple Ca2+ currents elicited by action potential waveforms in acutely isolated adult rat dorsal root ganglion neurons. *J. Neurosci.* 12, 1789–1801.

Serra, M. R., Biassoni, E. C., Richter, U., Minoldo, G., Franco, G., Abraham, S., et al. (2005). Recreational noise exposure and its effects on the hearing of adolescents. *Part I: an interdisciplinary long-term study. Int. J. Audiol.* 44, 65–73. doi: 10.1080/14992020400030010

Shupak, A., Tal, D., Sharoni, Z., Oren, M., Ravid, A., and Pratt, H. (2007). Otoacoustic emissions in early noise-induced hearing loss. *Otol. Neurotol.* 28, 745–752. doi: 10.1097/MAO.0b013e3180a726c9

Sliwinska-Kowalska, M., and Kotylo, P. (1997). [Is otoacoustic emission useful in the differential diagnosis of occupational noise-induced hearing loss?]. *Med. Pr.* 48, 613–620.

Sliwinska-Kowalska, M., and Kotylo, P. (2001). Otoacoustic emissions in industrial hearing loss assessment. *Noise Health* 3, 75–84.

Smith, P. A., Davis, A., Ferguson, M., and Lutman, M. E. (2000). The prevalence and type of social noise exposure in young adults in England. *Noise Health* 2, 41–56.

Sulaiman, A. H., Husain, R., and Seluakumaran, K. (2013). Evaluation of early hearing damage in personal listening device users using extended high-frequency audiometry and otoacoustic emissions. *Eur. Arch. Otorhinolaryngol.* 8, 710–715.

TigerSpeech Technology (2012). TigerSpeech Technology. Los Angeles: Innovative Speech Software.

Vanneste, S., and De Ridder, D. (2012). The auditory and non-auditory brain areas involved in tinnitus. *An emergent property of multiple parallel overlapping subnetworks. Front. Syst. Neurosci.* 6:31. doi: 10.3389/fnsys.2012.00031

Van Wieringen, A., and Wouters, J. (2008). LIST and LINT: sentences and numbers for quantifying speech understanding in severely impaired listeners for Flanders and the Netherlands. *Int. J. Audiol.* 47, 348–355. doi: 10.1080/14992020801895144

Weisz, N., Hartmann, T., Dohrmann, K., Schlee, W., and Norena, A. (2006). High-frequency tinnitus without hearing loss does not mean absence of deafferentation. *Hear. Res.* 222, 108–114. doi: 10.1016/j.heares.2006.09.003

Widen, S. E., and Erlandsson, S. I. (2004). Self-reported tinnitus and noise sensitivity among adolescents in Sweden. *Noise Health* 7, 29–40.

Yildirim, G., Berkiten, G., Kuzdere, M., and Ugras, H. (2010). High frequency audiometry in patients presenting with tinnitus. *J. Int. Adv. Otol.* 6, 401–407.

14

Biomarkers of Presbycusis and Tinnitus in a Portuguese Older Population

Haúla F. Haider[1]*, Marisa Flook[2], Mariana Aparicio[3], Diogo Ribeiro[1], Marilia Antunes[4], Agnieszka J. Szczepek[5], Derek J. Hoare[6], Graça Fialho[2], João C. Paço[1] and Helena Caria[2,7]

[1] ENT Department, Hospital Cuf Infante Santo, NOVA Medical School, Lisbon, Portugal, [2] Deafness Research Group, BTR Unit, BioISI, Faculty of Sciences, University of Lisbon (FCUL), Lisbon, Portugal, [3] Faculty of Sciences, University of Lisbon, Lisbon, Portugal, [4] Centro de Estatística e Aplicações, Faculty of Sciences, University of Lisbon, Lisbon, Portugal, [5] Department of Otolaryngology, Charite University Hospital, Berlin, Germany, [6] NIHR Nottingham Biomedical Research Centre, Division of Clinical Neuroscience, School of Medicine, University of Nottingham, Nottingham, United Kingdom, [7] ESS/IPS- Biomedical Sciences Department, School of Health, Polytechnic Institute of Setubal, Setubal, Portugal

***Correspondence:**
Haúla F. Haider
haula.f.haider@jmellosaude.pt;
hfhaider@gmail.com

Introduction: Presbycusis or age-related hearing loss (ARHL) is a ubiquitous health problem. It is estimated that it will affect up to 1.5 billion people by 2025. In addition, tinnitus occurs in a large majority of cases with presbycusis. Glutamate metabotropic receptor 7 (*GRM7*) and *N*-acetyltransferase 2 (*NAT2*) are some of the genetic markers for presbycusis.

Objectives: To explore patterns of hearing loss and the role of *GRM7* and *NAT2* as possible markers of presbycusis and tinnitus in a Portuguese population sample.

Materials and Methods: Tonal and speech audiometry, tinnitus assessment, clinical interview, and DNA samples were obtained from patients aged from 55 to 75 with or without tinnitus. *GRM7* analysis was performed by qPCR. Genotyping of single nucleotide polymorphisms (SNPs) in *NAT2* was performed by PCR amplification followed by Sanger sequencing or by qPCR.

Results: We screened samples from 78 individuals (33 men and 45 women). T allele at *GRM7* gene was the most observed (60.3% T/T and 33.3% A/T). Individuals with a T/T genotype have a higher risk for ARHL and 33% lower risk for tinnitus, compared to individuals with A/A and A/T genotype, respectively. Being a slow acetylator (53%) was the most common *NAT2* phenotype, more common in men (55.8%). Intermediate acetylator was the second most common phenotype (35.9%) also more frequent in men (82.6%). Noise exposed individuals and individuals with 'high frequency' hearing loss seem to have a higher risk for tinnitus. Our data suggests that allele AT of *GRM7* can have a statistically significant influence toward the *severity* of tinnitus.

Conclusion: For each increasing year of age the chance of HL increases by 9%. The risk for ARHL was not significantly associated with *GRM7* neither *NAT2*. However, we cannot conclude from our data whether the presence of T allele at *GRM7* increases the odds for ARHL or whether the A allele has a protective effect. Genotype A/T at *GRM7* could potentially be considered a biomarker of tinnitus severity. This is the first study evaluating the effect of *GRM7* and *NAT2* gene in tinnitus.

Keywords: presbycusis, *GRM7*, *NAT2*, tinnitus, markers, comorbidities

INTRODUCTION

Presbycusis [age-related hearing loss (ARHL)] is a universal feature of mammalian aging in which the auditory function is compromised, hearing thresholds increase, and frequency resolution gets poorer. As a result, in noisy environments speech-understanding deteriorates and temporal processing deficits in gap detection measures increase (Lee, 2013). In humans, this condition affects tens of millions of people world-wide (Yamasoba et al., 2013). Many people with hearing loss also experience tinnitus, which is the perception of a sound in one or both ears or in the head in the absence of an external sound source (Jastreboff and Hazell, 1993).

Presbycusis is complex in that it has repercussions at a physical, cognitive, emotional, and social level; quality of life can deteriorate, and for some people presbycusis could lead to depression, social isolation and lower self-esteem (Lee, 2013; Ciorba et al., 2015). Environmental factors such as diet, physical exercise, smoking, and intake of medications are some of the extrinsic factors predisposing to presbycusis. There are several auditory structures affected by presbycusis, such as hair cells, *stria vascularis,* afferent spiral ganglion neurons and the central auditory pathways (Fuentes-Santamaría et al., 2013). Based on results of audiometric tests and temporal bone pathology, Schuknecht and Gacek (1993) and later modified by Nelson and Hinojosa (2003), classified presbycusis as either sensory (downslope audiometry and cochlear degeneration), neural (downslope audiometry and very poor speech discrimination, spiral ganglion and nerve fibers degeneration), metabolic (audiometry in a platform and strial atrophy), cochlear conductive (downslope audiometry and thickening and stiffening of basilar membrane), mixed (mixture of the above), or undetermined (none of the above) types.

Depending on the type and severity of the hearing loss, several options are available to reduce the hearing difficulties and consequently improve quality of life. When patients are appropriately fitted and motivated, hearing aids and cochlear implants (CIs) are the most commonly used devices for treating mild-severe presbycusis. Electric-acoustic stimulation and active middle ear implants may also be suitable solutions for treating presbycusis (Sprinzl and Riechelmann, 2010).

Biological markers are widely used in oncology, hematology and in other medical disciplines to diagnose or to monitor various diseases. In otology, biological markers are not yet widely used, but once identified, they could provide a means of determining the time-course or most effective treatment for an individual with presbycusis or tinnitus. Potential biomarkers include mutations in mitochondrial DNA, chromosomal mutations, state of chronic inflammation, presence of certain diseases associated with earlier onset or progression of presbycusis (e.g., diabetes, hypertension) and metabolic diseases (Van Eyken et al., 2007; Verschuur et al., 2014). It was recently estimated that 35–55% of auditory aging could have a genetic background (Ruan et al., 2014). Of interest are genes coding for glutamate receptors as glutamate is the main excitatory neurotransmitter in the peripheral and central auditory pathways. It has been suggested that increased release of glutamate may be involved in the auditory aging and the generation and maintenance of tinnitus by causing "excitotoxicity." There are many types of glutamate receptors, such as *N*-methyl-D-aspartate (NMDA) and alfa-amine propionic acid (AMPA), the latter being the most relevant receptor in physiological neurotransmission at auditory pathways. NMDA receptors are not essential for the auditory transmission, but they have been shown to be expressed in the cochlea after induction of tinnitus. Moreover, it has been demonstrated that the application of NMDA antagonists directly into the cochlear fluid can block salicylate-induced tinnitus in animals (Figueiredo et al., 2008).

GRM7 encodes a metabotropic glutamate receptor subtype 7 (mGluR7), a G protein-coupled receptor regulating auditory nerve excitability. When bound by L-glutamate, mGluR7changes the configuration of adenylyl cyclase, which has implications in the metabolism of AMPc, control of cellular cycle, and normal functioning of central nervous pathways. mGluR7 plays a general role in glutamate synaptic transmission (Voytenko and Galazyuk, 2011). In the auditory periphery, mGluR7 is thought to mediate glutamate excitotoxicity (Pujol et al., 1993) and in the cochlea mGluR7 maintains the glutamate-dependent equilibrium between the inner hair cells and the spiral ganglion neurons (Newman et al., 2012). Its role in the higher auditory pathways remains unclear (Lu, 2014). Single nucleotide polymorphisms (SNPs) of *GRM7* have been demonstrated to be associated with auditory aging in European (Friedman et al., 2009) and American populations (Newman et al., 2012) but not of a Chinese population (Luo et al., 2013). Interestingly, Newman et al. (2012) have reported that certain SNP variants of *GRM7* associate with poorer speech recognition in the elderly. The importance of *GRM7* in the auditory system is supported by the detection of mGluR7 in the inner and outer hair cells and in the spiral ganglion nerve (Friedman et al., 2009).

Highly concentrated glutamate may affect membrane permeability in the hair cells, causing an increase in Cl^- influx, and consequently an osmotic imbalance and membrane disruption (Puel et al., 1998). In addition, glutamate excitotoxicity induces apoptotic cell death and inflammation (Sahley et al., 2013). This was demonstrated in an animal model to be directly responsible for the loss of inner hair cells in a time-, dose- and tonotopy-dependent manner (Hu et al., 2015). Interestingly, neonatal exposure to monosodium glutamate has been shown to induce neuronal atrophy and dysmorphia in the cochlear nucleus and in the superior olivary complex (Foran et al., 2017). The physiological effects of glutamate excitotoxicity therefore are concluded to include ARHL (Pujol et al., 1993) and tinnitus (Brozoski et al., 2012; Sahley et al., 2013; Yu et al., 2016).

Oxidative stress represents an imbalance between the production of reactive oxygen species (ROS) and their detoxification and has been postulated to play a major role in the overall aging process and to significantly contribute to the ARHL. Oxidative stress in the inner ear, secondary to impairments in defense mechanisms caused by certain polymorphisms related to a battery of antioxidant systems, could make individuals more susceptible to ARHL (Seidman et al., 2002; Fujimoto and Yamasoba, 2014).

In the adult inner ear, presence of several detoxification and antioxidant enzymes including catalase, superoxide dismutase, glutathione peroxidase, and glutathione *S*-transferases (GST) has been demonstrated.

One of the sources leading to accumulation of ROS are insufficiently acetylated drugs which accumulate and may be converted into reactive drug metabolites by oxidative enzymes. *N*-acetyltransferase (*NAT*) are enzymes responsible for the detoxification of exogenic substrates via *N*-acetylation or *O*-acetylation. In humans, the catalytic activity by *NAT* isoenzymes *NAT1* and *NAT2* may be regulate by these substrate concentration. Both isoenzymes are highly polymorphic and catalyze many aromatic amines and hydrazine substances important for the balance of the oxidative status. In addition, *NATs* are known to be involved in the detoxification of harmful xenobiotics (Vatsis and Weber, 1993; Hein, 2002; Ünal et al., 2005b).

Variation in *NAT2* alleles or haplotypes resulting from combination of SNPs is responsible for the *N*-acetylation polymorphism. Regarding the latter, rapid, intermediate, and slow acetylator phenotypes have been demonstrated. These phenotypes are associated with the rate of catalytic activity and accordingly predispose toward drug toxicity (Rajasekaran et al., 2011).

Because the individuals with the null genotype for *NAT2* may be more susceptible to effects of environmental toxins and oxidative free radical cellular damage, the presbycusis becomes an ideal model for evaluation of gene-environmental interaction (Ünal et al., 2005a,b). Although many individuals have been exposed to several environmental risk factors, the ARHL develops to a different degree in various age groups. This suggests genetic host factor(s) contributing to the degenerative mechanisms (Ünal et al., 2005b).

Previous studies demonstrated the association between the common human *NAT2* alleles and ARHL. Independent studies have showed a significant association between *NAT2* polymorphisms and presbycusis, namely *NAT2*6A* in the Turkish population (Ünal et al., 2005b) and in the European population (Van Eyken et al., 2007) with Caucasian subjects carrying a *NAT*6A* mutant allele having an increased risk to Presbycusis (Bared et al., 2010). Other studies considering different *NAT2* alleles reported negative associations with ARHL (Dawes et al., 2015) and with the shape of the audiograms (Angeli et al., 2012), when considering audiometric patterns of presbycusis in older individuals. However, most authors suggested that *NAT2* gene is a susceptibility factor for development of hearing impairment (Ünal et al., 2005b; Dawes et al., 2015).

Here we explore the relationships between presbycusis, tinnitus, co-morbidities, and the genotypes of *GRM7* and *NAT2*, in a sample of older Portuguese adults.

PATIENTS AND METHODS

Subjects

Inclusion criteria was the presence of sensory presbycusis, with or without tinnitus, in adults of any gender, aged between 55 and 75 years, from the Portuguese population.

Our sample included 78 older individuals ($n = 45$ women, $n = 33$ men).

For the purposes of inclusion presbycusis was defined as bilateral sensorineural deafness in downslope audiometric pattern, above 1000 Hz with poor speech discrimination (discrimination threshold > 40 dB SPL and 100% discrimination to 60 dB or worse). Although all included participants have presbycusis we will consider a subgroup with normal hearing because the adopted classification uses conversational frequencies.

Exclusion criteria were considered: inability to understand and sign the informed consent due to a significant cognitive impairment, an uncompensated medical disorder that requires urgent evaluation or if the individual has a serious psychiatric disorder. Also individuals over 55 years who presented possible factors that may overlap the variables under study were excluded [e.g., Ménière's disease, chronic otitis media, otosclerosis, tinnitus from disease of the outer ear (occlusive exostosis, outer otitis)], history of ototoxic drugs use, massive noise exposure, a history of previous malignancy with chemotherapy, history of autoimmune disorders and neurodegenerative and demyelinating diseases.

This study had the approval of the Ethical Committees from Hospital Cuf Infante Santo (November 26th, 2014), Nova Medical School (n°65/2014/CEFCM) and the National Department of Personal Data Protection (authorization number:1637/2016).

Accordingly we obtained the Institutional Scientific Review Board approval of the process for taking informed consent and overall study design. The study was conducted in accordance with the Declaration of Helsinki.

Clinical Evaluation

Written informed consent, clinical and familial history, audiological evaluation and a blood sample, using Whatman® FTA® card technology, was obtained from every subject.

A questionnaire concerning epidemiologic data (demographic, previous and present diseases, toxicological habits and noise exposure) was completed by the researcher through participant interview.

Audiological Assessment

Hearing thresholds were determined by pure tone audiometry (air and bone) according to ISO 8253 and 389. The exam was performed in a soundproof booth using an Interacoustics®, Assens, Denmark audiometer (Model: AC40, Serial No.: 98 019 046) and TDH39 headphones fitted with noise-excluding headset ME70 and bone conductor B-71. Audiometry was performed at frequencies from 0.25 to 16 kHz (standard tonal audiometry and extended high frequency). The category of Hearing Loss (HL) was defined according to the average threshold across 500, 1000, 2000, and 4000 Hz in the better ear as mild (21–40 dB), moderate (41–70 dB), severe (71–95 dB) or profound (>95 dB), from an average of thresholds at 500, 1000, 2000, and 4000 Hz in the better ear, according to the European Working Group Genetics of Hearing Impairment (After Liu and Xu, 1994; Parving and Newton, 1995).

Speech audiometry evaluation was obtained with headphones (using mp3 player), or in open field, where the evaluator was hiding his lips to prevent lip-reading. The number of disyllables that patient repeats correctly was recorded. This intelligibility threshold for two-syllable words intends to measure hearing sensitivity threshold through the intensity level identification in which the patient can correctly identify 50% or more of a disyllables list. On the other hand, the speech discrimination evaluates the lowest intensity level at which a listener can understand speech.

Tinnitus Assessment

Psychoacoustic assessment consisted of loudness match, pitch match, minimum masking level (MML) or Feldmann masking curves, residual inhibition, and loudness discomfort levels (LDL). The severity of tinnitus was evaluated using the Tinnitus Handicap Inventory (THI; Newman et al., 1996). THI comprises 25 questions concerning tinnitus, and the response options are "Yes," "Sometimes," and "No," respectively, corresponds to 4, 2, and 0, accounting for a total score that may vary between 0 and 100. The questionnaire comprehends three sub-scales or dimensions: Functional (11 items - contributing 0–44 for the final score), Emotional (9 items - contributing 0–36 for the final score) and Catastrophic (5 items - contributing 0–20 for the final score). This allow to verify which are the most affected aspects and accordingly choose the therapeutic interventions. The total score of the responses allows tinnitus classification according to its severity or impact in daily life - 0–16: Slight or no handicap (Grade 1), 18–36: Mild handicap (Grade 2), 38–56: Moderate handicap (Grade 3), 58–76: Severe handicap (Grade 4), 78–100: Catastrophic handicap (Grade 5).

Additionally THI is a self-administered instrument, easy to quote, to interpret and has good psychometrics properties (McCombe et al., 2001).

Genetic Analysis

Total genomic DNA was extracted from a blood sample on FTA cards using a commercial NZY Tissue gDNA Isolation Kit (NZYTech, Lisbon, Portugal), strictly according to the manufacturer's instructions. Molecular analysis of *GRM7* gene was assessed by qPCR for A/A, A/T, and T/T genotypes, at rs11928865 SNP. Concerning *NAT2* gene, rs1041983, rs1801280, rs1799929, rs1799930, rs108 and s1799931 were assessed by qPCR or by bidirectional sequencing of the target region in order to identify all the SNPs.

Statistical Analysis

We conducted a descriptive analysis for variables such as gender and age. The audiograms were analyzed considering the best ear (estimated based on the lowest average of frequencies of 0.5–4 kHz). We also evaluated the "high frequency" pure-tone average (PTA) at 2, 4, and 8 kHz (Newman et al., 2012). Chi-square Test or Fisher Exact Test for general association between two variables were used. Mann–Whitney or Kruskal–Wallis (for more than two groups) tests were employed to compare hearing thresholds. A Dunn's test with a Bonferroni correction was applied for multiple pairwise comparisons. The level of significance considered was $p = 0.05$.

All the results were analyzed through logistic regression model, where age and gender where considered as control for all other variables.

RESULTS

Participants in our study were 78 older adults aged 64.6 ± 5.58 years old (range = 55–75 years old). Most participants were female ($n = 45$, 57.7%), presenting an average age of 64.1 ± 5.35 years old. For men ($n = 33$, 42.3%), the mean age was 65.3 ± 5.89 years old (**Table 1**).

Hearing Thresholds

The average hearing threshold values (by gender and age) are shown in **Figure 1**. There were significant differences between the gender groups regarding average and median values of hearing thresholds at the frequencies of 4 kHz (p-value = 0.007) and 8 kHz ($p = 0.031$) when comparing male and female (**Figure 1**). There were significant differences between age groups regarding the average and median values of hearing thresholds at frequencies of 4 kHz ($p = 0.003$), 8 kHz ($p < 0.001$), 10 kHz ($p < 0.001$) and 12 kHz ($p < 0.001$) when comparing the different age groups (**Figure 1**).

When comparing hearing thresholds between the different age groups, we found significant differences in females at 4 kHz ($p = 0.009$), 8 kHz ($p = 0.011$), 10 kHz ($p = 0.018$) and 12 kHz ($p = 0.002$) (**Figure 2**). For males statistically significant differences were observed between age groups at 8 kHz ($p = 0.009$), 10 kHz ($p = 0.003$) and 12 kHz ($p = 0.004$) (**Figure 2**).

According to age and gender grouping and comparing males to females we found significant differences for hearing thresholds for the age group 55–60 years old for 1 kHz frequency ($p = 0.022$) and 4 kHz frequency ($p = 0.028$) (**Figure 2**).

Distribution of the individuals according to the hearing loss and tinnitus presence (**Table 1**) shows that in subgroup 1, 18 (23.1%) individuals who had normal hearing thresholds at speech frequencies (0.5–4 kHz) but not tinnitus; subgroup 2, 23 (29.5%) individuals who had normal hearing thresholds at speech frequencies and tinnitus; subgroup 3, 10 (12.8%) individuals who had hearing loss but not tinnitus; and subgroup 4, 27 (34.6%) individuals who had hearing loss and tinnitus (see also **Figure 3**). There are no statistical differences in age or gender between those four subgroups.

TABLE 1 | Distribution of the individuals by subgroups according to hearing loss, tinnitus presence (PTA = Pure Tone Average) and gender.

Subgroup	Audiological characteristic	Gender		*n*
		Male	**Female**	
1	PTA ≤ 20 without Tinnitus	5	13	18 (28%)
2	PTA ≤ 20 with Tinnitus	8	15	23 (29.5%)
3	PTA ≥ 20 without Tinnitus	6	4	10 (12.8%)
4	PTA ≥ 20 with Tinnitus	14	13	27 (34.6%)
Total		33	45	**78**

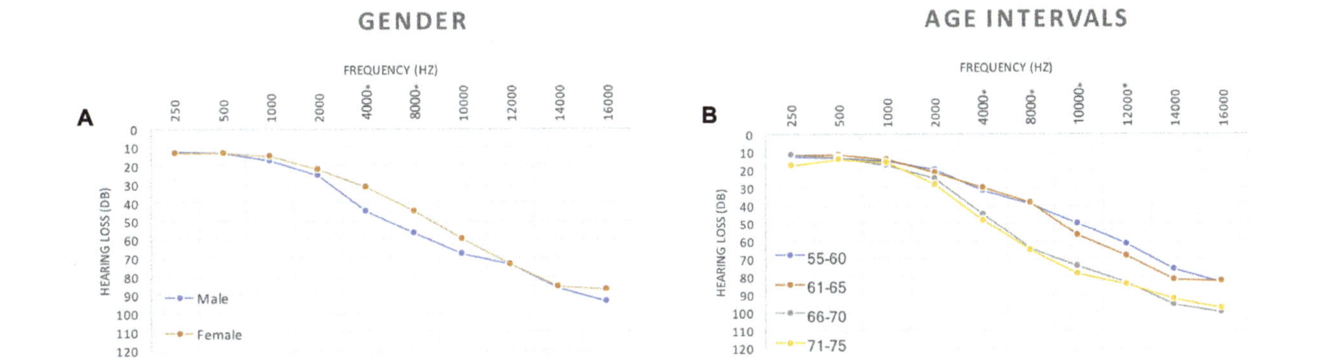

FIGURE 1 | Tonal audiogram curves showing differences between: **(A)** gender and **(B)** age intervals, for all the frequencies used to estimate HL status.

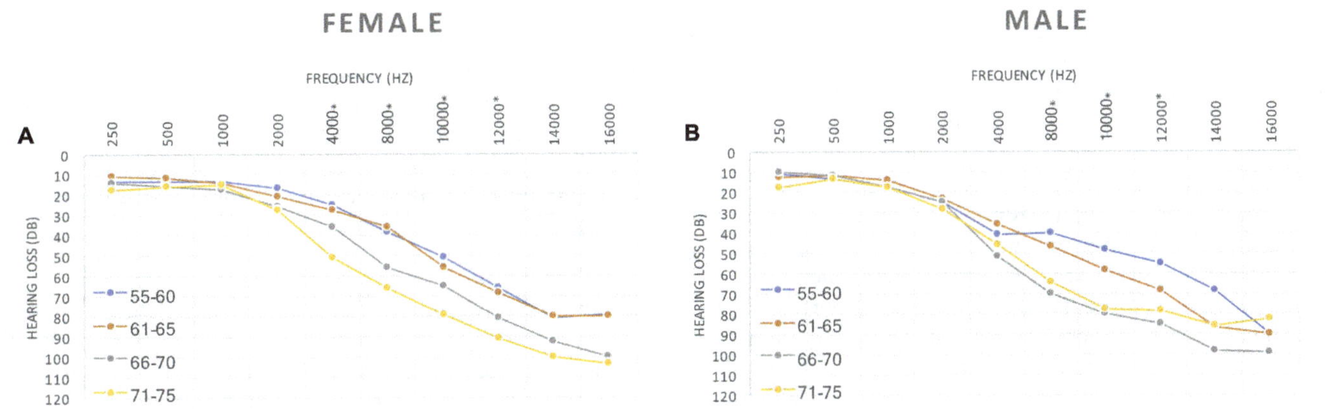

FIGURE 2 | (A) Female and **(B)** Male hearing thresholds between the different aging groups.

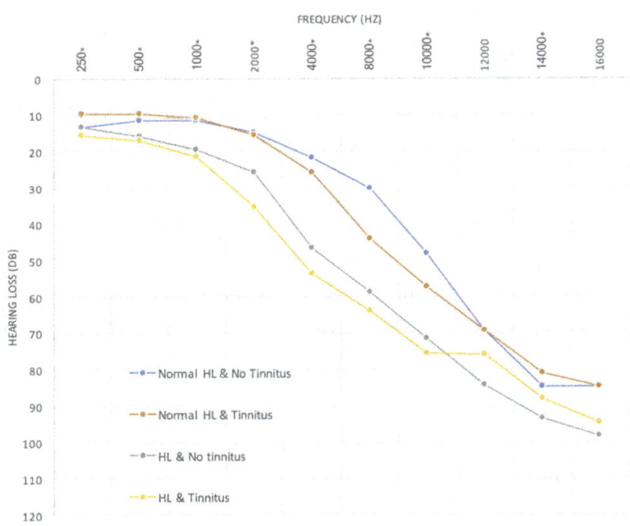

FIGURE 3 | Hearing thresholds between subgroups.

We found statistically relevant differences between the four described groups which corroborates the logical of having chosen this subdivision of our study population. (p < 0.001 at the majority of frequencies).

There were significant differences in speech audiograms (PTA, speech recognition threshold [SRT], 100%; p-value = <0.001; <0.001; <0.001, respectively) between subgroups, either for the right ear or for the left ear. The differences were found between subgroups 4 or 3 and the subgroups 1 and 2 for PTA (0%), SRT (50%) and (100%) (**Figure 4**).

Because our study population represents older adult individuals with sensory presbycusis we evaluated the "high frequency" pure-tone average (PTA) at 2, 4, and 8 kHz. We compared the groups of individuals with and without tinnitus and the four subgroups (**Table 1**). In respect to having or not tinnitus we found statistical differences between those groups (p = 0.003) (for more details see Appendix 1). We found statistically significant differences (p < 0.001) when comparing the four subgroups described in **Table 1** (for more details see Appendix 2).

Characterization of the considered comorbidities in our sample are presented in **Table 2**. Concerning hearing thresholds according to presence or not of the studied comorbidities, we found the following relevant significant differences: from 0.5 to 4 kHz for cholesterol; at 4 kHz for measles.

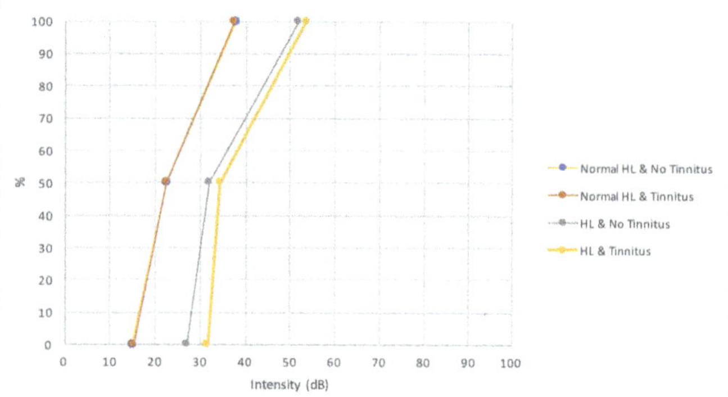

FIGURE 4 | Speech audiograms between subgroups.

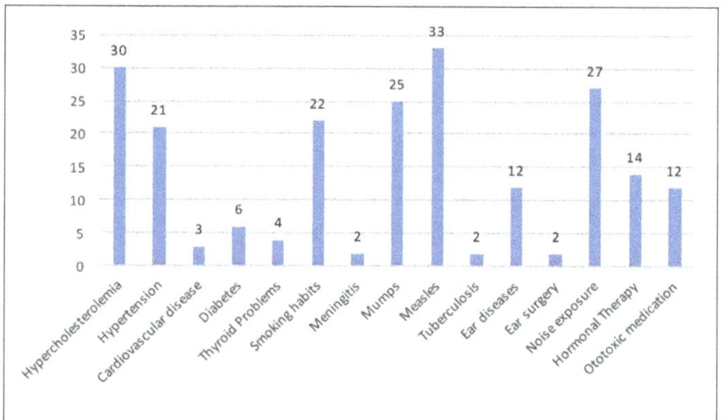

FIGURE 5 | Distribution of the most common comorbidities in the individuals with tinnitus.

When comparing the group of participants with and without tinnitus the most statistical relevant results were concerning 'high frequency' hearing loss and noise exposure. In our study population, 50 individuals (64.1%) had tinnitus.

We have determined the distribution of studied comorbidities in our tinnitus population (**Figure 5**). The most prevalent were measles, hypercholesterolemia, noise exposure, mumps, smoking and hypertension, in a descendent order of frequency.

In our sample, 49 participants (62.8%) reported to have high blood values of cholesterol. Of those, 27 individuals (55.1%) were taking medication (statins) (Appendix 3). There was a significant association between tinnitus and statins intake in those individuals reporting hypercholesterolemia ($\widehat{OR} = 0.28$, $p = 0.045$, $CI = 0.08 - 0.99$) (**Table 3**). We found no relevant association between statins intake and hearing loss.

TABLE 2 | Distribution of the most common comorbidities in the individual of the sample.

Comorbidities	*n*	
	Absent	**Present**
Cholesterol	29 (37.2%)	49 (62.8%)
Hypertension	43 (55.1%)	35 (44.9%)
Cardiovascular disease	73 (93.6%)	5 (6.4%)
Tinnitus	28 (35.8%)	50 (64.1%)
Diabetes	65 (83.3%)	13 (16.7%)
Thyroid problems	70 (89.7%)	8 (10.3%)
Smoking habits	44 (56.4%)	34 (43.6%)
Meningitis	77 (98.7%)	1 (1.3%)
Mumps	44 (56.4%)	34 (43.6%)
Measles	21 (26.9%)	57 (73.1%)
Tuberculosis	75 (96.2%)	3 (3.8%)
Ear diseases	62 (79.5%)	16 (20.5%)
Ear surgery	76 (97.4%)	2 (2.6%)
Noise exposure	51 (65.4%)	27 (34.6%)
Hormonal therapy	55 (70.5%)	23 (29.5%)
Ototoxic medication	58 (74.4%)	20 (25.6%)

Tinnitus Evaluation

Subgroups 2 and 4 included participants with tinnitus. Concerning tinnitus laterality, 33 of them reported to have a unilateral tinnitus (12 on the right ear and 21 on the left ear) and 17 participants have a bilateral tinnitus. According to THI score (**Figure 6**) for most participants tinnitus was bothersome, only 10 subjects had a slight handicap.

Modeling the data

All the results were analyzed through a logistic regression model age and gender were considered in all the models with the objective of controlling eventual confounding since these two factors are known to be related to hearing loss.

The regression logistic model was applied to HL considering female as reference (for more details see Appendix 4). The odds of developing presbycusis was significantly higher for males than for females ($\widehat{OR} = 2.9, p = 0.032$). When considering age as a covariate, the effect was slight but significant, being the odds of having hearing loss 9% higher for each increasing year ($\widehat{OR} = 1.09, p = 0.03$).

Using this statistical model for all the comorbidities considered and controlled for age the odds of having hearing loss was significantly lower for subjects with high cholesterol ($\widehat{OR} = 0.33, p = 0.034$).

We found no association between HL and high blood pressure or noise exposure.

In addition, using the regression logistic model for tinnitus considering men and the absence of tinnitus as reference, we found that noise exposure seems to influence the occurrence of tinnitus ($\widehat{OR} = 3.65, p = 0.026, CI = 1.2 - 11.4$), when considered isolated. This result is statistically very relevant.

There were no other statistically significant results concerning other comorbidities in this study (for more details see Appendix 5).

GRM7 and NAT2 genes

Results for *GRM7* gene at rs11928865 SNP refers to A or T alleles and contribute for three possible genotypes: A/A, A/T, or T/T. *GRM7* data are presented comparatively (**Table 4**) with data for Iberian Peninsula and Europe in order to compare our population with others.

TABLE 3 | Association between tinnitus and statins intake in individuals reporting hypercholesterolemia.

	Statins intake	Without Statins	$\widehat{OR}$	*p*-value (fisher test)	95% IC
Tinnitus	13	17	0.28	$p = 0.045$	[0.08 – 0.99]
Without tinnitus	14	5			

**p-value* < 0.05.

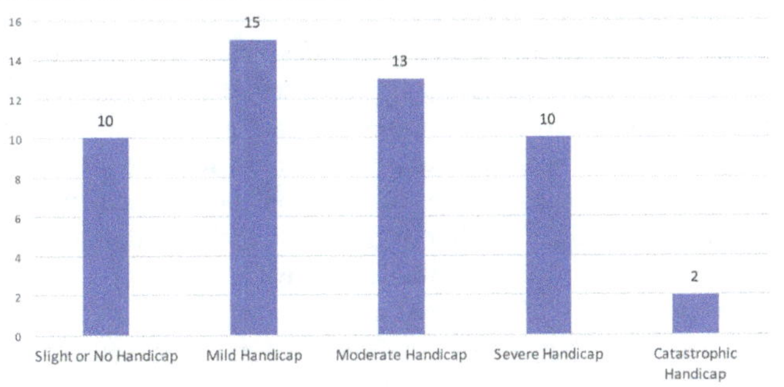

FIGURE 6 | Distribution of the individuals according to THI.

Some genetic specificity has been reported for different populations regarding deafness genes, and, interestingly, genotypes representativeness for the individuals of our sample were in accordance with values described in the European population as well as in the Iberian population.

Analyzing these results and considering the hearing thresholds, no significant differences were found in males or females when the three genotypes were compared, however, some differences in the pattern of the curves on the audiogram can be seen.

Considering the Tinnitus Handicap Inventory scores (please see **Figure 6**) the variable severe tinnitus ($n = 12$) joins the severe and catastrophic grades. We found relevant statistical association between the presence of *GRM7* and severe tinnitus (individuals having scored severe or catastrophic grade in THI). The results are present in the **Table 5**.

We found no relevant statistical differences considering *GRM7* when comparing the four sub groups already described in **Table 1**, evidencing no relation with this SNP and the presence of presbycusis with or without tinnitus.

When considering genetic data, *GRM7* genotype was found not to be associated with the risk of developing presbycusis ($p = 0.889$). However, the odds of HL is higher in individuals presenting A/T (29%) or T/T (2%) genotype, than in A/A genotype. The same results were observed when controlling for age and gender, however, in this case the odds of HL in A/T genotype individuals was nearly 39% higher than for A/A genotype individuals. The odds of HL in T/T genotype was 15% higher than in A/A genotype.

TABLE 4 | Comparative results for rs11928865 SNP on *GRM7* gene and comparison with other populations.

Genotypes	*N*	Frequency	Europe	United Kingdom	Iberian peninsula
A/A	5	0.064	0.087	0.055	0.065
A/T	26	0.333	0.382	0.473	0.393
T/T	47	0.603	0.531	0.473	0.542
Total	**78**	1	1	1	1

TABLE 5 | Association between THI score (tinnitus severity) and *GRM7* gene.

GRM7	Severe tinnitus	*p*-value	Fisher test
A/A	1		
A/T	7	**0.0233***	**0.0175**
T/T	4		

**p-value* < 0.05.

The relation between tinnitus and GRM7 gene was evaluated considering two groups, one defined as "having an A allele" (AA + AT) other defined as "not having an A allele" (TT). Results were not significant ($\widehat{OR} = 0.96$) however, since the estimated $\widehat{OR} < 1$, a decrease in the risk for tinnitus could be thought. The GRM7 genotype was not identified as a risk factor for tinnitus, neither when controlling for age ($\widehat{OR} = 0.94$) (OR = 0.94) for gender ($\widehat{OR} = 0.93$) or both simultaneously ($\widehat{OR} = 0.93$). Similar analysis was performed considering also two groups but defined as "having a T allele" (TT and AT genotypes). However, no significant association with tinnitus was found.

Genetic analysis of *NAT2* gene was performed in 65 individuals, 39 females (60%), and 26 males (40%). Rapid (R) phenotype was least common (12.3%, $n = 8$), followed by Intermediate (I) phenotype (35.4%, $n = 23$) and Slow (S) phenotype (52.3%, $n = 34$) (please see **Table 6**).

The genotype 4/4 (considered as wild type) was observed in 9.1% ($n = 6$) of the individuals being the allele 4 present in 56.9% ($n = 37$) of the genotypes. The genotype 6A/6A previously associated with presbycusis was found in 6.2% ($n = 4$) of the individuals being the allele 6A present in 23.1% ($n = 15$) of the individuals. The most common genotype is 5B/5B accounting for 50% ($n = 11$) of all the homozygous genotypes (33.9%, $n = 22$) the sample (Kuznetsov et al., 2009).

We found no statistical differences in *NAT2* gene expression across our four subgroups described in **Table 1**, evidencing no relation with the presence of presbycusis with or

TABLE 6 | Genotypes observed in the sample and their corresponding phenotypes.

Genotype	Phenotype
*NAT2*4/NAT2*5U; NAT2*6A/NAT2*6A; NAT2*5B/NAT2*5D; NAT2*6J/NAT2*13A; NAT2*5A/NAT2*5B; NAT2*6N/NAT2*6N; NAT2*6A/NAT2*6B; NAT2*5D/NAT2*5G; NAT2*5B/NAT2*5B; NAT2*5R/NAT2*12A; NAT2*4/NAT2*5J*	S
*NAT2*4/NAT2*4; NAT2*12A/NAT2*12C; NAT2*4/NAT2*12C*	R
*NAT2*4/NAT2*5B; NAT2*4/NAT2*6A; NAT2*4/NAT2*5B; NAT2*4/NAT2*5A; NAT2*5B/NAT2*12A; NAT2*4/NAT2*13A; NAT2*4/NAT2*5V; NAT2*6A/NAT2*13A; NAT2*5B/NAT2*13A*	I

without tinnitus. No significant association with ARHL was found, for the in the right and left ear or best or worst ear.

Considering the Tinnitus Handicap Inventory scores, we found significant association between severity of tinnitus (grades severe and catastrophic from THI) and the presence of *NAT2* gene (please see more details in the next sub-heading).

Modeling the Data - *GRM7* and *NAT2*

All the results were analyzed through logistic regression model (**Tables 7, 8**) where age, gender and noise exposure were considered in the models with the purpose of controlling for confounding. The independent variable in the model was severe tinnitus ($n = 12$), (the sum of severe and catastrophic grades from THI) (**Figure 6**).

We have considered the genotype T/T because after crossing the *GRM7* gene with the tinnitus population, we found that the T/T genotype is more frequent and it is the most representative so it was chosen as the reference category.

The odds of developing severe tinnitus was significantly higher in the presence of genotype A/T when compared to genotype T/T ($\widehat{OR} = 14.2$, $p = 0.009$, $CI = 2.0 - 97.8$). When considering the genotype A/A, no statistically significant difference was found ($\widehat{OR} = 2.9$, $p = 0.443$, $CI = 0.2 - 42.2$). The probability of severe tinnitus among individuals with genotype A/T is significantly higher when compared with individuals with the genotype T/T (for more details see Appendix 6).

When analyzing the presence of severe tinnitus through a logistic regression model considering *NAT2* as the independent variable and controlling for age, gender and noise exposure, the odds of developing severe tinnitus was significantly higher in the presence of slow acetylator phenotype when compared to intermediate acetylator ($\widehat{OR} = 5.7$, $p = 0.095$, $CI = 1.5 - 21.9$). No statistically significant difference was found with respect to rapid acetylator ($\widehat{OR} = 2.8$, $p = 0.504$, $CI = 0.4 - 20.8$) (for more details see Appendix 7).

TABLE 7 | Logistic regression model in the *GRM7* applied to severe tinnitus considering the genotype T/T as reference.

Variable*	$\widehat{OR}$	p-value (Wald test)	(95% IC)
GRM7			
A/A	2.9	0.443	(0.2, 42.2)
A/T	14.2	**0.009****	(2.0, 97.8)

**p-value < 0.05.

TABLE 8 | Logistic regression model in the *NAT2* applied to severe tinnitus considering intermediate acetylator as reference.

Variable*	$\widehat{OR}$	p-value (Wald test)	(90% IC)
NAT2			
Rapid acetylator	2.8	0.504	(0.4, 20.8)
Slow acetylator	5.7	0.095	(1.5, 21.9)

DISCUSSION

In the present research, we conducted a case history questionnaire, hearing evaluation and gene screening analysis for *GRM7* and *NAT2* in a sample of patients aged between 55 and 75 years, in an attempt to find factors that might contribute to the diagnosis of presbycusis and tinnitus, which could be useful for diagnosis and future therapeutic interventions.

Comorbidities Effect

Although in previous literature was described that individuals with thyroid problems present increased hearing thresholds, suggesting that thyroid hormones may act as regulators of the auditory system (Forrest et al., 1996) our results do not show any statistical relevance concerning this, one possible explanation is the sample size. Only 10% of our participants report thyroid problems which precludes statistical analysis.

Possibly for a similar reason our data doesn't show that individuals with high blood pressure may be at greater risk of presbycusis than the normotensive. Hypertension has previously been associated with increasing of the hearing threshold (Agarwal et al., 2013, p. 614). Since both presbycusis and hypertension are common and widespread disorders, the fact that hypertension may influence presbycusis strongly suggests adding cardiologists to the multidisciplinary team of professionals screening for presbycusis and improving the quality of life of positively identified individuals (Agarwal et al., 2013).

Our results found that hypercholesterolemic individuals had a lower risk of HL, probably this is due to the fact that the majority of them (67%) were having medication (statins) to control cholesterol levels. These results are in accordance with previous publications (Gopinath et al., 2011). In individuals with hypercholesterolemia the chance of occurring tinnitus is 72% lower in those who have statins intake. According to our results It seems like the statins have a protector effect.

Noise exposure and "high frequency" hearing loss seems to influence the occurrence of tinnitus, those were two of the most statistical relevant findings in our study population, which is in accordance with previous literature (Hoffman and Reed, 2004).

Gender and Age Effect

Significant differences on the HL degree were observed in different frequencies for different age groups (**Figure 2**). Our results show a significant age-dependent increase of hearing loss in about 13% for both genders, although the risk of developing presbycusis is about three times higher for men. This finding is consistent with a previous reports (Pearson et al., 1995) but contradicts another (Homans et al., 2016) where women were found to have more hearing loss.

According to our data, the risk of presbycusis increases 9% per year of life. Considering the increase in life expectancy of the population in industrialized countries, our result presents obvious consequences and must be considered for future clinical management guidelines.

In our sample tinnitus was present in 60.7% of the participants and men showed 53% more likelihood of developing tinnitus than women. This contradicts other results (Vielsmeier et al.,

2012) who reported higher tinnitus prevalence in women but in a much younger population.

According to our data, and in agreement with previous literature (Hoffman and Reed, 2004; Shargorodsky et al., 2010) age is not associated with the risk of developing tinnitus.

GRM7 and *NAT2* Effect

We did not find a significant relationship between *GRM7* genotype and either presbycusis or tinnitus. Especially for men, some differences concerning the pattern in the audiogram curves were observed in relation to *GRM7* phenotypes. For both genders, the T allele in *GRM7* gene is the most common allele in our sample of older adults with presbycusis and tinnitus, where genotypes A/T and T/T present higher level of hearing loss compared to A/A genotype. Perhaps in a larger population it could be demonstrated that the allele A of *GRM7* plays a protective role in presbycusis.

Hence, according to our results, *GRM7* genotype does not seem to be predictive of presbycusis since the odds to have ARHL is not significant ($p = 0.78$). Corroborating our results, Luo et al. (2013) studying an all-male population found that the T-allele frequency was significantly different from the genotype A/A+A/T comparing ARHL patients and healthy controls and that the *GRM7* SNP A > T was significantly different between the two groups (Luo et al., 2013). On the other hand, our findings differ from Friedman et al. (2009) most likely due to sample size (Luo et al., 2013). Moreover, the impact of the other variables - environmental, lifestyle, noise exposure, cholesterol levels and stochastic element - perhaps has prevailed over the genetic factor, declining the importance between *GRM7* gene and ARHL. Certainly multicenter studies with higher sample sizes would overcome these aspects.

Concerning *NAT2* gene, Rapid (R) phenotype was the least common, followed by the Intermediate (I) and Slow (S) phenotypes.

We found relevant statistical association between the presence of the allele A/T of *GRM7* and severe tinnitus. The chance for having a severe grade of tinnitus (severe or catastrophic grades in THI) is 14,2 higher for those carrying the allele A/T compared to T/T. Probably in larger scale studies could be demonstrated the role of allele A/A that is the less frequent in our sample.

The odds of developing severe tinnitus was relatively higher in the presence of slow acetylator phenotype of *NAT2* when compared to intermediate acetylator.

Our data suggests that allele A/T of *GRM7* can have a statistically significant influence toward the *severity* of tinnitus. As well slow acetylator phenotype of *NAT2* seems to have a similar influence (not statistically relevant in our results). Nevertheless, those results should be interpreted with caution and future studies in larger scale are necessary to confirm this correlation.

However, present data shows that genotype A/T and T/T present, respectively, a 70 and 33.3% lower risk of developing tinnitus, when compared to A/A genotype. No other studies were found relating *GRM7*, *NAT2* and tinnitus.

CONCLUSION

To the best of our knowledge, this is the first study on the association between *GRM7* and *NAT2* gene and the presbycusis and tinnitus in a population of Portuguese older adults.

Tinnitus was present in the majority of the presbycusis individuals.

Age and gender significantly influence the risk for presbycusis but not for tinnitus. Overall hearing thresholds rates increase exponentially with age (9% per year), and the increment rate and speed were gender-specific, but this increasing rate and velocity are different for women and men.

High blood pressure, thyroid diseases and hypercholesterolemia seem to have an effect on the hearing thresholds but no significant associations were found.

Our findings agree with previously observed correlations between tinnitus, noise exposure, and "high frequency" hearing loss.

No significant associations between presbycusis, tinnitus, and *GRM7* or *NAT2* were found in our sample. Our results precludes a definitive clarification about the role of *GRM7* as a possible genetic biomarkers for ARHL, although since the genotypes A/T and T/T have higher odds for HL than A/A genotypes, thus A allele could be pointed as protective biomarker for HL Nevertheless, the current state of knowledge regarding *GRM7* impact in presbycusis is insufficient to make conclusions, and so, further large-scale studies are necessary to clarify this relation.

Considering tinnitus severity (according to THI), our results bring-up very innovative conclusions.

Our data suggests the tracks that can lead to the pathway of a tinnitus severity biomarker. Potentially individuals carrying the allele A/T of *GRM7* and slow acetylator phenotype of *NAT2* (the later one with smaller statistic relevance) are prone to develop a more severe form of tinnitus, that requires specific therapeutic interventions and ideally personally tailored.

The occurrence of presbycusis is thought to be determined by genetic factors but can also be influenced by environmental or comorbidities effects, with a huge impact on quality of life and general health (Huang and Tang, 2010; Ciorba et al., 2015). However, there is still much research to explore and elucidate which risk factors contribute more to presbycusis and tinnitus, so this could help on therapeutic or preventive interventions (Huang and Tang, 2010).

Information on family history and clinical epidemiological data may help the design and development of future clinical management plans for an increasing presbycusis population.

AUTHOR CONTRIBUTIONS

HH conceived and designed this study and had contributions to all its stages. MAp and MA performed the statistical analysis. HH, MF, and HC contributed equally to all other stages of the manuscript development, drafted and revised the manuscript. DR worked with HH on interpretation of results and created appendices. DR created all audiometric figures. JP, MA, AS, DH, and GF provided consultative advice and revised the final manuscript.

FUNDING

HH, DH, AS, DR, and HC are members of COST Action (TINNET BM1306 - Better Understanding the Heterogeneity of Tinnitus to Improve and Develop New Treatments) a research program funded under the Biomedicine and Molecular Biosciences European Cooperation in Science and Technology (COST) Action framework. Travel, subsistence, and accommodation for them to participate in Tinnet meetings has been funded by Tinnet and that has been an opportunity to enhance networking collaboration between them. HH has received a Ph.D. Grant from Jmellosaude (20,000€). DH is funded by the National Institute for Health Research (NIHR) Biomedical Research Centre Program. The views expressed are those of the authors and not the funder.

REFERENCES

Agarwal, S., Mishra, A., Jagade, M., Kasbekar, V., and Nagle, S. K. (2013). Effects of hypertension on hearing. *Indian J. Otolaryngol. Head Neck Surg.* 65, 614–618.

Angeli, S., Lin, X., and Liu, X. Z. (2012). Genetics of hearing and deafness. *Anat. Rec.* 295, 1812–1829.

Bared, A., Ouyang, X., Angeli, S., Du, L. L., Hoang, K., Yan, D., et al. (2010). Antioxidant enzymes, presbycusis, and ethnic variability. *Otolaryngol. Head Neck Surg.* 143, 263–268. doi: 10.1016/j.otohns.2010.03.024

Brozoski, T., Odintsov, B., and Bauer, C. (2012). Gamma-aminobutyric acid and glutamic acid levels in the auditory pathway of rats with chronic tinnitus: a direct determination using high resolution point-resolved proton magnetic resonance spectroscopy (H-MRS). *Front. Syst. Neurosci.* 6:9. doi: 10.3389/fnsys.2012.00009

Ciorba, A., Hatzopoulos, S., Bianchini, C., Aimoni, C., Skarzynski, H., and Skarzynski, P. H. (2015). Genetics of presbycusis and presbystasis. *Int. J. Immunopathol. Pharmacol.* 28, 29–35. doi: 10.1177/0394632015570819

Dawes, P., Emsley, R., Cruickshanks, K. J., Moore, D. R., Fortnum, H., Edmondson-Jones, M., et al. (2015). Hearing loss and cognition: the role of hearing AIDS, social isolation and depression. *PLOS ONE* 10:e0119616. doi: 10.1371/journal.pone.0119616

Figueiredo, R. R., Langguth, B., de Oliveira, P. M., and de Azevedo, A. A. (2008). Tinnitus treatment with memantine. *Otolaryngol. Head Neck Surg.* 138, 492–496. doi: 10.1016/j.otohns.2007.11.027

Foran, L., Blackburn, K., and Kulesza, R. J. (2017). Auditory hindbrain atrophy and anomalous calcium binding protein expression after neonatal exposure to monosodium glutamate. *Neuroscience* 344, 406–417. doi: 10.1016/j.neuroscience.2017.01.004

Forrest, D., Erway, L. C., Ng, L., Altschuler, R., and Curran, T. (1996). Thyroid hormone receptor b is essential for development of auditory function. *Nat. Genet.* 13, 354–357.

Friedman, R. A., Van Laer, L., Huentelman, M. J., Sheth, S. S., Van Eyken, E., Corneveaux, J. J., et al. (2009). *GRM7* variants confer susceptibility to age-related hearing impairment. *Hum. Mol. Genet.* 18, 785–796. doi: 10.1093/hmg/ddn402

Fuentes-Santamaría, V., Alvarado, J. C., Gabaldón-Ull, M. C., and Manuel Juiz, J. (2013). Upregulation of insulin like growth factor and interleukin 1β occurs in neurons but not in glial cells in the cochlear nucleus following cochlear ablation. *J. Comp. Neurol.* 521, 3478–3499.

Fujimoto, C., and Yamasoba, T. (2014). Oxidative stresses and mitochondrial dysfunction in age-related hearing loss. *Oxid. Med. Cell. Longev.* 2014:582849.

Gopinath, B., Flood, V. M., Teber, E., McMahon, C. M., and Mitchell, P. (2011). Dietary intake of cholesterol is positively associated and use of cholesterol-lowering medication is negatively associated with prevalent age-related hearing loss. *J. Nutr.* 141, 1355–1361. doi: 10.3945/jn.111.138610

Hein, D. W. (2002). Molecular genetics and function of *NAT1* and *NAT2*: role in aromatic amine metabolism and carcinogenesis. *Mutat. Res.* 506, 65–77.

Hoffman, H. J., and Reed, G. W. (2004). "Epidemiology of tinnitus," in *Tinnitus: Theory and Management*, ed. J. B. Snow (Lewiston, NY: BC Decker Inc.), 16–41.

Homans, N. C., Metselaar, R. M., Dingemanse, J. G., van der Schroeff, M. P., Brocaar, M. P., Wieringa, M. H., et al. (2016). Prevalence of age-related hearing loss, including sex differences, in older adults in a large cohort study. *Laryngoscope* 127, 725–730. doi: 10.1002/lary.26150

Hu, Y., Zhou, L. Q., Lu, H. T., Yuan, K., and Gong, S. S. (2015). Excitotoxic effects of glutamate on cochlear organotypic cultures. *J. Huazhong Univ. Sci. Technol.* 35, 117–121. doi: 10.1007/s11596-015-1399-0

Huang, Q., and Tang, J. (2010). Age-related hearing loss or presbycusis. *Eur. Arch. Otorhinolaryngol.* 267, 1179–1191. doi: 10.1007/s00405-010-1270-7

Jastreboff, P. J., and Hazell, J. W. (1993). A neurophysiological approach to tinnitus: clinical implications. *Br. J. Audiol.* 27, 7–17.

Kuznetsov, I. B., McDuffie, M., and Moslehi, R. (2009). A web-server for inferring the human N-acetyltransferase-2 (*NAT2*) enzymatic phenotype from *NAT2* genotype. *Bioinformatics* 25, 1185–1186. doi: 10.1093/bioinformatics/btp121

Lee, K. Y. (2013). Pathophysiology of age-related hearing loss (peripheral and central). *Korean J. Audiol.* 17, 45–49. doi: 10.7874/kja.2013.17.2.45

Liu, X., and Xu, L. (1994). Nonsyndromic hearing loss: an analysis of audiograms. *Ann. Otol. Rhinol. Laryngol.* 103, 428–433. doi: 10.1177/000348949410300602

Lu, Y. (2014). Metabotropic glutamate receptors in auditory processing. *Neuroscience* 274, 429–445. doi: 10.1016/j.neuroscience.2014.05.057

Luo, H., Yang, T., Jin, X., Pang, X., Li, J., Chai, Y., et al. (2013). Association of *GRM7* variants with different phenotype patterns of age-related hearing impairment in an elderly male Han Chinese population. *PLOS ONE* 8:e77153. doi: 10.1371/journal.pone.0077153

McCombe, A., Baguley, D., Coles, R., McKenna, L., McKinney, C., and Windle-Taylor, P. (2001). Guidelines for the grading of tinnitus severity: the results of a working group commissioned by the British Association of Otolaryngologists, Head and Neck Surgeons. *Clin. Otolaryngol.* 26, 388–393.

Nelson, E. G., and Hinojosa, R. (2003). Presbycusis: a human temporal bone study of individuals with flat audiometric patterns of hearing loss using a new method to quantify stria vascularis volume. *Laryngoscope* 113, 1672–1686.

Newman, D. L., Fisher, L. M., Ohmen, J., Parody, R., Fong, C. T., Frisina, S. T., et al. (2012). *GRM7* variants associated with age-related hearing loss based on auditory perception. *Hear. Res.* 294, 125–132. doi: 10.1016/j.heares.2012.08.016

Newman, C. W., Jacobson, G. P., and Spitzer, J. B. (1996). Development of the tinnitus handicap inventory. *Arch. Otolaryngol. Head Neck Surg.* 122, 143–148.

Parving, A., and Newton, V. (1995). Guidelines for description of inherited hearing loss. *J. Audiol. Med.* 4, 2–5.

Pearson, J. D., Morrell, C. H., Gordon Salant, S., Brant, L. J., Metter, E. J., Klein, L. L., et al. (1995). Gender differences in a longitudinal study of age-associated hearing loss. *J. Acoust. Soc. Am.* 97, 1196–1205.

Puel, J. L., Ruel, J., d'Aldin, C. G., and Pujol, R. (1998). Excitotoxicity and repair of cochlear synapses after noise trauma induced hearing loss. *Neuroreport* 9, 2109–2114.

Pujol, R., Puel, J. L., D'aldin, C. G., and Eybalin, M. (1993). Pathophysiology of the glutamatergic synapses in the cochlea. *Acta Otolaryngol.* 113, 330–334.

Rajasekaran, M., Abirami, S., and Chen, C. (2011). Effects of single nucleotide polymorphisms on human N-acetyltransferase 2 structure and dynamics by molecular dynamics simulation. *PLOS ONE* 6:e25801. doi: 10.1371/journal.pone.0025801

Ruan, Q., Ma, C., Zhang, R., and Yu, Z. (2014). Current status of auditory aging and anti-aging research. *Geriatr. Gerontol. Int.* 14, 40–53. doi: 10.1111/ggi.12124

Sahley, T. L., Hammonds, M. D., and Musiek, F. E. (2013). Endogenous dynorphins, glutamate and N-methyl-d-aspartate (NMDA) receptors may participate in a stress-mediated Type-I auditory neural exacerbation of tinnitus. *Brain Res.* 1499, 80–108. doi: 10.1016/j.brainres.2013.01.006

Schuknecht, H. F., and Gacek, M. R. (1993). Cochlear pathology in presbycusis. *Ann. Otol. Rhinol. Laryngol.* 102(1 Pt 2), 1–16.

Seidman, M. D., Khan, M. J., Tan, W. X., and Quirk, W. S. (2002). Influence of lecithin on mitochondrial DNA and age-related hearing loss. *Otolaryngol. Head Neck Surg.* 127, 138–144.

Shargorodsky, J., Curhan, G. C., and Farwell, W. R. (2010). Prevalence and characteristics of tinnitus among US adults. *Am. J. Med.* 123, 711–718. doi: 10.1016/j.amjmed.2010.02.015

Sprinzl, G. M., and Riechelmann, H. (2010). Current trends in treating hearing loss in elderly people: a review of the technology and treatment options–a mini-review. *Gerontology* 56, 351–358. doi: 10.1159/000275062

Ünal, M., Tamer, L., Akbaş, Y., Pata, Y. S., Vayisoğlu, Y., Değirmenci, U., et al. (2005a). Genetic polymorphism of N-acetyltransferase 2 in the susceptibility to laryngeal squamous cell carcinoma. *Head Neck* 27, 1056–1060.

Ünal, M., Tamer, L., Doğruer, Z. N., Yildirim, H., Vayisoğlu, Y., and Çamdeviren, H. (2005b). N-acetyltransferase 2 gene polymorphism and presbycusis. *Laryngoscope* 115, 2238–2241.

Van Eyken, E., Van Camp, G., and Van Laer, L. (2007). The complexity of age-related hearing impairment: contributing environmental and genetic factors. *Audiol. Neurotol.* 12, 345–358.

Vatsis, K. P., and Weber, W. W. (1993). Structural heterogeneity of Caucasian N-acetyltransferase at the *NAT1* gene locus. *Arch. Biochem. Biophys.* 301, 71–76.

Verschuur, C., Agyemang-Prempeh, A., and Newman, T. A. (2014). Inflammation is associated with a worsening of presbycusis: evidence from the MRC national study of hearing. *Int. J. Audiol.* 53, 469–475. doi: 10.3109/14992027.2014.891057

Vielsmeier, V., Strutz, J., Kleinjung, T., Schecklmann, M., Kreuzer, P. M., Landgrebe, M., et al. (2012). Temporomandibular joint disorder complaints in tinnitus: further hints for a putative tinnitus subtype. *PLOS ONE* 7:e38887. doi: 10.1371/journal.pone.0038887

Voytenko, S. V., and Galazyuk, A. V. (2011). mGluRs modulate neuronal firing in the auditory midbrain. *Neurosci. Lett.* 492, 145–149. doi: 10.1016/j.neulet.2011.01.075

Yamasoba, T., Lin, F. R., Someya, S., Kashio, A., Sakamoto, T., and Kondo, K. (2013). Current concepts in age-related hearing loss: epidemiology and mechanistic pathways. *Hear. Res.* 303, 30–38. doi: 10.1016/j.heares.2013.01.021

Yu, H., Patil, K. V., Han, C., Fabella, B., Canlon, B., Someya, S., et al. (2016). GLAST deficiency in mice exacerbates gap detection deficits in a model of salicylate-induced tinnitus. *Front. Behav. Neurosci.* 10:158. doi: 10.3389/fnbeh.2016.00158

15

A Case of Acoustic Shock with Post-Trauma Trigeminal-Autonomic Activation

*Alain Londero[1], Nicolas Charpentier[2], Damien Ponsot[3], Philippe Fournier[4], Laurent Pezard[4] and Arnaud J. Noreña[4]**

[1] Service ORL et CCF, Hôpital Européen G. Pompidou, Paris, France, [2] Faculté de médecine de Nancy, Université de Lorraine, Nancy, France, [3] Lycée Germaine Tillion, Académie de Lyon, Sain-Bel, France, [4] Laboratoire Neurosciences Intégratives et Adaptatives, UMR CNRS 7260, Fédération 3C, Aix-Marseille Université, Marseille, France

***Correspondence:**
Arnaud J. Noreña
arnaud.norena@univ-amu.fr

This study reports the case of an acoustic shock injury (ASI), which did not result in a significant hearing loss, but was followed by manifold chronic symptoms both within (tinnitus, otalgia, tingling in the ear, tension in the ear, and red tympanum) and outside the ears (blocked nose, pain in the neck/temporal region). We suggest that these symptoms may result from a loop involving injury to middle ear muscles, peripheral inflammatory processes, activation and sensitization of the trigeminal nerve, the autonomic nervous system, and central feedbacks. The pathophysiology of this ASI is reminiscent of that observed in post-traumatic trigeminal-autonomic cephalalgia. This framework opens new and promising perspectives on the understanding and medical management of ASI.

Keywords: tinnitus and hyperacousis, otalgia, pain, trigeminal nerve, acoustic shock, inflammation, referred pain

INTRODUCTION

Acoustic shocks are brief exposure to loud sounds that do not cause substantial hearing loss but can trigger a cluster of debilitating symptoms, i.e., otalgia, ear fullness, ear tension, tinnitus, sound intolerance, dizziness and head, face or neck aches (1, 2). In most cases, these symptoms are temporary and disappear within a few hours or days following the acoustic incident. However, in certain cases, they can become chronic and seriously affect quality of life (1). The pathophysiological mechanisms underlying these symptoms remain unknown, even though some authors have hypothesized a dysfunction in the tensor tympani muscle (TTM) (1, 2). The patient described here was able to precisely report his symptoms, their temporal evolution, and take pictures of his eardrums over time during symptom severity fluctuations. The psychoacoustic characteristics of his tinnitus and the functional integrity of the middle ears were also investigated. This invaluable dataset provides critical insights into the pathophysiology of the acoustic shock injury (ASI) and beyond, i.e., tinnitus, hyperacusis, and otalgia.

METHODS

The patient (NC) was a 27-year-old Caucasian male working as a general medical practitioner at the time of the acoustic shock. Written informed consent was obtained from the participant for the publication of this case report. On November 10th 2013, in a leisure shooting stand, without wearing any hearing protection, he was exposed to a unique and unexpected gunfire at an approximate 7 m distance from his right side. As bothersome symptoms progressively emerged after this acoustic incident, he attended several ENT clinics. Audiograms at week 3 and 7 after ASI (thresholds <15 dBHL at all tested frequencies from 0.125 to 8 kHz) and all other exams (tympanometry, blood check, and cerebral MRI) were normal. Later, he was asked to assess the severity of his symptoms, using a 0–10 visual analog scale, for each ear several times a day (from May 1st to May 9th 2015). The symptoms were tingling, otalgia, ear tension, tinnitus loudness, neck pain/tension, temporal pain/tension, and pain/blocked nose. He also managed to photograph his eardrums using a video-otoscope (Firefly DE500 v1.1, 4 mm speculum). For analysis purpose, the images were transformed into numeric values estimating the "redness" of the eardrum. The number of red pixels was normalized according to the eardrum surface captured by the video-otoscope. In March 2017, NC visited our laboratory in Marseille to assess the psychoacoustic properties of his tinnitus and explored the middle ear function (Multifrequency Tympanometer Zodiac, Otometrics). Static admittance was obtained at four frequencies (226, 678, 800, and 1,000 Hz). Admittance variation while the patient voluntarily (but not forcefully) eye blinked was investigated over time both at the pressure at which the admittance is maximal and at ±50 daPa from this value. Symptom severity from each ear was analyzed using principal component analysis (PCA). The PCA was performed on all symptoms, excluding neck and temporal pain as these symptoms did not affect the left side.

RESULTS

In regard to the clinical course, immediately after ASI, the patient felt a clicking in the right ear and thereafter reported a subjective perception of ear tension and fullness. At week 2 emerged a bilateral high-pitched fluctuating tinnitus. These auditory symptoms were associated with an erratic acute pain (sting or electrical shock) located deep in either ear. More than 3 weeks after the acoustic shock, the patient reported additional painful sensations starting around the concha and irradiating to the mid-face (constriction, blocked nose, and clear nasal discharge) and to the temporal region or the neck. Interestingly, the laterality and severity of the pain was correlated with the amount of tension perceived in the ipsilateral (right) ear. The psychoacoustic properties of the tinnitus, its amplitude modulation (tremolo), also varied according to the ear tension level. From low to mid tension, the tremolo varied from low frequency ("morse code") to high frequency ("cricket-like sound"). For high tension, tinnitus was described as a high-pitched whistling. The pitch of this tinnitus was measured at 12 kHz and the tremolo, estimated from an amplitude modulated stimulus at the tinnitus frequency, was found at 32 Hz (the severity of ear tension and tinnitus loudness were 4 and 3, respectively). The loudness of this high-pitched tinnitus is reported in **Figure 1**. The patient also reported a low-pitched tinnitus associated with a sensation of fluttering in the ear. The low-pitched tinnitus was enhanced when something (earplug, stethoscope) was inserted in the ear canal. The high- and low-pitched tinnitus could be absent when the ear was completely relaxed. In contrast the tinnitus was not modulated by forceful head and neck contractions (3).

The temporal evolution of symptoms severity (**Figure 1**) was investigated using PCA. The first principal component (48% of the total variance) represents the severity of the symptoms and does not discriminate between them. On the other hand, the second principal component (18% of the total variance) separates two symptom clusters, namely "tension," "blocked nose," and "tympanum redness" for symptom cluster 1 and "tingling," "tinnitus," and "otalgia" for symptom cluster 2 (**Figure 2**, upper panels). The feeling of pain in the temporal region and the neck (plotted on the first two PCA axes) represent a third group of symptoms (symptom cluster 3), different from cluster 1 and 2. The symptom cluster 3 is reported in the right side only, is moderate in severity, and is present only occasionally compared to the other symptoms. The PCA indicates that the correlation between symptom cluster 3 and both symptom cluster 1 and 2 is low. **Figure 2** (middle panels) shows the multi-dimensional data (symptom severity) plotted on the new coordinate system defined by the first two principal components at each time point. The symptoms are usually more severe in the right ear than in the left ear, and the maximum severity is also greater in the right ear. Interestingly, the two symptom clusters are reported in the right ear, while only symptom cluster 1 is reported in the left ear. The temporal dynamics of symptom severity (first principal component) in the left and right ear (**Figure 2**, bottom panel) is also clearly anti-correlated across the two ears.

The sensation of tension in the ear was associated with tympanum hyperemia (**Figure 1**, also see Video S1 in Supplementary Material). This hyperemia was also present during jaw muscle contraction (hypothetically involving the mylohyoid muscle) and was associated with an increase of the high-pitch tinnitus (see Video S2 in Supplementary Material). This phenomenon was reported to be only present when the sensation of tension in the ear was high and coincidentally, the tympanum was always showing dilated vessels.

The tympanometry measurements demonstrated different middle ear function for the two ears (**Figure 3**). Indeed, for the right ear, the static admittance was larger (**Figure 3**, upper panel) and the resonant frequency (estimated from the frequency at which the susceptance is null) was abnormally low (<678 Hz) (**Figure 3**, middle panel). Moreover, the admittance was modulated by eyelid closure, especially in the right ear (**Figure 3**, bottom panel). Finally, the stapedial reflexes were present and clinically normal in both ears at 500 Hz and 4 kHz at 95–100 dB HL.

DISCUSSION

This report completes and adds to previous studies on acoustic shock (1). First, the symptoms reported after the acoustic shock, including their temporal dynamics and characteristics, have been described both qualitatively and quantitatively. This case reports all the symptoms that are commonly described after ASI, except vertigo and/or dizziness (1), and additional symptoms (nasal congestion, rhinorrhea, and tympanum hyperemia). Second, the functional integrity of the middle ears was also investigated

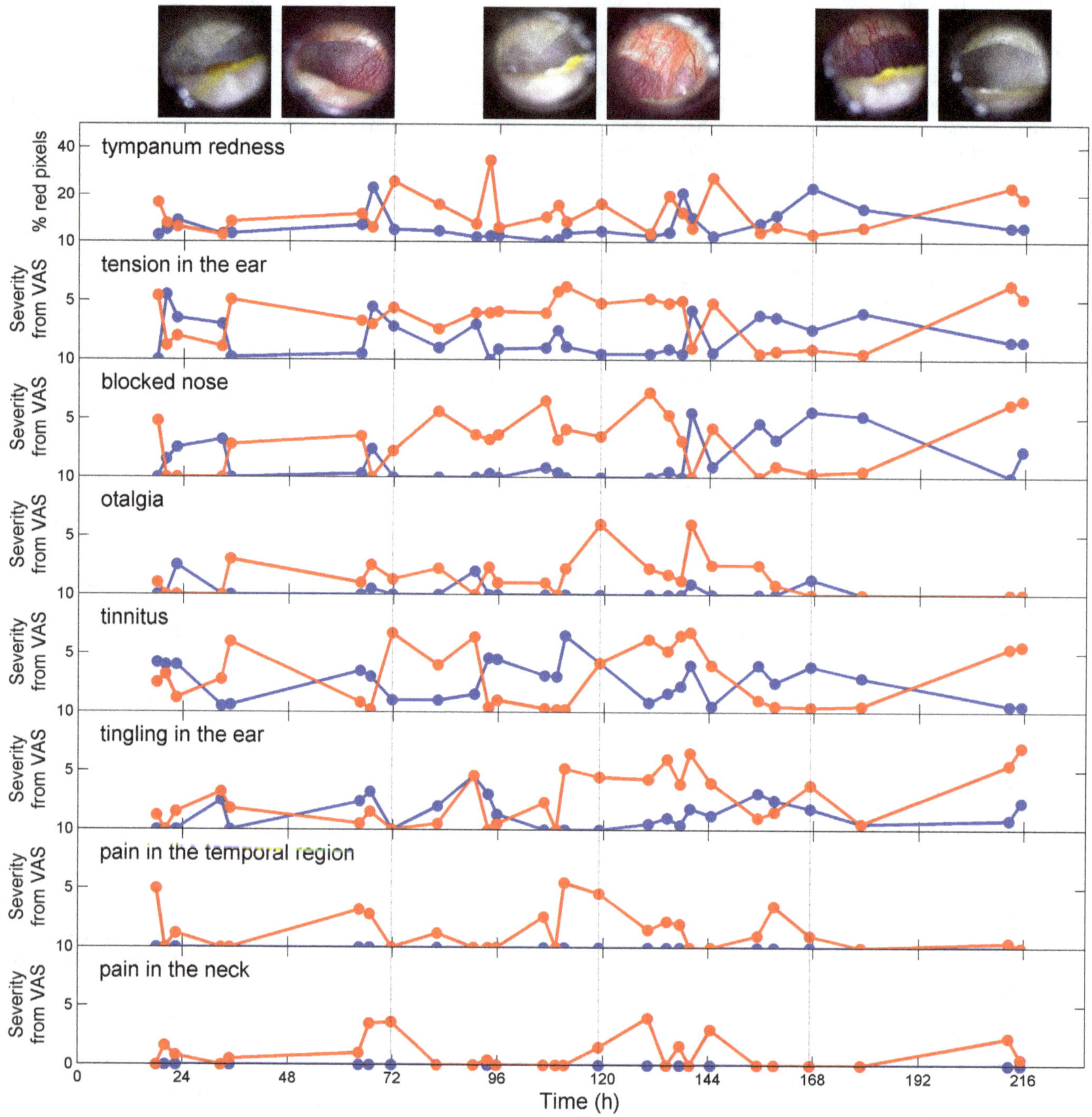

FIGURE 1 | Severity of acoustic shock symptoms (assessed by VAS) as a function of time. The blue line represents the left ear and the red line represents the right ear. Examples of tympanum pictures are shown at the top (left images: left ear; right images: right ear, the vertical lines corresponds to the time at which the pictures were taken).

using multifrequency tympanometry and direct examination of the eardrums. Our findings provide further insights into the mechanisms involved in ASI, and in particular they question and extend the framework previously developed by others (1, 2).

This study is the first to provide experimental support suggesting that middle ear muscles (MEM) can behave abnormally after ASI. Indeed, middle ear admittance is changed by simple eyelid closure, eardrum movements in the right ear can be large enough to be visible by the naked eye and the fluttering sensation (likely accompanying MEM contraction) is enhanced by cutaneous stimulation of the ear canal (4–7). This abnormal behavior of MEM may result from a dysfunction and/or injury of MEM caused by an exaggerated contraction in response to the acoustic incident. While stapedius muscle contraction is activated by loud

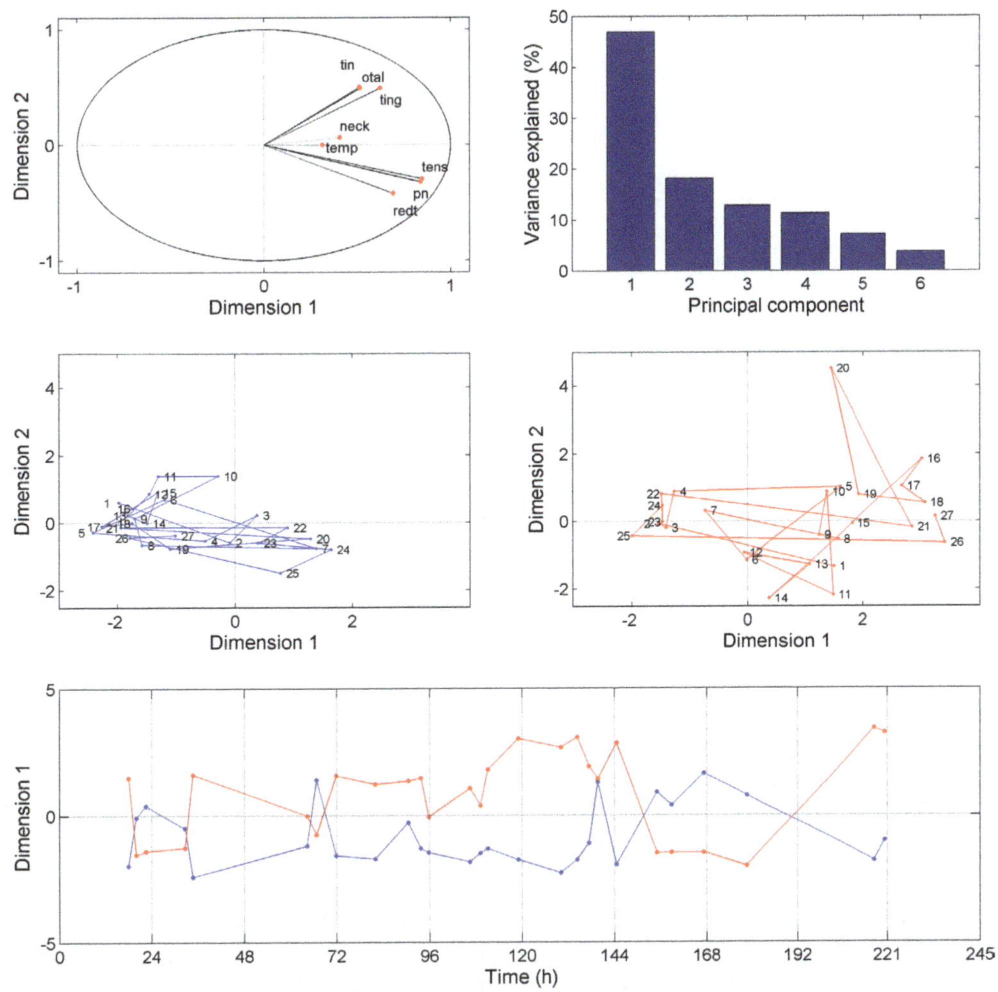

FIGURE 2 | Results obtained from the principal component analysis (PCA). The upper left panel represents each symptom as a function of the first two principal components derived from the PCA. The upper right panel shows the percentage of variance explained by the different principal components. The middle panels (left: left ear, right: right ear) show the symptoms plotted at each time point as a function the first two principal components. The bottom panel shows the first principal component for each ear (blue line: left ear, red line: right ear) as a function of time.

sounds, TTM contraction can be triggered by unexpected sounds through the general startle reflex (8). The low resonant frequency and large admittance in the most symptomatic (right) ear may reflect an abnormal ossicle arrangement, possibly caused by the exaggerated contraction of the MEM. The sensation of tension in the ear reported immediately after the acoustic shock may result from an abnormal contraction of the MEM signaled by the muscle spindles (9) and tympanum mechanoreceptors due to eardrum deformation (10). The traumatic acoustic episode may lead to anxiety and sensory hypersensitivity, which may in turn reduce the startle reflex threshold and/or potentiate the startle reflex (11), possibly through a descending serotoninergic innervation (12). This central feedback may facilitate tonic and phasic TTM contraction.

The putative exaggerated contraction of the MEM, eventually followed by tonic contraction, may be associated with MEM injury and inflammatory processes. In particular, the TTM is innervated by fibers containing substance P and calcitonin gene-related peptide, which may play a key role in the noise-induced inflammation of the middle ear (13–15). Inflammation can then diffuse from the MEM to the tympanum and middle ear mucosa and can even become neurogenic as these tissues are rich in mastocytes (16–18). The diverse pain feelings in the ear (otalgia and tingling) likely result from middle ear inflammation and activation of the trigeminal nerve (TGN), which innervates the middle ear mucosa, the eardrum, and the TTM (15, 19). Intriguingly, tinnitus loudness is correlated to the severity of otalgia and tingling in the ear, suggesting that middle ear inflammation plays a role in tinnitus generation and/or severity. One can propose that antidromic activation of the TGN may change the vascular permeability of the blood vessels in the stria vascularis (20), which may eventually increase the endocochlear potential and produce tinnitus.

The MEM dysfunction/injury and the chronic inflammatory processes following ASI may be associated with neural hyperactivity in the trigeminal pathways. This neural hyperactivity may

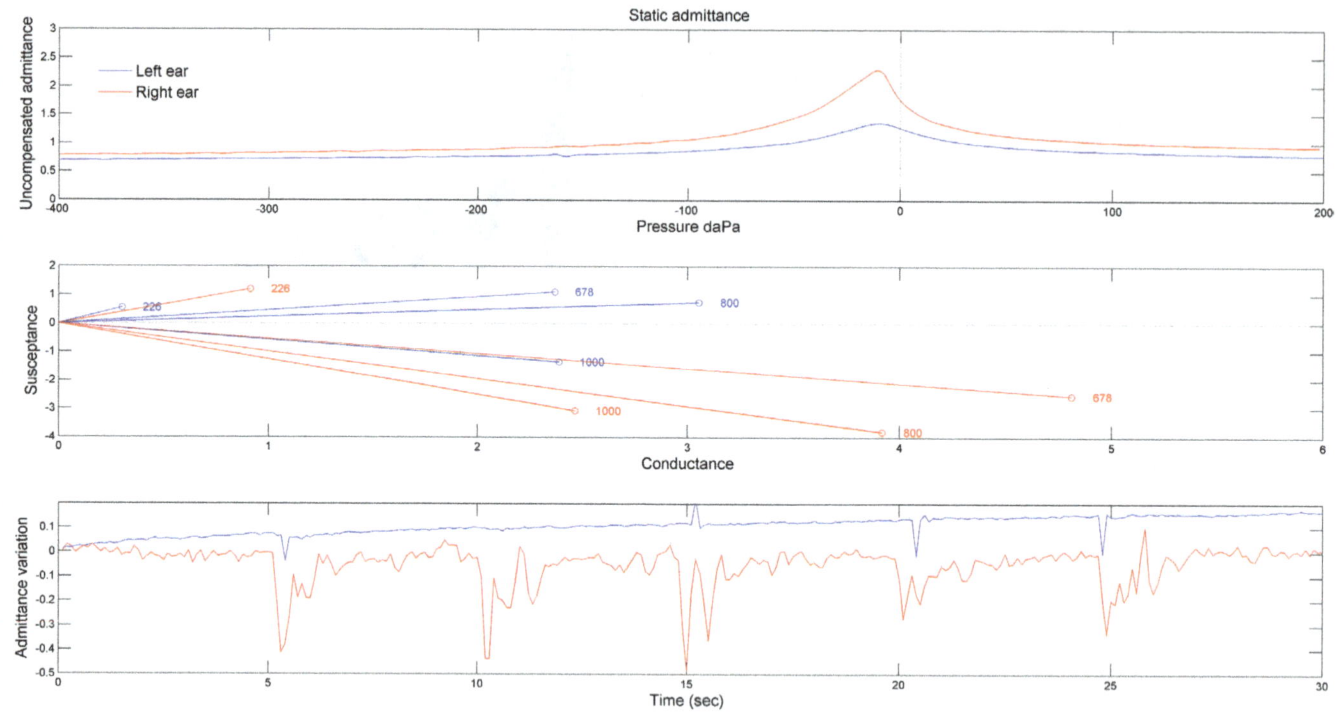

FIGURE 3 | Results obtained by tympanometry measurements. The upper panel shows the static admittance for the two ears obtained for a 226 Hz probe. The middle panel shows the susceptance as a function of the conductance at four frequencies of probe tone stimulation (226, 678, 800, and 1,000 Hz). The bottom panel shows the admittance variation when the patient blinked voluntarily (but not forcefully) his eyes. The patient was asked to do so every 5 s (blue line: left ear, red line: right ear).

in turn lead to plastic changes (sensitization) at several levels of the trigeminal pathways (21). Pain in the neck and the temporal region may result from referred pain as a consequence of central sensitization, possibly at the trigemino-cervical complex (TCC) level where multimodal neurons are present (22). Sensitization may also contribute to shift the pathophysiology from acute to chronic (21).

Finally, the PCA suggests that the symptoms from cluster 1 originate from tightly coupled mechanisms. The trigeminal sensory inputs from regions of the head, including middle ear mucosa, eardrums, and the TTM (14, 15, 19), are collected by the TCC that has a reflex connection with the superior salivatory nucleus (SSN). Interestingly, the SSN provides a parasympathetic innervation to the head region *via* the sphenopalatine ganglion. This reflex loop between the TGN and the parasympathetic pathway of the head has been suggested to account for the autonomic symptoms associated with trigeminal-autonomic cephalalgia (TAC) (23). The activation of the trigeminal-autonomic reflex in this case may account for the nasal congestion, rhinorrhea, and the tympanic hyperemia. The autonomic nervous system, which innervates the middle ear (18, 24–26), may also contribute to enhance the MEM tonus and the feeling of tension and aural fullness (27).

In summary, this case suggests that a complex pathophysiology can be involved in ASI. Initially, the acoustic shock may trigger an exaggerated MEM response causing muscle dysfunction/injury and inflammatory processes, which may later diffuse to the tympanum and middle ear mucosa. The activation of the trigeminal pathways due to inflammation may account for the diverse pain feelings in the ear and tinnitus (symptom cluster 2) and also for referred pain in the neck and the temporal region (symptom cluster 3) after induction of central sensitization. Finally, nasal congestion and tympanum hyperemia, which are tightly coupled to the feeling of ear tension (symptom cluster 1), may result from the activation of a trigeminal-autonomic reflex. Interestingly, the pathophysiology of ASI is strongly reminiscent of that of post-traumatic TAC (28). In this context, the case reported here may define a new clinical entity that we suggest calling post-traumatic trigeminal-autonomic otalgia. The clinical picture presented here, i.e., with numerous, diverse, and severe symptoms, could be an extreme form of this clinical entity and may be relatively rare. However, the prevalence of this clinical entity may be more prevalent than expected at first sight, as less symptomatic forms may also exist. Many patients with tinnitus and/or hyperacusis report one or more additional symptoms such as ear fullness, otalgia, tympanic flutter, and/or pain in the neck (2). This framework opens new and promising perspectives on the understanding and medical management of ASI and beyond, i.e., tinnitus and hyperacusis (23).

ETHICS STATEMENT

The case reported in the study gave written informed consent in accordance with the Declaration of Helsinki.

AUTHOR CONTRIBUTIONS

AL, NC, DP, PF, LP, and AN collected data. LP and AN analyzed data and made figures. AN wrote a first version of the manuscript. All authors contributed to the final version of the manuscript.

ACKNOWLEDGMENTS

The authors would like to thank Dirk De Ridder, Anne Donnet, and Lénaic Monconduit for their useful comments on earlier versions of the manuscript. We also wish to thank Otometrics for their help and support. This work has been conducted with the financial assistance of CNRS, Aix-Marseille Université, B2V, and the supplementary pension institution of Klesia.

SUPPLEMENTARY MATERIAL

VIDEO S1 | The video shows the right eardrum when the feeling of tension in the ear is high and when it is low.

VIDEO S2 | The video shows the right eardrum, when the tension in the ear is high, before, during, and after the mylohyoid muscle contraction.

REFERENCES

Westcott M. Acoustic shock injury (ASI). *Acta Otolaryngol Suppl* (2006) 556:54–8. doi:10.1080/03655230600895531

Westcott M, Sanchez TG, Diges I, Saba C, Dineen R, McNeill C, et al. Tonic tensor tympani syndrome in tinnitus and hyperacusis patients: a multi-clinic prevalence study. *Noise Health* (2013) 15:117–28. doi:10.4103/1463-1741. 110295

Levine RA, Abel M, Cheng H. CNS somatosensory-auditory interactions elicit or modulate tinnitus. *Exp Brain Res* (2003) 153:643–8. doi:10.1007/ s00221-003-1747-3

Klockhoff IH, Anderson H. Recording of the stapedius reflex elicited by cutaneous stimulation; preliminary report. *Acta Otolaryngol* (1959) 50:451–4. doi:10.3109/00016485909129218

Ellenstein A, Yusuf N, Hallett M. Middle ear myoclonus: two informative cases and a systematic discussion of myogenic tinnitus. *Tremor Other Hyperkinet Mov (N Y)* (2013) 3. doi:10.7916/D8RX9BS1

Salomon G, Starr A. Electromyography of middle ear muscles in man during motor activities. *Acta Neurol Scand* (1963) 39:161–8. doi:10.111 1/j.1600-0404.1963.tb05317.x

Watanabe I, Kumagami H, Tsuda Y. Tinnitus due to abnormal contraction of stapedial muscle. An abnormal phenomenon in the course of facial nerve paralysis and its audiological significance. *ORL J Otorhinolaryngol Relat Spec* (1974) 36:217–26. doi:10.1159/000275177

Klockhoff I, Anderson H. Reflex activity in the tensor tympani muscle recorded in man; preliminary report. *Acta Otolaryngol* (1960) 51:184–8. doi:10.3109/00016486009124480

Kierner AC, Zelenka I, Lukas JR, Aigner M, Mayr R. Observations on the number, distribution and morphological peculiarities of muscle spindles in the tensor tympani and stapedius muscle of man. *Hear Res* (1999) 135:71–7. doi:10.1016/S0378-5955(99)00092-1

Nagai T, Tono T. Encapsulated nerve corpuscles in the human tympanic membrane. *Arch Otorhinolaryngol* (1989) 246:169–72. doi:10.1007/BF00456661

Grillon C. Models and mechanisms of anxiety: evidence from startle studies. *Psychopharmacology (Berl)* (2008) 199:421–37. doi:10.1007/ s00213-007-1019-1

Thompson AM, Thompson GC, Britton BH. Serotoninergic innervation of stapedial and tensor tympani motoneurons. *Brain Res* (1998) 787:175–8. doi:10.1016/S0006-8993(97)01020-2

Yamazaki M, Sato I. Distribution of substance P and the calcitonin gene-re- lated peptide in the human tensor tympani muscle. *Eur Arch Otorhinolaryngol* (2014) 271:905–11. doi:10.1007/s00405-013-2469-1

Kierner AC, Mayer R, Adunka O. Is there a double innervation of the tensor tympani muscle in humans? *Ann Otol Rhinol Laryngol* (2003) 112:1056–8. doi:10.1177/000348940311201211

Uddman R, Grunditz T, Larsson A, Sundler F. Sensory innervation of the eardrum and middle-ear mucosa: retrograde tracing and immunocytochemistry. *Cell Tissue Res* (1988) 252:141–6. doi:10.1007/BF00213835

Ebmeyer J, Furukawa M, Pak K, Ebmeyer U, Sudhoff H, Broide D, et al. Role of mast cells in otitis media. *J Allergy Clin Immunol* (2005) 116:1129–35. doi:10.1016/j.jaci.2005.07.026

Ylikoski J, Panula P. Neuropeptides in the middle ear mucosa. *ORL J Otorhinolaryngol Relat Spec* (1988) 50:176–82. doi:10.1159/ 000275987

Nagaraj BS, Linthicum FH. Autonomic innervation of the human middle ear: an immunohistochemical study. *Am J Otolaryngol* (1998) 19:75–82. doi:10.1016/S0196-0709(98)90099-0

Oyagi S, Ito J, Honjo I. The trigeminal sensory innervation to the middle ear, eustachian tube, and pharynx: a study by the horseradish peroxidase tracer method. *Laryngoscope* (1990) 100:873–7. doi:10.1288/00005537-199008000- 00014

Vass Z, Steyger PS, Hordichok AJ, Trune DR, Jancsó G, Nuttall AL. Capsaicin stimulation of the cochlea and electric stimulation of the trigeminal ganglion mediate vascular permeability in cochlear and vertebro-basilar arteries: a potential cause of inner ear dysfunction in headache. *Neuroscience* (2001) 103:189–201. doi:10.1016/S0306-4522(00)00521-2

Bernstein C, Burstein R. Sensitization of the trigeminovascular pathway: perspective and implications to migraine pathophysiology. *J Clin Neurol* (2012) 8:89–99. doi:10.3988/jcn.2012.8.2.89

Piovesan EJ, Kowacs PA, Oshinsky ML. Convergence of cervical and trigeminal sensory afferents. *Curr Pain Headache Rep* (2003) 7:377–83. doi:10.1007/ s11916-003-0037-x

Eller M, Goadsby PJ. Trigeminal autonomic cephalalgias. *Oral Dis* (2016) 22:1–8. doi:10.1111/odi.12263

Ogawa T, Rutka J. The presence of ganglion cells in the human mid- dle ear: a histological survey. *Acta Otolaryngol Suppl* (1999) 540: 38–41.

Oyagi S, Ito J, Honjo I. The origin of autonomic nerves of the middle ear as studied by the horseradish peroxidase tracer method. *Acta Otolaryngol* (1987) 104:463–7. doi:10.3109/00016488709128275

Ito J, Oyagi S, Honjo I. Autonomic innervations in the middle ear and pharynx. *Acta Otolaryngol Suppl* (1993) 506:90–3. doi:10.3109/ 00016489309130249

Yuasa R, Kambayashi J, Saijo S, Hozawa K, Iino Y, Kaneko Y. Sensation of aural fullness and its treatment with an autonomic nerve block- ing agent. *Acta Otolaryngol Suppl* (1987) 435:122–9. doi:10.3109/ 00016488709107361

Charney L, Rubino A, Cohen JM. Acaseofbarotrauma-inducedpost-traumatic headache with a cluster headache phenotype. *Headache* (2016) 56:769–72. doi:10.1111/head.12727

16

Misophonia and Potential Underlying Mechanisms

*Devon B. Palumbo[1], Ola Alsalman[1], Dirk De Ridder[2], Jae-Jin Song[3] and Sven Vanneste[1]**

[1] Lab for Clinical and Integrative Neuroscience, School of Behavioral and Brain Sciences, The University of Texas at Dallas, Richardson, TX, United States, [2] Department of Surgical Sciences, Section of Neurosurgery, Dunedin School of Medicine, University of Otago, Dunedin, New Zealand, [3] Department of Otorhinolaryngology-Head and Neck Surgery, Seoul National University Bundang Hospital, Seongnam, South Korea

***Correspondence:**
Sven Vanneste
sven.vanneste@utdallas.edu

There is a growing research interest in the diagnosis rate of misophonia, a condition characterized by a negative emotional/autonomic reaction to specific everyday sounds. Diagnosis of misophonia requires a thorough case history and audiological test procedures. Associative and non-associative learning models for understanding the underlying mechanisms of misophonia have been presented. Currently, there is no cure or pharmaceutical agent for misophonia; however, therapy programs addressing misophonia and its characteristics do exist. Investigation of comorbid conditions and other psychological therapy strategies might help to reveal more about the underlying mechanisms and potentially lead to a successful treatment method.

Keywords: misophonia, auditory system, limbic system, associative learning, classical conditioning, sensitization

INTRODUCTION

Misophonia is a condition where patients experience a negative emotional reaction and dislike (e.g., anxiety, agitation, and annoyance) to specific sounds (e.g., ballpoint pen clicking (repeatedly), tapping, typing, chewing, breathing, swallowing, tapping foot, etc.) (Jastreboff and Jastreboff, 2002). Misophonia is a derivate from the Greek words misos (hate) and phónè (voice), and means hate of sound. Each patient's reaction is unique as it depends on the specific conditions under which the sound was experienced and any previous evaluations of that sound. Prior to Jastreboff introducing the term misophonia, there have been different terms to describe the condition, such as soft sound sensitivity symptom, select sound sensitivity syndrome, decreased sound tolerance, and sound-rage (Schwartz et al., 2011; Neal and Cavanna, 2013). A patient's negative reaction and dislike may occur in response to sound at any level. Although hyperacusis and misophonia can coexist, hyperacusis refers specifically to an increased sensitivity to certain frequencies and volume ranges of sound (Song et al., 2014). Misophonia can be distinguished from hyperacusis by its sensitivity to the subjective response provoked (Pienkowski et al., 2014). A subtype of misophonia is phonophobia, when fear to a specific sound is the dominant factor (Jastreboff and Hazell, 1999; Henry et al., 2002; Jastreboff and Jastreboff, 2015). It is important to recognize that "subtype" implies that the class of sounds that elicit phonophobia are drawn from misophonic sounds or that they share a similar mechanism, neither of which is necessarily true. From a phenomenological viewpoint, while fear is the dominant emotion in phonophobia, anger is the dominant emotion in misophonia. However, more recent research suggest that other than anger there is at least four other dominant emotions present in misophonia (i.e., irritation, stress and anxiety, aggravation, feeling trapped, and impatience) (Rouw and Erfanian, 2018).

INCIDENCE

In a recent study, Wu et al. (2014) investigated the incidence, correlates, and impairments associated with misophonia in a student population. Out of 483 undergraduate students (mean age = 21.4 years), 22.8% were often or always sensitive to or annoyed by specific sounds (e.g., eating, repetitive tapping, or nasal noises). Dislike of throat sounds, rustling papers, and environmental sounds were reported by 19.5, 16.1, and 14% of respondents, respectively. Literature suggests that 60% of patients with tinnitus also have misophonia (Jastreboff and Jastreboff, 2002; Jastreboff and Hazell, 2004) and 86% of tinnitus patients have hyperacusis, 25–30% of which requiring treatment (Anari et al., 1999; Jastreboff and Jastreboff, 2006). Jastreboff deduced that 1.75% of the general population has hyperacusis without tinnitus, but it is still difficult to differentiate those who have hyperacusis alone, misophonia alone, and those who have both (Jastreboff, 2015).

CHARACTERISTICS

Misophonia usually begins during childhood or adolescence, sometimes affecting academic performance (Edelstein et al., 2013; Schroder et al., 2013). An intense negative emotional reaction is usually triggered by bodily sounds (e.g., chewing, breathing, swallowing, and foot tapping, etc.) and may be connected to a particular person creating that sound (Edelstein et al., 2013; Schroder et al., 2013). In addition to the emotional aversion, patients sometimes report physical pressure building in the chest, the desire to stop the person from making the sound, and other autonomic reactions (Moller, 2011). Sometimes patients will mimic the sound to cancel it out. Rarely do physical reactions, such as assaulting the person making the sound, occur. However, because the patient is never sure when the trigger sound might be heard, the patient often lives in a perpetual state of anxiety. Patients are hyper-focused on listening for that trigger; they will avoid certain situations, people, and foods that they think will cause the sound (Edelstein et al., 2013). Overall, patients may suffer physical and emotional discomfort, contributing to a reduced quality of life (Edelstein et al., 2013).

According to Jastreboff and Jastreboff (2015), only 7 cases (2.2%) out of 318 misophonic patients exhibited a psychiatric disorder. Some researchers argue that misophonia and psychiatric disorders are unrelated. However, others tend to believe that psychiatric disorders and misophonia might coexist. Schroder et al. (2013) conducted a study to classify misophonia as its own form of psychiatric disorder. Their results showed a pattern of intense reactions to specific stimuli, avoidance, and worry that matched with traits of other psychiatric disorders, i.e., social phobia, post-traumatic stress disorder, personality disorders with impulsive aggression, intermittent explosive disorder, autism spectrum disorder, sensory processing disorders, antisocial personality disorder, and phonophobia (Schroder et al., 2013). Although the nosological nature of misophonia is still a topic of debate, Schroder's findings seem to call for misophonia to be classified as a subtype of a discrete psychiatric disorder.

DIAGNOSIS

Clinically, diagnosing misophonia requires a detailed case history to determine onset, triggers, reactions, and co-morbid conditions. Questionnaires may also be useful when determining the severity and uniqueness of each patient's case. Although certain questionnaires have been proposed to evaluate the severity of misophonia (Khalfa et al., 2002; Dauman and Bouscau-Faure, 2005), their validity needs to be confirmed. On the other hand, no one questionnaire has been consistently used across studies for the evaluation of misophonia. Examples of some of the questionnaires currently being used to evaluate misophonia are: (1) the Misophonia Questionnaire (MQ), which is a three-part self-report questionnaire developed by Wu et al. (2014) to assess the presence of misophonia symptoms as well as related emotions and behaviors; and (2) the Amsterdam Misophonia Scale (A-MISO-S), a concept scale based on the already validated Yale-Brown Obsessive-Compulsive Scale (Y-BOCS) (Schroder et al., 2013). The A-MISO-S is a six-item scale that evaluates different areas affected by misophonia such as: the time spent focusing on misophonia; interference with social functions; level of anger; impulse control; control over thoughts and anger; and time spent avoiding situations contributing to misophonia.

The audiological assessment of misophonia is complex. To date there is no agreement on a specified protocol to assess misophonia. However, audiological assessment includes pure tone thresholds and loudness discomfort levels (LDL). Patients with misophonia may have hearing loss or normal hearing. LDLs have been reported at normal and reduced levels (Jastreboff and Jastreboff, 2013). There is no precise description of how to test LDLs in patients with misophonia. It is therefore possible that variations can occur in the results obtained due to the specific method administrated and differences in the way patients are instructed (Hawkins et al., 1987; Sherlock and Formby, 2005; Jastreboff and Jastreboff, 2015). Nevertheless, Jastreboff and Jastreboff (2015) indicated that when misophonia is present with hyperacusis, LDL values can range from 30 to 120 dB HL. This further emphasizes that LDLs alone are insufficient to accurately diagnose hyperacusis and/or misophonia (Jastreboff and Jastreboff, 2015). Differences in auditory late potentials may be present when patients are tested using an oddball paradigm. Schroder et al. (2014) concluded that the deviant tone evoked a smaller N100 in misophonia patients than in healthy controls. Such responses might have been because of deficits in processing auditory information at low intensities or because of coexisting mood and psychiatric conditions. This study supports the recommendation of a thorough case history and use of questionnaires to understand all aspects of the patient's life that may contribute to misophonia (Ferreira et al., 2013; Schroder et al., 2013).

Anecdotal Cases in the Literature

A 36-year-old woman, Ms. A, raised in foster homes, had a mother suffering from depression and a father who did not provide support and affection (Veale, 2006). At the time that she visited the clinic, she was married and had one son.

Ms. A was a solitary person who desired to be deaf. Her desire was so intense that she would block her ears with cotton balls soaked in oil. Veale (2006) had the patient complete a series of questionnaires and found that she was extremely averse to sounds of any kind and fulfilled criteria for multiple personality disorders. In this case, repeated avoidance of sound might have led to increased auditory gain and worsening of symptoms.

Neal and Cavanna (2013) offered a case study of a 52-year-old man suffering from Tourette syndrome and misophonia. Neuropsychiatric examination revealed multiple motor ticks (e.g., facial grimacing and shoulder shrugging) and phonic ticks (e.g., yelping and barking) since age 11. The man also had mild obsessive-compulsive behaviors, depression, and sleep problems. Interestingly, this man noticed his aversion to sounds (e.g., father chewing food, sounds when riding a bus) developed about 1 year before his tics started. The authors thus speculated that there may be a pathophysiological association between the two conditions.

Webber et al. (2014) reported a pediatric case of misophonia and Tourette syndrome. The young female patient was also diagnosed with comorbid obsessive-compulsive spectrum disorder (OCD) and attention deficit hyperactivity disorder (ADHD). At 6 years of age, she developed frequent motor and vocal tics. During an interview, the young girl reacted strongly to certain auditory and visual stimuli and demanded that the sound stop. These findings are like those reported by Neal and Cavanna (2013), i.e., obsessive compulsive tendencies, an early age of onset, and the presence of both motor and vocal tics. The neural circuitry involved in OCD and Tourette syndrome may be similar to that of misophonia (Husted et al., 2006; Neal and Cavanna, 2013). A methodical screening for misophonia in disorders such as Tourette syndrome and OCD might uncover a pathophysiological connection between sounds and anomalies within the limbic system and its connections with the auditory cortex and the autonomic nervous system.

Kluckow et al. (2014) interviewed 15 patients being treated for eating disorders about possible misophonia symptoms. Three of the 15 patients met the criteria for misophonia. The first patient recalled her misophonia trigger to high-pitched voices starting around age six. Hearing the sound would cause her to binge eat. Coping mechanisms included ear plugs, music for distraction, and digging her fingernail into her hand to cause pain but not draw blood. The second patient had misophonia triggered by the eating habits of family friends. Following the development of her aversion, the patient started to increase exercise and decrease eating. The third patient presented with misophonia caused by the sound of family members eating cereal out of a bowl; she found the clinking spoon in the bowl and the sound of cereal being chewed repulsive. Aversion to these stimuli was so strong that she was unable to eat. In all three cases, severe aversion to eating sounds preceded the development of an eating disorder. Kluckow et al. (2014) suggested that the co-presentation of misophonia and eating disorders should be investigated during a thorough case history.

TREATMENT

Currently, there are no research studies that have investigated pharmaceutical options to treat misophonia. Anecdotal information suggests the prescription of antidepressants and anxiolytics to address the reactions and co-morbid conditions associated with misophonia. Despite the lack of pharmaceutical remedies, a variety of therapies have been considered, with some showing signs of potential success.

Tinnitus retraining therapy (TRT) is a therapy program designed by Jastreboff to manage tinnitus and, as a secondary effect, hyperacusis and misophonia (Jastreboff and Jastreboff, 2006). TRT assumes that altering conditioned reflexes at the subconscious level will reduce or eliminate the connection between the auditory system and the limbic and autonomic nervous systems (Kiessling, 1980). Relating these auditory conditions to conditioned reflexes also helps to understand how loudness correlates with severity (Tyler et al., 2007). The connection is reinforced by the two stimuli and the auditory characteristics are of less importance. The therapy protocol consists of directive counseling and sound therapy, tailored to each patient's specific situation. This model emphasizes the need for the patient to understand the underlying mechanisms of the condition. The patient will adhere to the treatment assigned and make conscious efforts to alter the underlying mechanisms once s/he understands how they operate. A clear review of TRT and individual goals between patient and clinical provider will ensure the patient has realistic expectations. For sound therapy, TRT works to reinforce positive sounds and reduce exposure to sounds causing a negative reaction. Exposure to background noise and avoidance of silence work to desensitize certain sounds. If the patient also has hearing loss, s/he may benefit from ear-level combination devices, which provide amplification and tranquil background sounds. Overall, TRT should take about 9–18 months to complete (Jastreboff and Jastreboff, 2002). If the patient is suffering from hyperacusis and misophonia, Jastreboff and Jastreboff (2015) recommend first treating hyperacusis. Once misophonia is isolated, the goal is to change the relationship between the auditory, limbic, and autonomic nervous systems and to eliminate the conditioned reflex. Although the conditioned-reflex model of TRT has been challenged in theory (Tyler et al., 2006), TRT should work better with misophonia patients than with tinnitus patients because misophonia involves an external trigger, which can be manipulated to potentially eliminate the conditioned response (Jastreboff and Jastreboff, 2002). Misophonia patients undergoing TRT are encouraged to avoid silence and ear overprotection. Decreasing patients' reactions to their trigger sounds by introducing pleasant sounds and constant low intensity sounds is thought to improve these patients' conditions. Reclassifying the sounds plus heavy counseling are recommended to help these patients. TRT outcomes were reported by Jastreboff et al., as 152 out of 184 patients with misophonia with hyperacusis, and patients with misophonia without hyperacusis (139 patients out of 167) showed improvements after TRT (Jastreboff and Jastreboff, 2015).

Although the development of a therapeutic approach such as TRT often applied it has not proven to be clinically effective. This has led to some controversy regarding the application of this theory as a therapeutic approach, partially because the underlying mechanism of misophonia is not well understood. Besides TRT, other neuropsychiatric therapies might be effective for misophonia patients. Schneider and Arch (Schneider and Arch, 2015) reviewed potential treatments for misophonia based on specific characteristics of the condition. Since one of the common responses to a misophonia trigger is anger, they suggested focusing on therapies that work to decrease anger, such as cognitive restructuring and stress inoculation training (Blake and Hamrin, 2007). A literature review of therapy and training programs for anger in youth populations indicated that Cognitive-Relaxation Coping Skills Training and Multicomponent Cognitive-Behavioral Therapy (CBT) were able to reduce anger-related behaviors and improve control over the expression of anger (Blake and Hamrin, 2007). Similarly, a stress inoculation training program for high school students significantly decreased negative stress events and reduced overall anger (Hains, 1992). Since misophonic symptoms often arise in adolescence, these anger therapies may also apply to the misophonia population.

Other ways to address misophonia could be through compassion training, distress-tolerance, and acceptance-based treatments (Schneider and Arch, 2015). Mindfulness (moment-to-moment awareness) may enhance traditional CBT programs in psychologically distraught patients (Hofmann et al., 2011). In a group of moderately to severely distressed tinnitus patients, internet-based CBT and acceptance and commitment therapy (ACT) were both shown to reduce the negative impact of tinnitus on quality of life, as measured by tinnitus severity and tinnitus-related distress (Hesser et al., 2014). Techniques used in these programs included applied relaxation, positive imagery, attention training, cognitive restructuring, exposure, and background sounds to cope with tinnitus. There are only two case studies reported in the literature that show the effects of CBT for youths with misophonia (McGuire et al., 2015). After completing psychoeducation, reviewing how to appropriately respond when a trigger is present, and gradually increasing exposure to the trigger sounds, the two female patients had reduced symptoms and expressed that they now had the tools to cope. Although two case studies alone do not constitute concrete evidence that CBT will work with misophonia patients, it does invite further research to determine the efficacy of such a therapy program.

The potential therapies listed above look to address emotional reactions caused by misophonia triggers. In order to have a truly effective treatment, more research is needed to better define a diagnostic protocol, rule out comorbid conditions, and to provide evidence for the underlying mechanisms of misophonia (Webber and Storch, 2015). Since misophonia triggers can be from many sources, people, and situations, it is likely that one therapy program will not address every manifestation of misophonia, indicating a need for individualized therapy.

UNDERLYING MECHANISMS

Auditory information ascends through the brainstem to the cerebral cortices in two parallel pathways, mainly known as the classical and non-classical auditory pathways (Moller and Rollins, 2002). The anatomy of the non-classical pathway differs from that of the classical pathway mainly in the thalamic relay nuclei (Moller and Rollins, 2002). The classical pathway is intermittent in the ventral portion of the medial geniculate body, while the non-classical pathway is interrupted in nuclei located in the medial and dorsomedial geniculate body (Moller and Rollins, 2002; Moller et al., 2005). Recall that misophonia is described as a negative reaction to sound results from enhanced limbic and autonomic responses without abnormal enhancement of the auditory system (Jastreboff, 1999; Jastreboff and Hazell, 1999). Since it is known that classical and non-classical auditory pathways interact with the limbic system, a breakdown in such processes may contribute to an increased association between auditory stimuli and emotional and autonomic reactions (Jastreboff and Hazell, 2004; Langguth and Landgrebe, 2011).

The literature suggests that the majority of patients with misophonia have normal hearing sensitivity (Schroder et al., 2014), while the limbic and autonomic nervous systems are in a heightened state of excitation and thus react abnormally to normal auditory input (Moller, 2011). A recent functional and structural MRI study has revealed that trigger sounds elicited increased responses in the anterior insular cortex (AIC) and abnormal functional connectivity between the AIC and medial frontal, medial parietal, and medial temporal regions (Kumar et al., 2017). The findings of Kumar et al. (2017) implied that there was abnormal myelination in the medial frontal cortex that shows abnormal functional connectivity, and that the aberrant neural response mediates the emotional coloring and physiological arousal that accompany misophonic experiences.

A focal point of rebuttal by the Kumar et al. (2017), study lies in their experimental designs where general annoyance elicited by one stimulus condition (i.e., baby crying, a person screaming) was disassociate from a specifically misophonic reaction elicited by another stimulus condition (i.e., eating and breathing sounds). In a commentary (Schroder et al., 2017), Schroder et al. argued that it was unclear whether the subjects in the Kumar et al. (2017) study actually suffered from misophonia, as Schroder et al. promote the idea that misophonia is a distinct form of a psychiatric disorder with specific and well-defined diagnostic criteria (Schroder et al., 2013). Secondly, the validity of the questionnaire used to select subjects with misophonia were put into question. In addition, anger, which is an essential component in the diagnosis of misophonia, was overlooked and instead the focus was on annoyance. As such, part of Schroder et al.'s argument was that the observed brain differences in the Kumar et al. (2017) study might be correlated to general annoyance rather than anger specifically. A final comment was about the design of the study and how it might have put subjects at risk of sensitization to sound by repeated exposure (Kumar and Griffiths, 2017; Schroder et al., 2017).

In response, Kumar et al. (2017) stated that, to date, there are no diagnostic criteria for misophonia in ICD 10 or DSM-5, as subjects were selected based on having stable typical response to trigger sounds over years which are usually anger but can also come in the form of anxiety. This argument was supported by findings of a large scale study involving more than 300 subjects with misophonia, who primary reported emotional responses in the form of irritation/annoyance and not anger (Kumar and Griffiths, 2017). Finally, regarding Schroder et al.'s last comment, Kumar argued that it was not clear how re-exposure to sounds that have been producing a typical misophonic reaction for years might have any bearing on the reaction produced (Kumar and Griffiths, 2017). Despite the controversy surrounding these findings, the AIC is one of the core components of limbic and autonomic nervous system activity control.

Learning involves associating events happening at different times, a process that is of fundamental importance for a number of perceptual and cognitive processes (Wallenstein et al., 1998; Fuster et al., 2000). There are two forms of learning, associative and non-associative, which we will briefly describe and then use to elucidate misophonia. Associative learning involves one stimulus presented simultaneously with another stimulus, creating a specific reaction. Conditioning to stimuli can be either through classical or operant conditioning (Vlaeyen, 2015). Non-associative learning is a change in behavior after repeated presentations of a stimulus, but there is no reinforcement via a second stimulus like there is in associative learning. In response to a single stimulus, an individual can either experience habituation or sensitization. Habituation is a decrease in response to a stimulus following multiple identical presentations (Ursin, 2014). In healthy systems, habituation and sensitization counteract one another and allow the individual to stay in a neutral state (Ursin, 2014). Associative learning, particularly classical conditioning, and non-associative learning, particularly sensitization, may help to explain the underlying mechanisms of misophonia.

Associative and Non-associative Learning

Jastreboff and Jastreboff (2002) developed a model to explain the neural mechanisms governing tinnitus, hyperacusis, and misophonia (Jastreboff and Jastreboff, 2002). Associative learning via classical conditioning supports their theory. Since classical conditioning works in anticipation of a change to the environment (Vlaeyen, 2015), they hypothesized that patients suffering from one or all three of these problems have enhanced connections between their auditory system and their limbic and autonomic nervous systems (Jastreboff and Hazell, 2004). Misophonia is a form of conditioned behavior that develops as a physical reflex through classical conditioning with a misophonia trigger (e.g., eating noises, lip-smacking, pen clicking, tapping and typing . . .) as the conditioned stimulus, and anger, irritation or stress the unconditioned stimulus. The involvement of the limbic system helps to explain the emotional component to this condition and suggests that the connection is controlled by a conditioned reflex. Three components of the limbic system (the amygdala, parahippocampus, and insula) have been shown to activate more strongly in other conditions such as tinnitus (Song et al., 2013, 2015; Carpenter-Thompson et al., 2014). Moller (2013) also suggested that the amygdala's control of fear, depression, and anxiety may explain a connection to the auditory system in patients with phonophobia.

Activating the limbic and autonomic nervous systems triggers irrational reactions to stimuli (Molini et al., 2014). Hyperacusis patients have increased auditory sensitivity, which is passed on to the autonomic nervous system and results in increased activation (Jastreboff and Jastreboff, 2015). Similarly, misophonia patients have an increase in activation between the auditory pathways and autonomic nervous system, resulting in negative emotional reaction to sound. Similarly, pain processing involves an association with intrusion, long-term exposure, depression, anxiety, defensive responses, and prolonged avoidance (Vlaeyen, 2015). Misophonia patients have triggers that cause annoyance, anxiety, and depression. They respond by trying to ignore or escape the stimulus. Prolonged avoidance can exacerbate the condition. Misophonia patients may plug their ears with cotton balls or live a life of silence (Veale, 2006; Edelstein et al., 2013). As in pain, the trigger is not life-threatening, and yet it leads to worry, fear, and anxiety. Although these points should not be treated as specific to misophonia, further investigation into tinnitus, hyperacusis, and pain mechanisms may also help to understand misophonia.

This begs the question of why some people learn this type of association (classical conditioning) and not others. Classical conditioning or associative learning elicits reflexive, automatic, and involuntary behavior (Jarius and Wildemann, 2015; Kotchoubey and Pavlov, 2017). The only responses that can be elicited out of classical conditioning are those that rely on responses that are naturally made by the individual with misophonia or, for that matter, any other condition. These responses are often involuntary and occurring below the level of conscious awareness (Jarius and Wildemann, 2015). The hallmark of misophonia is an extreme emotional response to the trigger stimulus. As a result, for misophonic patients, these emotional responses might create a classical conditioning paradigm that maintains or strengthens the misophonic physical reflex (Schroder et al., 2013). With that said, individual differences in associative learning do exist, in part due to psychological and individual personality variables (Murphy and Msetfi, 2014).

On the other hand, non-associative learning can result in habituation or sensitization. The symptoms of misophonia arise from enhanced sensitized functional connections or shortcuts between the limbic, auditory, and autonomic nervous system (Schwartz et al., 2011). Sensitization is defined as increased neuronal activity in response to a stimulus (Jimenez et al., 2017). Before stimuli or neural activity reach the brain, they are classified and evaluated by complex neuronal pathways. If the signal becomes actively connected to previous emotions or memories, there will be an overlap in the auditory signal and emotions, creating a complex neural signal. That complex neural signal is what finally reaches the level of conscious awareness; hence, the anxiety and stress related to the auditory signal are incorporated subconsciously and revealed at the conscious level. After repeated cycles of this process, the neuronal reaction threshold decreases and allows the complex hyper-responses to reach the brain more easily (Zenner et al., 2006). The underling mechanism for sensitization in misophonia is unknown, but has typical been associated to strengthening of synaptic signals, a process known as long-term potentiation, or "kindling," repeated stimulation of specific neurons in the limbic system. In a recent publication showed that misophonia patients can have enhanced autonomic reactivity to a sound, but not to other sensory stimuli (Edelstein et al., 2013). The subjective experiences described by these misophonia patients to trigger sounds share qualitative features with the sensory symptoms reported by patients with tic disorders such as Tourette syndrome. Recent reports have also suggested that misophonic symptoms can be found in the context of two of the most common psychiatric comorbidities of Tourette syndrome, in addition to obsessive-compulsive disorder, generalized anxiety disorder, and schizotypal personality disorder (Ferreira et al., 2013; Neal and Cavanna, 2013; Cavanna and Martino, 2014). Overall, although there is preliminary evidence supporting the suggestion that the underlying mechanism can occur in misophonia due to sensitization more research is needed.

Association Between Misophonia and Synesthesia

The brain constantly integrates signals across different modalities. To that extent, a defining aspect of misophonia occurs when the disturbing sound produced by others provoke an emotional response. This emotional response exhibits a marked connection between the auditory system and other limbic and autonomic systems (Bruxner, 2016). This process resembles another phenomenon: synesthesia which is the occurrence of a particular sensory stimulus can evoke additional sensations and associations (Galton, 1883; Harrison and Baron-Cohen, 1995; Baron-Cohen et al., 1996; Barnett et al., 2008; Edelstein et al., 2013). It is proposed that synesthesia results from an increase of neural connections and interactions between different sensory modalities (Brang and Ramachandran, 2011; Mylopoulos and Ro, 2013).

There may be a connection between misophonia and synesthesia. In synesthesia, as in misophonia, a pathological distortion of connections between the auditory cortex and limbic structures can cause a form of sound-emotion synesthesia (Edelstein et al., 2013). Furthermore, in both phenomena, an external sound can produce internal perceptual and sensational experiences (Barratt and Davis, 2015). There are also reports suggesting that the two phenomena are linked by their affective components, in addition to their perceptual similarities (Edelstein et al., 2013). For example, negative autonomic reactions are associated with the experience of misophonia. Specifically, sufferers report that noises of any volume made by others such as breathing, swallowing, or foot tapping can elicit feelings of disgust, anger, or hatred (Schroder et al., 2013). Misophonic experiences are also similar to synesthetic associations in that they are both automatic and cross-modal. Further exploration of the similarities between these two conditions is needed to discover whether and how these two phenomena are related.

CONCLUSION

Certain characteristics of misophonia that follow rules from both associative and non-associative learning principles could possibly be used to better understand the underlying mechanisms. If non-associative learning does help to explain the underlying mechanisms of misophonia, then there needs to be research investigating this connection. To date, research has made only weak speculation, with little evidence to support the theory. TRT seems to be an effective treatment option for patients with sound sensitivity disorders such as misophonia. Although the majority of patients do find relief through TRT, there are still cases that receive no relief. Finally, Vlaeyen (2015) suggested a connection between non-associative and associative learning. The anxiety evoked by a stimulus may induce negative effects, causing sensitization. Perhaps this is the key to a successful misophonia treatment. By combining TRT and sensitization strategies, those few patients who do not receive relief via either method alone might benefit from a combined method. Future studies should focus on further examining the relationship between associative and non-associative learning and misophonia.

AUTHOR CONTRIBUTIONS

All authors listed have made a substantial, direct and intellectual contribution to the work, and approved it for publication.

REFERENCES

Anari, M., Axelsson, A., Eliasson, A., and Magnusson, L. (1999). Hypersensitivity to sound–questionnaire data, audiometry and classification. *Scand. Audiol.* 28, 219–230. doi: 10.1080/010503999424653

Barnett, K. J., Finucane, C., Asher, J. E., Bargary, G., Corvin, A. P., Newell, F. N., et al. (2008). Familial patterns and the origins of individual differences in synaesthesia. *Cognition* 106, 871–893. doi: 10.1016/j.cognition.2007.05.003

Baron-Cohen, S., Burt, L., Smith-Laittan, F., Harrison, J., and Bolton, P. (1996). Synaesthesia: prevalence and familiality. *Perception* 25, 1073–1079. doi: 10.1068/p251073

Barratt, E. L., and Davis, N. J. (2015). Autonomous Sensory Meridian Response (ASMR): a flow-like mental state. *PeerJ* 3:e851. doi: 10.7717/peerj.851

Blake, C. S., and Hamrin, V. (2007). Current approaches to the assessment and management of anger and aggression in youth: a review. *J. Child Adolesc. Psychiatr. Nurs.* 20, 209–221. doi: 10.1111/j.1744-6171.2007.00102.x

Brang, D., and Ramachandran, V. S. (2011). Survival of the synesthesia gene: why do people hear colors and taste words? *PLoS Biol.* 9:e1001205. doi: 10.1371/journal.pbio.1001205

Bruxner, G. (2016). 'Mastication rage': a review of misophonia - an under-recognised symptom of psychiatric relevance? *Australas. Psychiatry*24, 195–197. doi: 10.1177/1039856215613010

Carpenter-Thompson, J. R., Akrofi, K., Schmidt, S. A., Dolcos, F., and Husain, F. T. (2014). Alterations of the emotional processing system may underlie preserved rapid reaction time in tinnitus. *Brain Res.* 1567, 28–41. doi: 10.1016/j.brainres.2014.04.024

Cavanna, A. E., and Martino, D. (2014). How many Gilles de la Tourette syndromes? *Eur. J. Neurol.* 21, 685–686. doi: 10.1111/ene.12282

Dauman, R., and Bouscau-Faure, F. (2005). Assessment and amelioration of hyperacusis in tinnitus patients. *Acta Otolaryngol.* 125, 503–509. doi: 10.1080/00016480510027565

Edelstein, M., Brang, D., Rouw, R., and Ramachandran, V. S. (2013). Misophonia: physiological investigations and case descriptions. *Front. Hum. Neurosci.* 7:296. doi: 10.3389/fnhum.2013.00296

Ferreira, G. M., Harrison, B. J., and Fontenelle, L. F. (2013). Hatred of sounds: misophonic disorder or just an underreported psychiatric symptom? *Ann. Clin. Psychiatry* 25, 271–274.

Fuster, J. M., Bodner, M., and Kroger, J. K. (2000). Cross-modal and cross-temporal association in neurons of frontal cortex. *Nature* 405, 347–351. doi: 10.1038/35012613

Galton, F. (1883). *Inquiries into Human Faculty and its Development*. London: Macmillan. doi: 10.1037/14178-000

Hains, A. A. (1992). A stress inoculation training program for adolescents in a high school setting: a multiple baseline approach. *J. Adolesc.* 15, 163–175. doi: 10.1016/0140-1971(92)90045-7

Harrison, J., and Baron-Cohen, S. (1995). Synaesthesia: reconciling the subjective with the objective. *Endeavour* 19, 157–160. doi: 10.1016/0160-9327(96)82878-X

Hawkins, D. B., Walden, B. E., Montgomery, A., and Prosek, R. A. (1987). Description and validation of an LDL procedure designed to select SSPL90. *Ear Hear.* 8, 162–169. doi: 10.1097/00003446-198706000-00006

Henry, J. A., Jastreboff, M. M., Jastreboff, P. J., Schechter, M. A., and Fausti, S. A. (2002). Assessment of patients for treatment with tinnitus retraining therapy. *J. Am. Acad. Audiol.* 13, 523–544.

Hesser, H., Westin, V. Z., and Andersson, G. (2014). Acceptance as a mediator in internet-delivered acceptance and commitment therapy and cognitive behavior therapy for tinnitus. *J. Behav. Med.* 37, 756–767. doi: 10.1007/s10865-013-9525-6

Hofmann, S. G., Grossman, P., and Hinton, D. E. (2011). Loving-kindness and compassion meditation: potential for psychological interventions. *Clin. Psychol. Rev.* 31, 1126–1132. doi: 10.1016/j.cpr.2011.07.003

Husted, D. S., Shapira, N. A., and Goodman, W. K. (2006). The neurocircuitry of obsessive-compulsive disorder and disgust. *Prog. Neuropsychopharmacol. Biol. Psychiatry* 30, 389–399.

Jarius, S., and Wildemann, B. (2015). And Pavlov still rings a bell: summarising the evidence for the use of a bell in Pavlov's iconic experiments on classical conditioning. *J. Neurol.* 262, 2177–2178. doi: 10.1007/s00415-015-7858-5

Jastreboff, M., and Jastreboff, P. (2002). Decreased sound tolerance and tinnitus retraining therapy (TRT). *Aust. N. Z. J. Audiol.* 24, 74–84. doi: 10.1375/audi.24.2.74.31105

Jastreboff, P., and Hazell, J. (2004). *Tinnitus Retraining Therapy: Implementing the Neurophysiological Model*. Cambridge: Cambridge University Press. doi: 10.1017/CBO9780511544989

Jastreboff, P., and Jastreboff, M. (2013). Using TRT to treat hyperacusis, misophonia and phonophobia. *ENT Audiol. News* 21, 88–90.

Jastreboff, P. J. (1999). Tinnitus retraining therapy. A clinical implementation of the neurophysiological model of tinnitus. *Verhaltenstherapie* 9:33. doi: 10.1007/s00106-014-2979-1

Jastreboff, P. J. (2015). 25 years of tinnitus retraining therapy. *HNO* 63, 307–311. doi: 10.1007/s00106-014-2979-1

Jastreboff, P. J., and Hazell, W. P. J. (1999). Tinnitus retraining therapy. *Br. J. Audiol.* 33, 68–69.

Jastreboff, P. J., and Jastreboff, M. M. (2006). Tinnitus retraining therapy: a different view on tinnitus. *ORL J. Otorhinolaryngol. Relat. Spec.* 68, 23–29; discussion 29–30. doi: 10.1159/000090487

Jastreboff, P. J., and Jastreboff, M. M. (2015). Decreased sound tolerance: hyperacusis, misophonia, diplacousis, and polyacousis. *Handb. Clin. Neurol.* 129, 375–387. doi: 10.1016/B978-0-444-62630-1.00021-4

Jimenez, X. F., Aboussssouan, A., Mandell, D., and Huffman, K. L. (2017). Additional evidence supporting the central sensitization inventory (CSI) as an outcome measure among chronic pain patients in functional restoration program care. *Spine J.* 17:1765. doi: 10.1016/j.spinee.2017.08.225

Khalfa, S., Dubal, S., Veuillet, E., Perez-Diaz, F., Jouvent, R., and Collet, L. (2002). Psychometric normalization of a hyperacusis questionnaire. *ORL J. Otorhinolaryngol. Relat. Spec.* 64, 436–442. doi: 10.1159/000067570

Kiessling, J. (1980). [Masking of tinnitus aurium by maskers and hearing aids (author's transl)]. *HNO* 28, 383–388.

Kluckow, H., Telfer, J., and Abraham, S. (2014). Should we screen for misophonia in patients with eating disorders? A report of three cases. *Int. J. Eat. Disord.* 47, 558–561. doi: 10.1002/eat.22245

Kotchoubey, B., and Pavlov, Y. G. (2017). Name conditioning in event-related brain potentials. *Neurobiol. Learn. Mem.* 145, 129–134. doi: 10.1016/j.nlm.2017.09.009

Kumar, S., and Griffiths, T. D. (2017). Response: commentary: the brain basis for misophonia. *Front. Behav. Neurosci.* 11:127. doi: doi: 10.3389/fnbeh.2017.00127 doi: 10.3389/fnbeh.2017.00127

Kumar, S., Tansley-Hancock, O., Sedley, W., Winston, J. S., Callaghan, M. F., Allen, M., et al. (2017). The brain basis for misophonia. *Curr. Biol.* 27, 527–533. doi: 10.1016/j.cub.2016.12.048

Langguth, B., and Landgrebe, M. (2011). "Tinnitus and depression," in *Textbook of Tinnitus*, eds A. R. Moller, B. Langguth, D. De Ridder, and T. Kleinjung (New York, NY: Springer), 493–498. doi: 10.1007/978-1-60761-145-5_63

McGuire, J. F., Wu, M. S., and Storch, E. A. (2015). Cognitive-behavioral therapy for 2 youths with misophonia. *J. Clin. Psychiatry* 76, 573–574. doi: 10.4088/JCP.14cr09343

Molini, E., Faralli, M., Calzolaro, L., and Ricci, G. (2014). Impact of identifying factors which trigger bothersome tinnitus on the treatment outcome in tinnitus retraining therapy. *ORL J. Otorhinolaryngol. Relat. Spec.* 76, 81–88. doi: 10.1159/000360994

Moller, A. R. (2011). "Misophonia, phonophobia, and "exploding head" syndrome," in *Textbook of Tinnitus*, eds A. R. Moller, B. Langguth, D. De Ridder, and T. Kleinjung (New York, NY: Springer), 25–26. doi: 10.1007/978-1-60761-145-5_4

Moller, A. R. (2013). *Hearing: Anatomy, Physiology, and Disorders of the Auditory System*. San Diego, CA: Plural Publishing, Inc.

Moller, A. R., Kern, J. K., and Grannemann, B. (2005). Are the non-classical auditory pathways involved in autism and PDD? *Neurol. Res.* 27, 625–629.

Moller, A. R., and Rollins, P. R. (2002). The non-classical auditory pathways are involved in hearing in children but not in adults. *Neurosci. Lett.* 319, 41–44. doi: 10.1016/S0304-3940(01)02516-2

Murphy, R. A., and Msetfi, R. M. (2014). Individual differences in associative learning. *Front. Psychol.* 5:466. doi: doi: 10.3389/fpsyg.2014.00466 doi: 10.3389/fpsyg.2014.00466

Mylopoulos, M. I., and Ro, T. (2013). Synesthesia: a colorful word with a touching sound? *Front. Psychol.* 4:763. doi: 10.3389/fpsyg.2013.00763

Neal, M., and Cavanna, A. E. (2013). Selective sound sensitivity syndrome (misophonia) in a patient with Tourette syndrome. *J. Neuropsychiatry Clin. Neurosci.* 25:E01. doi: 10.1176/appi.neuropsych.11100235

Pienkowski, M., Tyler, R. S., Roncancio, E. R., Jun, H. J., Brozoski, T., Dauman, N., et al. (2014). A review of hyperacusis and future directions: part I Measurement, I., mechanisms, and treatment. *Am. J. Audiol.* 23, 420–436. doi: 10.1044/2014_AJA-13-0037

Rouw, R., and Erfanian, M. (2018). A large-scale study of misophonia. *J. Clin. Psychol.* 74, 453–479. doi: 10.1002/jclp.22500

Schneider, R. L., and Arch, J. J. (2015). Letter to the editor: potential treatment targets for misophonia. *Gen. Hosp. Psychiatry* 37, 370–371. doi: 10.1016/j.genhosppsych.2015.03.020

Schroder, A., van Diepen, R., Mazaheri, A., Petropoulos-Petalas, D., Soto de Amesti, V., Vulink, N., et al. (2014). Diminished n1 auditory evoked potentials to oddball stimuli in misophonia patients. *Front. Behav. Neurosci.* 8:123. doi: 10.3389/fnbeh.2014.00123

Schroder, A., van Wingen, G., Vulink, N. C., and Denys, D. (2017). Commentary: the brain basis for misophonia. *Front. Behav. Neurosci.* 11:111. doi: 10.3389/fnbeh.2017.00111

Schroder, A., Vulink, N., and Denys, D. (2013). Misophonia: diagnostic criteria for a new psychiatric disorder. *PLoS One* 8:e54706. doi: 10.1371/journal.pone.0054706

Schwartz, P., Leyendecker, J., and Conlon, M. (2011). Hyperacusis and misophonia: the lesser-known siblings of tinnitus. *Minn. Med.* 94, 42–43.

Sherlock, L. P., and Formby, C. (2005). Estimates of loudness, loudness discomfort, and the auditory dynamic range: normative estimates, comparison of procedures, and test-retest reliability. *J. Am. Acad. Audiol.* 16, 85–100. doi: 10.3766/jaaa.16.2.4

Song, J. J., De Ridder, D., Schlee, W., Van de Heyning, P., and Vanneste, S. (2013). "Distressed aging": the differences in brain activity between early- and late-onset tinnitus. *Neurobiol. Aging* 34, 1853–1863. doi: 10.1016/j.neurobiolaging.2013.01.014

Song, J. J., De Ridder, D., Weisz, N., Schlee, W., Van de Heyning, P., and Vanneste, S. (2014). Hyperacusis-associated pathological resting-state brain oscillations in the tinnitus brain: a hyperresponsiveness network with paradoxically inactive auditory cortex. *Brain Struct. Funct.* 219, 1113–1128. doi: 10.1007/s00429-013-0555-1

Song, J. J., Vanneste, S., Schlee, W., Van de Heyning, P., and De Ridder, D. (2015). Onset-related differences in neural substrates of tinnitus-related distress: the anterior cingulate cortex in late-onset tinnitus, and the frontal cortex in early-onset tinnitus. *Brain Struct. Funct.* 220, 571–584. doi: 10.1007/s00429-013-0648-x

Tyler, R. S., Coelho, C., and Noble, W. (2006). Tinnitus: standard of care, personality differences, genetic factors. *ORL J. Otorhinolaryngol. Relat. Spec.* 68, 14–19; discussion 20–22. doi: 10.1159/000090486

Tyler, R. S., Oleson, J., Noble, W., Coelho, C., and Ji, H. (2007). Clinical trials for tinnitus: study populations, designs, measurement variables, and data analysis. *Prog. Brain Res.* 166, 499–509. doi: 10.1016/S0079-6123(07)66048-8

Ursin, H. (2014). Brain sensitization to external and internal stimuli. *Psychoneuroendocrinology* 42, 134–145. doi: 10.1016/j.psyneuen.2014.01.008

Veale, D. (2006). A compelling desire for deafness. *J. Deaf Stud. Deaf Educ.* 11, 369–372. doi: 10.1093/deafed/enj043

Vlaeyen, J. W. (2015). Learning to predict and control harmful events: chronic pain and conditioning. *Pain* 156(Suppl. 1), S86–S93. doi: 10.1097/j.pain.0000000000000107

Wallenstein, G. V., Eichenbaum, H., and Hasselmo, M. E. (1998). The hippocampus as an associator of discontiguous events. *Trends Neurosci.* 21, 317–323. doi: 10.1016/S0166-2236(97)01220-4

Webber, T. A., Johnson, P. L., and Storch, E. A. (2014). Pediatric misophonia with comorbid obsessive-compulsive spectrum disorders. *Gen. Hosp. Psychiatry* 36.e1–2. doi: 10.1016/j.genhosppsych.2013.10.018

Webber, T. A., and Storch, E. A. (2015). Toward a theoretical model of misophonia. *Gen. Hosp. Psychiatry* 37, 369–370. doi: 10.1016/j.genhosppsych.2015.03.019

Wu, M. S., Lewin, A. B., Murphy, T. K., and Storch, E. A. (2014). Misophonia: incidence, phenomenology, and clinical correlates in an undergraduate student sample. *J. Clin. Psychol.* 70, 994–1007. doi: 10.1002/jclp.22098

Zenner, H. P., Pfister, M., and Birbaumer, N. (2006). Tinnitus sensitization: sensory and psychophysiological aspects of a new pathway of acquired centralization of chronic tinnitus. *Otol. Neurotol.* 27, 1054–1063. doi: 10.1097/01.mao.0000231604.64079.77

17

Different Patterns of Hearing Loss among Tinnitus Patients: A Latent Class Analysis of a Large Sample

Berthold Langguth[1,2], Michael Landgrebe[1,3], Winfried Schlee[1,2], Martin Schecklmann[1,2], Veronika Vielsmeier[2,4], Thomas Steffens[2,4], Susanne Staudinger[2], Hannah Frick[5] and Ulrich Frick[1,6]*

[1] Department of Psychiatry and Psychotherapy, University of Regensburg, Regensburg, Germany, [2] Interdisciplinary Tinnitus Center of the University of Regensburg, Regensburg, Germany, [3] kbo Lech-Mangfall-Klinik Agatharied, Hausham, Germany, [4] Department of Otorhinolaryngology, University of Regensburg, Regensburg, Germany, [5] Department of Statistical Science, University College London, London, UK, [6] HSD University of Applied Sciences, Cologne, Germany

Correspondence:
Berthold Langguth
berthold.langguth@medbo.de

Background: The heterogeneity of tinnitus is a major challenge for tinnitus research. Even if a complex interaction of many factors is involved in the etiology of tinnitus, hearing loss (HL) has been identified as the most relevant etiologic factor. Here, we used a data-driven approach to identify patterns of hearing function in a large sample of tinnitus patients presenting in a tinnitus clinic.

Methods: Data from 2,838 patients presenting at the Tinnitus Center of the University Regensburg between 2007 and 2014 have been analyzed. Standard audiometric data were frequency-wise categorized in four categories [a: normal hearing (0–20 dB HL); b: moderate HL (25–50 dB HL; representing outer hair cell loss); c: severe HL (>50 dB HL; representing outer and inner hair cell loss); d: no data available] and entered in a latent class analysis, a statistical method to find subtypes of cases in multivariate categorical data. To validate the clinical relevance of the identified latent classes, they were compared with respect to clinical and demographic characteristics of their members.

Results: The classification algorithm identified eight distinct latent classes with an excellent separation. Patient classes differed with respect to demographic (e.g., age, gender) and clinical characteristics (e.g., tinnitus location, tinnitus severity, gradual, or abrupt onset, etc.).

Discussion: Our results demonstrate that data-driven categorization of hearing function seems to be a promising approach for profiling tinnitus patients, as it revealed distinct subtypes that reflect prototypic forms of HL and that differ in several relevant clinical characteristics.

Keywords: chronic tinnitus, hearing loss, cluster analysis, latent classes, audiometry

INTRODUCTION

Tinnitus, the perception of sound in the absence of a corresponding auditory stimulus, is a frequent disorder (1). Clinically, tinnitus can be very heterogeneous with respect to the perceived sound characteristics (e.g., tonal vs. broadband noise), its localization (in one or both ears, in the head, etc.), its time course (continuous, intermittent, fluctuating), its modifying factors (e.g., reduction by masking), and its comorbidities (hyperacusis, depression, insomnia). This clinical heterogeneity is paralleled by heterogeneity in tinnitus pathophysiology. Recent pathophysiological models assume that tinnitus emerges as a clinical symptom as result of abnormal activation of different overlapping and interacting brain networks (2). Abnormally activated networks in tinnitus patients include the auditory, attention, salience, and distress networks. The activation pattern varies from patient to patient and reflects the individuals' symptoms (3, 4). As an example, distressed and not distressed tinnitus patients differ in their activation of the cortical stress-related network (5).

Among other factors, the large heterogeneity of the tinnitus patient population represents a major barrier for the development of effective tinnitus treatments [see, e.g., Ref. (4) for a review]. The heterogeneity of tinnitus can be described on various dimensions such as its etiology, perceptual characteristics of the sound (i.e., pitch and loudness), time since onset, continuous or intermittent, levels of conscious awareness and perceived distress, and comorbidities (6). One approach to address this challenge is the establishment of large databases for enabling data-driven identification of subtypes (7–9).

Even if current etiologic models assume a complex interplay of various factors, several lines of evidence indicate that hearing loss (HL) is the most relevant etiologic factor for tinnitus development (10, 11). First, epidemiological studies have identified HL as a major risk factor for tinnitus (12). Second, induction of HL in animals induces reliably increased neuronal activity and synchronicity (11, 13) as well as behavioral evidence of tinnitus (14). Third, the tinnitus spectrum of most tinnitus patients is clearly related to their pattern of HL (15, 16). If, for example, somebody experiences tinnitus at 4 kHz at the left ear, typically a HL at 4 kHz on the left ear can be detected in the audiogram.

Because of the high etiological relevance of HL for tinnitus, hearing function is presumably one of the relevant criteria for classifying tinnitus patients. Currently, this factor is not receiving major attention in the classification of tinnitus patients. In the description of study samples in tinnitus research rarely details are given about the hearing function of participants. If anything, the mean audiogram (averaged over all participants) is displayed. Whenever statistical analyses are performed relating hearing function to other aspects of tinnitus, typically either HL averaged over both ears and all measured frequencies or the maximum HL is used to characterize patients' incapacities.

Both indicators are of only limited value, as there exist different patterns of the quantity of HL, e.g., related to outer or inner hair cell damage, which might be highly relevant for a comprehensive characterization of a tinnitus patient. However, the information about specific patterns of HL quantity is getting lost, if the audiograms of participants are averaged.

Here, we used a data-driven approach to identify patterns of hearing function in a large sample of tinnitus patients presenting in a specialized Tinnitus Center. The goal of the study was to clarify, whether specific patterns of HL quantity can be established from patients' audiograms and how stable different tinnitus patients can be classified using these patterns of HL. In case, this data-driven approach for pattern identification reveals a statistically sound and medically well interpretable solution, one could assume that this new categorization of hearing function would be a reasonable alternative to current approaches to deal with audiogram data in the characterization of tinnitus patients.

MATERIALS AND METHODS

Patient Assessment

The analysis has been based on data from all patients who presented between 2007 and 2014 at the Interdisciplinary Tinnitus Center at the University of Regensburg, Regensburg, Germany and who gave informed consent for data collection in the Tinnitus Research Initiative database (TRI Database). The TRI Database is an international patient database that has been established for facilitating research efforts toward the identification of tinnitus subtypes and outcome predictors (8). For these purposes, patients presenting in tinnitus clinics and undergoing specific, well-defined treatment interventions, both in clinical trials or in clinical routine, are systematically assessed and their data are preprocessed for plausibility in standardized protocols (8). In addition to audiometric data, the database includes demographic and clinical data, data about tinnitus handicap, tinnitus severity, and quality of life [for a detailed description of the datasets, see Ref. (8)]. Collection of data for the TRI Database has been approved by the local ethics committee of the University of Regensburg, Germany. All patients completed various tinnitus questionnaires, underwent a microscopy of the ear and received an audiological examination including pure-tone audiometry (125–8,000 Hz). Sample size for this classificatory part of our analysis thus reached $n = 2{,}838$.

Due to item-wise missing values of the 17 variables used to describe demographic or clinical characteristics of patients beyond the results of the audiometry, effective sample sizes in comparisons of emerging latent classes (see below) vary. Most variables reach effective sample sizes clearly above 2,000 patients. Only Beck Depression Inventory (BDI) ($n = 1{,}544$) and TBF-total score ($n = 1{,}464$), which both were added later to the assessment program, and patients' CGI-ratings ($n = 807$), which were assessed only in patients entering a treatment program at their first day of treatment, reached smaller sample sizes.

Classification of Hearing Function

As HL presenting at different threshold levels can be linked to different possible pathological mechanisms (17), patients' audiogram data were not treated as a "naive" continuous metric of intensity of HL, but classified into four different states. At each of seven pre-specified frequencies (125 Hz, 250 Hz, 500 Hz, 1 kHz, 2 kHz, 4 kHz, and 8 kHz) the measured grade of HL was classified into one of the following four categories: (1) normal hearing (0–20 dB HL); (2) mild/moderate HL (25–50 dB HL), representing mostly outer hair cell loss; (3) severe/profound HL (>50 dB HL), representing outer and inner hair cell damage; and (4) no data available (either due to technical restrictions or because of physician based abbreviations of the audiogram assessment). This categorization tries to better reflect the physiological condition of patients' hearing and to avoid a potentially misleading interpretation of HL as homogenously quantifiable risk factor (18). Additionally, by introducing a fourth category of "not measured" into the analysis, a potential selection bias due to technical equipment or due to physicians' practices in assessing HL can be avoided.

Statistical Methods

Latent class analysis (LCA) is a statistical approach for identifying groups of cases in multivariate categorical data. These groups are called latent classes. Our assumption is that HL of the left ear does not predetermine HL for the right side, and *vice versa*. Therefore, a vector of 14 variables (each frequency with 4 HL categories) per patient defines the starting point of statistical analysis. Theoretically, over 250 million combinations (exactly 4**14 = 268,435,456) are possible. Observed were 590 answering vectors in 2,838 patients. LCA tries to reproduce the empirical frequencies of these answering vectors by estimating two different kinds of model parameters: π_g, i.e., the relative sizes of G latent classes (G has to be determined *a priori*), and the probability π_{isg} for an answer s ($s = 1, \ldots, 4$) on each item i ($i = 1, \ldots, 14$), given the membership in a certain latent class g. The class-specific answering probabilities $\pi_{ix|g}$ thus indicate the nearness between this specific answer and membership in the respective latent class g. LCA therefore results in G membership probabilities per person to each of the latent classes (see Supplementary Material for further details). Strong solutions with little overlap between different latent profiles provide for each person one unequivocal high membership probability and $m - 1$ very low membership probabilities. Classification then is based on the modal value of these probabilities.

Visualization of membership probabilities is an intuitively appealing method of model evaluation. Alternatively, so-called fit indices can be calculated for each number of latent classes chosen. Clearly, a perfect model fit must be reached, if (in our case) 590 classes are introduced to the model. By introducing a penalty term for adding new latent classes, a decision for the optimal number of classes can be drawn choosing the model with the best fit. We used the BIC index as criteria to decide on the number of latent classes. Calculations were performed using WinMIRA by von Davier (19).

Differences between latent classes on continuous variables (like age) were assessed using SAS PROC GLM to perform analysis of variance for unequal cell sizes. Differences on qualitative variables (like sex) were assessed using chi-square test (SAS PROC FREQ). Due to the exploratory character of this study, no adjustment for type-I error inflation was performed.

RESULTS

The sample comprised 2,838 patients (mean age 51.7 ± 12.9 years, 67.6% male). In 1,925 of them, audiometric data were available.

In order to avoid local maxima of the estimation function, 50 starting values for parameter estimation were randomly chosen for each model covering 2 up to 12 latent classes. According to the BIC fit index, eight latent classes represent an optimal solution for the given data set. Posterior probabilities of class membership display excellent separation of groups of HL as indicated by a mean membership probability above 0.9 for all latent classes (**Table 1**) (see Supplementary Material for details about the calculation of latent classes). Detailed clinical and demographic data of the sample are given in **Table 2**.

The largest class (LC1; **Figure 1** upper left chart) comprises nearly one-third (32.2%) of the sample and represents patients with lacking audiometry. By holding these untested patients in a separate group it is possible to scrutinize potential selection biases between clinical characteristics and audiometry. Therefore, it is meaningful to analyze these patients as a specific "pattern of hearing loss."

The 21.6% of the sample suffers from mild to moderate HL probably due to primarily outer hair cell damage especially for frequencies above 4 kHz (LC2; **Figure 1**, upper right chart). This group was entitled "bilateral high frequency (HF) hearing loss." Tinnitus patients with nearly normal audiogram (LC3; **Figure 1**, lower left chart) comprise about 20.6% of the total sample. Here, in rare cases (about 10% of this group), only frequencies above 4 kHz are involved with mild/moderate HL for both ears. A large proportion of patients with at least moderate HL in higher frequencies (2 kHz and above) for both ears can be observed in LC4. Twenty to thirty percent of this latent class were measured with thresholds over 50 dB above 4 kHz. Lower frequencies (below 500 Hz) are mostly not affected by HL. The proportion of this group is 13% of the total sample. The group was entitled "bilateral medium-high frequency HL."

Figure 2 displays patterns of HL with much smaller proportion among tinnitus patients (all <5%). LC5 (upper left chart in **Figure 2**) was called "severe pantonal HL" and is characterized by high proportions of at least moderate HL at all measured frequencies. Almost half of the patients of this group have thresholds over 50 dB above 4 kHz. Both ears are concerned quite similarly.

By contrast, latent classes 6, 7, and 8 all display asymmetric patterns of HL. In LC6 (3.8% of total sample; upper right chart in **Figure 2**), most patients have normal hearing at the right ear below 4 kHz but severely impaired hearing at their left ear at all frequencies. Damage on the left ear is mostly a HL between 25 and 50 dB ("mild to moderate"). We therefore named this group "left-sided pantonal medium HL."

It is noteworthy, that LC7 (2.9%, lower left chart of **Figure 2**) is not a symmetrical counterpart to LC6, though in this group mostly the right ear is affected by HL. But whereas LC6 members displayed mild to moderate HL at their affected left ear, members of LC7 have a broadband severe HL at their right ears. Already at 125 Hz, more than 20% of this group suffer from threshold elevations above 50 dB. This proportion is continuously increasing with increasing frequencies up to nearly 60% at 8 kHz. We therefore called this group of patients "right-sided pantonal severe HL."

The smallest group of patients isolated by LCA can be depicted from the lower right chart of **Figure 2** (LC8). In 1.2% of all patients, a pattern was observed with considerable proportion of normal hearing at the right ear in lower frequencies (e.g., 66% at 125 kHz), continuously decreasing to 20% at 8 kHz. But at patients' left ears, nearly nobody was measured with normal hearing at any frequency: mostly, a severe HL (thresholds >50 dB) could be observed across all frequencies, or the left ear was not assessed (especially at higher frequencies). As practically, all patients had a full examination of the right ear, it can be assumed that missing values for left ears in this group do not mean "unknown" degree of HL, but represent a physician's or audiologist's decision to stop the assessment, because complete deafness of the left ear impede

TABLE 1 | Mean membership probabilities for latent classes.

Patient is classified into		Mean membership probabilities for latent classes							
Class no.	**Relative class size**	**LC1**	**LC2**	**LC3**	**LC4**	**LC5**	**LC6**	**LC7**	**LC8**
LC1	0.322	1.000	0.000	0.000	0.000	0.000	0.000	0.000	0.000
LC2	0.216	0.000	0.910	0.058	0.030	0.000	0.001	0.000	0.000
LC3	0.206	0.000	0.054	0.943	0.003	0.000	0.001	0.000	0.000
LC4	0.133	0.000	0.057	0.004	0.914	0.009	0.012	0.004	0.000
LC5	0.048	0.000	0.000	0.000	0.018	0.967	0.009	0.003	0.004
LC6	0.037	0.000	0.002	0.000	0.019	0.012	0.963	0.004	0.000
LC7	0.029	0.000	0.006	0.000	0.009	0.013	0.004	0.968	0.000
LC8	0.011	0.000	0.000	0.000	0.000	0.002	0.000	0.000	0.998

a full measurement of all frequencies at the left side. This group therefore was named "left-sided pantonal severe HL."

Latent class 1 (lacking audiometry) during all statistical comparisons of clinical and demographic parameters yielded results very similar to the total average or proportions of the total sample (see **Table 2**). Therefore, no hints are present that the lack of an audiometric test was related to a certain subgroup of tinnitus patients. The relative size of the remaining seven HL-patterns thus could be adjusted to the proportions given in **Table 2**. These reflect the expected latent class sizes in our patient sample, if all patients had received threshold measurements.

Mean age of patients (see **Table 2**) was 51.7 years (SD 12.9) with the youngest patients presenting in LC3 (normal hearing) and the oldest patients in LC5 (severe pantonal HL). Female patients (total: 32.4%, see **Table 2**) were under-represented in LC2 (bilateral HF HL) and LC4 (bilateral medium-HF HL), and at largest over-represented in LC5 (severe pantonal HL) and LC6 (left-sided pantonal medium HL).

Age at onset of tinnitus was on average 43.2 years (SD 13.9; **Table 2**). Thus, there was a mean delay of nearly 9 years until presenting at the Regensburg Tinnitus Center. Patients with more or less normal hearing (LC3) had virtually no delay in help seeking. The small difference between age at onset as compared to biographical mean age (41.7 vs. 41.9 years) is probably confounded by missing values about the onset. Patients with bilateral medium-to severe HF HL (LC4) and with severe pantonal HL (LC5) reported the latest onset of tinnitus.

Symptom load as measured by the Tinnitus Questionnaire (TQ, 20) was highest in LC5 (severe pantonal HL), and lowest in LC3 (normal hearing). Signs of depression as measured by BDI were also most prominent in LC5, and quite lenient in all other patient groups. For the TBF Questionnaire, a short form of the Tinnitus Handicap Inventory, mean scores 2 points above the total average were found for LC5 and LC8 (left-sided pantonal severe HL). Whereas patients' self-ratings of tinnitus severity on the clinical global impression scale of tinnitus (CGI self-rating) revealed no significant differences between the different latent classes, the answers to the question "How much of a problem is your tinnitus?" differed significantly. But this effect was very small with membership in latent classes of HL explaining only less than 3% of the variance of patients' ratings.

Characteristics of tinnitus manifestation over groups of HL are also given in **Table 2**. The different latent classes differed in most but not all characteristics (see **Table 2**). Whether or not tinnitus started abruptly, differed most between LC4 (43% abrupt start) and LC5 (40%) on the one side, and over 60% for latent classes 6 (left-sided pantonal medium HL) and 7 (right-sided pantonal severe HL). A non-pulsatile tinnitus was in total reported by 79.6% of all patients. Only in LC7 (right-sided pantonal severe HL) this proportion was considerably smaller (66%).

Handedness of patients could not be shown to covary with patterns of HL (and therefore was also not connected to side of HL). On which side patients experienced their tinnitus (exclusively on one side or with dominance of one side vs. bilateral symptoms) was clearly connected to the asymetrical patterns of HL. Members of LC6 (left-sided pantonal HL) as well as members of LC8 (left-sided pantonal severe HL) reported tinnitus more often for their left side. Accordingly, patients in LC7 (right-sided pantonal severe HL) clearly reported more often to experience their tinnitus on the right side (48% as compared to 12.3% in the total sample).

For LC8 (left-sided pantonal severe HL), their tinnitus was more frequently experienced as constant over time. If patients suffered from HF HL (LC2) or had quite normal audiometric results (LC3), they tended more often to describe their tinnitus as a tonal event. Patients with severe pantonal HL (LC5) by contrast had much higher proportions of tinnitus experienced as a kind of noise. The tinnitus pitch did not differ too much across the LCs except a smaller proportion of very high pitch (19% as compared to 28% for the whole sample) in LC7 (right-sided pantonal severe HL), and more prominence of low pitch tinnitus in LC3 (normal hearing) and LC6 (left-sided pantonal medium HL) with 4.4 and 6.3% (total sample: 2.5%).

DISCUSSION

In the present study, we performed a data-driven analysis of a large sample to identify clinically meaningful subtypes of HL patterns among tinnitus patients. Information about hearing function was derived from standard pure-tone audiograms, which were all performed in the context of clinical routine assessment according to standard procedures in one clinical center.

A potential limitation of our study is the limited sensitivity of the standard audiogram. The database only contained audiogram data from air conduction measurements, which made it impossible to differentiate cochlear from conductive HL. Moreover measurement of otoacoustic emissions might provide a more exact measurement of outer hair cell function than audiometric

TABLE 2 | Patterns of HL and related demographic and clinical data.

Description of patterns of HL											
Variable	**Pattern of hearing loss (HL)**	**LC2: bilateral high frequency (HF) HL**	**LC3: normal hearing**	**LC4: bilateral medium-HF HL**	**LC5: severe pantonal HL**	**LC6: left-sided pantonal medium HL**	**LC7: right-sided pantonal severe HL**	**LC8: left-sided pantonal severe HL**	**LC1: lacking audiometry**	**Total**	**Prob. *F*-test**
	N[a]	614	581	378	135	104	81	32	913	2.838	
Prevalence (adjusted)	(without LC1)	0.319	0.302	0.196	0.070	0.054	0.042	0.017	n.a.	1.00	n.a.
Age	Mean	53.099	41.878	58.706	61.186	53.799	57.026	57.372	51.763	51.694	$p < 0.0001$
	SD	9.76	11.32	10.94	12.78	10.92	12.51	12.69	13.00	12.94	
Age at onset	Mean	45.201	41.726	47.869	47.944	45.765	46.908	44.630	43.053	43.213	$p < 0.0001$
	SD	11.92	11.98	13.51	16.61	10.92	14.66	16.91	14.08	13.85	
Tinnitus Questionnaire total score (at screening)	Mean	40.178	36.813	41.894	50.944	44.768	42.519	46.500	41.639	40.910	$p < 0.0001$
	SD	17.35	17.[illegible]9	16.83	17.09	17.35	17.95	17.88	18.31	17.76	
Beck Depression Inventory total score (at screening)	Mean	10.117	10.835	10.086	14.356	10.970	11.188	11.409	11.532	10.905	$p < 0.01$
	SD	8.04	8.62	7.70	9.84	10.11	7.95	8.74	9.05	8.60	
TBF-12 total score (at screening)	Mean	12.772	11.970	13.158	14.971	13.563	13.083	14.733	12.706	12.801	$p < 0.01$
	SD	5.10	5.58	5.28	4.90	0.96	5.76	5.20	5.68	5.42	
Severity rating (patient, at screening)	Mean	3.407	3.219	3.548	3.813	3.437	3.472	3.567	3.486	3.431	$p < 0.0001$
	SD	0.84	0.90	0.81	0.83	0.84	0.87	0.82	0.90	0.88	
CGI rating (patient, at first visit)	Mean	3.880	3.978	3.769	3.800	4.094	3.920	4.133	3.909	3.901	n.s.
	SD	0.79	0.78	0.80	0.94	0.96	0.91	0.92	0.80	0.82	
Categorical variables											**Prob. chi-square test**
Sex	% Female	24.9	36.7	27.0	50.4	50.0	46.9	46.9	30.6	32.4	$p < 0.001$
Handedness	% Right hand	83.3	84.1	83.1	87.9	80.6	73.8	78.1	83.8	83.3	n.s.
Abrupt beginning of tinnitus	% Abrupt	48.8	56.8	43.1	40.0	60.4	60.3	57.1	52.3	51.1	$p < 0.001$
Tinnitus pulsation	% No	82.2	80.0	82.3	72.7	81.5	66.2	75.0	77.9	79.6	$p < 0.01$
Location of tinnitus[b]	% Right	8.6	14.3	10.0	9.9	4.0	48.2	6.3	12.9	12.3	$p < 0.001$
	% Left	18.2	13.1	15.2	15.2	37.6	11.1	37.5	17.7	17.1	
	% Both sides (worse left)	18.2	22.6	26.3	21.2	21.8	6.2	34.4	18.7	20.6	
	% Both sides (worse right)	16.7	13.6	17.6	21.2	12.9	23.5	6.3	17.2	17.1	
	% Both sides equally	27.8	24.5	20.6	24.2	13.9	8.6	6.3	23.8	23.4	
Tinnitus manifestation over time	% Constant	87.9	82.8	88.8	92.0	88.5	80.8	93.3	84.4	86.1	$p < 0.05$

(Continued)

TABLE 2 | Continued

Description of patterns of HL

Variable	Pattern of hearing loss (HL)	LC2: bilateral high frequency (HF) HL	LC3: normal hearing	LC4: bilateral medium-HF HL	LC5: severe pantonal HL	LC6: left-sided pantonal medium HL	LC7: right-sided pantonal severe HL	LC8: left-sided pantonal severe HL	LC1: lacking audiometry	Total	Prob. *F*-test
Loudness variation	% Yes	60.4	61.1	55.5	64.0	63.8	59.2	63.3	61.5	60.4	n.s.
Tonal characteristic of tinnitus[c]	% Tone	64.8	65.6	58.3	45.2	50.5	53.3	33.3	63.7	61.3	$p < 0.001$
	% Noise	5.7	10.6	11.0	32.5	19.0	23.4	33.3	11.3	11.9	
	% Crickets	21.5	15.6	20.7	12.7	15.8	13.0	16.7	16.1	17.7	
Tinnitus pitch	% Very high	30.8	27.8	23.6	27.4	28.1	18.7	30.0	29.1	27.9	$p < 0.001$
	% High	56.1	51.8	55.8	53.0	42.2	41.3	46.7	52.0	52.8	
	% Medium	11.9	16.0	19.4	16.2	22.9	40.0	20.0	16.6	16.8	
	% Low	1.3	4.4	1.2	3.4	6,3	0.0	3.3	2.3	2.5	

[a]*Due to missing values, sample sizes might vary.*
[b]*Lacking categories to 100% are "inside head," "elsewhere."*
[c]*Lacking category is "other."*

thresholds and it also remains to be determined whether the cut-offs for categorization of HL used in this study (<20 dB HL, 25–50 dB HL, >50 dB HL) are most appropriate. Finally, cochlear damage in the HF range above 8 kHz (21), dead regions between tested frequencies (22) and synaptopathy of high-threshold fibers (23) can all be relevant for tinnitus development but are not detected by the standard audiogram.

Presumably the different forms of "hidden hearing loss" are particularly relevant in LC3, the group with normal audiogram. However, in spite of the fact that patient categorization was only based on the audiogram which represents a rather rough information of cochlear function, our analysis revealed several relevant findings.

First, the classification algorithm identified eight distinct latent classes with an excellent separation. This means that all patients could be almost unambiguously allocated to a given class.

Second, the HL patterns of the different classes reflected typical clinical patterns of HL: bilateral normal hearing (LC3), bilateral HF HL (LC2), bilateral medium to HF HL (LC4), bilateral pantonal HL (LC5), medium (LC6), severe (LC8) pantonal HL left, and medium-to-severe pantonal HL right (LC7).

Third, patients of the various latent classes differed in most demographic and clinical tinnitus characteristics indicating the clinical relevance of our categorization and confirming HL as a relevant criterion for profiling of tinnitus patients.

As expected from the fact that bilateral HL frequently develops over the life span, patients with normal audiogram (LC3) were younger, whereas patients with pantonal pronounced HL (LC5) were older than average. This fits with the pattern of HL in LC5 which is typical for age-related HL. Another expected finding was that tinnitus laterality was related to the side of unilateral HL (LC6, LC7, LC8). Patients with unilateral HL (LC6, LC7) reported also more frequently abrupt tinnitus onset, which fits with sudden HL as a frequent cause of unilateral hearing impairment. By contrast, bilateral hearing impairment (LC4, LC5), which is typically developing slowly over time, was more often related to gradual onset.

Patients with HL exclusively in the HF range (LC2) and patients with normal audiogram (LC3), who frequently have hearing impairment in the extended HF range (21) had more often tonal tinnitus, which fits with their circumscribed hearing impairment. Accordingly, noise-like tinnitus was more frequently observed in patients with pantonal hearing impairment (LC5). Patients with pantonal impairment (LC5) were also characterized by higher tinnitus severity and more depressive symptoms, as reflected by increased scores in TQ, TBF-12, and BDI. This finding is in line with earlier investigations demonstrating that the degree of HL is associated with tinnitus severity (24).

In summary, our findings revealed distinct subtypes that reflect prototypic forms of HL and that differ in several relevant clinical characteristics. Further research should aim at further refinement by taking into account more detailed audiological informations. Finally, other possible approaches for cluster analyses should be tested and compared. One possible approach would be to weight differences between adjacent frequencies, as they might be particularly relevant for tinnitus generation (25). Such an approach may help to better identify relevant characteristics of hearing function (for example, the 4 kHz dip as a typical pattern of HL

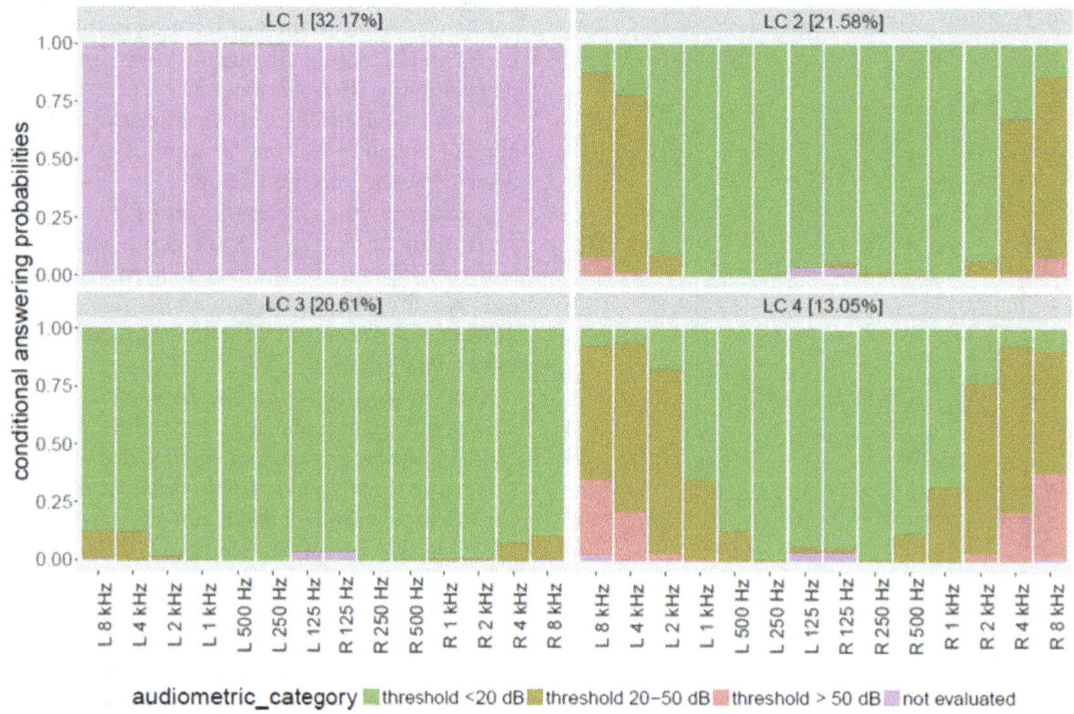

FIGURE 1 | Patterns of hearing loss with high prevalence in tinnitus patients.

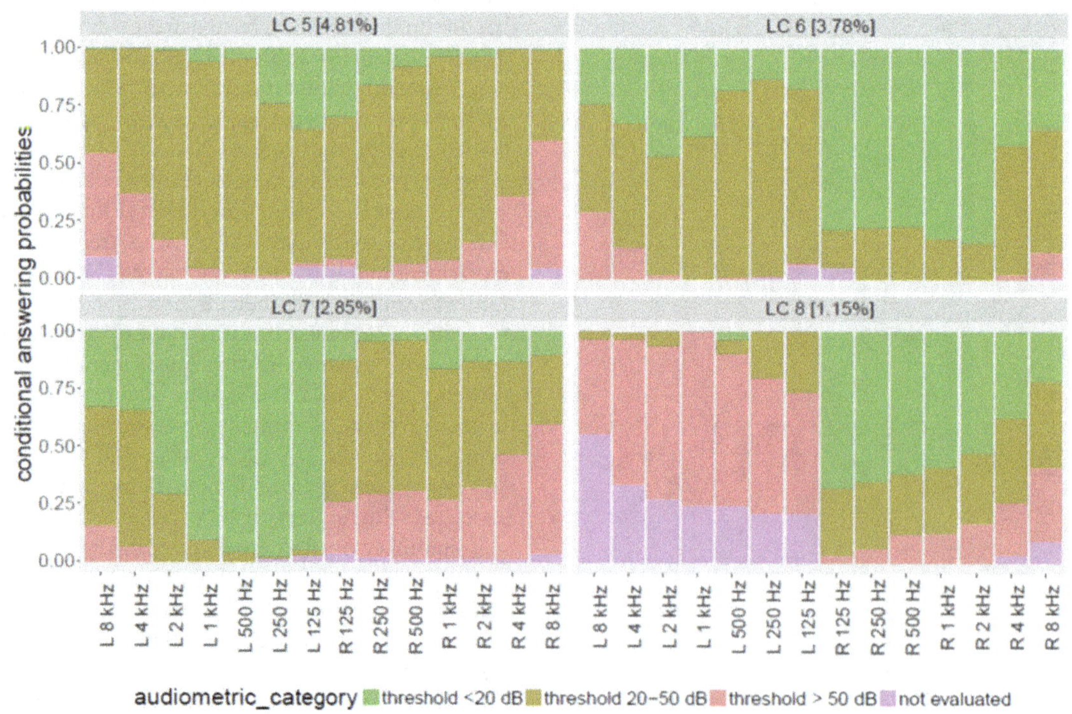

FIGURE 2 | Patterns of hearing loss with low prevalence in tinnitus patients.

among tinnitus patients), which may remain insufficiently represented by a classification algorithm in which all tested frequencies are weighted equally.

AUTHOR CONTRIBUTIONS

BL, ML, HF, and UF designed the study; ML, MS, VV, TS, and SS were responsible for data management; HF and UF performed the statistical analysis; BL, ML, WS, and ML interpreted the results; BL and UF drafted the manuscript; all the authors contributed to the manuscript and approved first final version.

ACKNOWLEDGMENTS

We thank Sandra Pfluegl, Ulrike Stadler, Helene Niebling, and Jarmila Gerxhaliu-Holan for their assistance in data management. Most of all, we want to thank our patients for participating in our studies and allowing us to use their data for analyses.

FUNDING

The study has been financially supported by Otonomy. Otonomy had no influence on study conduct, data analysis, decision to publish, or on the submitted manuscript. The authors have no further conflicts of interest, financial or otherwise, related directly or indirectly to the submitted work.

REFERENCES

Gallus S, Lugo A, Garavello W, Bosetti C, Santoro E, Colombo P, et al. Prevalence and determinants of tinnitus in the Italian adult population. *Neuroepidemiology* (2015) 45:12–9. doi:10.1159/000431376

De Ridder D, Elgoyhen AB, Romo R, Langguth B. Phantom percepts: tinnitus and pain as persisting aversive memory networks. *Proc Natl Acad Sci U S A* (2011) 108:8075–80. doi:10.1073/pnas.1018466108

De Ridder D, Vanneste S, Weisz N, Londero A, Schlee W, Elgoyhen AB, et al. An integrative model of auditory phantom perception: tinnitus as a unified percept of interacting separable subnetworks. *Neurosci Biobehav Rev* (2014) 44C:16–32. doi:10.1016/j.neubiorev.2013.03.021

Elgoyhen AB, Langguth B, De Ridder D, Vanneste S. Tinnitus: perspectives from human neuroimaging. *Nat Rev Neurosci* (2015) 16(10):632–42. doi:10.1038/nrn4003

Vanneste S, Plazier M, Van der Loo E, Van de Heyning P, Congedo M, De Ridder D. The neural correlates of tinnitus-related distress. *Neuroimage* (2010) 52:470–80. doi:10.1016/j.neuroimage.2010.04.029

Baguley D, McFerran D, Hall D. Tinnitus. *Lancet* (2013) 382:1600–7. doi:10.1016/S0140-6736(13)60142-7

Tyler R, Coelho C, Tao P, Ji H, Noble W, Gehringer A, et al. Identifying tinnitus subgroups with cluster analysis. *Am J Audiol* (2008) 17:S176–84. doi:10.1044/1059-0889(2008/07-0044)

Landgrebe M, Zeman F, Koller M, Eberl Y, Mohr M, Reiter J, et al. The Tinnitus Research Initiative (TRI) database: a new approach for delineation of tinnitus subtypes and generation of predictors for treatment outcome. *BMC Med Inform Decis Mak* (2010) 10:42. doi:10.1186/1472-6947-10-42

Witsell DL, Schulz KA, Moore K, Tucci DL. Implementation and testing of research infrastructure for practice-based research in hearing and communication disorders. *Otolaryngol Head Neck Surg* (2011) 145:565–71. doi:10.1177/0194599811406369

Langguth B, Kreuzer PM, Kleinjung T, De Ridder D. Tinnitus: causes and clinical management. *Lancet Neurol* (2013) 12:920–30. doi:10.1016/ S1474-4422(13)70160-1

Shore SE, Roberts LE, Langguth B. Maladaptive plasticity in tinnitus – triggers, mechanisms and treatment. *Nat Rev Neurol* (2016) 12:150–60. doi:10.1038/nrneurol.2016.12

Hoffman HJ, Reed GW. Epidemiology of tinnitus. In: Snow JB, editor. *Tinnitus: Theory and Management*. London: BC Decker (2004). p. 16–41.

Eggermont JJ, Roberts LE. The neuroscience of tinnitus. *Trends Neurosci* (2004) 27:676–82. doi:10.1016/j.tins.2004.08.010

Turner JG. Behavioral measures of tinnitus in laboratory animals. *Prog Brain Res* (2007) 166:147–56. doi:10.1016/S0079-6123(07)66013-0

Norena A, Micheyl C, Chery-Croze S, Collet L. Psychoacoustic characterization of the tinnitus spectrum: implications for the underlying mechanisms of tinnitus. *Audiol Neurootol* (2002) 7:358–69. doi:10.1159/000066156

Schecklmann M, Vielsmeier V, Steffens T, Landgrebe M, Langguth B, Kleinjung T. Relationship between audiometric slope and tinnitus pitch in tinnitus patients: insights into the mechanisms of tinnitus generation. *PLoS One* (2012) 7:e34878. doi:10.1371/journal.pone.0034878

Shekhawat GS, Searchfield GD, Stinear CM. The relationship between tinnitus pitch and hearing sensitivity. *Eur Arch Otorhinolaryngol* (2014) 271:41–8. doi:10.1007/s00405-013-2375-6

Stebbins WC, Hawkins JE Jr, Johnson LG, Moody DB. Hearing thresholds with outer and inner hair cell loss. *Am J Otolaryngol* (1979) 1:15–27. doi:10.1016/ S0196-0709(79)80004-6

von Davier M. *WINMIRA—A Program System for Analyses with the Rasch-Model, with the Latent Class Analysis and with the Mixed-Rasch Model*. Kiel: IPN (1999).

Goebel G, Hiller W. [The tinnitus questionnaire. A standard instrument for grading the degree of tinnitus. Results of a multicenter study with the tinnitus questionnaire]. *HNO* (1994) 42(3):166–72. German.

Vielsmeier V, Lehner A, Strutz J, Steffens T, Kreuzer PM, Schecklmann M, et al. The relevance of the high frequency audiometry in tinnitus patients with normal hearing in conventional pure-tone audiometry. *Biomed Res Int* (2015) 2015:302515. doi:10.1155/2015/302515

Weisz N, Hartmann T, Dohrmann K, Schlee W, Norena A. High-frequency tinnitus without hearing loss does not mean absence of deafferentation. *Hear Res* (2006) 222:108–14. doi:10.1016/j.heares.2006.09.003

Kujawa SG, Liberman MC. Synaptopathy in the noise-exposed and aging cochlea: primary neural degeneration in acquired sensorineural hearing loss. *Hear Res* (2015) 330:191–9. doi:10.1016/j.heares.2015.02.009

Mazurek B, Olze H, Haupt H, Szczepek AJ. The more the worse: the grade of noise-induced hearing loss associates with the severity of tinnitus. *Int J Environ Res Public Health* (2010) 7:3071–9. doi:10.3390/ ijerph7083071

Konig O, Schaette R, Kempter R, Gross M. Course of hearing loss and occurrence of tinnitus. *Hear Res* (2006) 221:59–64. doi:10.1016/j.heares.2006. 07.007

18

Impact of Multiple Factors on the Degree of Tinnitus Distress

Petra Brüggemann[1†], Agnieszka J. Szczepek[2*†], Matthias Rose[3], Laurence McKenna[4], Heidi Olze[2] and Birgit Mazurek[1*]

[1] Tinnitus Center, Universitätsmedizin Berlin, Berlin, Germany, [2] Department of Otorhinolaryngology, Universitätsmedizin Berlin, Berlin, Germany, [3] Department of Internal Medicine and Psychosomatics, Universitätsmedizin Berlin, Berlin, Germany, [4] Royal National Throat Nose and Ear Hospital, University College Hospitals, London, UK

***Correspondence:**
Agnieszka J. Szczepek
agnes.szczepek@charite.de;
Birgit Mazurek
birgit.mazurek@charite.de

Objective: The primary cause of subjective tinnitus is a dysfunction of the auditory system; however, the degree of distress tinnitus causes depends largely on the psychological status of the patient. Our goal was to attempt to associate the grade of tinnitus-related distress with the psychological distress, physical, or psychological discomfort patients experienced, as well as potentially relevant social parameters, through a simultaneous analysis of these factors.

Methods: We determined the level of tinnitus-related distress in 531 tinnitus patients using the German version of the tinnitus questionnaire (TQ). In addition, we used the Perceived Stress Questionnaire (PSQ); General Depression Scale Allgemeine Depression Skala (ADS), Berlin Mood Questionnaire (BSF); somatic symptoms inventory (BI), and SF-8 health survey as well as general information collected through a medical history.

Results: The TQ score significantly correlated with a score obtained using PSQ, ADS, BSF, BI, and SF-8 alongside psychosocial factors such as age, gender, and marital status. The level of hearing loss and the auditory properties of the specific tinnitus combined with perceived stress and the degree of depressive mood and somatic discomfort of a patient were identified as medium-strong predictors of chronic tinnitus. Social factors such as gender, age, or marital status also had an impact on the degree of tinnitus distress. The results that were obtained were implemented in a specific cortical distress network model.

Conclusions: Using a large representative sample of patients with chronic tinnitus permitted a simultaneous statistical measurement of psychometric and audiological parameters in predicting tinnitus distress. We demonstrate that single factors can be distinguished in a manner that explains their causative association and influence on the induction of tinnitus-related distress.

Keywords: the grade of tinnitus-related distress, the psychological distress, physical or psychological discomfort, social parameters, multi-level analyses

INTRODUCTION

Multi-Dimensional Causes of Tinnitus

Tinnitus distress is a multidimensional phenomenon that can be associated with problems such as difficulties with concentration, insomnia, or negative thinking which can amplify it in vicious cycles (Zirke et al., 2013; McKenna et al., 2014). Complex relationships between tinnitus, other stressors, and social factors such as education, age, and gender have been reported in the literature (Nondahl et al., 2012; Seydel et al., 2013). Furthermore, tinnitus distress seems to be more commonly reported by patients from lower social classes. Tinnitus percept results from an imbalance between excitatory and inhibitory functions in the auditory pathway (Eggermont and Roberts, 2012). Cortical mental hyperactivity can exacerbate tinnitus distress and turn it into a chronic condition. Sub-cortical structures that participate in the emotional processing of auditory signals may contribute to negative interpretations of the noise and can amplify it in response to stress, anxiety, or other factors (Leaver et al., 2011). Tinnitus can also be worsened by various orthopedic conditions (Biesinger et al., 2008).

Influence of Psychological and Somatic Complaints

A patient's level of awareness of tinnitus depends on multiple sound-processing mechanisms (Hesse, 2008) and is considered a result of selective attention combined with an absence of habituation (Hallam et al., 2004). From a psychological point of view, reducing negative interpretations of the noise and changing certain types of behavior will generally reduce emotional distress while increasing habituation, to render the tinnitus less intrusive (Wallhausser-Franke et al., 2012; McKenna et al., 2014). The neurophysiological model of tinnitus assumes that it originates in the inner ear, followed by detection to the subcortex and further steps of processing, perception, and evaluation to various cortical areas (Jastreboff, 1999). A current model views specific thalamic nuclei as filters or gates where decisions about the conscious processing of tinnitus are made (Rauschecker et al., 2010). While these psychological and neurophysiological models appear similar, they emphasize different conscious and unconscious processes in attempting to explain the experience of tinnitus distress and the treatments they propose, reflecting differences in their philosophical underpinnings (Hallam et al., 2004).

Whatever the mechanism that generates tinnitus distress, it is widely thought to involve a link between overly negative thoughts and emotions and auditory stimuli. Patients recite a common litany of despair, persecution, hopelessness, a loss of enjoyment in life, a desire for peace and quiet, and often beliefs that others do not understand (Wilson and Henry, 1998). Tinnitus distress often leads to negative thinking about the disease itself and its role in a patient's life (Henry and Wilson, 1995; Andersson and Westin, 2008). In advanced stages, tinnitus distress amplifies negative thoughts about the disease itself, starting a cycle that can lead to an even greater emotional decline. At some point 65% of tinnitus patients are diagnosed with depression, anxiety, or another mental condition (Hiller and Goebel, 1992; Andersson and Kaldo, 2004; Zirke et al., 2013).

Recently these links were highlighted in a report on the association between catastrophic thinking, high subjective judgments of the loudness of the tinnitus, poorer coping, the appearance of symptoms of depression, and more frequent medical visits (Weise et al., 2013). Catastrophic interpretations of tinnitus were also associated with fear (Cima et al., 2011; Pattyn et al., 2016). Several other studies have suggested a link between a poor emotional state and increased tinnitus distress (Halford and Anderson, 1991; Zoger et al., 2006; Wallhausser-Franke et al., 2012; Milerova et al., 2013). The overall process appears to include an increase in stress arousal, culminating in selective attention, and more monitoring of tinnitus, which in turn increases its detection and creates a vicious cycle (McKenna et al., 2014). This is consistent with observations that catastrophic interpretations lead to fear, increased attention devoted to the tinnitus, and a decrease in quality of life (Cima et al., 2011). Another result is that patients change their behavior in ways that are intended to reduce the threat, but in fact perpetuate it or increase negative thinking even more (Hesser and Andersson, 2009; Kleinstauber et al., 2013).

Such observations have strengthened the notion that links between limbic and auditory areas of the brain play a significant role in processing tinnitus and generating accompanying distress. The perception of tinnitus must follow from some neurophysiological process that sensitizes cognitive areas (Zenner, 2003). This model suggests that neuronal plasticity lowers normal perceptual thresholds and makes tinnitus audible, and the neural network responds by making subject, emotional, and somatic/motoric functions hyper-reactive. In the diathesis-stress model and similar frameworks, tinnitus is regarded as a stressor and may be aggravated by the elevated levels of stress associated with a vulnerable constitution (Andersson and McKenna, 1998; Kroner-Herwig et al., 2006).

Comorbidity

Many polygenic diseases with high rates of comorbidity are considered to incorporate a significant stress component (Chrousos, 2009). The influence of stress on the auditory system has been detected on molecular and cellular levels (Ma et al., 1995; Horner, 2003; Mazurek et al., 2010a, 2012; Kraus and Canlon, 2012). Stress can arise from a number of sources, including an individual's general disposition or psychological coping mechanisms. The severity of tinnitus has been related to the personality traits of perfectionism (Andersson et al., 2005) and anxiety sensitivity (Andersson and Kaldo, 2004; Hesser and Andersson, 2009). Optimism, as might be expected, is negatively associated with tinnitus distress (Vollmann et al., 2013).

Establishing a causal relationship between such personality variables and tinnitus distress is challenging. The appearance of traits of anxiety shortly after the onset of tinnitus has been used as a predictor that the distress will be greater 6 months later (Langenbach et al., 2005) suggesting that people who are already emotionally strained are more likely to be distressed by tinnitus. An additional relationship has been found between distress, quality of life, and Type D personalities (marked by a generally sad and gloomy view of life and social inhibition) (Bartels et al., 2010a,b). The influence of this personality type on the severity of distress was partly mediated by anxiety and depression (also possibly reactions to tinnitus). Cognitive variables such as dysfunctional thoughts (Lee et al., 2004), particularly catastrophization could also influence this relationship (Weise et al., 2013), as could tinnitus-specific perceptions of illness (Vollmann et al., 2013). Dysfunctional coping strategies are related to an increase in tinnitus distress (Budd and Pugh, 1996; Scott and Lindberg, 2000). An increase in suspicions about external control reinforces the psychiatric symptoms associated with tinnitus (Budd et al., 1998).

The presence of a formal psychological disorder is another source of stress for the person. While psychiatric disturbance may be a reaction to tinnitus, it has also been proposed as a trigger for tinnitus (Henry et al., 2005). In 64% of cases, the onset of tinnitus is preceded by other mental disorders (Goebel and Floezinger, 2008). Studies point to a link between problematic tinnitus and depression (Wilson et al., 1991; Goebel and Floezinger, 2008), connecting the severity of tinnitus to that of depression or anxiety (Budd and Pugh, 1996; Andersson et al., 2005; Zoger et al., 2006). Accordingly, an improvement in depressive symptoms has been associated with a reduction of tinnitus distress (Folmer, 2002).

The literature offers the overall impression of a diathesis-stress interaction in which the diathesis is a patient's vulnerability to distress, and the stress is the level of tinnitus, an idea supported by Andersson and McKenna (1998); Kroner-Herwig et al. (2006). Patients who find tinnitus highly distressing often exhibit additional somatic conditions or comorbidities including autoimmune diseases, cardiovascular, endocrine, or metabolic diseases (Stobik et al., 2003). Increased tension of the head and neck muscles and other functional impairments have been described in tinnitus patients (Rubinstein et al., 1990; Peroz, 2003). These factors have raised clinical interest in a classification of tinnitus distress that takes into account not only the degree of tinnitus, hearing loss, and the audiological characteristics of the conditions but also psychosocial variables and comorbid factors (i.e., a biopsychosocial model) (Seydel et al., 2010).

Prior studies have linked single mental and physical factors to tinnitus distress; in the present study we carry out *simultaneous analyses* of its association with many factors, hoping to develop a broader view. The literature shows that stress, anxiety or depression contribute to tinnitus-related distress; here, we wanted to know if this distress is affected by *individual but networked conditions* that can be assessed by the subscales of psychometric instruments. Using a large data set, we also aimed to determine *where* such conditions overlap with tinnitus, as well as ways in which tinnitus-induced distress *differs* from the experience of other types of stress and emotions. Finally, we used quantitative methods to assign weights to the factors in terms of their relative contributions to tinnitus impairment.

METHODS

Patients

Five hundred and thirty one patients with chronic tinnitus were recruited to this study, which was carried out between January 2008 and March 2010. The patients originated from a routine flow of individuals consecutively admitted to day ward of Tinnitus Center for treatment. The study sample consisted of 251 (47%) men and 280 (53%) women with a mean age of 49 years (SD 13.29 + Min 16 Max 59). All patients were informed of the purpose for which the data was being collected and gave their consent. This study was approved by the local Ethics Committee.

Audiometry

Pure tone audiometry was performed on both ears of each patient to determine the degree and nature of any hearing loss. A discomfort threshold was used to determine the possible presence of hyperacusis; (data not included in the evaluation). We used tinnitus matching (frequency and loudness) to detect and provide an audiometric description of each patient's tinnitus.

Psychometric Evaluation

The study employed the self-reporting psychometric instruments shown in **Table 1**, chosen on the basis of clinical experience and representative cross-reference data from the Department of Psychosomatic Medicine, Charité, Universitätsmedizin Berlin (scores obtained from tinnitus patients are compared with those of patients with psychosomatic disorders in Zirke et al., 2013 and Devine et al., 2016).

- The degree of tinnitus distress was measured using the German version of tinnitus questionnaire TQ (Goebel and Hiller, 1994). The subscales include emotional and cognitive stress, intrusiveness of tinnitus, hearing problems, sleep disorders, and somatic symptoms associated with tinnitus.
- The Perceived Stress Questionnaire (Fliege et al., 2005) registers a subject's level and perception of stress (tension, worry, joy).
- Depressive symptoms were measured using the validated German version of the Center for Epidemiologic Studies Depression Scale, abbreviated here as ADS—Allgemeine Depression Skala (Radloff, 1991).
- Additional measurements were made of "anxious depression," "annoyance," and "positive mood" with the Berlin mood questionnaire (BSF) (Hoerhold and Klapp, 1993).
- Subjects' quality of life and mental and physical functions were assessed with the Short Form Health Survey (SF-36) (Morfeld et al., 2005).
- The Somatic Symptoms Inventory was used to characterize somatic symptoms considered independent of tinnitus.

Computational support included the use of a personal digital assistant (PDA) and data analysis, permitting physicians to provide subjects with an immediate interpretation of the results of their survey (Rose et al., 1999).

Statistical Evaluation

The analysis was performed with SPSS Statistics (version 15). First, the data were examined to determine the relationship between psychometric and audiological data and tinnitus distress (total tinnitus distress-score from TQ and its corresponding subscales). Correlations were calculated to provide initial values for the strength of each connection, followed by multiple regressions to examine cause and effect relationships. The dependent variable was TQ score whereas independent variables were the scores of remaining instruments and audiometric values. In addition to the psychometric tests, social data (age, sex, marital status, education, employment), and audiometric parameters such as hearing loss, tinnitus loudness, and frequency were included. This produced multiple regression model, which achieved a high level of significance, with an overall regression

TABLE 1 | Psychometric tests used during the study.

Questionnaire	Item example	Measured domain
Tinnitus questionnaire by Goebel and Hiller (TQ, 51 items)	**Emotional stress:** to be worried sick **Cognitive stress:** thoughts on prognosis **Intrusiveness:** distraction of tinnitus **Hearing problems:** distortion of voices **Sleep disorders:** falling asleep **Somatic symptoms:** severe headache	Tinnitus distress
Questionnaire to tinnitus localization and quality (TLQ, 10 Items)	**Localization:** left, **quality**: rustle	Tinnitus
Visual analog scales (VAS, 3 items)	**Loudness of tinnitus** **Frequency of perception**: Affected by tinnitus	Tinnitus
Perceived stress questionnaire (PSQ; 20 items)	**General requirements:** They feel under deadline pressure **Tension:** You feel tense **Worries:** Your problems seem to pile up in front of you **Joy:** You are a light hearted	Stress amount Stress perception
General depression scale (ADS-L; 20 Items)	**Depressive affect:** self-devaluation **Somatic symptoms**: drive **Interpersonal experiences**: Rejection by others **Positive affect:** zest for life	Depression
Berlin mood questionnaire (BSF; 30 Items)	**Anxious depression:** I feel worried **Anger:** I feel aggressive **Elation**: I feel solved **Engagement:** I feel included	Mood
Somatic symptoms inventory (BI; 24 Items)	**Fatigue:** fatigue **Stomach complaints:** bloating **Limb pain:** neck pain **Heart disease:** shortness of breath	Somatic symptoms
Short form—8 health survey (SF8; 8 Items)	How much have you physical health or emotional problems in the past 4 weeks, limiting your normal contacts with family members or friends?	Quality of life
Total: 175 items		

coefficient $R = 0.993$ (ANOVA: $F = 24.753$, $p < 0.000$). Due to limited capacity of SPSS version 15, the predictor importance was computed with a stochastically defined, randomly chosen by software subset of the sample ($N = 140$). In addition, multiple regression model was performed separately for the subset of 140 patients chosen for predictor importance computing. That model has also achieved high level of significance with regression coefficient $R = 0.890$ (ANOVA: $F = 4.896$, $p < 0.000$). All correlations that were significant for the whole sample remained significant in the subset and no new correlations were identified, indicative of sample homogeneity.

RESULTS

Based on the tinnitus distress score TQ, 400 patients (75%) were classified as having a compensated, moderate tinnitus response (TQ-score < 46), while 131 patients (25%) exhibited decompensated, severe tinnitus reactions (TQ score>, 47). The first interview recorded stress, depressive symptoms, disease-related fears, patients' medication and drug use, alongside audiometric measurements, and a medical history.

Dependence of the Degree of Tinnitus Distress (TQ) on Somatic Factors

Hearing

The audiometric examination revealed a moderate hearing loss of 23.53 dB/HL for the left ear and 22.96 dB/HL for the right ear in the study population.

Hearing Loss

The correlation between hearing loss and tinnitus distress (TQ-score) was significant both for the total value of the TQ and the subscales "hearing problems" and "intrusiveness of tinnitus" (**Table 3**).

Multiple regressions (linear model, all variables) found no significant association between hearing loss, specific

TABLE 2 | Patients' description.

	Number of patients	Mean value	Standard deviation	Minimum	Maximum
Age	531	48.88	13.29	16	79
Mean total score TQ	531	34.73	16.38	2	79
TQ emotional	531	9.53	5.49	0	23
TQ cognitive	531	6.13	3.90	0	16
TQ intrusiveness	531	9.51	3.55	0	16
TQ acoustic	531	4.70	3.55	0	14
TQ sleep	531	3.07	2.57	0	8
TQ somatic symptoms	531	1.79	1.74	0	6
PSQ worries	531	36.13	22.20	0	100
PSQ tension	531	50.83	22.88	0	100
PSQ joy	531	52.24	22.61	0	100
PSQ demands	531	44.91	24.17	0	100
Mean score ADSL	531	16.11	11.03	0	53
Tinnitus frequency right (Hz)	279	5058.17	2758.00	125	10,000
Tinnitus frequency left (Hz)	292	5380.14	2776.07	125	10,000
Tinnitus loudness right (dB)	276	36.09	21.17	-4	100
Tinnitus loudness left (dB)	290	37.42	20.97	2	93
Mean hearing loss right (dB)	531	23.00	16.73	1.9	130.0
Mean hearing loss left (dB)	530	23.28	15.01	0.6	86.4

characteristics of tinnitus and the level of distress it caused. A tendency for a significant negative regression was found between hearing loss on the right and TQ-total value ($t = -1.793$, $p = 0.075$).

Tinnitus Loudness

The loudness of tinnitus (dB HL, separated for unilateral and bilateral tinnitus), but not its frequency (**Table 2**), correlated with the scores of the TQ (Spearman correlation). Significant correlations were found between tinnitus loudness and the subscales "hearing problems" and "intrusiveness" and, with lower significance, for the total value of the TQ (**Table 3**). In the regression model, neither the loudness nor frequency of the tinnitus (respectively right/left) achieved significance.

Somatic Symptoms Inventory (*BI*)

A significant correlation was found between somatic symptoms measured by Somatic Symptoms Inventory, all subscales of TQ, and the total value (**Table 3**).

The regression analysis revealed a significant regression of fatigue with tinnitus distress (TQ total) with$t = 2.038$ ($p = 0.043$).

Dependence of Tinnitus Distress (from TQ) on Psychological Burden

Stress (PSQ) Related to Tinnitus Distress (TQ)

The level of perceived stress was significantly associated with tinnitus distress (TQ-scores) and correlated with the following PSQ subscales: demands, worry, tension, and joy (**Table 3**).

The regression analysis revealed no significant correlation in the overall model.

Depression Score (ADS) Correlates with Tinnitus Distress (TQ)

The total score for the Depression-Scale, which mainly focuses on cognitive aspects of depression such as a tendency to worry and negative thought circuits, correlated to the total TQ score as well as with its all separate subscales at a high level of significance (**Table 3**).

The multiple regression model revealed a significant regression with $t = 2.98$ ($p = 0.003$).

Mood Scores (BSF) are Related to Tinnitus Distress (TQ)

Symptoms of anxiety and depression, which were evaluated with the BSF, correlated significantly with the total TQ score and all its separate subscales, as was the case for "annoyance." The positive moods, commitment and joy, had significant negative correlations with the total value and all subscales (**Table 3**).

Multiple regression found a significant relationship for anxious depression and total TQ with $t = -2.20$ ($p = 0.029$).

Dependence of Tinnitus Distress (TQ) on Social Stress

Quality of Life (SF-8) is Significantly Affected by Tinnitus Distress (TQ)

A significant negative correlation was found between physical and mental health as measured by the SF-8 and the total TQ score as well as all TQ subscales (**Table 3**). In the regression model, no significant correlations were found.

TABLE 3 | Results of correlation analysis in the study population ($n = 531$).

		Tinnitus distress total score	Emotional and cognitive stress	Hearing problems	Somatic symptoms	Intrusiveness	Sleep problems
1. HEARING							
Hearing loss right	r_s	0.173*	0.090	0.247*	0.088	0.197*	−0.006
Hearing loss left	r_s	0.235**	0.135*	0.384**	0.095	0.269*	0.064
2. TINNITUS							
Tinnitus loudness right	r_s	0.176*	0.092	0.247*	0.083	0.227**	0.094
Tinnitus loudness left	r_s	0.111*	0.027	0.239**	0.041	0.158*	0.039
Tinnitus frequency right	r_s	0.008	−0.003	0.010	0.351**	0.426**	0.385**
Tinnitus frequency left	r_s	−0.029	−0.018	−0.054	−0.065	−0.022	0.022
3. SOMATIC SYMPTOMS INVENTORY BI							
Fatigue	r_s	0.535**	0.498**	0.359**	0.397**	0.424**	0.325**
Stomach	r_s	0.403**	0.368**	0.359**	0.313**	0.283**	0.239**
Limbs	r_s	0.478**	0.384**	0.403**	0.538**	0.373**	0.273**
Heart	r_s	0.401**	0.358**	0.320**	0.330**	0.303**	0.225**
BI_total score	r_s	0.588**	0.520**	0.449*	0.513**	0.452**	0.345**
4. PSQ							
Worries	r_s	0.444**	0.472**	0.254**	0.226*	0.342**	0.208**
Joy	r_s	−0.388**	−0.376**	−0.296**	−0.269**	−0.306**	−0.151*
Tension	r_s	0.485**	0.442**	0.320**	0.328**	0.449**	0.270**
General requirements	r_s	0.216**	0.196*	0.189*	0.162*	0.173*	0.083
PSQ_ total score	r_s	0.463**	0.449**	0.322**	0.298**	0.382**	0.214**
5. GENERAL DEPRESSION SCALE AND BERLIN MOOD QUESTIONNAIRE BSF, ADS							
Engagement	r_s	0.335**	−0.306**	−0.258**	0.239**	−0.269**	−0.178*
Joy	r_s	−0.409**	−0.396**	−0.249**	−0.272**	−0.347**	−0.217**
Annoyance	r_s	0.512**	0.518**	0.306**	0.311**	0.396**	0.275**
Anxious depression.	r_s	0.586**	0.637**	0.283**	0.344**	0.426**	0.302**
ADS_ total score	r_s	0.579**	0.572**	0.349**	0.351**	0.426**	0.385**
6. SHORT FORM - 8 HEALTH SURVEY SF 8							
Physical health	r_s	−0.446**	0.417**	0.323**	−0.270**	−0.363**	−0.258**
Mental health	r_s	−0.455**	−0.464**	0.295**	−0.249**	−0.339**	−0.240**
SF8_ total score	r_s	−0.388**	−0.370**	−0.315**	−0.201*	−0.299**	−0.199*

r_s, correlation coefficient.
**, significance $p < 0.05$.*
***, significance $p < 0.01$.*

Age, Gender, and Marital Status are Related to Tinnitus Distress (TQ)

Patients who lived alone had a higher hearing loss on both sides and greater hearing problems than those living with a partner, as indicated by scores of the respective subscales (TQ). A similar trend was found for tinnitus loudness, judged higher by people living alone. The regression analysis showed a significant positive correlation with age $t = 2.23$ ($p = 0.027$).

Weighting of Each Component in Relation to Tinnitus Distress (TQ) in the Regression Analysis

The multiple regression analysis [evaluating the effects of tinnitus distress (TQ) for other psychometric data] showed that depression and stress scores had particularly high predictor values (**Figures 1, 2**).

The analysis of social variables revealed significant correlations with age, education, employment, and the number of physicians a patient had consulted. Additionally, a correlation, between hearing loss and tinnitus distress was found.

Summary of Results

- There was a clear association between physical symptoms and tinnitus distress TQ, particularly seen in correlations with the TQ subscales "hearing problems" and "somatic symptoms," and to some degree with "emotional stress."
- Quality of life and tinnitus distress are negatively correlated, as indicated by the negative influence of the subscales "emotional stress," "somatic symptoms," and "hearing problems" on mental health.
- Tinnitus distress (TQ total score) correlated significantly with perceived stress and (depressive) mood. For perceived stress (PSQ), the TQ subscales "emotional stress" and "hearing problems" proved to be especially significant. The subscales "emotional stress," "sleep problems" and, to a lesser

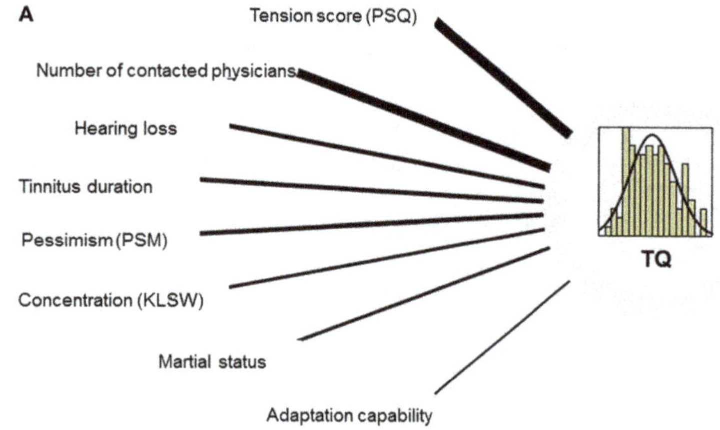

B

Source	Significance level (*p*)	Predictor importance
Tension score (PSQ)	0.000	0.434
Number of contacted physicians	0.000	0.216
Hearing loss	0.025	0.079
Tinnitus duration	0.039	0.066
Pessimism (PSM)	0.046	0.062
Concentration (KLSW)	0.054	0.058
Martial status	0.072	0.050
Adaptation capability	0.129	0.036

FIGURE 1 | (A) Regression analysis graphical model [overall model: $R = 0.993$ (ANOVA: $F = 322.97$, $p < 0.000$)] calculated with subset of the data ($n = 140$). **(B)** Computed predictor importance and significance.

degree, "tinnitus intrusiveness" significantly correlated with the depression grade.

DISCUSSION

The aim of our study was to simultaneously measure associations between tinnitus distress and other mental and physical conditions in a single group of patients. Previous studies have linked distress to a number of individual factors, but their relative contributions to the outcome of tinnitus distress have not been ranked in a single model. Our efforts found a number of correlations between measurements of tinnitus distress (TQ) and physical symptoms, the quality of life, perceived stress, and depressive symptoms.

Psychometric methods have been established as a means of expressing tinnitus distress. A number of studies have concluded that psychoacoustic features of tinnitus, such as loudness, cannot be used to predict a patient's degree of distress (Henry and Meikle, 2000; Hiller and Goebel, 2007). Here we demonstrate that acoustic variables such as the loudness and frequency of tinnitus correlate only marginally with the overall tinnitus-related burden experienced by patients. Tinnitus loudness could only be correlated with the TQ subscales "hearing problems" and "intrusiveness of tinnitus." The louder the tinnitus, the more penetrating is its perception. However, our study revealed no correlation was found between tinnitus frequency and the TQ total score.

Past studies have reported some correlations between auditory processing and patient mood. A representative study recently conducted in Sweden concluded that the strongest predictor for the *occurrence* of tinnitus was hearing loss. A patient's subjective *experience* of tinnitus, however, was more dependent on the presence of a depressive co-morbidity (Hebert et al., 2012; Kraus and Canlon, 2012).

In earlier work (Mazurek et al., 2010b), we determined that tinnitus-induced distress is positively correlated with hearing loss, and the present study corroborates this finding.

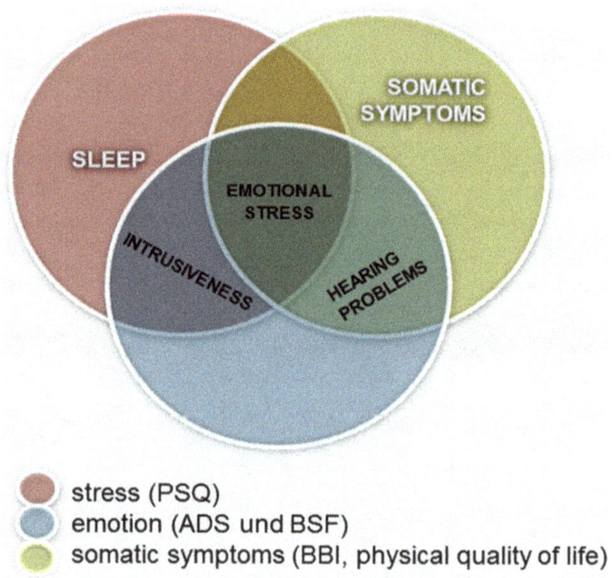

FIGURE 2 | Measurements of constructs related to tinnitus distress: graphical summary of the overlapping and not covering areas.

We also found that age has a significant impact on tinnitus distress. This confirms findings from single-factor association studies that have linked distress to hearing problems and sleep disorders, which also increase with age. Similar findings from other recent studies demonstrate that older patients find tinnitus more stressful (Schlee et al., 2011a). Previous work by our group has shown that age influences various aspects of tinnitus distress; starting at the age of 60, patients report more distress (Seydel et al., 2013).

Here our computing of predictor importance identifies only two factors that account for a significant amount of the variance of tinnitus distress: the side on which patients experience tinnitus, and the overall status of their hearing.

No significant correlations were found based on age or gender.

We have shown that tinnitus distress is closely related to more general types of stress, a negative mood, and hearing loss. Increasing age is generally accompanied by poorer hearing and other somatic symptoms, which then amplify tinnitus distress. Age-related changes in tinnitus have been reported in the literature (see a review Henry et al., 2005) and in detail by our group (Seydel et al., 2013, 2015). The correlations that emerge, however, are multidimensional. Causal relationships seem to be indicated for gender, the duration of tinnitus, hearing impairment, age, and psychosocial variables (such as employment, education level, and use of the health system).

An analysis of the influence of marital status of tinnitus patients revealed a trend toward greater hearing loss in people who live alone. They perceive tinnitus louder than patients who live with a partner. Somatic symptoms and general physical health (quality of life-SF 8) are co-morbidities whose effects vary significantly in association with hearing, and partly in relation to age and sex. A decline in hearing had a significant influence on other symptoms captured in the somatic symptoms inventory (BI). As people age, they generally report a decline in aspects of the quality of life linked to physical health. For tinnitus patients, the loss of hearing likely has an additive effect on these negative perceptions.

A review of associations that have been made between tinnitus and subjective tinnitus distress in the literature yielded high correlations with "somatic problems" and "intrusiveness." This association seems to depend on a patient's perception of tinnitus and its additive effects on other somatic problems, some of which may have a physiological basis. Liotti and Mayberg have proposed that a negative mood or depressive emotions, which chiefly originate in the limbic system, can lead to down-regulations of activity in the inferior parietal cortex and dorsolateral prefrontal cortex (Liotti and Mayberg, 2001). These regions include the auditory cortex, where acoustic stimuli are processed. The effects may extend to a wider network involved in attention and spatial orientation (Sturm et al., 2004; Schonwiesner et al., 2007; McKenna et al., 2014). By modulating processes and brain areas involved in attention, negative moods may also influence activity in the auditory or somatosensory areas of the brain.

Previous studies have reported high correlations between the total score for tinnitus distress (as determined by the -TQ) with stress and stress perception (Olderog et al., 2004), with depression and negative mood (Andersson and Kaldo, 2004), and even with physical complaints and perceptions of a decline in quality of life (Cima et al., 2011). Bi-directional interference has been observed between tinnitus perception and stress, pain, sleep, and fatigue Hebert et al. (2012). Langguth (2011) suggest that there are similarities in the pathophysiology of depression and tinnitus, especially in regard to associated distress factors (Langguth, 2011). Here we confirm a strong correlation between tinnitus distress and other forms of stress and depression. However, the regression analysis offers a multi-dimensional view of these relationships, suggesting that other forms of somatic stress and depression contribute to total tinnitus distress (TQ) in distinct ways. The stress scales (PSQ) showed correlations to all subscales of TQ; correlation coefficients were particularly high for emotional stress, intrusiveness and tinnitus-induced hearing problems. Depression, on the other hand, was predominantly correlated with the TQ-subscales "emotional stress," "intrusiveness," and "sleep."

So far these studies have exposed a number of factors that play some role in the development of tinnitus and the ways patients cope, but they have not turned up a specific association that correlates with a high-distress response reliably enough to serve as a predictor. This will come as no surprise to clinicians, who are familiar with the diverse symptoms and responses of patients. What has been missing is a more complex model that integrates these findings, reveals combinations of factors that influence the facets of tinnitus, and assigns weights to components that reflect their contributions to various processes.

Our approach involved a large cohort of tinnitus patients, from whom we simultaneously captured a wide range of psychological and somatic parameters. We used computational methods to detect associations between high tinnitus distress and various combinations of psychological, biological, and lifestyle factors. The analysis revealed a network of associations linking aspects of tinnitus distress to other aspects of patients' lives and health. In some cases we could assess the contributions of each component and distinguish crucial factors from weak contributors.

We anticipated that our combined approach would reveal new, more precise associations between subscales of tinnitus distress and diverse aspects of patients' lives; these, in turn, could provide new insights into causal mechanisms that linked them. Finding a strong correlation between tinnitus perception and depression and negative moods, for example, is evidence of a connection between acoustic perception and the regulation of emotions, thus implicating specific regions of the brain and possibly suggesting something about their coordination.

The Global Brain Model of Tinnitus proposes a scenario in which acoustic input to the brain falls, which can be caused by various types of damage to the auditory system (Schlee et al., 2011b). This leads to a change in the central auditory system, where inhibitory mechanisms usually dampen the strength of acoustic signals; now those mechanisms become less active, resulting in more excitation of cortical areas.

The activity of auditory areas is modulated by a fronto-parietal-cingular network, where higher activity is associated with high levels of patient distress. The particularly important structures in this network are the dorsolateral prefrontal cortex, the orbitofrontal cortex, the anterior cingulum, and the precuneus/posterior cingulate. De Ridder et al. (2011) describes a network of ACC, amygdala, and anterior insula (tested by EEG data) and claims that it is responsible for tinnitus distress. This network is also activated in pain-associated distress (Moisset and Bouhassira, 2007). Recent epidemiological studies suggest that similar or related symptoms might account for the relationship between tinnitus distress and depression, but they may also have common etiologies (Hebert et al., 2012). These ideas are interesting in light of the observation that either depression or a high general level of stress leads to a more pronounced perception of tinnitus symptoms by patients (Bartels et al., 2010b).

The diverse models that have been proposed for tinnitus distress may indicate that it might be reached through several routes that depend on different mechanisms. Clinical experience would tend to support this view, given the diversity of patients affected by tinnitus and their subjective experiences of it. Ultimately, hypotheses and models of tinnitus mechanisms must be validated in patient studies, and ideally they should be designed with an eye to clinical benefits and new, effective types of treatment.

Further studies will be necessary to clarify how different processing mechanisms interact to produce the complex symptoms of tinnitus. At least three types of components are involved: somatic (generators, influenced by a range of somatosensory stimuli), psychological (emotional "depressive" processing, attention, stress), and social. The unique features of tinnitus might trigger a unique "Distress Network"; this might explain the increased level of stress and other physical and psychological symptoms observed in patients with chronic decompensated tinnitus (De Ridder et al., 2011). Helping patients become habituated to tinnitus and find healthy ways to compensate will probably require therapies that address and reduce combinations of symptoms related to stress and depression.

AUTHOR CONTRIBUTIONS

PB: study conception and design; data acuisition; analysis and interpretation of data; drafting of manuscript. AS: analysis and interpretation of data; drafting of manuscript. MR: analysis and interpretation of data. LM: critical revision; drafting of manuscript. HO: critical revision. BM: study design; data acuisition; analysis and interpretation of data.

REFERENCES

Andersson, G., Airikka, M., Buhrman, M., and Kaldo, V. (2005). Dimensions of perfectionism and tinnitus distress. *Psychol. Health Med.* 10, 78–87. doi: 10.1080/13548500512331315389

Andersson, G., and Kaldo, V. (2004). Internet-based cognitive behavioral therapy for tinnitus. *J. Clin. Psychol.* 60, 171–178. doi: 10.1002/jclp.10243

Andersson, G., and McKenna, L. (1998). Tinnitus masking and depression. *Audiology* 37, 174–182. doi: 10.3109/00206099809072971

Andersson, G., and Westin, V. (2008). Understanding tinnitus distress: introducing the concepts of moderators and mediators. *Int. J. Audiol.* 47(Suppl. 2), S106–S111. doi: 10.1080/14992020802301670

Bartels, H., Middel, B., Pedersen, S. S., Staal, M. J., and Albers, F. W. (2010a). The distressed (Type D) personality is independently associated with tinnitus: a case-control study. *Psychosomatics* 51, 29–38. doi: 10.1176/appi.psy.51.1.29

Bartels, H., Pedersen, S. S., Van Der Laan, B. F., Staal, M. J., Albers, F. W., and Middel, B. (2010b). The impact of Type D personality on health-related quality of life in tinnitus patients is mainly mediated by anxiety and depression. *Otol. Neurotol.* 31, 11–18. doi: 10.1097/MAO.0b013e3181bc3dd1

Biesinger, E., Reisshauer, A., and Mazurek, B. (2008). [The role of the cervical spine and the craniomandibular system in the pathogenesis of tinnitus. Somatosensory tinnitus]. *HNO* 56, 673–677. doi: 10.1007/s00106-008-1721-2

Budd, R. J., Oles, G., and Hughes, I. C. (1998). The relationship between coping style and burden in the carers of relatives with schizophrenia. *Acta Psychiatr. Scand.* 98, 304–309. doi: 10.1111/j.1600-0447.1998.tb10088.x

Budd, R. J., and Pugh, R. (1996). Tinnitus coping style and its relationship to tinnitus severity and emotional distress. *J. Psychosom. Res.* 41, 327–335. doi: 10.1016/S0022-3999(96)00171-7

Chrousos, G. P. (2009). Stress and disorders of the stress system. *Nat. Rev. Endocrinol.* 5, 374–381. doi: 10.1038/nrendo.2009.106

Cima, R. F., Crombez, G., and Vlaeyen, J. W. (2011). Catastrophizing and fear of tinnitus predict quality of life in patients with chronic tinnitus. *Ear Hear.* 32, 634–641. doi: 10.1097/AUD.0b013e31821106dd

De Ridder, D., Elgoyhen, A. B., Romo, R., and Langguth, B. (2011). Phantom percepts: tinnitus and pain as persisting aversive memory networks. *Proc. Natl. Acad. Sci. U.S.A.* 108, 8075–8080. doi: 10.1073/pnas.1018466108

Devine, J., Fliege, H., Kocalevent, R., Mierke, A., Klapp, B. F., and Rose, M. (2016). Evaluation of Computerized Adaptive Tests (CATs) for longitudinal monitoring of depression, anxiety, and stress reactions. *J. Affect. Disord.* 190, 846–853. doi: 10.1016/j.jad.2014.10.063

Eggermont, J. J., and Roberts, L. E. (2012). The neuroscience of tinnitus: understanding abnormal and normal auditory perception. *Front. Syst. Neurosci.* 6:53. doi: 10.3389/fnsys.2012.00053

Fliege, H., Rose, M., Arck, P., Walter, O. B., Kocalevent, R. D., Weber, C., et al. (2005). The Perceived Stress Questionnaire (PSQ) reconsidered: validation and reference values from different clinical and healthy adult samples. *Psychosom. Med.* 67, 78–88. doi: 10.1097/01.psy.0000151491.80178.78

Folmer, R. L. (2002). Long-term reductions in tinnitus severity. *BMC Ear Nose Throat Disord.* 2:3. doi: 10.1186/1472-6815-2-3

Goebel, G., and Floezinger, U. (2008). Pilot study to evaluate psychiatric co-morbidity in tinnitus patients with and without hyperacusis. *Audiol. Med.* 6, 78–84. doi: 10.1080/16513860801959100

Goebel, G., and Hiller, W. (1994). [The tinnitus questionnaire. A standard instrument for grading the degree of tinnitus. Results of a multicenter study with the tinnitus questionnaire]. *HNO* 42, 166–172.

Halford, J. B., and Anderson, S. D. (1991). Anxiety and depression in tinnitus sufferers. *J. Psychosom. Res.* 35, 383–390. doi: 10.1016/0022-3999(91)90033-K

Hallam, R. S., McKenna, L., and Shurlock, L. (2004). Tinnitus impairs cognitive efficiency. *Int. J. Audiol.* 43, 218–226. doi: 10.1080/14992020400050030

Hebert, S., Canlon, B., Hasson, D., Magnusson Hanson, L. L., Westerlund, H., and Theorell, T. (2012). Tinnitus severity is reduced with reduction of depressive mood–a prospective population study in Sweden. *PLoS ONE* 7:e37733. doi: 10.1371/journal.pone.0037733

Henry, J. A., Dennis, K. C., and Schechter, M. A. (2005). General review of tinnitus: prevalence, mechanisms, effects, and management. *J. Speech Lang. Hear. Res.* 48, 1204–1235. doi: 10.1044/1092-4388(2005/084)

Henry, J. A., and Meikle, M. B. (2000). Psychoacoustic measures of tinnitus. *J. Am. Acad. Audiol.* 11, 138–155.

Henry, J. L., and Wilson, P. H. (1995). Coping with tinnitus: two studies of psychological and audiological characteristics of patients with high and low tinnitus-related distress. *Int. Tinnitus J.* 1, 85–92.

Hesse, G. (2008). [Neurootologic and psychosomatic habituation therapy. Treatment approaches in chronic tinnitus]. *HNO* 56, 686–693. doi: 10.1007/s00106-008-1723-0

Hesser, H., and Andersson, G. (2009). The role of anxiety sensitivity and behavioral avoidance in tinnitus disability. *Int. J. Audiol.* 48, 295–299. doi: 10.1080/14992020802635325

Hiller, W., and Goebel, G. (1992). A psychometric study of complaints in chronic tinnitus. *J. Psychosom. Res.* 36, 337–348. doi: 10.1016/0022-3999(92)90070-I

Hiller, W., and Goebel, G. (2007). When tinnitus loudness and annoyance are discrepant: audiological characteristics and psychological profile. *Audiol. Neurootol.* 12, 391–400. doi: 10.1159/000106482

Hoerhold, M., and Klapp, B. (1993). Testing the invariance and hierarchy of a multidimensional model of mood by means of repeated measurement with student and patient samples. *Z. Med. Psychol.* 2, 27–35.

Horner, K. C. (2003). The emotional ear in stress. *Neurosci. Biobehav. Rev.* 27, 437–446. doi: 10.1016/S0149-7634(03)00071-X

Jastreboff, P. J. (1999). Tinnitus retraining therapy. *Br. J. Audiol.* 33, 68–70.

Kleinstauber, M., Jasper, K., Schweda, I., Hiller, W., Andersson, G., and Weise, C. (2013). The role of fear-avoidance cognitions and behaviors in patients with chronic tinnitus. *Cogn. Behav. Ther.* 42, 84–99. doi: 10.1080/16506073.2012.717301

Kraus, K. S., and Canlon, B. (2012). Neuronal connectivity and interactions between the auditory and limbic systems. Effects of noise and tinnitus. *Hear. Res.* 288, 34–46. doi: 10.1016/j.heares.2012.02.009

Kroner-Herwig, B., Zachriat, C., and Weigand, D. (2006). Do patient characteristics predict outcome in the outpatient treatment of chronic tinnitus? *Psychosoc. Med.* 3:Doc07.

Langenbach, M., Olderog, M., Michel, O., Albus, C., and Kohle, K. (2005). Psychosocial and personality predictors of tinnitus-related distress. *Gen. Hosp. Psychiatry* 27, 73–77. doi: 10.1016/j.genhosppsych.2004.08.008

Langguth, B. (2011). A review of tinnitus symptoms beyond 'ringing in the ears': a call to action. *Curr. Med. Res. Opin.* 27, 1635–1643. doi: 10.1185/03007995.2011.595781

Leaver, A. M., Renier, L., Chevillet, M. A., Morgan, S., Kim, H. J., and Rauschecker, J. P. (2011). Dysregulation of limbic and auditory networks in tinnitus. *Neuron* 69, 33–43. doi: 10.1016/j.neuron.2010.12.002

Lee, S. Y., Kim, J. H., Hong, S. H., and Lee, D. S. (2004). Roles of cognitive characteristics in tinnitus patients. *J. Korean Med. Sci.* 19, 864–869. doi: 10.3346/jkms.2004.19.6.864

Liotti, M., and Mayberg, H. S. (2001). The role of functional neuroimaging in the neuropsychology of depression. *J. Clin. Exp. Neuropsychol.* 23, 121–136. doi: 10.1076/jcen.23.1.121.1223

Ma, Y. L., Gerhardt, K. J., Curtis, L. M., Rybak, L. P., Whitworth, C., and Rarey, K. E. (1995). Combined effects of adrenalectomy and noise exposure on compound action potentials, endocochlear potentials and endolymphatic potassium concentrations. *Hear. Res.* 91, 79–86. doi: 10.1016/0378-5955(95)00172-7

Mazurek, B., Haupt, H., Joachim, R., Klapp, B. F., Stover, T., and Szczepek, A. J. (2010a). Stress induces transient auditory hypersensitivity in rats. *Hear. Res.* 259, 55–63. doi: 10.1016/j.heares.2009.10.006

Mazurek, B., Haupt, H., Klapp, B. F., Szczepek, A. J., and Olze, H. (2012). Exposure of Wistar rats to 24-h psycho-social stress alters gene expression in the inferior colliculus. *Neurosci. Lett.* 527, 40–45. doi: 10.1016/j.neulet.2012.08.019

Mazurek, B., Olze, H., Haupt, H., and Szczepek, A. J. (2010b). The more the worse: the grade of noise-induced hearing loss associates with the severity of tinnitus. *Int. J. Environ. Res. Public Health* 7, 3071–3079. doi: 10.3390/ijerph7083071

McKenna, L., Handscomb, L., Hoare, D. J., and Hall, D. A. (2014). A scientific cognitive-behavioral model of tinnitus: novel conceptualizations of tinnitus distress. *Front. Neurol.* 5:196. doi: 10.3389/fneur.2014.00196

Milerova, J., Anders, M., Dvorak, T., Sand, P. G., Koniger, S., and Langguth, B. (2013). The influence of psychological factors on tinnitus severity. *Gen. Hosp. Psychiatry* 35, 412–416. doi: 10.1016/j.genhosppsych.2013.02.008

Moisset, X., and Bouhassira, D. (2007). Brain imaging of neuropathic pain. *Neuroimage* 37(Suppl. 1), S80–S88. doi: 10.1016/j.neuroimage.2007.03.054

Morfeld, M., Bullinger, M., Nantke, J., and Brahler, E. (2005). [The version 2.0 of the SF-36 health survey: results of a population-representative study]. *Soz. Praventivmed.* 50, 292–300. doi: 10.1007/s00038-005-4090-6

Nondahl, D. M., Cruickshanks, K. J., Huang, G. H., Klein, B. E., Klein, R., Tweed, T. S., et al. (2012). Generational differences in the reporting of tinnitus. *Ear Hear.* 33, 640–644. doi: 10.1097/AUD.0b013e31825069e8

Olderog, M., Langenbach, M., Michel, O., Brusis, T., and Kohle, K. (2004). [Predictors and mechanisms of tinnitus distress - a longitudinal analysis]. *Laryngorhinootologie* 83, 5–13. doi: 10.1055/s-2004-814235

Pattyn, T., Van Den Eede, F., Vanneste, S., Cassiers, L., Veltman, D. J., Van De Heyning, P., et al. (2016). Tinnitus and anxiety disorders: a review. *Hear. Res.* 333, 255–265. doi: 10.1016/j.heares.2015.08.014

Peroz, I. (2003). [Dysfunctions of the stomatognathic system in tinnitus patients compared to controls]. *HNO* 51, 544–549. doi: 10.1007/s00106-002-0750-5

Radloff, L. S. (1991). The use of the Center for Epidemiologic Studies Depression Scale in adolescents and young adults. *J. Youth Adolesc.* 20, 149–166. doi: 10.1007/BF01537606

Rauschecker, J. P., Leaver, A. M., and Muhlau, M. (2010). Tuning out the noise: limbic-auditory interactions in tinnitus. *Neuron* 66, 819–826. doi: 10.1016/j.neuron.2010.04.032

Rose, M., Hess, V., Horhold, M., Brahler, E., and Klapp, B. F. (1999). [Mobile computer-assisted psychometric diagnosis. Economic advantages and results on test stability]. *Psychother. Psychosom. Med. Psychol.* 49, 202–207.

Rubinstein, B., Axelsson, A., and Carlsson, G. E. (1990). Prevalence of signs and symptoms of craniomandibular disorders in tinnitus patients. *J. Craniomandib. Disord.* 4, 186–192.

Schlee, W., Kleinjung, T., Hiller, W., Goebel, G., Kolassa, I. T., and Langguth, B. (2011a). Does tinnitus distress depend on age of onset? *PLoS ONE* 6:e27379. doi: 10.1371/journal.pone.0027379

Schlee, W., Lorenz, I., Hartmann, T., Müller, N., Schulz, H., and Weisz, N. (2011b). "A global brain model of tinnitus," in *Textbook of Tinnitus*, eds A. R. Møller, B. Langguth, D. De Ridder, and T. Kleinjung (New York, NY: Springer New York), 161–169.

Schonwiesner, M., Novitski, N., Pakarinen, S., Carlson, S., Tervaniemi, M., and Naatanen, R. (2007). Heschl's gyrus, posterior superior temporal gyrus, and mid-ventrolateral prefrontal cortex have different roles in the detection of acoustic changes. *J. Neurophysiol.* 97, 2075–2082. doi: 10.1152/jn.01083.2006

Scott, B., and Lindberg, P. (2000). Psychological profile and somatic complaints between help-seeking and non-help-seeking tinnitus subjects. *Psychosomatics* 41, 347–352. doi: 10.1176/appi.psy.41.4.347

Seydel, C., Haupt, H., Olze, H., Szczepek, A. J., and Mazurek, B. (2013). Gender and chronic tinnitus: differences in tinnitus-related distress depend on age and duration of tinnitus. *Ear Hear.* 34, 661–672. doi: 10.1097/AUD.0b013e31828149f2

Seydel, C., Haupt, H., Szczepek, A. J., Hartmann, A., Rose, M., and Mazurek, B. (2015). Three years later: report on the state of well-being of patients with chronic tinnitus who underwent modified tinnitus retraining therapy. *Audiol. Neurootol.* 20, 26–38. doi: 10.1159/000363728

Seydel, C., Haupt, H., Szczepek, A. J., Klapp, B. F., and Mazurek, B. (2010). Long-term improvement in tinnitus after modified tinnitus retraining therapy enhanced by a variety of psychological approaches. *Audiol. Neurootol.* 15, 69–80. doi: 10.1159/000231632

Stobik, C., Weber, R. K., Munte, T. F., and Frommer, J. (2003). [Psychosomatic stress factors in compensated and decompensated tinnitus]. *Psychother. Psychosom. Med. Psychol.* 53, 344–352. doi: 10.1055/s-2003-40947

Sturm, W., Longoni, F., Fimm, B., Dietrich, T., Weis, S., Kemna, S., et al. (2004). Network for auditory intrinsic alertness: a PET study. *Neuropsychologia* 42, 563–568. doi: 10.1016/j.neuropsychologia.2003.11.004

Vollmann, M., Scharloo, M., Langguth, B., Kalkouskaya, N., and Salewski, C. (2013). Illness representations as mediators of the relationship between dispositional optimism and depression in patients with chronic tinnitus: a cross-sectional study. *Psychol. Health* 29, 81–93. doi: 10.1080/08870446.2013.828294

Wallhausser-Franke, E., Brade, J., Balkenhol, T., D'amelio, R., Seegmuller, A., and Delb, W. (2012). Tinnitus: distinguishing between subjectively perceived loudness and tinnitus-related distress. *PLoS ONE* 7:e34583. doi: 10.1371/annotation/96f457f9-3f48-4f88-a7f0-1d5e6067e7a5

Weise, C., Hesser, H., Andersson, G., Nyenhuis, N., Zastrutzki, S., Kroner-Herwig, B., et al. (2013). The role of catastrophizing in recent onset tinnitus: its nature and association with tinnitus distress and medical utilization. *Int. J. Audiol.* 52, 177–188. doi: 10.3109/14992027.2012.752111

Wilson, P. H., Henry, J., Bowen, M., and Haralambous, G. (1991). Tinnitus reaction questionnaire: psychometric properties of a measure of distress associated with tinnitus. *J. Speech Hear. Res.* 34, 197–201. doi: 10.1044/jshr.3401.197

Wilson, P. H., and Henry, J. L. (1998). Tinnitus cognitions questionnaire: development and psychometric properties of a measure of dysfunctional cognitions associated with tinnitus. *Int. Tinnitus J.* 4, 23–30.

Zenner, H. P. (2003). [Cognitive tinnitus desensitization: evidence-based and guideline-adherent habituation therapy for chronic tinnitus sensitization]. *HNO* 51, 687–689. doi: 10.1007/s00106-003-0939-2

Zirke, N., Seydel, C., Szczepek, A. J., Olze, H., Haupt, H., and Mazurek, B. (2013). Psychological comorbidity in patients with chronic tinnitus: analysis and comparison with chronic pain, asthma or atopic dermatitis patients. *Qual. Life Res.* 22, 263–272. doi: 10.1007/s11136-012-0156-0

Zoger, S., Svedlund, J., and Holgers, K. M. (2006). Relationship between tinnitus severity and psychiatric disorders. *Psychosomatics* 47, 282–288. doi: 10.1176/appi.psy.47.4.282

19

Auditory Brainstem Responses in Tinnitus: A Review of Who, How and What?

Victoria Milloy[1], Philippe Fournier[2], Daniel Benoit[1], Arnaud Noreña[2] and Amineh Koravand[1]*

[1] *School of Rehabilitation Sciences, University of Ottawa, Ottawa, ON, Canada,*

[2] *Centre National de la Recherche Scientifique, Aix-Marseille University, Marseille, France*

***Correspondence:**
Victoria Milloy
vmilloy@uottawa.ca

The auditory brainstem response (ABR) in tinnitus subjects has been extensively investigated over the last decade with the hopes of finding possible abnormalities related to the pathology. Despite this effort, the use of the ABR for tinnitus diagnosis or as an outcome measure is under debate. The present study reviewed published literature on ABR and tinnitus. The authors searched PubMed, MedLine, Embase, PsycINFO, and CINAHL, and identified additional records through manually searching reference lists and gray literature. There were 4,566 articles identified through database searching and 151 additional studies through the manual search (4,717 total): 2,128 articles were removed as duplicates, and 2,567 records did not meet eligibility criteria. From the final 22 articles that were included, ABR results from 1,240 tinnitus subjects and 664 control subjects were compiled and summarized with a focus on three main areas: the participant characteristics, the methodology used, and the outcome measures of amplitude and/or latency of waves I, III, and V. The results indicate a high level of heterogeneity between the studies for all the assessed areas. Amplitude and latency differences between tinnitus and controls were not consistent between studies. Nevertheless, the longer latency and reduced amplitude of wave I for the tinnitus group with normal hearing compared to matched controls was the most consistent finding across studies. These results support the need for greater stratification of the tinnitus population and the importance of a standardized ABR method to make comparisons between studies possible.

Keywords: tinnitus, ABR, review, brainstem, synaptopathy, meta-analysis, hearing loss

INTRODUCTION

Tinnitus is known as a phantom sound that is perceived in the absence of an acoustic stimulation. It is described by patients in a variety of ways that can be as simple as a single pure tone and as complex as a combination of different sounds (Stouffer and Tyler, 1990). It can also be perceived differently in one ear, both ears or in the head, and can be modulated in some individuals by orofacial movements (Levine, 1999), touch, background noise, stress, anxiety, depression, and attention (Tyler et al., 2008).

Although, the pathophysiology of tinnitus is still not clear, various origins, and mechanisms have been described in the literature (Henry et al., 2014). The fact that tinnitus is not always suppressed when the cochlear nerve is sectioned suggests there are, at least, two distinct tinnitus sub-types:

cochlear tinnitus and central tinnitus (House and Brackmann, 1981; Berliner et al., 1992). Cochlear tinnitus can be defined as a tinnitus subtype that results from aberrant activity in the cochlear nerve (Noreña, 2011). Central tinnitus can be defined as a tinnitus subtype that does not result from an increase of activity (or synchrony) in the cochlear nerve but rather at cortical levels within the central auditory pathways (Noreña, 2011). In this latter subtype, the tinnitus perception may result from cortical changes associated with the reduction of sensory inputs due to hearing loss.

One technique used to assess the activation along the neural pathways between the eighth peripheral nerve of the cochlear nucleus up to the inferior colliculus is the Auditory Brainstem Response (ABR) (Melcher and Kiang, 1996). Auditory Brainstem Responses (ABRs) are acoustically stimulated signals that represent the synchronized neural activation along the neural pathways. A study investigating the generation sites of ABRs in cats revealed the first wave (I) of the ABR reflects activity of the spiral ganglion cells at the distal part of the eighth auditory nerve, wave II is predominantly from the globular cells in the cochlear nucleus, wave III is generated by the cochlear nucleus spherical cells and globular cells, and waves IV and V generate from the medial superior olive and its projections to the nuclei in the lateral lemniscus and the inferior colliculus (Melcher and Kiang, 1996). These electrophysiological responses are typically less than a microvolt in amplitude (Burkard and Secor, 2002; Chalak et al., 2013). The success of revealing true and reliable responses relies heavily on averaging techniques employed to reduce noise contamination thereby improving the signal to noise ratio (Burkard and Secor, 2002). ABRs have been used clinically for two main purposes: hearing threshold estimations and neurodiagnostics. Indeed, the ABR is a well known cost-effective test that is routinely used in clinical practice as an objective diagnostic measure for determining the presence of hearing loss in infants, young children and patients that are difficult to test behaviorally. More so, the ABR is an important clinical tool for identifying the presence of retrocochlear lesions, acoustic neuromas, and vestibular schwannomas (Kotlarz et al., 1992; Rupa et al., 2003). This is achieved by identifying waves I, III, and V peaks and comparing the absolute latency values to normative ranges for each wave. For example, the presence of an acoustic neuroma at the level of the auditory nerve could significantly delay neural conduction. As a result, the latency between waves I and V is usually extended from the normative value by more than 0.2 ms (Wilson et al., 1992). Normative ABR latency values, for clicks at 70 dB nHL, collected on the most reliable waves I, III, and V are, respectively, 1.66, 3.68, and 5.64 ms for the left ear, and 1.66, 3.65, and 5.59 ms for the right ear (Chalak et al., 2013). When comparing between genders of the same age, the latencies are shorter and the amplitudes are larger in women compared to men (Hultcrantz et al., 2006). Hearing loss of different configurations affect the ABR: high frequency hearing losses show a delayed wave V at low intensities and a greater degree of wave I delay at all intensities, low frequency hearing losses show an earlier wave V at low intensities (Keith and Greville, 1987; Watson, 1996). Furthermore, elevated hearing thresholds also reduce the amplitude of waves I and V using the click-ABR (Sand and Saunte, 1994) and wave V using tone-burst ABR when the tone-burst characteristic frequency falls within the frequency region of the hearing loss (Lewis et al., 2015). The ABR sensitivity and specificity for both hearing threshold estimations and neurodiagnostics, have been shown to be very high with values of 100 and 91% for the former (Hyde et al., 1990) and 88 and 92% for the latter (Bauch et al., 1996). ABR assessment is also used for the diagnosis of auditory neuropathy (Starr et al., 1996). In such a case, the function of the outer hair cell of the cochlea is mostly normal, irrespective of hearing thresholds, even though the ABR waves are absent due to a lack of synchronized neural activity or excessive auditory fatigue (see Giraudet and Avan, 2012). The ABR technique thus provides information about the integrity of the central auditory system and can be a valuable diagnostic tool. Moreover, ABRs are relatively easy to obtain from only a few electrodes and are mostly insensitive to cognitive states (e.g., attention or arousal) or even consciousness (Burkard and Secor, 2002).

In tinnitus research, ABRs have been used in a variety of ways in humans. ABRs have been used to differentiate peripheral from central lesion sites in patients (Kehrle et al., 2008), and to investigate tinnitus treatment efficacy following drug administration (Shulman and Seitz, 1981; Milicic and Alcada, 1999; Bayar et al., 2001; Gopal et al., 2015). ABRs have also been used to identify noise-induced hidden hearing loss. In brief, Kujawa and Liberman found that the ABR wave I amplitude of mice significantly decreased at moderately-high levels (above 70 dB) up to 2 months following noise exposure even when the auditory thresholds had recovered to normal values (Kujawa and Liberman, 2006, 2009). In addition to the amplitude reduction, damage to the synaptic ribbons of the inner hair cells and spiral ganglion cells were revealed, suggesting that reduced wave I amplitude may be indicative of auditory nerve deafferentation. The term "cochlear synaptopathy" was further proposed to describe damage at the cochlear synapse without loss of hair cells resulting in "hidden hearing loss," a functional hearing deficit without an elevation of audiometric thresholds (Liberman and Kujawa, 2017). In tinnitus patients with normal hearing (≤20 dB HL, Freq: 0.25–8 kHz), Schaette and McAlpine (2011) and Gu et al. (2012) showed similar reduced wave I amplitudes at high levels (80–90 dB SPL) compared to non-tinnitus matched controls, which were both interpreted as diminished activity of the low spontaneous rate auditory nerve fibers (LSR). Interestingly, the amplitude of wave V (measured baseline to peak) was reported to be significantly higher in only Gu et al. (2012). Schaette and McAlpine (2011) suggest the normal wave V amplitude, despite a reduction in wave I, is due to the central auditory system increasing its neural responsiveness to compensate for the reduced activity of the auditory nerve. Conversely, Gu et al. (2012) suggest that the higher amplitude of wave V is an artifact from the use of a lower frequency filter cutoff. Based on these findings, people suffering from tinnitus with normal audiometric thresholds show ABR amplitude changes that may be indicative of cochlear synaptopathy (reduced wave I) and the compensated responses of central/cortical regions (normal or elevated wave V). The increased responsiveness of central regions would generate increased spontaneous activity leading to tinnitus generation. Hickox and Liberman (2014) attempted to link synaptopathy to the generation of tinnitus in noise-exposed mice. The mice exposed to loud noise displayed the typical auditory nerve degeneration (determined by ribbon counts), reduced wave I amplitude/enhanced wave V ABR responses, and subtle changes in the behavioral response of tinnitus that did not reached significance (using the gap prepulse inhibition acoustic startle reflex or GPIAS). Low efficacy of this particular behavioral technique (GPIAS) in CBA-mice might explain the failure of significant results (Yu et al., 2016). Using another strain with better GPIAS could maximize these effects and link wave I reduction to a behavioral measure of tinnitus in animals. Another animal study (Rüttiger et al., 2013), exposed animals to loud noise and separated them based on tinnitus behavior. They found that although the ABR waveform was generally reduced after the trauma for both groups, wave I did not significantly change amplitude after recovery. Interestingly, the tinnitus group showed reduced wave IV and V amplitude after recovery, which the authors proposed to arise from a failure to compensate for the cochlear loss at the central levels of the auditory system.

It is noteworthy that ABR wave amplitude may be altered by the number of neural components activated by the stimulation and/or the level of synchronization between them. As amplitude of wave I is mostly due to tightly synchronized activity at the level of the cochlear nerve, the reduction in amplitude noted previously at high intensities might indicate not only a loss of neural fibers but also a decrease of synchronization. Conversely, increased neural synchrony has been proposed as a potential mechanism of tinnitus generation (Eggermont, 1984; Moeller, 1984). It was postulated that increased synchrony of the spontaneous firing rate even at the peripheral level of the auditory nervous system could be sufficient to produce a perception of a sound in the absence of external stimulation. The higher wave V amplitude reported in tinnitus subjects might reflect increased neural synchronization at higher levels of the auditory system. In brief, changes in wave I might reflect damage to the periphery and the following wave modifications might reflect compensation mechanisms such as higher increased neural synchrony in tinnitus. Still, modifications of wave III and wave V amplitude might occur without being related to wave I alterations. In a recent study, decreases in the amplitude of waves III and V were not adequately explained by changes in wave I in older participants compared to younger ones (Konrad-Martin et al., 2012). In this study, the reduction of the peak amplitudes of waves III and V, seemed to be linked to the effects of aging, instead of wave I amplitude reduction (and latency shift), which is believed to be the consequence of reduced auditory nerve inputs.

The current purpose of the study was to review ABR findings on tinnitus to assess any consistencies across studies in terms of absolute wave amplitudes and latencies. As ABR waves are affected by hearing loss (Don et al., 1998), and tinnitus mechanisms may differ between normal hearing and hearing loss participants (Henry et al., 2014), studies were separated based on this variable. A potential decrease in wave I amplitude in tinnitus subjects with normal hearing is expected to be one of the most consistent findings across studies (Schaette and McAlpine, 2011; Gu et al., 2012). The current review might also bring insight on possible modifications of the other waves such as wave III and wave V, in populations reporting tinnitus. A careful analysis of studies on tinnitus and ABR from 1980 to 2016 was made and convergent evidence was extracted based on the population/sample (who?), the methodology (how?), and the outcome (what?). The investigated outcomes were related to the latency and amplitude of waves I, III, and V.

METHODS

Database Search

A scoping review of the literature was conducted using the method described by Arksey and O'Malley (2005). This approach uses a five stage framework that includes (1) identifying the research question, (2) identifying relevant studies, (3) selecting the study, (4) charting the data, and (5) collating, summarizing, and reporting the results. Statistics for each level of data collection are tabulated in the PRISMA schema (Moher et al., 2009; **Figure 1**).

A team approach to the process of the review was used to eliminate the level of error produced by a single individual and a second reviewer was used to independently analyze all the abstracts for inclusion (Levac et al., 2010). Given the high volume of articles yielded from the comprehensive search strategy, a "liberal accelerated" approach was used: the second reviewer analyzed only articles excluded by the first reviewer instead of the entire yield (Khangura et al., 2012).

The primary outcome of interest is measurement of the absolute peak amplitudes (peak to following trough) and latencies of the ABR waveform in tinnitus patients with and without hearing loss. Searches were conducted, between April 2015 and August 2016, by the principal investigator (V.M.) using the strategies detailed in Supplementary Table 1. In brief, the search terms (and their variations) used alone or in combination referring to tinnitus were: tinnitus, ear, buzz, ring, roar, click, pulsate, or pulse, and referring to the auditory brainstem measurements were: brainstem, brain, stem, auditory, response, potential, ABR, BAER, BSER, and evoked. The databases PubMed, CINAHL, Medline, PsycInfo, and Embase were searched separately and results were compiled in a Microsoft Excel (2011) spreadsheet where the search strategy yields were dated and organized (Supplementary Table 1). Gray literature which includes conference papers, master dissertations, and doctoral theses was also searched (October 2016) using ProQuest Dissertations and Theses Global and Conference Papers Index and added to the compiled list of articles. No conference papers, master dissertations, or doctoral theses were included in the final compilation as all those found were later published. Articles were limited to those published after 1980 as the waveforms were only just described in the 1970s by Jewett and colleagues and not yet applied to subjects with tinnitus (Jewett et al., 1970; Jewett and Williston, 1971). Any articles assessing populations with tinnitus due to underlying medical conditions were excluded for the purposes of this review (i.e., acoustic neuroma, otitis media, otitis externa, etc.). Excluding various comorbidities ensured the ABR outcomes

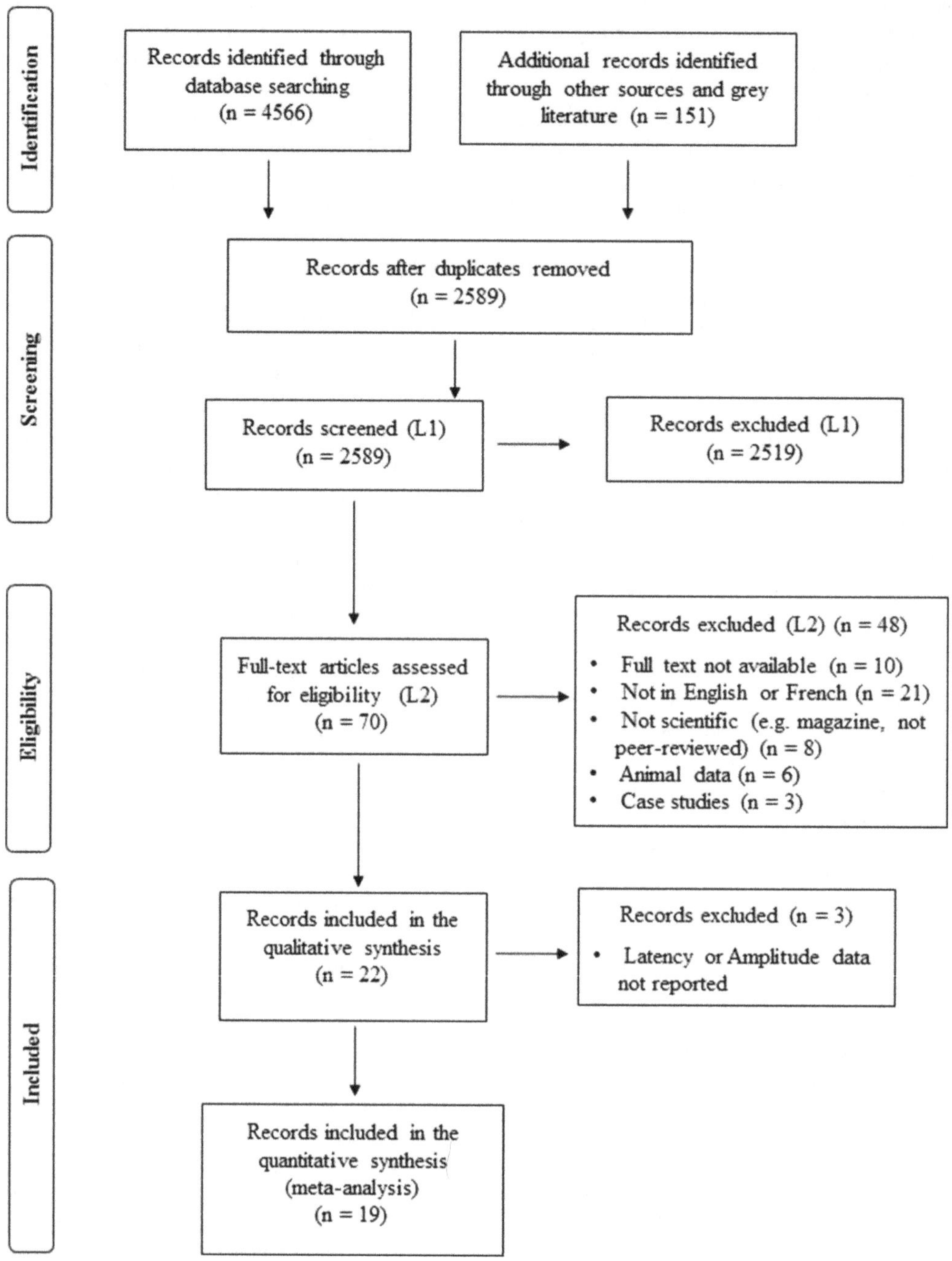

FIGURE 1 | Flowchart of study selection (PRISMA diagram).

reported were not due to known covariables. Any articles discussing ABRs for the purpose of measuring hearing loss such as threshold searching and newborn hearing screenings were also excluded. Preoperative and intraoperative ABRs were not included in this review as clinical populations with other underlying conditions, such as acoustic neuromas, or vascular abnormalities, are typically involved in these studies and are known covariables of ABR (Berliner et al., 1992; De Ridder et al., 2015).

The first screening (L1) consisted of excluding the articles that did not meet the criteria described in **Table 1** based on the analysis of title and abstract of the article. The second reviewer screened the articles rejected by the first reviewer. Both reviewers completed the second screening (L2) where eligibility was based on the analysis of the full text. The use of a language translator was not feasible for this study, therefore all texts written in languages other than French or English were eliminated. Three case-report studies, where a single participant was reported

TABLE 1 | Inclusion and exclusion criteria applied to the scoping review search.

	Inclusion criteria	Exclusion criteria
Population	Subjective tinnitus with or without hearing loss. This includes individuals with noise-induced hearing loss.	Subjective tinnitus with a history of ontological conditions (i.e., hypertension, tumors, demylenation, multiple sclerosis, Meniere's disease, auditory neuropathy, otitis media, otitis externa, middle ear pathologies etc.). Individuals with cochlear implants, CAPD, head trauma, psychological disorders, sudden hearing loss. Individuals with objective tinnitus or pulsatile tinnitus. Studies with a sample size of 1.
Evaluation	Auditory evoked potentials of the brainstem.	Long Latency Auditory Evoked Potentials (P1, N1, P2, N2); Event Related Potentials (MMN, P300, N400, P600 etc.). Auditory Steady State Responses, intraoperative ABR, preoperative monitoring, newborn hearing screening.
Publication type	Peer-reviewed journals only with articles published after 1980 in English or French.	Any unscientific papers: Magazine articles, conference proceedings, editorials, and manuals.
Outcomes	Measured peak amplitudes and latencies of the ABR wave.	

(Shulman and Seitz, 1981; Milicic and Alcada, 1999; Gopal et al., 2015), were removed from the remaining yield. The sample size was too small to significantly contribute to the analysis, and the purpose of these studies was mostly to measure the responsiveness to treatment.

After the two levels of title and abstract screening (L1) and full-text screening (L2) were completed, a narrative synthesis was used to organize key points of the data into two charts. Key points of interest included population (i.e., age, tinnitus etiology, tinnitus localization, and hearing status), technical information (i.e., transducer used, ABR system used, stimulus type, presentation levels, tinnitus characterization, and recording filters), and results.

Meta-Analysis of the Compiled Data

The results were compiled in Microsoft Excel (2011) for a meta-analysis of the data using two different methodologies. The first method (meta-analysis 1) consisted of compiling the latency and amplitude values from Waves I, III, and V for all the subjects, with or without tinnitus, from all the studies reporting these values. The mean values for absolute latency and amplitude, standard deviations, and sample size for each study were organized in a table as a function of the ABR waves. The results were also separated based on hearing status and reported tinnitus. For example, the results of the four groups were determined based on the participants having (a) normal hearing without tinnitus, (b) normal hearing with tinnitus, (c) hearing loss without tinnitus, and (d) hearing loss with tinnitus. In these cases, we used the normal hearing and hearing loss definitions established within each article. These definitions varied from one study to the other (see Section Results and Discussion). Meta-analysis calculations were carried out on these data to determine (a) the total number of subjects for all the studies separated by hearing status; (b) the total mean latency/amplitudes weighted according to sample size of each study; (c) the composite standard deviation calculated as a combination of all the groups from all the studies; (d) the 95% confidence interval (CI) determined based on the composite standard deviation; (e) the mean difference latency/amplitude (i.e., the mean latency/amplitude of the tinnitus group subtracted by the mean latency/amplitude of the non-tinnitus group) again weighted according to the sample size. The confidence interval was calculated using Microsoft Excel software and consisted of adding or subtracting the confidence value from the weighted mean. The confidence value was calculated based on the composite standard deviation and the total number of observations of the pooled data grouped in one of the categories: normal hearing, normal hearing and tinnitus, hearing loss, or hearing loss and tinnitus. Confidence intervals were chosen because the interval estimate obtained from this method is more informative for data comparison of future studies than a sample mean and *T*-test. The confidence level of the confidence intervals was set at 95%, which is the equivalent of $p < 0.05$.

The second method (meta-analysis 2) consisted of calculating the difference of the mean amplitude and latency for waves I, III, and V (and the 95% CI) between the tinnitus and control groups, only for studies with at least matched age and hearing status. This method was added to minimize the risk of identifying differences in population variables, assessment techniques or methodologies between tinnitus and control groups. The differences found with the second methodology are thus presumed to be the result of group differences as both groups were tested with very similar protocols.

RESULTS

Study Selection

A total of 4,566 articles were retrieved from the databases PubMed, MedLine, Embase, PsycINFO, and CINAHL. An additional 133 articles were found by manually searching citations from the reference lists of articles that met the eligibility criteria and another 18 from gray literature (i.e., doctoral theses and conference papers). After the duplicates were removed, 2,589 articles were screened by title and abstract and 70 of those articles were analyzed by reading the full text. Of the remaining articles, 22 were included in the qualitative narrative synthesis and 19 in the meta-analysis (see **Figure 1**). The most common objective of the studies is the assessment of possible changes to the ABR of tinnitus patients compared to those without tinnitus ($n = 19$)

TABLE 2 | Demographics include the number of subjects, the mean age, the tinnitus etiology, and localization and the hearing status criteria.

Study	Subjects	Mean age in years (Range)	Tinnitus characterization	Tinnitus localization	Hearing status criteria	Results: latency	Results: amplitude
NOISE-INDUCED ETIOLOGY							
Attias et al., 1993	Tinnitus ($n = 12$) Controls ($n = 12$) Matched: Age, HL severity and configuration	Not mentioned (26-45) Not mentioned (26-45)	Pitch Matching Loudness Matching	Bilateral ($n = 12$)	Audiometrically matched, No definition Noise induced hearing loss	No differences	No differences
Attias et al., 1996	Tinnitus ($n = 13$) Controls ($n = 11$) Matched: Age and Hearing	35 (21-45) Not mentioned (age and hearing matched)	Pitch Matching Loudness Matching Tinnitus severity profile	Unilateral ($n = 8$) Bilateral ($n = 5$)	Normal hearing: ≤20 dB HL, Freq: 0.25–2 kHz Hearing loss: 20–45 dB HL, Freq: 2–8 kHz	No differences	Enhanced Wave III amplitude
Gilles et al., 2016	Tinnitus ($n = 19$) Controls ($n = 23$) Matched: Age, Sex, and Hearing	~23 (SD: 2.4)	VAS–Loudness TQ	Head ($n = 1$) Unilateral ($n = 2$) Bilateral ($n = 16$)	Normal hearing (<25 dB HL, Freq: 0.25–16 kHz?) Hearing loss (>25 dB HL, Freq: 0.25–16 kHz?) HF tested (up to 16 kHz)	No differences	No differences
Santos-Filha et al., 2014	Tinnitus ($n = 30$) Controls ($n = 30$) Matched: Age, Sex, Hearing	41 (27-50) 41.6 (27-50)	VAS—Severity	Bilateral (67%) Unilateral (33%)	Normal hearing (<25 dB HL, Freq: 0.25–8 kHz)	No differences	Not reported
IDIOPATHIC ETIOLOGY							
Cartocci et al., 2012	Tinnitus ($n = 10$) Controls ($n = 14$) Matched: Age, Sex, Hearing	43.9 (SD: 11.0) 45.1 (SD: 11.9)	Not reported	Unilateral ($n = 5$) Bilateral ($n = 5$)	Normal hearing (≤20 dB HL, Freq: 0.125–8 kHz)	Longer Wave V and III–V	Not reported
Mahmoudian et al., 2013	Tinnitus ($n = 44$) No Controls	43.45 (18-65)	Not reported	Unilateral ($n = 19$) Bilateral ($n = 25$)	Included Hearing levels (≤30 dB HL, Freq: 0.5–2 kHz and <60 dB HL, Freq: 4–8 kHz)	No latency changes	III/V and I/V ratio modifications following electrical RI
Maurizi et al., 1985	Tinnitus ($n = 54$) No Controls	Not mentioned (23-78)	Residual Inhibition	Unilateral ($n = 54$)	Classification of hearing loss: 1) ≤20 dB HL, Freq: 0.5–4 kz 2) 21–49 dB HL, Freq: 0.5–4 kHz and >50 dB HL, Freq: 0.5–4 kHz	Prolonged Wave V in tinnitus ears vs. control ears	Not reported
McKee and Stephens, 1992	Tinnitus ($n = 18$) Controls ($n = 19$) Matched: Age and Hearing	26 (18-37) 27.5 (17-38)	Not reported	Head ($n = 2$) Unilateral ($n = 2$) Bilateral ($n = 14$)	Normal hearing (≤20 dB HL, Freq: 0.25–8 kHz) HF tested (up to 18 kHz)	No differences	Not reported
Nemati et al., 2014	Tinnitus ($n = 25$) Controls ($n = 16$) Matched: Age, Sex, Hearing	34.4 (20-57) Not mentioned (matched)	Not reported	Unilateral ($n = 19$) Bilateral ($n = 6$)	Normal hearing (<25 dB HL, Freq: 0.25–8 kHz)	No differences	Amplitude ratio V/I larger
Singh et al., 2011	Tinnitus ($n = 25$) Controls ($n = 20$) Matched: Age, Sex, Hearing	32 (18-45) Not mentioned (matched)	Not reported	Unilateral ($n = 19$) Bilateral ($n = 6$)	Normal hearing (<25 dB HL, Freq: 0.25–8 kHz)	Longer Wave I Shorter Wave V Shorter I–II and I–V	Not reported

(Continued)

TABLE 2 | Continued

Study	Subjects	Mean age in years (Range)	Tinnitus characterization	Tinnitus localization	Hearing status criteria	Results: latency	Results: amplitude
HETEROGENEOUS ETIOLOGY							
Kim et al., 2016	Tinnitus ($n = 123$) No Controls	53.5 (SD: 13.4)	VAS–Discomfort Minimum masking level Residual inhibition THI Pitch matching	Unilateral ($n = 79$) Bilateral ($n = 44$)	Audiometric configurations: 1) Flat 2) High frequency gently sloping 3) High frequency steeply sloping	Prolonged latencies I, III and V for steeply high frequency hearing loss group	Not reported
ETIOLOGY NOT MENTIONED							
Barnea et al., 1990	Tinnitus ($n = 12$) Controls (n = ??) Matched: Age, Sex, Hearing	35 (21-45) Not mentioned (matched)	Pitch matching Loudness matching	Unilateral (60%) Bilateral (40%)	Normal hearing (≤20 dB HL, Freq: 0.25–8 kHz) HF tested (up to 20 kHz)	No difference	No differences
De Lavernhe-Lemaire and Beutter, 1989	Tinnitus ($n = 164$) Controls ($n = 57$) Not Matched	Not mentioned	Not reported	Unilateral ($n = 112$) Bilateral ($n = 52$)	Not mentioned	Longer Wave I, but decreased inter-peak I–V	Not reported
De Lavernhe-Lemaire and Beutter, 1990	Tinnitus ($n = 139$) Controls ($n = 20$) Not Matched	27-74	Not reported	Unilateral ($n = 93$) Bilateral ($n = 46$)	Not mentioned	Not reported	Decrease wave I and III amplitude
Gerken et al., 2001	Tinnitus ($n = 9$) Controls with normal hearing ($n = 11$) Controls with hearing loss ($n = 8$) Controls-elderly ($n = 7$) Not Matched	45.7 (26-68) 28 (22-37) 40.9 (23-53) 63.6 (60-68)	Pitch matching Loudness matching Minimum masking level	Not mentioned	Normal hearing (≤15 dB HL, Freq: 0.5–8 kHz) Hearing loss (>15 dB HL, Freq: 0.5–8 kHz)	Problem tinnitus group longer wave VII	No differences
Gu et al., 2012	Tinnitus ($n = 15$) Controls ($n = 21$) Matched: Age, Sex, Hearing	42 (SD: 6) 43 (SD: 7)	Pitch matching Loudness matching Minimum masking level Residual inhibition	Head ($n = 4$) Unilateral ($n = 2$) Bilateral ($n = 9$)	Normal hearing (≤20 dB HL, Freq: 0.25–8 kHz) HF tested (up to 16 kHz)	No latency differences	Reduced wave I and enhanced wave V
Ikner and Hassen, 1990	Tinnitus ($n = 35$) Controls ($n = 35$) Matched: Age, Sex, Hearing	40 36	Not reported	Not mentioned	Normal hearing (<20 dB HL, Freq: 1–4 kHz)	Longer wave I, III, V, and III–V interval	Not reported
Kehrle et al., 2008	Tinnitus ($n = 37$) Controls ($n = 38$) Matched: Age, Sex, Hearing	36 (SD: 7.2) Not mentioned (matched)	Not reported	Unilateral ($n = 13$) Bilateral ($n = 24$)	Normal hearing (<25 dB HL, Freq: 0.5–8 kHz)	Longer Wave I, III, V, and III–V	Ratio V/I
Kehrle et al., 2016	Tinnitus ($n = 84$) Controls ($n = 47$) Matched: Age, Sex, Hearing	37.2 (18-48) 35.7 (18-48)	VAS– severity Pitch matching Loudness matching THI	Unilateral ($n = 26$) Bilateral ($n = 58$)	Normal hearing (≤25 dB HL, Freq: 0.25–8 kHz)	Abnormal for wave I, wave III, wave V, inter-peak I–III, inter-peak III–V, Inter-peak I–V	Not reported

(Continued)

TABLE 2 | Continued

Study	Subjects	Mean age in years (Range)	Tinnitus characterization	Tinnitus localization	Hearing status criteria	Results: latency	Results: amplitude
Lemaire and Beutter, 1995	Tinnitus ($n = 355$) Controls ($n = 129$) Not matched	52.1 (SD: 16.4) <25	Pitch matching Loudness matching	Unilateral ($n = 220$) Bilateral ($n = 135$)	Normal hearing (<20 dB HL, Freq: ??)	Longer for 0–I and I–V on the tinnitus affected side	Reduced Wave I, III, and sometimes V
Rosenhall and Axelsson, 1994	Tinnitus with hearing loss ($n = 57$) Tinnitus with normal hearing ($n = 56$) Controls with hearing loss ($n = 166$) Controls with normal hearing ($n = 54$) Matched: Age, Sex, Hearing	57.2 (SD: 10.6) 42.1 (SD: 13.8) Not mentioned (matched) Not mentioned (matched)	Not reported	Unilateral ($n = 30$) Bilateral ($n = 83$)	Normal hearing (<20 dB HL, Freq: 0.125–2 kHz and <35 dB HL, Freq: 4–8 kHz) Hearing loss (45-60 dB HL, Freq: 4 kHz)	Longer Wave I, III, and V	Not reported
Schaette and McAlpine, 2011	Tinnitus ($n = 15$) Controls ($n = 18$) Matched: Age, Sex, Hearing	36.3 (SD: 2.6) 33.2 (SD: 1.9)	Modified tinnitus spectrum	Not mentioned	Normal hearing (≤20 dB HL, Freq: 0.25–8 kHz) HF tested (up to 16 kHz)	Not reported	Reduced Wave I, No change Wave V

SD, Standard deviation; dB, decibels; HL, hearing loss; Freq, frequency; n, number of subjects; VAS, visual analog scale; TQ, Tinnitus Questionnaire; THI, Tinnitus Handicap Inventory; HF, high frequency thresholds above 8 kHz.

for the purpose of distinguishing between peripheral and central tinnitus or identifying lesions or deafferentation of the auditory nerve. Other objectives were to compare the ABR to tinnitus perception ($n = 1$), emotions ($n = 1$), and the behavioral effects of residual inhibition ($n = 1$).

Population Characteristics

Characteristics of the populations tested in the 22 studies are shown in **Table 2**. Nineteen out of the 22 studies had a control group. The matching procedures varied between the studies, if mentioned at all. In 12 studies subjects were matched by sex, age, and hearing status, in three studies by age and hearing only and in four studies not matched (see **Table 2**). The mean age of the tinnitus and control groups was 40.1 and 38.0 years old, respectively, but varied widely between the studies ranging from 18 to 78-year-old participants. Since the data were not reported for smaller age groups, this data could not be separated into more narrowly defined age divisions. The tinnitus etiology was characterized as noise-induced for five of the studies, idiopathic for six studies, and not mentioned for the remaining 11 studies. Seventeen studies assessed patients with both bilateral or unilateral tinnitus, two studies used either bilateral tinnitus (Attias et al., 1993) or unilateral tinnitus exclusively (Maurizi et al., 1985) and three studies did not mention the lateralization of the tinnitus. Gender of the population was reported in 19 of the 22 studies of which five separated ABR data for males and/or females.

Hearing status was reported in all except two studies (De Lavernhe-Lemaire and Beutter, 1989, 1990). Among the studies that evaluated hearing, 17 studies used hearing status as a way to match controls to the tinnitus group. Three articles (Maurizi et al., 1985; Mahmoudian et al., 2013; Kim et al., 2016) did not have a control group and focused their comparisons on subgroups of tinnitus patients based on the configuration of the audiogram. These 17 studies either ensured that they used only a normal hearing population for both the tinnitus and control groups ($n = 12$), or a mixture of normal hearing and hearing loss for the control and tinnitus groups, matched based on the degree of hearing loss ($n = 5$). These studies used average audiometric thresholds of ≤15 dB HL ($n = 1$), <20 dB HL ($n = 3$), ≤20 dB HL ($n = 6$), <25 dB HL ($n = 5$), ≤25 dB HL ($n = 1$) as the criteria for normal hearing for the standard clinical frequencies. One study did not mention the criteria used to define normal hearing (Attias et al., 1993). Still, the frequency by which the audiometric criteria for normal hearing were applied varied from one study to the other. Indeed, there were typically defined from 0.25 to 8 kHz ($n = 9$), 0.125 to 8 kHz ($n = 1$), or 0.5 to 8 kHz ($n = 2$). Some studies limited the frequencies to a narrower range ($n = 5$). Of the five studies that used hearing loss populations, hearing loss was either undefined (Ikner and Hassen, 1990; Attias et al., 1993), defined within a limited range (i.e., 20-45, 21-49, 31-60, or 45-60 dB HL), or an unlimited range (i.e., above 15, 25 or 50 dB HL). A small number of studies ($n = 5$) tested frequencies above 8 kHz (Barnea et al., 1990; McKee and Stephens, 1992; Schaette and McAlpine, 2011; Gu et al., 2012; Gilles et al., 2016) (see also **Table 2**).

Characteristics of the Assessment and ABR Technique

Tinnitus was characterized in only 12 of the studies (see **Table 2**). Of these studies, four used a visual analog scale to determine either loudness ($n = 1$), severity ($n = 2$), or discomfort ($n = 1$), and eight used matching psychoacoustic procedures for loudness and pitch or a variation called the modified tinnitus spectrum procedure where pitch and loudness are rated (see **Table 2**). Residual inhibition was measured in three studies. The characteristics of the assessment and the ABR technique can be found in **Table 3**. The most commonly reported systems used to acquire the ABR were the Nicolet CA-1000 ($n = 4$) and the Bio-Logic NavPro or Traveler Express ($n = 5$). Transducers used were typically the supra-auricular headphones TDH-39(P) ($n = 6$) and TDH-49 ($n = 4$), or the insert headphones ER-3(A) ($n = 3$) with the exception of one study that used high frequency Sennheiser HDA-200 circumauricular headphones (Gu et al., 2012). The stimulus type was largely broadband clicks ($n = 19$) with a typical duration of 0.1 ms ($n = 16$) presented at a rate of 10–31 clicks per second. Exceptionally, one study used 0.05 ms clicks (Schaette and McAlpine, 2011) and another study used 3 ms tone bursts (Gerken et al., 2001). Presentation levels were generally high (>80 dB) and were either expressed in HL ($n = 8$), nHL ($n = 6$), or SPL ($n = 7$). Of the six studies reporting stimulus level in dB nHL, three reported using their own subjects to determine the minimum click intensity in dB SPL that elicited a behavioral response (Maurizi et al., 1985; Gu et al., 2012; Mahmoudian et al., 2013). When filter characteristics were reported ($n = 16$), the cutoff frequency of the high-pass filters ranged from 5 to 200 Hz and from the 1,500 to 5,000 Hz for the low-pass filters. Contralateral masking was used in 5 studies, all of which used a white noise at an intensity of 55 dB nHL (Gilles et al., 2016) or 50 dB HL (De Lavernhe-Lemaire and Beutter, 1989, 1990; Lemaire and Beutter, 1995; Kehrle et al., 2008).

Latency was reported in all studies except for De Lavernhe-Lemaire and Beutter (1990) and Schaette and McAlpine (2011). The most common outcome was no change in latency ($n = 9$) or an increase in the latency of waves I ($n = 8$), III ($n = 5$), and V ($n = 7$) for the tinnitus group (See **Table 2**). Only one study reported a decrease in wave V latency. Other latency changes for the tinnitus group varied considerably from increased interlatencies between waves III–V ($n = 4$), I–V ($n = 1$), and I–III ($n = 1$) to decreased interlatencies between waves I–II ($n = 1$) and I–V ($n = 3$). Out of the 12 studies that reported amplitude, four did not report any changes. The others reported the tinnitus group amplitudes either increased for waves III ($n = 1$), or decreased for waves I ($n = 4$), III ($n = 2$) and V ($n = 2$). Amplitude ratios were reported in four studies: V/III ($n = 1$) and V/I ($n = 3$). Gilles et al. (2016) was the sole study that reported the latency and amplitude of waves II and IV.

Meta-Analysis 1: Quantitative Analysis of ABR Latency and Amplitude Changes Separated by Hearing Status

The data of the 19 studies were compiled: a total of 1,240 subjects included in the tinnitus population and 664 control subjects were found. Three studies were not included because they have not reported any amplitude or latency data in format suitable for the analysis (see **Figure 1**). A summary of the mean latency and amplitude pooled from all studies is presented in **Table 4**. Each ear was treated as a separate data point when available in the literature. The raw latency and amplitude values for all the studies are available in Supplementary Table 2. **Table 4** shows that for the normal hearing populations, there is no significant difference between the tinnitus and non-tinnitus groups. The difference in mean latency for the normal hearing tinnitus group was 0, 0.01, and 0.03 ms higher than the control group for waves I, III, and V, respectively. For the hearing loss populations, the tinnitus group lower limit (95% CI) values of 1.75 (I), 3.83 (III), and 5.80 (V) ms were significantly higher than the upper limit (95% CI) values of 1.62 (I), 3.76 (III), and 5.68 (V) ms for the non-tinnitus groups. When comparing hearing loss groups, the tinnitus groups were 0.21, 0.15, and 0.22 ms delayed for waves I, III, and V compared to the group without tinnitus. Amplitudes for the normal hearing population were 0.04 μV lower for the wave I, and 0.02 and 0.01 μV higher for waves III, and V, respectively, for the tinnitus group. The hearing loss population showed 0.1, 0.09, and 0.06 μV lower wave I, III, and V amplitudes for the tinnitus group. Amplitudes were significantly different for the hearing loss population but not significantly different for normal hearing populations. Nevertheless, the wave I amplitude reduction in the tinnitus with normal hearing compared to the normal hearing controls was close to significance with a higher limit of the 95% CI of 0.24 μV compared to 0.23 μV 95% CI lower limit for the controls.

Meta-Analysis 2: Quantitative Analysis of ABR Latency and Amplitude Mean Difference between Tinnitus and Matched Control Groups Separated by Hearing Status

The mean differences in latencies and amplitudes between the tinnitus group and the matched controls (age and hearing status) were extracted when possible. For the latencies, the extraction of the mean difference was possible for only 10 out of the 15 studies that minimally matched their controls for age and hearing status. From the five excluded studies, one study did not report latencies (Schaette and McAlpine, 2011) and four studies provided insufficient information for data extraction (i.e., only the tinnitus data were presented, standard deviation was omitted, etc.; Barnea et al., 1990; McKee and Stephens, 1992; Rosenhall and Axelsson, 1994; Nemati et al., 2014). To note, only two studies out of the 10 studies that were kept for the latency meta-analysis did not include gender in their matching procedure (Attias et al., 1993, 1996). Interestingly, they were also the two studies with the highest degree of variability for both latency and amplitude analysis. For amplitudes, the number of included studies is even lower with five studies included in the second meta-analysis. Given that the amplitudes of waves III and V are poorly reported, the analysis was made on wave I only. Overall, similar problems extracting sufficient information were found for both the amplitude and latency data.

TABLE 3 | Characteristics of the Auditory Brainstem Responses methodologies used including the latency and amplitude outcome results.

Study	ABR system	Transducer	Polarity	Stimulus type	Presentation level(s)	Recording filters (Hz)
Attias et al., 1993	Microshev-4000 System	Not reported	Alternating	Broadband clicks, (0.1 ms duration 10 clicks/s)	120 dB SPL	200–3,000
Attias et al., 1996	Not mentioned	TDH-49	Alternating	Broadband clicks, (0.1 ms duration 10.3 clicks/s)	120 dB peSPL	100–2,000
Barnea et al., 1990	Microshev-2000	TDH-49	Alternating	Broadband clicks, (0.1 ms duration, 10 clicks/s)	120 dB SPL	200–2,000
Cartocci et al., 2012	Epic Plus	Not reported	Alternating	Broadband clicks, (0.1 ms duration, 11 clicks/s)	90 dB HL 80 dB HL	150–1,500
De Lavernhe-Lemaire and Beutter, 1989	Nicolet CA-1000	TDH-39P	Alternating	Broadband clicks, (0.1 ms duration, 11.1 clicks/s)	90 dB HL	150–1,500
De Lavernhe-Lemaire and Beutter, 1990	Nicolet CA-1000	TDH-39P	Alternating	Broadband clicks, (0.1 ms duration, 11.1 clicks/s)	90 dB HL	150–1,500
Gerken et al., 2001	Tucker-davis FT5 Grass P511k	ER2 inserts	Not reported	Tone bursts (1–8 kHz) (3 ms duration, 9.7 clicks/s)	112.5 peak dB SPL	1–3,000
Gilles et al., 2016	Bio-Logic with Nav Pro	ER-3A	Alternating	Broadband clicks, (0.1 ms duration, 31 clicks/s)	80 dB nHL	100–3,000
Gu et al., 2012	Tucker-Davis Medusa	HDA-200	Condensation	Broadband clicks, (0.1 ms duration, 11 clicks/s)	30, 50, 70, 80 dB nHL	5–5,000
Ikner and Hassen, 1990	Nicolet CA-1000	TDH-39	Condensation	Broadband clicks, (0.1 ms duration, 21.9 clicks/s)	75 dB nHL	Not reported
Kehrle et al., 2008	Amplaid Mk-15	TDH-50P	Alternating	Broadband clicks, (0.1 ms duration, 12 clicks/s)	80 dB HL	100–2,500
Kehrle et al., 2016	Biologic Navigator Pro AEP	E-A-RTONE 3A	Rarefaction	Broadband clicks, (0.1 ms duration, 21.1 clicks/s)	80 dB HL	100–3,000
Kim et al., 2016	Not reported	Not reported	Not reported	Not reported	Not reported	Not reported
Lemaire and Beutter, 1995	Nicolet CA-1000	TDH-39P	Alternating	Broadband clicks, (0.1 ms duration, 11.1 clicks/s)	90 dB HL	150–1,500
Mahmoudian et al., 2013	Bio-Logic with Nav Pro	ER-3	Alternating	Broadband clicks, (0.1 ms duration, 11.1 clicks/s)	20 dB over the AEP threshold level	30–3,000
Maurizi et al., 1985	Amplaid MK 6	TDH-49	Rarefaction	Broadband clicks, (0.1 ms duration, 21 clicks/s)	60 dB nHL	200–2,000
McKee and Stephens, 1992	Biologic Evoked Potential System	Not reported	Not reported	Broadband clicks, (0.1 ms duration, 19.1 clicks/s)	85 dB HL	Not reported
Nemati et al., 2014	ICS CHARTR	Not reported	Alternating	Broadband clicks, (duration not reported, 11.1 clicks/s)	90 dB SPL	Not reported
Rosenhall and Axelsson, 1994	Madsen 2250 ERA	Not reported	Rarefaction	Broadband clicks, (duration not reported, 20 clicks/s)	80 dB nHL	150–2,000
Santos-Filha et al., 2014	Bio-Logic Traveler Express	TDH-39	Rarefaction	Broadband clicks (0.1 ms duration 19 clicks/s)	80 dB HL	Not mentioned
Schaette and McAlpine, 2011	Medelec Synergy T-EP system	TDH-49	Not reported	Broadband clicks, (0.05 ms duration, 11 clicks/s)	90 and 100 dB SPL	100–1,500
Singh et al., 2011	Not reported	Not reported	Not reported	Not reported	Not reported	Not reported

dB, Decibels; HL, hearing loss; SPL, sound pressure level; TDH, Telephonics supraauricular headphones; ER, Etymonic insert earphones; HAD, Sennheiser circumauricular headphones.

TABLE 4 | Summary table of the meta-analysis (1) of the mean latency and amplitude of waves I, III, and V for tinnitus and non-tinnitus groups separated by hearing status.

	Tinnitus			No tinnitus		
	I	III	V	I	III	V
NORMAL HEARING						
Mean latency (ms)	1.59	3.73	5.61	1.59	3.72	5.58
Standard error	0.02	0.02	0.02	0.01	0.02	0.02
95% CI	1.55–1.62	3.69–3.76	5.56–5.65	1.58–1.61	3.68–3.75	5.53–5.62
N-value	142	142	152	490	118	132
Mean Amplitude (μV)	0.21	0.34	0.43	0.25	0.32	0.42
Standard error	0.01	0.01	0.02	0.008	0.009	0.01
95% CI	0.19–0.24	0.31–0.36	0.39–0.48	0.23–0.26	0.30–0.34	0.40–0.44
N-value	105	75	75	248	212	212
HEARING LOSS						
Mean latency (ms)	1.77	3.86	5.84	1.56	3.71	5.62
Standard error	0.007	0.02	0.02	0.03	0.03	0.03
95% CI	**1.75**–1.78	**3.83**–3.89	**5.80**–5.88	1.5–**1.62**	3.66–**3.76**	5.57–**5.68**
N-value	1,407	369	385	69	69	69
Mean Amplitude (μV)	0.15	0.19	0.33	0.25	0.28	0.39
Standard error	0.004	0.004	0.005	0.04	0.03	0.03
95% CI	0.14–**0.16**	0.18–**0.20**	0.32–**0.34**	**0.17**–0.32	**0.23**–0.34	**0.34**–0.45
N-value	831	919	919	34	34	34

Confidence intervals (CI) and number of observations (n-value) are presented for each group. Bolded values are significant (comparing the limits of the 95% CI of the tinnitus to the no tinnitus group). Number of observations was obtained by adding the reported number of subjects or ears of each study within the group.

For the latency mean differences, the meta-analysis revealed that only three studies out of 10 found a significantly prolonged wave I in the tinnitus group compared to controls and two other studies were close to significance (**Figure 2**). To note, two of the studies that are not close to significance were the only ones that tested participants (tinnitus and controls) with hearing loss (**Figure 2**, white diamonds), all the other studies used normal hearing individuals for both the tinnitus and control groups (**Figure 2**, black diamonds). As previously mentioned, they were also the two only studies that did not match their groups on the basis of gender. For wave III and V latencies, significantly prolonged latencies were found in three studies for the former and four for the latter. Kehrle et al. (2008, 2016) were the only studies that showed all three waves were significantly prolonged although Ikner and Hassen (1990) reported a similar trend. Interestingly, none of the studies with a specific noise induced tinnitus etiology inclusion criteria reported a significant latency effect for any of the waves (**Figure 2**, studies in Bold).

For the mean amplitude differences, the second meta-analysis revealed that only two studies out of five found a significant reduction of wave I (see **Figure 3**). Two of the studies that did not report significant reduction of wave I amplitude tested noise-induced hearing loss participants with and without tinnitus (**Figure 3**, white diamonds). Gilles et al. (2016) reported a tendency of the wave I amplitude to be increased in the tinnitus group, although this did not reach significance (**Figure 3**).

DISCUSSION

The aim of the present scoping review was to investigate whether consistent ABR abnormalities are prevalent in populations with tinnitus. Although there is increasing interest in the use of ABRs for measuring auditory function in tinnitus individuals, the present scoping review found that the evidence of abnormalities within this population is sparse. Only 22 studies corresponding to the broad inclusion and exclusion criteria were found. Of these 22 studies, only 19 used control groups to make their comparisons. The present review unfortunately indicates that the tested tinnitus populations (i.e., *who*) are typically poorly defined across ABR studies as the vast majority did not report tinnitus etiology, assess and/or report the psychoacoustic properties of tinnitus, did not measure high frequency thresholds (above 8 kHz) and used various definitions of normal hearing and/or hearing loss. In regards to the methodology used (i.e., *how*), the ABR system, the type of transducer, the presentation level and the filtering strategies varied significantly across the studies. Still, the results of these studies (i.e., *what*) showed significant changes in amplitude and/or latency for high intensity stimulation levels as the current review did not assess low stimulation levels. In addition to this, longer latency and reduced amplitude of wave I for the normal hearing tinnitus group compared to hearing matched controls was consistently shown across numerous studies. Since high sound levels of stimulation were used in most studies, these results might indicate cochlear nerve fiber degeneration, a loss of neural synchrony, or both. These results will be further discussed by looking at the population characteristics, the various techniques and assessments, and the outcomes of the included studies. Based on these results, recommendations for future studies will be made as well as a description of the future direction of electrophysiology in tinnitus research.

Heterogeneous Population Characteristics

One of the issues found by the current review is the poorly defined and undefined tinnitus population tested. Many of the studies reported the tinnitus from their test groups were either subjective or idiopathic. The vast majority did not report the tinnitus etiology at all. Only four studies chose noise-induced tinnitus as their sample population of which two included sensorineural hearing loss participants. Interestingly, none of the studies on noise-induced tinnitus reported any significant effects on wave latencies and amplitudes with the only exception being Attias et al. (1996) who found higher wave III amplitude in the tinnitus group compared to age and hearing matched controls. These null results contrast the findings by Gu et al. (2012) and Schaette and McAlpine (2011) showing reduced wave I amplitude in human tinnitus subjects, as well as animal studies showing decrease ABR wave I amplitudes at high stimulation levels after noise exposure without significant hearing threshold shifts (Kujawa and Liberman, 2006, 2009). Still, these human studies did not mention the etiology of the tinnitus nor did they classify their subjects as having noise-induced tinnitus. Conversely, the

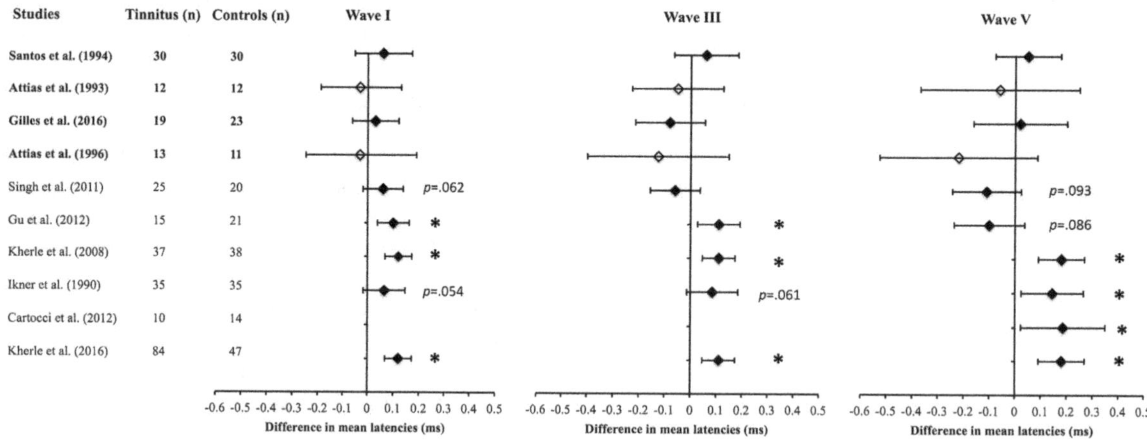

FIGURE 2 | Meta-analysis (2) of the net difference in latencies for Wave I, III, and V (95% CI) between tinnitus and control groups when matched for hearing status. Black diamonds represent studies with normal hearing participants and white diamonds studies with hearing loss participants. The studies in bold included only noise-induced tinnitus. *Asterisks represent significant differences ($p < 0.05$).

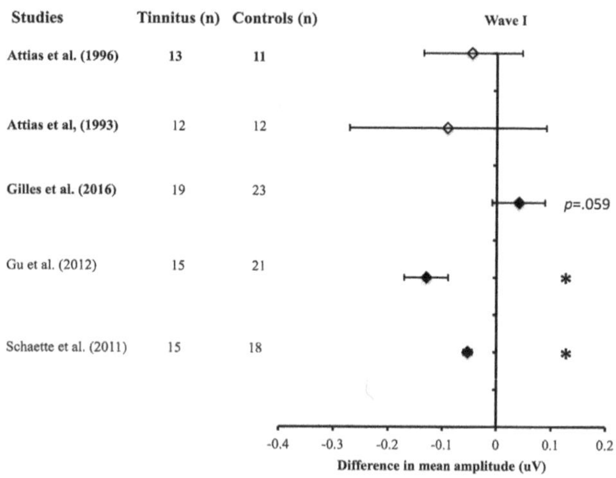

FIGURE 3 | Meta-analysis (2) of the net difference in amplitudes for Wave I (95% CI) between tinnitus and control groups when matched for hearing status. Black diamonds represent studies with normal hearing participants and white diamonds studies with hearing loss participants. The studies in bold included only noise-induced tinnitus. *Asterisks represent significant differences ($p < 0.05$).

Kujawa and Liberman (2006, 2009) animal studies did not assess tinnitus. Thus, the direct link between ABR abnormalities obtained in noise-induced animals and humans is not completely elucidated. Indeed, a recent study investigating ABRs in a young adult cohorts with normal audiograms but exposed to noise, did not find any significant reductions of wave I (Prendergast et al., 2017). More so, a recent study on a young adult sample (early 20's) of noise-induced tinnitus found no differences in the amplitude and latency of any of the ABR waves (Gilles et al., 2016). In that study, the ABR was assessed only on a subgroup of tinnitus and controls subjects. Their participants were matched for age, sex, and hearing thresholds for pure tones of 1–4 kHz only. Since a measure of synaptopathy such as the AP/SP ratio of the electrocochleography and very high frequency thresholds have been shown to be correlated (Liberman et al., 2016), it is thus possible that the tinnitus group had better thresholds at very high frequencies (>8 kHz) than the controls, and less synaptopathy. Still, this would be very unlikely considering that tinnitus subjects usually display more hearing loss than controls for those high frequencies when matched for normal thresholds at conventional frequencies (Fournier and Hébert, 2013). One possible interpretation of these results is that it takes some time, maybe years, for the nerve fibers to degenerate and therefore to effect the ABR responses. Another possibility is that ABRs are not sensitive enough to reveal synaptopathy and/or that synaptopathy loss is not necessary to develop tinnitus. Also, differences across species have been noted in the development of synaptopathy (Prendergast et al., 2017): losses of cochlear synapses have been shown to be irreversible in rodents but not in guinea pigs (although their function remained abnormal) (Liu et al., 2012; Shi et al., 2013; Song et al., 2016). Thus, one has to be cautious when comparing results from different animal species and, even more cautious, when translating such results to human listeners.

Very few studies assessed ABR wave characteristics between tinnitus and controls with hearing loss. Considering that tinnitus is often associated with hearing loss and remains rare in individuals with normal hearing, why have so few studies assessed ABR abnormalities in tinnitus participants with significant hearing loss? It is well known that two of three individuals with hearing loss will go on to develop tinnitus (Hoffman and Reed, 2004). It is possible these studies purposefully avoided recruiting participants with hearing loss in order to prevent known confounding effects of hearing loss on the ABR. However, ABR abnormalities in individuals with hearing loss might nevertheless help reveal certain underlying neural mechanisms responsible for tinnitus generation. To date, the only reported significant effect in this specific population is higher wave III amplitude (Attias et al., 1996).

We conducted the first meta-analysis to demonstrate the effects of tinnitus within a large clinical population separated based on hearing loss. The advantage of such an approach is that the population is more comparable to what would be seen in a clinical setting, and the higher power, due to the large sample size, increases the chances of revealing tinnitus-related cofactors, such as hearing loss, whilst reducing the effects of random variables not related to tinnitus (i.e., gender, thickness of the scalp, transducer frequency response). This analysis shows increased latencies and reduced amplitudes for all three waves (I, III, and V) for tinnitus subjects compared to controls (**Table 4**) with hearing loss. However, these results must be interpreted cautiously as the number of subjects with tinnitus was five to 20 times higher than the number of controls depending on the wave. This imbalance of the number of subjects is the result of compiling all the data available from the entire yield of studies even though four studies did not report a control group. These ABR effects did not survive the second meta-analysis where only studies with matched control groups were used: the only two studies that used matched hearing loss control groups did not report any significant changes (Attias et al., 1993, 1996). It can be argued that the longer latencies and lower amplitudes found in the first meta-analysis may be the result of the compiled tinnitus group having a greater degree of hearing loss than controls (for amplitude: Sand and Saunte, 1994; for latency: Keith and Greville, 1987). The possibility of a gender and/or an aging bias could also account for the differences obtained in meta-analysis one.

The present review highlighted some variability in the criteria used to define normal hearing and an even larger variability in defining hearing loss. Future studies should define normal hearing as thresholds of less or equal to 15 dB HL minimally at all standard clinical frequencies thus from 250 to 8,000 Hz (Clark, 1981). More so, the measurements of high frequency thresholds (>8 kHz) need to be undertaken as significant threshold elevation for those frequencies (10–16 kHz) have been recently shown and interpreted as an early sign of synaptopathy in humans (Liberman et al., 2016). More so, high frequency hearing loss (>8 kHz) in tinnitus patients with conventional normal hearing (250– 8,000 Hz) have been reported (Fournier and Hébert, 2013; Vielsmeier et al., 2015). It is thus crucial to control for high frequency thresholds, at least up to 16 kHz, when comparing tinnitus subjects to controls in order to distinguish with confidence the presence of synaptopathy. Participants should be separated and grouped based on the presence of hearing loss. In addition to this, the degree (mild, moderate, severe, or profound), the origin (cochlear vs. neural), and the configuration (flat, high, or low frequency slope, notch) of the hearing loss should be clearly defined and reported.

One other recommendation is to recruit tinnitus participants based on tinnitus etiology (or report etiology) and/or psychoacoustic measurements in order to separate the test groups. This in turn might show ABR related patterns within each subgroup that would be otherwise masked by the heterogeneity of the sample. Few studies used characteristics of the tinnitus perception, such as pitch and loudness matching of the tinnitus percept or residual inhibition, as a means to separate various tinnitus subtypes. For instance, Noreña et al. (1999) classified the late auditory evoked potentials in three tinnitus subgroups based on their self-reported changes of tinnitus perception in relation to noise. They were classified as having decreased, increased, or unchanged tinnitus perception in the presence of noise. Based on this classification, they found that patients with decreased tinnitus perception in noise had greater intensity-dependence and longer N1 latency than the subgroup that reported increased tinnitus perception. Within the included ABR articles for this review, Maurizi et al. (1985) used residual inhibition (RI); a known phenomenon where a temporary reduction in the loudness or even disappearance of tinnitus follows the cessation of a masking noise, to stratify unilateral tinnitus into positive or no RI subgroups. They found wave I was prolonged for the positive RI group and wave V was prolonged for the no RI group of the tinnitus ear compared to the contralateral ear. They also performed ABR testing before and after treatment for each group. Interestingly, they found that after masking, the positive RI group's longer wave I latency had disappeared but the no RI group's wave V latency did not change. Stratification of the tinnitus test population based on psychoacoustic methods and added information on the tinnitus etiology would be crucial for future studies on auditory evoked potentials.

To note, only one study reported a potential adverse effect of the ABR on tinnitus subject. Indeed, Gu et al. (2012) reported that they could not complete the ABR assessment in 10 participants because they did not tolerate the stimulus intensity level. The co-occurrence of hyperacusis, which is defined as a hypersensivitity to moderate to loud sounds, and tinnitus have been shown to be very high (Hébert et al., 2004, 2013; Dauman and Bouscau-Faure, 2005). Still, the Gu and colleagues group is the only one to have reported that the hypersensitivity was detrimental for the assessment. From all the studies found in the current review, four measured hyperacusis in different ways within their sample: one used the Khalfa questionnaire (Gilles et al., 2016) and the others used loudness discomfort levels (LDL) (Gerken et al., 2001; Cartocci et al., 2012; Gu et al., 2012). It is not known whether hyperacusis was detrimental for the ABR assessment in those studies, as none reported it. Future studies should address the potential adverse effects of ABR testing such as discomfort or pain on tinnitus patients with and without hyperacusis. A potential cut-off on a hyperacusis questionnaire or on a psychophysical method such as LDL could be used to triage those participants for which the procedure is judged to be safe from those at risk of discomfort.

Various Techniques and Assessments

Several techniques and assessments revealed by the review may have impacted the ABR results. One suspect issue occurs with the type of transducer. Out of the studies that reported the type of transducer used, 11 used various types of supra-auricular headphones while only four used insert earphones. According to Van Campen et al. (1992), insert earphones such as the ER-3A insert earphones can increase interaural attenuation, ambient noise attenuation, patient comfort, and eliminate ear canal collapse. Their study measured the acoustic output of TDH 39P, TDH 49P, and ER-3A inserts earphones on a KEMAR mannequin and used the same transducers for measuring click ABRs on normal hearing adults. One of the main differences they showed was that both TDH earphones had greater ringing than ER-3As for stimulus intensities down to 15 dB nHL. In addition to this, when tested on normal hearing adults, the insert earphones elicited a wave V that was significantly more delayed by 1.15 and 1 ms when stimulated at 40 dB nHL than the TDH earphones. Additionally, ER-3A earphones produced a significantly smaller wave I but similar wave V amplitude at 80 dB nHL than the TDH earphones, resulting in a greater V/I amplitude ratio. Given these differences, comparing data between insert and TDH earphones may be problematic.

Another potential issue comes from the frequency response of using various transducers with different response bandwidths. For example, the frequency response of an ER-3A earphone to a 500 Hz tone at 118.5 dB SPL is flat up to 4 kHz (E-A-R® Tone™ calibration specification sheet). This contrasts the Sennheiser HDA-200 headphones used by Gu et al. (2012) that was reported to have a bandwidth up to 8 kHz or the TDH 49 headphones that stimulate up to 7.1 kHz (Guest et al., 2016). Derived band measurements of the ABR to click stimuli show that wave I is mostly generated by characteristic frequencies above 2 kHz however wave V can be evoked by lower frequencies (Don and Eggermont, 1978; Abdala and Folsom, 1995). This may mean that the frequency response of the transducers used may influence the intensity of certain frequencies that may differ between studies. This variability may also contribute to the differences in latencies and amplitudes reported.

Heterogeneous Outcomes

The results found from the 22 studies were quite heterogeneous. For latencies, nine studies reported no change for any of the waves compared to nine who reported increased latency for waves I, V, and VII. Still, most well-controlled studies with appropriate matching procedures reported longer latencies for tinnitus compared to controls with wave I being the most consistently affected wave (**Figure 2**). A significant latency shift for all the three waves was found in Kehrle et al. (2008, 2016) and close to significance in Ikner and Hassen (1990) study. In these cases, the latency shift seen for waves III and V are not likely to be the result of the delayed wave I latency (due to neural damage) following through the other waves because the inter-peaks (I–V, III–V) were reported as abnormal in those same studies (see **Table 3**). These results might be related to a lack of central compensation in tinnitus individuals as suggested by Rüttiger et al. (2013).

Similar discordances were found within the amplitude data: four studies did not find any changes in amplitude for tinnitus, four reported decreased wave I, and either a decreased, an increased or even no modifications of the following amplitudes of waves III and V. Overall, only two of the five well-controlled studies reported decreased wave I amplitude. In addition to this, two well-controlled studies reported a higher V/I ratio (Kehrle et al., 2008; Nemati et al., 2014). More well-controlled studies are thus needed to clarify the presence of synaptopathy, as measured by wave I amplitude, in tinnitus patients. The large variability within the two studies with hearing loss tinnitus subjects prevent any conclusions that the trend towards lower wave I amplitude is due to an actual effect in tinnitus.

These mixed amplitude results may be related to the relative contribution of each type of nerve fibers (i.e., low-, medium-, and high-spontaneous rate) on the ABR signal. All the reviewed studies used high intensity stimuli that can be presumed to saturate the HSR fibers revealing potential difference linked only to LSR fibers. However, the specific contribution of each neural population (i.e., low-, medium-, and high- spontaneous rate) on the ABR waveform is not known. Substantial damage, for example to LSR fibers, may contribute to changes in the ABR amplitude in addition to the high spontaneous rate fibers. Bourien et al. (2014) have recently demonstrated that LSR fibers might have a negligible contribution to wave I ABR by measuring the compound action potential after selective damage to the LSR auditory nerve fibers of gerbils. They suggested that wave I reduction might be the result of damage to medium spontaneous rate fibers, which are usually mixed with LSR fibers in previous studies. It is also possible that damage to the LSR and MSR fibers varies across the length of the basilar membrane in such a way that the regions corresponding to certain frequencies have less damage than other areas. One way to target regions specifically affected by synaptopathy is to use specific frequencies or tone bursts, however narrowing the stimulus to include fewer frequencies may further reduce the number of responding fibers. For example, Gerken et al. (2001) used 10 tone bursts (1, 1.5, 2, 2.5, 3, 3.5, 4, 5, 6, and 8 kHz) at a level of 112 dB SPL to elicit the ABR in a tinnitus and non-tinnitus population with and without hearing loss. They found no significant differences for the ABR amplitude and latencies (Wave I, III, V) of the tinnitus group compared to the non-tinnitus subjects. Still, they did not use any matching procedures to compose their groups and included only nine tinnitus subjects with hearing loss. It may be interesting to replicate the Gerken et al. (2001) study on normal hearing populations (for all frequencies up to 16 kHz) with and without tinnitus, and with appropriate matching procedures (gender, age, and hearing status) for different intensity levels, for different frequencies (from low to high, including tinnitus pitch) in order to compare the response of the HSR, MSR, and LSR fibers.

Since the search for this review was conducted, two more articles on ABR and tinnitus populations have been published: Ravikumar and Murthy (2016) and Guest et al. (2016). Both studies compared tinnitus populations with normal hearing to normal hearing matched controls. Normal hearing was not defined in the former, and was defined as pure tone thresholds of $\leq$20 dB HL at 0.25–8 kHz for the latter. Latencies of wave I, III, and V were significantly ($p = 0.05$) prolonged (Ravikumar and Murthy, 2016) and wave V amplitude was higher but not significant (Guest et al., 2016). The latter study also reported no differences in the amplitude of wave I and found there was no correlation between the amplitude of wave I and history of noise exposure.

Recommendations for Future Studies on ABR

Clear and simple recommendations for future ABR investigations on tinnitus can be determined from these findings with the aim of improving future reviews on the subject, showing more reliable evidence of tinnitus, and making it easier to replicate previous studies. Most imperatively, it is highly encouraged that researchers report all the data collected including latencies and amplitudes of all the waves in a format that is suitable for meta-analysis. The meta-analysis of the current study was difficult particularly when latency or amplitude data was left unreported. From 22 studies found on ABR investigations of tinnitus in humans, only 10 studies could be used for the second meta-analysis to compare the mean difference of latencies between tinnitus and controls. Unfortunately, this represented <50% of all the studies found. For amplitude, even fewer studies were retained ($n = 5$), which represents <25% of all the studies. The mean and standard deviation of the latencies and amplitudes of the waves found within their paradigm for the tinnitus and control groups should be reported separately. Negative and non-significant results should always be reported in a similar fashion.

Secondly, all future ABR protocols should at least include control groups matched for gender, age and hearing status for sufficient control over these covariables. As mentioned previously, the two studies displaying the greatest variability for latencies and amplitudes in the second meta-analysis (Attias et al., 1993, 1996) did not match for gender between groups. Still, when comparing more recent studies to older ones, there appears to be a clear trend toward the use of more restrictive matching procedures. It is further suggested that hearing be assessed and matched for frequencies up to at least 16 kHz between groups. Studies should recruit participants with similar tinnitus etiologies (e.g., noise trauma) and include psychoacoustic measurements such as pitch and loudness matching, minimum masking level and residual inhibition. Future research should also consider separating participants into narrower age bands or at least separate younger and older subjects into two different groups. The two studies reporting reduced wave I in tinnitus (Schaette and McAlpine, 2011; Gu et al., 2012) tested participants approximately 10 years older on average than the study of Gilles et al. (2016) which included only participants below the age of 30. The absence of synaptopathy using wave I amplitude has also been reported in a study on noise-exposed young adults (mean age of 23, ranging from 18 to 36 years old), however tinnitus was not assessed (Prendergast et al., 2017). It is thus recommended that an age cut-off around 30 years old be used for future work. A sample size of at least 30 subjects per group is also recommended in order to reduce variability of the measures and to increase statistical power. Regarding the technical aspects of ABR measurement, insert headphones are preferred over circumauricular ones in order to optimize interaural attenuation, ambient noise attenuation, and to reduce the risk of ear canal collapsing. The frequency response of the transducer should also include as many frequencies above 2 kHz as possible.

Future Directions

Since the key publication of animal research demonstrating evidence of cochlear synaptopathy after noise exposure (Kujawa and Liberman, 2006, 2009), there has been a growing interest in improving ABR measurements in humans. Reliable ABR waveforms can sometimes be difficult to obtain mostly because of high inter-subject variability due to factors such as small signal to noise ratios, head shape, sex, as well as the various methodological concerns described above. Many research groups have attempted to address these issues by either improving the methodology of the click or tone-burst ABR method or by proposing new methods of assessment. For example, one study used an electrode placed on the tympanic membrane (TM) in order to improve the signal to noise ratio (Stamper and Johnson, 2015). Using a similar electrode tip on the TM, another group used electrocochleography instead of ABR to show significant differences in the SP/AP ratio between high and low noise exposure risk groups of participants (Liberman et al., 2016). This finding still needs to be replicated, but electrocochleography could potentially become a standard measure of synaptopathy instead of the classical ABR. Another group showed delayed wave V ABRs when responding to clicks in background noise as evidence of the presence of synaptopathy in animals and humans (Mehraei et al., 2016). The use of envelope following responses (EFR) with amplitude-modulated tones in notched noise with varying modulation depth have also shown deficits that are consistent with synaptopathy (Bharadwaj et al., 2015). All these new techniques could easily be applied to tinnitus participants. This in turn can bring new insight on a possible role, if any, played by cochlear synaptopathy in the generation of tinnitus. More so, the application of a paradigm to desynchronize neural activity may help reveal potential tinnitus mechanisms. Indeed, when click-rate is increased, the nerve fibers appear to have more difficulty synchronizing their discharge to the stimulus, resulting in smaller ABR amplitudes and prolonged wave V latencies (Konrad-Martin et al., 2012). Higher synchronous activity at higher levels of the auditory system related to tinnitus might thus only be revealed when using high click-rates.

Finally, ABRs have more recently been used not only to understand the pathophysiology of tinnitus but also objectify its presence in individuals. The gap-in-noise ABR (or GIN-ABR) has been used in animal subjects with different background noise frequencies before and after tinnitus induction by salicylate (Lowe and Walton, 2015). Using this method, they found a significant reduction in gap detection after salicylate treatment for only the 16 kHz background noise condition. The authors concluded that since salicylate is known to produce a 16 kHz tinnitus percept that appears to fill the gap, the GIN-ABR may be effective for objectifying the presence of tinnitus in animals. This in turn may be a promising new avenue for future auditory brainstem research applied to humans with tinnitus.

AUTHOR CONTRIBUTIONS

All the authors contributed to this work. VM and AK provided the original conception and design of the study. VM and PF worked on data acquisition, analysis, and interpretation. They both wrote the manuscript. DB, AN, and AK provided intellectual feedback and revised the content of several previous versions of the manuscript. All authors (VM, PF, DB, AN, and AK) approved the final version of the manuscript.

ACKNOWLEDGMENTS

This research was made possible thanks to a University of Ottawa internal grant to AK, and a post-doctoral fellow studentship from the Canadian Institute of Health Research (CIHR) and the Fonds de recherche du Québec—Santé (FRQS) to PF.

REFERENCES

Abdala, C., and Folsom, R. C. (1995). Frequency contribution to the click-evoked auditory-brain-stem response in human adults and infants. *J. Acoust. Soc. Am.* 97, 2394–2404. doi: 10.1121/1.411961

Arksey, H., and O'Malley, L. (2005). Scoping studies: towards a methodological framework. *Int. J. Soc. Res. Methodol.* 8, 19–32. doi: 10.1080/1364557032000119616

Attias, J., Pratt, H., Reshef, I., Bresloff, I., Horowitz, G., Polyakov, A., et al. (1996). Detailed analysis of auditory brainstem responses in patients with noise-induced tinnitus. *Audiology* 35, 259–270. doi: 10.3109/00206099609071946

Attias, J., Urbach, D., Gold, S., and Shemesh, Z. (1993). Auditory event related potentials in chronic tinnitus patients with noise induced hearing loss. *Hear. Res.* 71, 106–113. doi: 10.1016/0378-5955(93)90026-W

Barnea, G., Attias, J., Gold, S., and Shahar, A. (1990). Tinnitus with normal hearing sensitivity: extended high-frequency audiometry and auditory-nerve brain-stem-evoked responses. *Audiology* 29, 36–45. doi: 10.3109/00206099009081644

Bauch, C. D., Olsen, W. O., and Pool, A. F. (1996). ABR indices: sensitivity, specificity, and tumor size. *Am. J. Audiol.* 5, 97–104. doi: 10.1044/1059-0889.0501.97

Bayar, N., Böke, B., Turan, E., and Belgin, E. (2001). Efficacy of amitriptyline in the treatment of subjective tinnitus. *J. Otolaryngol.* 30, 300–303. doi: 10.2310/7070.2001.19597

Berliner, K., Shelton, C., and Hitselberger, W. (1992). Acoustic tumors: effect of surgical removal on tinnitus. *Otol. Neurotol.* 13, 13–17. doi: 10.1097/00129492-199201000-00005

Bharadwaj, H. M., Masud, S., Mehraei, G., Verhulst, S., and Shinn-Cunningham, B. G. (2015). Individual differences reveal correlates of hidden hearing deficits. *J. Neurosci.* 35, 2161–2172. doi: 10.1523/JNEUROSCI.3915-14.2015

Bourien, J., Tang, Y., Batrel, C., Huet, A., Lenoir, M., Ladrech, S., et al. (2014). Contribution of auditory nerve fibers to compound action potential of the auditory nerve. *J. Neurophysiol.* 112, 1025–1039. doi: 10.1152/jn.00738.2013

Burkard, R., and Secor, C. (2002). "Overview of auditory evoked potentials," in *Handbook of Clinical Audiology*, ed T. L. Julet (Baltimore, MD: Lippincott Williams and Wilkins), 233–248.

Cartocci, G., Attanasio, G., Fattapposta, F., Locuratolo, N., Mannarelli, D., and Filipo, R. (2012). An electrophysiological approach to tinnitus interpretation. *Int. Tinnitus J.* 17, 152–157. doi: 10.5935/0946-5448.20120027

Chalak, S., Kale, A., Deshpande, V. K., and Biswas, D. A. (2013). Establishment of normative data for monaural recordings of auditory brainstem response and its application in screening patients with hearing loss: a cohort study. *J. Clin. Diagn. Res.* 7, 2677–2679. doi: 10.7860/jcdr/2013/6768.3730

Clark, J. (1981). Uses and abuses of hearing loss. *ASHA* 23, 493–500.

Dauman, R., and Bouscau-Faure, F. (2005). Assessment and amelioration of hyperacusis in tinnitus patients. *Acta Otolaryngol.* 125, 503–509. doi: 10.1080/00016480510027565

De Lavernhe-Lemaire, M. C., and Beutter, P. (1989). Potentiels évoqués auditifs dans la distinction entre acouphènes périphériques et centraux. *Arch. Int. Physiol. Biochim.* 97, 135–144. doi: 10.3109/13813458909104533

De Lavernhe-Lemaire, M. C., and Beutter, P. (1990). Modifications des amplitudes des potentiels évoques auditifs précoces observées dans les acouphènes. *Arch. Int. Physiol. Biochim.* 98, 403–409. doi: 10.3109/13813459009114002

De Ridder, D., Vanneste, S., Langguth, B., and Llinas, R. (2015). Thalamocortical dysrhythmia: a theoretical update in tinnitus. *Front. Neurol.* 6:124. doi: 10.3389/fneur.2015.00124

Don, M., and Eggermont, J. J. (1978). Analysis of the click-evoked brainstem potentials in man using high-pass noise masking. *J. Acoust. Soc. Am.* 63, 1084–1092. doi: 10.1121/1.381816

Don, M., Ponton, C. W., Eggermont, J. J., and Kwong, B. (1998). The effects of sensory hearing loss on cochlear filter times estimated from auditory brainstem response latencies. *J. Acoust. Soc. Am.* 104, 2280–2289. doi: 10.1121/1.423741

Eggermont, J. J. (1984). Tinnitus: some thoughts about its origin. *J. Laryngol. Otol.* 98, 31–37. doi: 10.1017/S1755146300090089

Fournier, P., and Hébert, S. (2013). Gap detection deficits in humans with tinnitus as assessed with the acoustic startle paradigm: does tinnitus fill in the gap? *Hear. Res.* 295, 16–23. doi: 10.1016/j.heares.2012.05.011

Gerken, G. M., Hesse, P. S., and Wiorkowski, J. J. (2001). Auditory evoked responses in control subjects and in patients with problem-tinnitus. *Hear. Res.* 157, 52–64. doi: 10.1016/S0378-5955(01)00277-5

Gilles, A., Schlee, W., Rabau, S., Wouters, K., Fransen, E., and Van de Heyning, P. (2016). Decreased speech-in-noise understanding in young adults with tinnitus. *Front. Neurosci.* 10:288. doi: 10.3389/fnins.2016.00288

Giraudet, F., and Avan, P. (2012). Auditory neuropathies. *Curr. Opin. Neurol.* 25, 50–56. doi: 10.1097/WCO.0b013e32834f0351

Gopal, K. V., Thomas, B. P., Mao, D., and Lu, H. (2015). Efficacy of carnitine in treatment of tinnitus: evidence from audiological and MRI measures—a case study. *J. Am. Acad. Audiol.* 26, 311–324. doi: 10.3766/jaaa.26.3.10

Gu, J. W., Herrmann, B. S., Levine, R. A., and Melcher, J. R. (2012). Brainstem auditory evoked potentials suggest a role for the ventral cochlear nucleus in tinnitus. *J. Assoc. Res. Otolaryngol.* 13, 819–833. doi: 10.1007/s10162-012-0344-1

Guest, H., Munro, K. J., Prendergast, G., Howe, S., and Plack, C. J. (2016). Tinnitus with a normal audiogram: relation to noise exposure but no evidence for cochlear synaptopathy. *Hear. Res.* 344, 265–274. doi: 10.1016/j.heares.2016.12.002

Hébert, S., Fournier, P., and Noreña, A. (2013). The auditory sensitivity is increased in tinnitus ears. *J. Neurosci.* 33, 2356–2364. doi: 10.1523/JNEUROSCI.3461-12.2013

Hébert, S., Paiement, P., and Lupien, S. J. (2004). A physiological correlate for the intolerance to both internal and external sounds. *Hear. Res.* 190, 1–9. doi: 10.1016/S0378-5955(04)00021-8

Henry, J. A., Roberts, L. E., Caspary, D. M., Theodoroff, S. M., and Salvi, R. J. (2014). Underlying mechanisms of tinnitus: review and clinical implications. *J. Am. Acad. Audiol.* 25, 5–22. doi: 10.3766/jaaa.25.1.2

Hickox, A. E., and Liberman, M. C. (2014). Is noise-induced cochlear neuropathy key to the generation of hyperacusis or tinnitus? *J. Neurophysiol.* 111, 552–564. doi: 10.1152/jn.00184.2013

Hoffman, H., and Reed, G. (2004). "Epidemiology of tinnitus," in *Tinnitus: Theory and Management*, ed J. B. Snow (Lewiston, NY: BC Decker), 16–41.

House, J. W., and Brackmann, D. E. (1981). "Tinnitus: surgical treatment," in *Ciba Foundation Symposium 85: Tinnitus*, eds D. Evered and G. Lawrens (London: Pitman), 204–212.

Hultcrantz, M., Simonoska, R., and Stenberg, A. E. (2006). Estrogen and hearing: a summary of recent investigations. *Acta Otolaryngol.* 126, 10–14. doi: 10.1080/00016480510038617

Hyde, M. L., Riko, K., and Malizia, K. (1990). Audiometric accuracy of the click ABR in infants at risk for hearing loss. *J. Am. Acad. Audiol.* 1, 59–66.

Ikner, C. L., and Hassen, A. H. (1990). The effect of tinnitus on ABR latencies. *Ear Hear.* 11, 16–20. doi: 10.1097/00003446-199002000-00005

Jewett, D., Romano, M., and Williston, J. (1970). Human auditory evoked potentials: possible brain stem components detected on the scalp. *Science* 167, 1517–1518. doi: 10.1126/science.167.3924.1517

Jewett, D., and Williston, J. S. (1971). Auditory-evoked far fields averaged from the scalp of humans. *Brain* 94, 681–696. doi: 10.1093/brain/94.4.681

Kehrle, H. M., Granjeiro, R. C., Sampaio, A. L. L., Bezerra, R., Almeida, V. F., and Oliveira, C. A. (2008). Comparison of auditory brainstem response results in normal-hearing patients with and without tinnitus. *Arch. Otolaryngol. Head Neck Surg.* 134, 647–651. doi: 10.1001/archotol.134.6.647

Kehrle, H. M., Sampaio, A. L., Granjeiro, R. C., De Oliveira, T. S., and Oliveira, C. A. (2016). Tinnitus annoyance in normal-hearing individuals: correlation with depression and anxiety. *Ann. Otol. Rhinol. Laryngol.* 125, 185–194. doi: 10.1177/0003489415606445

Keith, W. J., and Greville, K. A. (1987). Effects of audiometric configuration on the auditory brain stem response. *Ear Hear.* 8, 49–55. doi: 10.1097/00003446-198702000-00009

Khangura, S., Konnyu, K., Cushman, R., Grimshaw, J., and Moher, D. (2012). Evidence summaries: the evolution of a rapid review approach. *Syst. Rev.* 1:10. doi: 10.1186/2046-4053-1-10

Kim, S. I., Kim, M. G., Kim, S. S., Byun, J. Y., Park, M. S., and Yeo, S. G. (2016). Evaluation of tinnitus patients by audiometric configuration. *Otolaryngol. Head Neck Surg.* 37, 1–5. doi: 10.1016/j.amjoto.2015.08.009

Konrad-Martin, D., Dille, M. F., McMillan, G., Griest, S., McDermott, D., Fausti, S. A., et al. (2012). Age-related changes in the auditory brainstem response. *J. Am. Acad. Audiol.* 23, 18–35. doi: 10.3766/jaaa.23.1.3

Kotlarz, J. P., Eby, T. L., and Borton, T. E. (1992). Analysis of the efficiency of retrocochlear screening. *Laryngoscope* 102, 1108–1112. doi: 10.1288/00005537-199210000-00004

Kujawa, S. G., and Liberman, M. C. (2006). Acceleration of age-related hearing loss by early noise exposure: evidence of a misspent youth. *J. Neurosci.* 26, 2115–2123. doi: 10.1523/JNEUROSCI.4985-05.2006

Kujawa, S. G., and Liberman, M. C. (2009). Adding insult to injury: cochlear nerve degeneration after "temporary" noise-induced hearing loss. *J. Neurosci.* 29, 14077–14085. doi: 10.1523/JNEUROSCI.2845-09.2009

Lemaire, M. C., and Beutter, P. (1995). Brainstem auditory evoked responses in patients with tinnitus. *Audiology* 34, 287–300. doi: 10.3109/00206099509071919

Levac, D., Colquhoun, H., and O'Brien, K. K. (2010). Scoping studies: advancing the methodology. *Implement. Sci.* 5:69. doi: 10.1186/1748-5908-5-69

Levine, R. A. (1999). Somatic (craniocervical) tinnitus and the dorsal cochlear nucleus hypothesis. *Am. J. Otolaryngol.* 6, 351–362. doi: 10.1016/S0196-0709(99)90074-1

Lewis, J. D., Kopun, J., Neely, S. T., Schmid, K. K., and Gorga, M. P. (2015). Tone-burst auditory brainstem response wave V latencies in normal-hearing and hearing-impaired ears. *J. Acoust. Soc. Am.* 138, 3210–3219. doi: 10.1121/1.4935516

Liberman, M. C., Epstein, M. J., Cleveland, S. S., Wang, H., and Maison, S. F. (2016). Toward a differential diagnosis of hidden hearing loss in humans. *PLoS ONE* 11:e0162726. doi: 10.1371/journal.pone.0162726

Liberman, M. C., and Kujawa, S. G. (2017). Cochlear synaptopathy in acquired sensorineural hearing loss: manifestations and mechanisms. *Hear. Res.* 349, 138–147. doi: 10.1016/j.heares.2017.01.003

Liu, L., Wang, H., Shi, L., Almuklass, A., He, T., Aiken, S., et al. (2012). Silent damage of noise on cochlear afferent innervation in guinea pigs and the impact on temporal processing. *PLoS ONE* 7:e49550. doi: 10.1371/journal.pone.0049550

Lowe, A. S., and Walton, J. P. (2015). Alterations in peripheral and central components of the auditory brainstem response: a neural assay of tinnitus. *PLoS ONE* 10:e0117228. doi: 10.1371/journal.pone.0117228

Mahmoudian, S., Lenarz, M., Esser, K.-H., Salamat, B., Alaeddini, F., Dengler, R., et al. (2013). Alterations in early auditory evoked potentials and brainstem transmission time associated with tinnitus residual inhibition induced by auditory electrical stimulation. *Int. Tinnitus J.* 18, 63–74. doi: 10.5935/0946-5448.20130009

Maurizi, M., Ottaviani, F., Paludetti, G., Almadori, G., and Tassoni, A. (1985). Contribution to the differentiation of peripheral versus central tinnitus via auditory brain stem response evaluation. *Audiology* 24, 207–216. doi: 10.3109/00206098509070104

McKee, G. J., and Stephens, S. D. G. (1992). An investigation of normally hearing subjects with tinnitus. *Audiology* 31, 313–317. doi: 10.3109/00206099209072919

Mehraei, G., Hickox, A. E., Bharadwaj, H. M., Goldberg, H., Verhulst, S., Liberman, M. C., et al. (2016). Auditory brainstem response latency in noise as a marker of cochlear synaptopathy. *J. Neurosci.* 36, 3755–3764. doi: 10.1523/JNEUROSCI.4460-15.2016

Melcher, J. R., and Kiang, N. Y. (1996). Generators of the brainstem auditory evoked potential in cat III: identified cell populations. *Hear. Res.* 93, 52–71. doi: 10.1016/0378-5955(95)00200-6

Milicic, D., and Alcada, M. N. (1999). A tinnitus objectivization: how we do it. *Int Tinnitus J.* 5, 5–15.

Moeller, A. R. (1984). Pathophysiology of tinnitus. *Ann. Otol. Rhinol. Laryngol.* 93, 39–44. doi: 10.1177/000348948409300110

Moher, D., Liberati, A., Tetzlaff, J., and Altman, D. G. (2009). Academia and clinic annals of internal medicine preferred reporting items for systematic reviews and meta-analyses: the PRISMA statement. *Ann. Intern. Med.* 151, 264–269. doi: 10.7326/0003-4819-151-4-200908180-00135

Nemati, S., Habibi, A. F., Panahi, R., and Pastadast, M. (2014). Cochlear and brainstem audiologic findings in normal hearing tinnitus subjects in comparison with non-tinnitus control group. *Acta Med. Iran.* 51, 822–826.

Noreña, A., Cransac, H., and Chéry-Croze, S. (1999). Towards an objectification by classification of tinnitus. *Clin. Neurophysiol.* 110, 666–675.

Noreña, A. J. (2011). An integrative model of tinnitus based on a central gain controlling neural sensitivity. *Neurosci. Biobehav. Rev.* 35, 1089–1109. doi: 10.1016/j.neubiorev.2010.11.003

Prendergast, G., Guest, H., Munro, K. J., Kluk, K., Léger, A., Hall, D. A., et al. (2017). Effects of noise exposure on young adults with normal audiograms I: electrophysiology. *Hear. Res.* 344, 68–81. doi: 10.1016/j.heares.2016.10.028

Ravikumar, G., and Murthy, V. A. (2016). A study of brainstem auditory evoked responses in normal hearing patients with tinnitus. *Indian J. Otolaryngol. Head Neck Surg.* 68, 429–433. doi: 10.1007/s12070-015-0917-5

Rosenhall, U., and Axelsson, A. (1994). Auditory brainstem response latencies in patients with tinnitus. *Scand. Audiol.* 24, 97–100. doi: 10.3109/01050399509047521

Rupa, V., Job, A., George, M., and Rajshekhar, V. (2003). Cost-effective initial screening for vestibular schwannoma: auditory brainstem response or magnetic resonance imaging? *Otolaryngol. Head Neck Surg.* 128, 823–828. doi: 10.1016/S0194-5998(03)00358-9

Rüttiger, L., Singer, W., Panford-Walsh, R., Matsumoto, M., Lee, S. C., Zuccotti, A., et al. (2013). The reduced cochlear output and the failure to adapt the central auditory response causes tinnitus in noise exposed rats. *PLoS ONE* 8:e57247. doi: 10.1371/journal.pone.0057247

Sand, T., and Saunte, C. (1994). ABR amplitude and dispersion variables: relation to audiogram shape and click polarity. *Scand. Audiol.* 23, 7–12. doi: 10.3109/01050399409047482

Santos-Filha, V., Samelli, A., and Matas, C. (2014). Noise-induced tinnitus: auditory evoked potential in symptomatic and asymptomatic patients. *Clinics* 69, 487–490. doi: 10.6061/clinics/2014(07)08

Schaette, R., and McAlpine, D. (2011). Tinnitus with a normal audiogram: physiological evidence for hidden hearing loss and computational model. *J. Neurosci.* 31, 13452–13457. doi: 10.1523/JNEUROSCI.2156-11.2011

Shi, L., Liu, L., He, T., Guo, X., Yu, Z., Yin, S., et al. (2013). Ribbon synapse plasticity in the cochleae of Guinea pigs after noise-induced silent damage. *PLoS ONE* 8:e81566. doi: 10.1371/journal.pone.0081566

Shulman, A., and Seitz, M. R. (1981). Central tinnitus- diagnosis and treatment. Observations simultaneous binaural auditory brain responses with monaural stimulation in the tinnitus patient. *Laryngoscope* 91, 2025–2036. doi: 10.1288/00005537-198112000-00005

Singh, S., Munjal, S. K., Panda, N. K., Munjal, K., S., Panda, K., N., Munjal, S. K., et al. (2011). Comparison of auditory electrophysiological responses in normal-hearing patients with and without tinnitus. *J. Laryngol. Otol.* 125, 668–672. doi: 10.1017/S0022215111000569

Song, Q., Shen, P., Li, X., Shi, L., Liu, L., Wang, J., et al. (2016). Coding deficits in hidden hearing loss induced by noise: the nature and impacts. *Sci. Rep.* 6:25200. doi: 10.1038/srep25200

Stamper, G. C., and Johnson, T. A. (2015). Auditory function in normal-hearing, noise-exposed human ears. *Ear Hear.* 36, 172–184. doi: 10.1097/AUD.0000000000000107

Starr, A., Picton, T. W., Sininger, Y., Hood, L. J., and Berlin, C. I. (1996). Auditory neuropathy. *Brain* 119, 741–753. doi: 10.1093/brain/119.3.741

Stouffer, J. L., and Tyler, R. S. (1990). Characterisation of tinnitus by tinnitus patients. *J. Speech Hear. Disord.* 55, 439–453. doi: 10.1044/jshd.5503.439

Tyler, R., Coelho, C., Tao, P., and Ji, H. (2008). Identifying tinnitus subgroups with cluster analysis. *Am. J. Audiol.* 17, S176–S184. doi: 10.1044/1059-0889(2008/07-0044)

Van Campen, L. E., Sammeth, C. A., Hall, J. W., and Peek, B. F. (1992). Comparison of Etymotic insert and TDH supra-aural earphones in auditory brainstem response measurement. *J. Am. Acad. Audiol.* 3, 315–323.

Vielsmeier, V., Lehner, A., Strutz, J., Steffens, T., Kreuzer, P. M., Schecklmann, M., et al. (2015). The relevance of the high frequency audiometry in tinnitus patients with normal hearing in conventional pure-tone audiometry. *Biomed. Res. Int.* 2015:302515. doi: 10.1155/2015/302515

Watson, D. R. (1996). The effects of cochlear hearing loss. *Audiology* 35, 246–258. doi: 10.3109/00206099609071945a

Wilson, D. F., Hodgson, R. S., Gustafson, M. F., Hogue, S., and Mills, L. (1992). The sensitivity of auditory brainstem response testing in small acoustic neuromas. *Laryngoscope* 102, 961–964. doi: 10.1288/00005537-199209000-00001

Yu, H., Patil, K. V., Han, C., Fabella, B., Canlon, B., Someya, S., et al. (2016). GLAST deficiency in mice exacerbates gap detection deficits in a model of salicylate-induced tinnitus. *Front. Behav. Neurosci.* 10:158. doi: 10.3389/fnbeh.2016.00158

20

Gender-Specific Differences in Patients with Chronic Tinnitus—Baseline Characteristics and Treatment Effects

Uli Niemann[1], Benjamin Boecking[2], Petra Brueggemann[2], Birgit Mazurek[2] and Myra Spiliopoulou[1]*

[1] *Faculty of Computer Science, Otto von Guericke University Magdeburg, Magdeburg, Germany,*

[2] *Tinnitus Center, Charité Universitaetsmedizin Berlin, Berlin, Germany*

Correspondence:
Uli Niemann
uli.niemann@ovgu.de

Whilst some studies have identified gender-specific differences, there is no consensus about gender-specific determinants for prevalence rates or concomitant symptoms of chronic tinnitus such as depression or anxiety. However, gender-associated differences in psychological response profiles and coping strategies may differentially affect tinnitus chronification and treatment success rates. Thus, understanding gender-associated differences may facilitate a more detailed identification of symptom profiles, heighten treatment response rates, and help to create access for vulnerable populations that are potentially less visible in clinical settings. Our research questions are: RQ1: how do male and female tinnitus patients differ regarding tinnitus-related distress, depression severity, and treatment response, RQ2: to what extent are answers to questionnaires administered at baseline associated with gender, and RQ3: which baseline questionnaire items are associated with tinnitus distress, depression, and treatment response, while relating to one gender only? In this work, we present a data analysis workflow to investigate gender-specific differences in N = 1,628 patients with chronic tinnitus (828 female, 800 male) who completed a 7-day multimodal treatment encompassing cognitive behavioral therapy (CBT), physiotherapy, auditory attention training, and information counseling components. For this purpose, we extracted 181 variables from 7 self-report questionnaires on socio-demographics, tinnitus-related distress, tinnitus frequency, loudness, localization, and quality as well as physical and mental health status. Our workflow comprises (i) training machine learning models, (ii) a comprehensive evaluation including hyperparameter optimization, and (iii) post-learning steps to identify predictive variables. We found that female patients reported higher levels of tinnitus-related distress, depression and response to treatment (RQ1). Female patients indicated higher levels of tension, stress, and psychological coping strategies rates. By contrast, male patients reported higher levels of bodily pain associated with chronic tinnitus whilst judging their overall health as better (RQ2). Variables measuring depression, sleep problems, tinnitus frequency, and loudness were associated with tinnitus-related distress in both genders and indicators of mental health and subjective stress were found to be associated with depression in both genders (RQ3). Our results suggest that gender-associated differences in symptomatology and treatment response profiles suggest clinical and conceptual needs for differential diagnostics, case conceptualization and treatment pathways.

Keywords: gender, tinnitus, distress, depression, treatment response, gender-influence on diagnostics, machine learning, variable importance

1. INTRODUCTION

Tinnitus refers to the perception of sound, such as ringing, whistling, hissing, or rustling in absence of an external sound stimulus (Eggermont and Roberts, 2004) and is experienced by 12–30% of the general population (McCormack et al., 2016). A subset of 1–2% of all people report considerable impairment with respect to quality of life associated with the tinnitus percept (Langguth et al., 2013). Due to its clinical heterogeneity in cause, perception and accompanying symptoms (Langguth et al., 2013), a treatment gold standard that is effective for every patient has not been established yet, despite scientifically proven efficacy of cognitive behavioral approaches in reducing tinnitus-related distress for some patients (Andersson and Lyttkens, 1999; Andersson, 2002; Cima et al., 2012, 2014).

Tinnitus is often accompanied by comorbid symptoms including agitation, anxiety, depression, insomnia, irritability, and stress (Langguth et al., 2009). For example, in between 14 and 80% of tinnitus patients (Langguth et al., 2011), tinnitus is associated with high levels of interacting anxiety and depression levels. Whereas, female gender was identified as one important risk factor of psychological comorbidities in many studies (Piccinelli and Wilkinson, 2000; Nolen-Hoeksema, 2001; Matud, 2004; Jaussent et al., 2011; McLean et al., 2011; Langguth et al., 2013; Asher et al., 2017), the relationship between gender and tinnitus is not well-understood yet. Previous studies have presented contradictory results about the relationship between gender and tinnitus severity and/or distress: Erlandsson et al. (1992) found no difference between genders in tinnitus severity measured by their Tinnitus Severity Questionnaire (TSQ) in 186 tinnitus patients. Pinto et al. (2010) concluded no influence of gender on tinnitus annoyance using the Tinnitus Handicap Inventory (THI; Newman et al., 1996) in 68 tinnitus patients. Further, Meric et al. (1998) found no difference between female and male tinnitus patients ($N = 281$) with respect to the scores of the Tinnitus Handicap Questionnaire (THQ; Kuk et al., 1990), the Tinnitus Reaction Questionnaire (Wilson et al., 1991) and the Subjective Tinnitus Severity Scale (Halford and Anderson, 1991). In contrast, Seydel et al. (2013) reported differences in tinnitus distress measured by the German version of the Tinnitus Questionnaire (TQ; Goebel and Hiller, 1998) between genders in 1,180 tinnitus patients although the manifestation of accompanying symptoms partly depended on age. Hiller and Goebel (2006) found higher levels of tinnitus loudness and annoyance for men measured by the TQ in 4,971 volunteers of the German Tinnitus League (Hiller and Goebel, 2006). Lugo et al. (2019) showed that severe tinnitus was associated with suicide attempts only in women among 71,542 participants of the Stockholm Public Health Cohort (Svensson et al., 2012). Han et al. (2019) revealed that significant associations between tinnitus severity with quality of life, depressivity, and stress prevail only among the male subjects of 248 patients with tinnitus complaints.

Overall, there is no consensus about gender-specific determinants for prevalence rates or concomitant symptoms of chronic tinnitus such as depression or anxiety. However, gender-associated differences in psychological response profiles and coping strategies may differentially affect tinnitus chronification and treatment success rates. Thus, understanding gender-associated differences may facilitate a more detailed identification of symptom profiles, heighten treatment response rates, and help to create access for vulnerable populations that are potentially less visible in clinical settings. In this work, our research questions were: RQ1: how do male and female tinnitus patients differ with respect to tinnitus-related distress, depression severity, and treatment response, RQ2: to what extent are answers to questionnaires administered at baseline associated with gender, and RQ3: which baseline questionnaire items are associated with tinnitus distress, depression, and treatment response, while relating to one gender only? For that purpose, we developed a hypothesis-free data analysis workflow that aimed to identify determinants of gender-specific differences in patients with chronic tinnitus based on data extracted from multiple questionnaires at baseline using machine learning.

2. MATERIALS AND METHODS

2.1. Patient Data

This study is based on retrospective data from 4,103 tinnitus patients who had been treated at the Tinnitus Center of Charité Universitaetsmedizin Berlin between January 2011 and October 2015, were 18 years of age or older and had been suffering from tinnitus for at least 3 months. Exclusion criteria were presence of an acute psychotic illness or addiction disorder (abstinence not ensured during treatment), deafness (untreated), and insufficient knowledge of the German language. Treatment comprised multimodal 7-day program that included intensive and daily informational counseling, detailed ear-nose-throat (ENT) as well as psychological diagnostics, cognitive behavior therapy interventions, hearing exercises with aspects of mindfulness-based stress reduction, progressive muscle relaxation and physiotherapy. At baseline (T0; before therapy commencement) and after treatment (T1), patients were asked to complete multiple self-report questionnaires assessing socio-demographics, tinnitus-related distress, tinnitus localization, quality, frequency and loudness, as well as physical and mental health status, including levels of depression and perceived stress. All patients gave informed written consent prior to data collection. The study has been approved by the ethics committee of the Charité Universitaetsmedizin Berlin.

In total, we used data from seven questionnaires: (a) General Depression Scale-long form (Allgemeine Depressionsskala; ADSL; Radloff, 1977; Hautzinger and Bailer, 2002), (b) Perceived Stress Questionnaire (PSQ; Fliege et al., 2005), (c) Short Form-8 Health Survey (SF8; Bullinger and Morfeld, 2008), (d) a sociodemographics questionnaire (SOZK; Brueggemann et al., 2016), (e) the German version of the Tinnitus Questionnaire (TQ; Goebel and Hiller, 1998), (f) visual analogue scales measuring tinnitus loudness, frequency, and impairment (TINSKAL), and (g) the Tinnitus Localization and Quality Questionnaire (TLQ; Goebel and Hiller, 1992). These questionnaires were selected to obtain a comprehensive assessment of tinnitus, comorbid conditions (e.g., depressivity), general quality of life and sociodemographic data. Most questionnaire items comprised multiple-choice questions with answers on a Likert scale. The corresponding ordinal variables were handled as continuous variables in the analysis. Categorical variables, as reported sex, marital status, and education level were encoded as dummy variables. For data analysis, a total of 181 variables from the baseline measurements were used as predictors, including the answers to single questionnaire items, subscale scores, total scores and, for each questionnaire, the average time needed to fill in an item. A brief overview of all variables is provided in **Table S1**.

Tinnitus-related distress was measured by the TQ total score (TQ_distress). Depression severity was obtained using the ADSL depression score (ADSL_depression). For TQ_distress and ADSL_depression, treatment effects were calculated as differences between T0 and T1 (denoted as teffect_TQ_distress and teffect_ADSL_depression). Hence, a negative (positive) score indicates that the patient exhibited a lower (higher) score in T1 (after therapy) than in T0 (before therapy).

Patients with incomplete data were excluded, resulting in a total number of 1,628 patients, with clinical data summarized in **Figure 1**. These 828 female (50.9%) and 800 male (49.1%) patients were between 18 and 83 years of age, with an average of 50.2 years (SD = 12.0). Approximately a third (33%) had been suffering from tinnitus (bilateral: 41%, unilateral left: 32%, unilateral right: 26%) for more than 5 years.

2.2. Data Analysis Workflow

Our data analysis workflow consisted of three components, (i) building machine learning models that are capable of separating between female and male patients and building gender-specific models with either tinnitus-related distress, depression severity, or treatment effect of each of these two as target variable, (ii) tuning the models via a hyperparameter grid in a cross-validation scheme, and (iii) identifying variables (questionnaire answers) that contributed most to the models' predictive performances, i.e., were highly associated with the target variables.

2.2.1. Building Classification and Regression Models

We used machine learning classification and regression algorithms to train models on gender, tinnitus-related distress, depression, and treatment response. More specifically, we defined five *learning tasks* (LT) for the following target variables (dependent variables) and data subsets, respectively:

- LT1—target: gender; all patients
- LT2—target: TQ_distress (tinnitus distress) in T0; LT2a: female patients; LT2b: male patients
- LT3—target: ADSL_depression (depression) in T0; LT3a: female patients; LT3b: male patients
- LT4—target: teffect_TQ_distress (treatment effect); LT4a: female patients; LT4b: male patients
- LT5—target: teffect_ADSL_depression; LT5a: female patients; LT5b: male patients.

LT1 has the goal of separating the data on gender and identifying the questionnaire answers and scores that contribute to this separation, i.e., are characteristic of one of the genders. For every learning task, we used variables from baseline (T0) as predictors. Furthermore, we removed variables derived from the same questionnaire as the task's target variable. For example, for LT2, all variables from the TQ questionnaire were excluded since the target variable was calculated from them. The learning tasks LT2, LT3, LT4, and LT5 build models over female patients only and models over male patients only. We denote these models as "F_model," resp. "M_model" hereafter; the learning task is given explicitly, if it cannot be concluded from the context.

We utilized the following five learning algorithms: least absolute shrinkage and selection operator (LASSO; Friedman et al., 2010), RIDGE (Hoerl and Kennard, 1970), support vector machine (SVM; Boser et al., 1992), random forest (RF; Breiman, 2001), and gradient boosted trees (GBT; Friedman, 2001).

2.2.2. Model Evaluation and Parameter Tuning

We used 10-fold stratified cross-validation to evaluate model generalization performance. In k-fold cross-validation, the data is randomly split into k approximately equally-sized partitions. The performance of a model trained on (k-1) partitions is measured by the remaining partition which serves as test set. Finally, the k single performance results are averaged into an overall estimate. For some algorithms, the predictive performance of their models depend substantially on the selection of appropriate hyperparameter values. Therefore, we employed a grid search for hyperparameter selection (cf. listing of parameter candidates in **Table S2**).

For LT1, we used accuracy as primary performance measure and sensitivity as secondary performance measure. Accuracy measures the number of observations that were correctly classified by the model. Sensitivity quantifies the true *positive* rate, i.e., the number of positive observations that were correctly classified as positive. We calculated sensitivity for each gender, respectively. For the remaining learning tasks with quantitative target variables, root mean squared error (RMSE) served as primary performance measure, defined as $RMSE = \sqrt{\frac{1}{N}\sum_{i=1}^{N}(\hat{y}_i - y_i)^2}$, where N is the total number of observations,

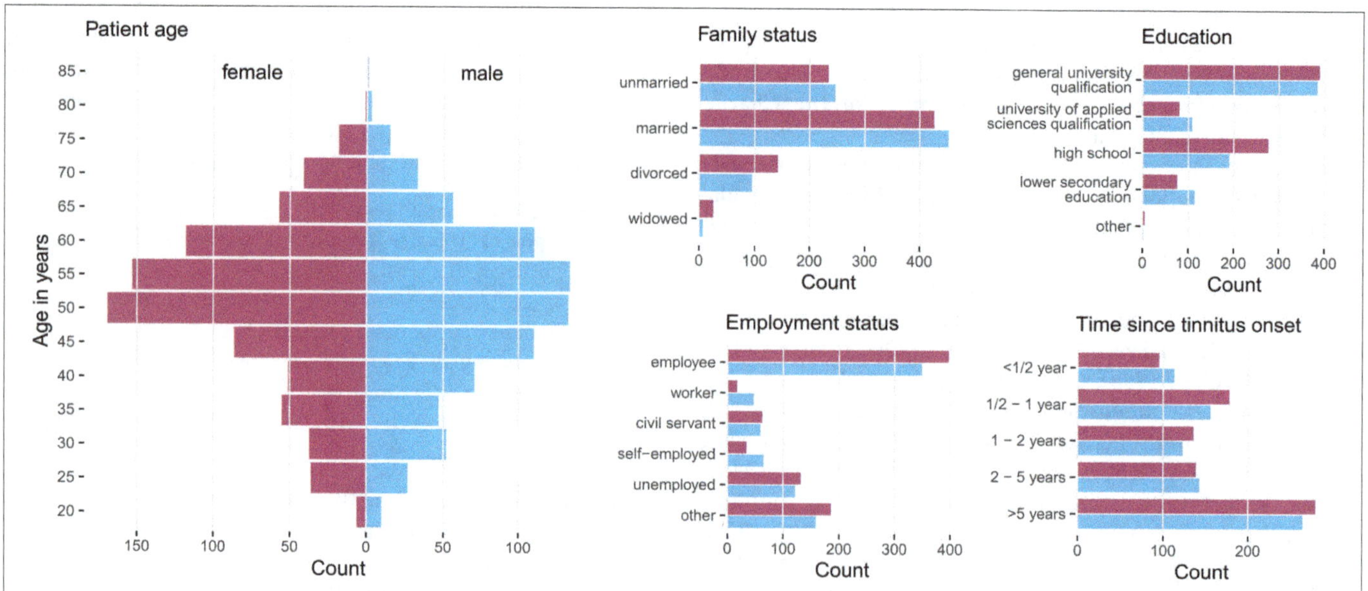

FIGURE 1 | Patient characteristics by gender. Histograms summarizing basic socio-demographic properties and years since tinnitus onset of the patients stratified by gender. Data from 828 female (50.9%) and 800 male (49.1%) patients with chronic tinnitus were considered for data analysis.

$\hat{y}_i$ is the predicted and y_i is the actual value of the target variable for observation i. The secondary performance measure was the coefficient of determination R^2, defined as $R^2 = 1 - \frac{\sum_{i=1}^{N}(\hat{y}_i - y_i)^2}{\sum_{i=1}^{N}(\bar{y} - y_i)^2}$, where $\bar{y}$ is the average predicted value of the model. Higher values are better for all measures except RMSE. Each model was compared against a *baseline*. For the classification problem of LT1, the baseline model always predicted the majority class over all training observations. Similarly, for the regression problems of LT2-5, the average value of a target variable over all training observations was used as prediction for every test instance.

2.2.3. Variable Importance

For each learning task, individual variable attributions toward model prediction were computed using model reliance (MR; Fisher et al., 2018). MR is a permutation-based variable importance measure that calculates the increase in model error when the values of the variable of interest are randomly shuffled within the training set. Suppose f is a variable, m is a model, e_{orig} is the model error on the original training data and e_{perm} is the model error on the training data where the values of f are randomly permuted. Then, the model reliance MR is defined as ratio of $MR(f, m) = \frac{e_{perm}}{e_{orig}}$. If f is important for the prediction of m, $MR(f, m) > 1$. If random permutation of the feature values leads to a higher performance of the model, then the feature's attribute to model quality is low (whereupon $MR < 1$).

For LT1, we identified the questionnaire answers and scores that contributed to separation. For LT2-5, we focused on the variables (i.e., questionnaire items and scales) themselves. To highlight these variables, we used scatterplot diagrams (see **Figure 2**) that express the contribution of a feature (as MR value) to an F_model (x-axis) and M_model (y_axis): features that contribute to both models equally are on a diagonal line, while features with higher MR on the one model are far away from the diagonal. The variables with highest average MR score or highest magnitude in difference between gender-specific MR scores were highlighted with red color.

2.3. Statistical Analysis

Psychometric scores and target variable scores were compared between female and male patients using two-tailed Wilcoxon rank-sum test. Additionally, for treatment effects, it was checked whether the scores were significantly under 0 using left-tailed Wilcoxon rank-sum test. To summarize the distribution of each continuous target variable, median, median absolute deviation, and basic, non-parametric 95% confidence interval using bootstrap sampling (DiCiccio and Efron, 1996) with 2,000 samples was computed. For each model, it was checked whether cross-validation scores of the primary performance measure were significantly better than the ones of the baseline using independent one-tailed Student's t-test (right-tailed for accuracy; left-tailed for RMSE). A significance level of $\alpha = 0.05$ was used for all statistical tests. All p-values were adjusted for multiple comparison using Benjamini-Hochberg correction.

3. RESULTS

Female and male patients ware compared with total scores and subscales of TQ, PSQ, SF8, ADSL, and TINSKAL (cf. **Table 1**). Female patients reported higher tinnitus distress than the male patients, as measured by the TQ total score and its subscales "auditory perceptual difficulties," "sleep disturbances," and "somatic complaints." Further, female patients had higher levels of stress, as measured by the PSQ total score and its subscales "worries," "tension," and "demand." Men scored higher on the mental and physical component of SF8, respectively.

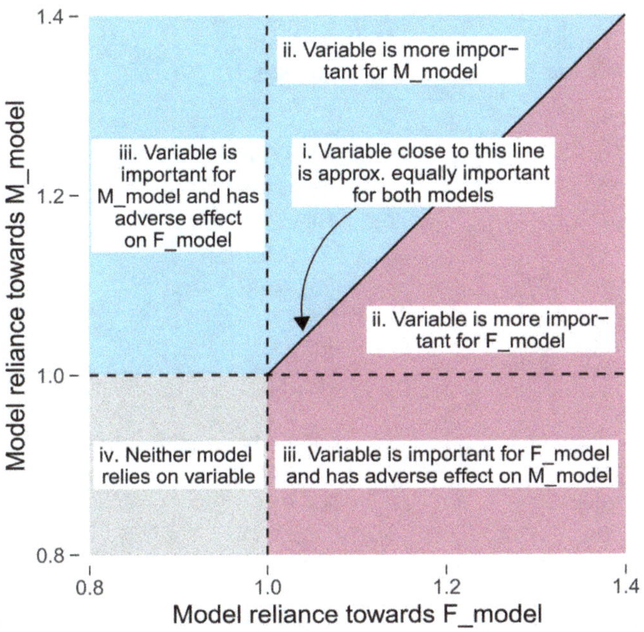

FIGURE 2 | Comparison of gender-specific variable importance. The position of a point represents the model reliance score of a variable with respect to the best model trained on the female patient subset (F_model; x-axis) and the best model trained on the male patient subset (M_model; y-axis). Higher values represent a higher attribution of a variable toward the model prediction. There are four characteristic areas: (i) important variables with similar attributions toward F_model and M_model; (ii) important variables with higher attribution toward one of the gender-specific models; (iii) variables that are important for *either* F_model *or* M_model, but adversarial for the other model; (iv) variables that are adversarial for both models.

Women showed higher levels of depression as measured by ADSL. Women also reported higher tinnitus frequency.

Table 2 provide an overview of all learning tasks (LT), distributions of the target variables, and the models' predictive performances.

3.1. Female Tinnitus Patients Reported Higher Levels of Tinnitus-Related Distress, Depression Severity, and Associated Treatment Effects (RQ1)

At baseline, female patients reported higher tinnitus-related distress (Median 39.00 vs. 35.50, $p < 0.01$) and depression severity (18.00 vs. 14.00, $p < 0.01$) (cf. **Table 2**). Using the TQ cutoff for tinnitus distress (>46; Goebel and Hiller, 1998), 34.1% of female and 30.8% of male subjects exhibited decompensated tinnitus. Using the ADSL cutoff for depression severity (>15; Hautzinger and Bailer, 2002), 57.4% of female and 45.0% of male subjects showed a clinical depression. Both patient subgroups improved from multi-modal treatment with respect to tinnitus distress: the median increase in TQ_distress score from T0 to T1 was −6.00 ($p < 0.01$) in female and −5.00 ($p < 0.01$) in male patients. For depression severity, both patient groups improved significantly (female: −4.00, $p < 0.01$; male: -3.00, $p < 0.01$). There were significant differences between female and male patients in treatment effects of tinnitus-related distress (median: −1.00, $p = 0.04$) and depression (median: −1.00, $p < 0.01$), respectively.

3.2. Learning Task 1: Female Patients Reported Higher Levels of Stress and Tension; Gender Differences in Tinnitus Quality (RQ2)

We compared the five classifiers in **Table 2** (LT1) and found that RIDGE achieves best cross-validation accuracy (72.19 ± 2.94%), with a sensitivity of 71.41 ± 5.46% for female patients and 73.02 ± 4.30% for male patients. **Figure 3** depicts item answer frequencies for the variables with the highest attribution toward model prediction quality: we show the variables in the top-5% of model reliance (MR). There are eight such variables, depicted in **Figures 3A–E**, ordered by MR value. For each variable, the horizontal legend depicts the text of the questionnaire item corresponding to this variable and the vertical axis shows the answers to this item. The horizontal axis shows the relative frequency per gender. These frequencies are shown as horizontal bars, red-violet for female patients and blue for male ones. A difference in the length of the two bars for the same answer means that the likelihood of giving this answer was different for each gender, and thus it contributes to class separation. ADSL_adsl17 (**Figure 3A**) was found to be the most discriminatory variable for the model (MR = 1.167): whereas 16% of female patients reported to had crying spells either "mostly" or "occasionally" during the previous week, the same number was just 4% in male patients, who predominantly gave the answer "rarely" (86.2%). Female patients tended to express higher levels of worries (cf. **Figures 3B,F**) and subjective stress (cf. **Figure 3H**). Furthermore, differences in tinnitus quality were found: more than half (52.4%) of all male patients reported the tinnitus sound (MR = 1.056) to be "whistling," which was considerably higher than in female patients (35.6%) who described their tinnitus as a "rustling" noise more often (33.3%) than male patients (22.9%).

3.3. Learning Task 2: Variables Measuring Depression, Sleep Problems, Tinnitus Frequency, and Loudness Were Associated With Tinnitus-Related Distress in Both Genders (RQ3)

We ran the five algorithms once for the female patients (block LT2a in **Table 2**) and once for the male patients (block LT2b in **Table 2**), classifying on tinnitus distress at baseline. **Table 2** shows RMSE and R^2 for each algorithm. For LT2a (female patients) and LT2b (male patients), GBT had best performance with respect to RMSE (LT2a: 10.92 ± 0.68, LT2b: 10.11 ± 1.12) and R^2 (LT2a: 0.55 ± 0.04, LT2b: 0.68 ± 0.06). We found that GBT and all other models were slightly more accurate for male patients than for female ones. The highest variable attribution according to model reliance (MR) was achieved by TINSKAL_impairment,

TABLE 1 | Comparison of psychometric scores between female and male patients.

Scale	Total (*N* = 1,628)	Female (*n* = 828)	Male (*n* = 800)	p-value
TQ				
Total score	38.53 ±17.18	39.95 ±16.34	37.06 ±17.89	<0.01*
Emotional distress	10.70 ± 5.68	10.88 ± 5.47	10.52 ± 5.88	0.136
Cognitive distress	6.82 ± 4.08	6.97 ± 3.99	6.67 ± 4.16	0.099
Psychological distress	17.53 ± 9.33	17.85 ± 9.01	17.19 ± 9.65	0.099
Intrusiveness	10.31 ± 3.67	10.49 ± 3.47	10.12 ± 3.87	0.130
Auditory perceptual difficulties	5.12 ± 3.70	5.41 ± 3.63	4.82 ± 3.74	<0.01*
Sleep disturbances	3.43 ± 2.54	3.74 ± 2.50	3.11 ± 2.54	<0.01*
Somatic complaints	2.15 ± 1.93	2.46 ± 1.94	1.82 ± 1.86	<0.01*
PSQ				
Total score	0.46 ± 0.18	0.48 ± 0.18	0.43 ± 0.19	<0.01*
Worries	0.39 ± 0.23	0.41 ± 0.22	0.37 ± 0.23	<0.01*
Tension	0.57 ± 0.23	0.61 ± 0.22	0.53 ± 0.24	<0.01*
Demand	0.49 ± 0.24	0.53 ± 0.24	0.46 ± 0.24	<0.01*
Joy	0.49 ± 0.23	0.48 ± 0.23	0.49 ± 0.23	0.182
SF8				
Mental component	41.34 ±12.10	40.16 ±11.80	42.55 ±12.29	<0.01*
Physical component	45.42 ± 9.71	44.44 ± 9.79	46.42 ± 9.53	<0.01*
ADSL				
Depressivity	17.93 ±11.60	19.33 ±11.44	16.48 ±11.59	<0.01*
TINSKAL				
Tinnitus impairment	4.99 ± 2.59	4.97 ± 2.66	5.02 ± 2.52	0.992
Tinnitus loudness	5.03 ± 2.62	4.95 ± 2.72	5.11 ± 2.51	0.486
Tinnitus frequency	8.09 ± 3.00	7.82 ± 3.24	8.37 ± 2.69	<0.01*

Values are reported as mean ± SD. p-values were calculated using independent two-tailed Wilcoxon test adjusted for multiple comparison using Benjamini-Hochberg correction. Asterisks denote significant differences between female and male patients with a significance level of $\alpha = 0.05$. ADSL: General Depression Scale-long form (Radloff, 1977; Hautzinger and Bailer, 2002); PSQ: Perceived Stress Questionnaire (Fliege et al., 2005); SF8: Short Form-8 Health Survey (Bullinger and Morfeld, 2008); TINSKAL: visual analogue scales measuring tinnitus loudness, frequency and impairment; TQ: German version of the Tinnitus Questionnaire (Goebel and Hiller, 1998).

tinnitus impairment measured by the TINSKAL visual analogue scale, with higher attribution toward the model on male patients (MR = 1.42 vs. 1.24; cf. **Figure 4A**). Further, the variables ADSL_depression (depressivity), ADSL_adsl11 (sleep problems), and TINSKAL_loudness (tinnitus loudness) were found to be important for both models. Only 8 out of all 120 variables were found with a substantial attribution of $MR > 1.05$ for either of the gender-specific models.

3.4. Learning Task 3: Indicators of Mental Health, Stress, and Worries Associated With Depression in Both Genders (RQ3)

For depression severity at T0 (cf. **Table 2** block LT3a and 3b), LASSO yielded the best model for both female patients (RMSE = 5.80 ± 0.73; R^2 = 0.74 ± 0.06) and male patients (RMSE = 5.10 ± 0.38; R^2 = 0.81 ± 0.03). Similarly to LT2, RMSE, and R^2 estimates were better for the models on the subset of male patients. **Figure 4B** shows that SF8_mentalhealth (mental health score) was the most important predictor for both F_model and M_model. Further, indicators of subjective stress (PSQ_stress05: "You feel lonely or isolated."), worries (PSQ_worries) and vitality (SF8_sf05: "During the past 4 weeks, how much energy did you have?") contributed considerably to prediction of both genders' models.

3.5. Learning Tasks 4 and 5: Treatment Effect Cannot Be Reliably Predicted Using Baseline Data Only

Models trained to predict treatment effects yielded low generalization performance. Comparison of the regression algorithms in **Table 2** (LT4a and LT4b) showed that the random forest model performed best predicting treatment effect on tinnitus-related distress in female patients (RMSE = 9.55 ± 0.84) as well as in male patients (RMSE = 9.34 ± 1.31). For the prediction of the treatment effect of depression LASSO (LT5a; RMSE = 8.21 ± 0.77) and GBT (LT5b; RMSE = 6.79 ± 0.73) performed best. All four models were just marginally better than the second-best models, respectively (**Table 2**). As for the other learning tasks, model performance on the male subset was better.

While all models of LT 1, 2a, 2b, 3a, and 3b outperformed the baselines, neither of the models predicting the treatment effect of tinnitus-related distress (LT4a and LT4b) or depressivity (LT5a and LT5b) was significantly better than the baselines. Hence, due

TABLE 2 | Performance of classification and regression models for each learning task (LT).

LT	Target	Target distribution	Method	Accuracy [%]	Sens. ♀[%]	Sens. ♂[%]
1	Gender	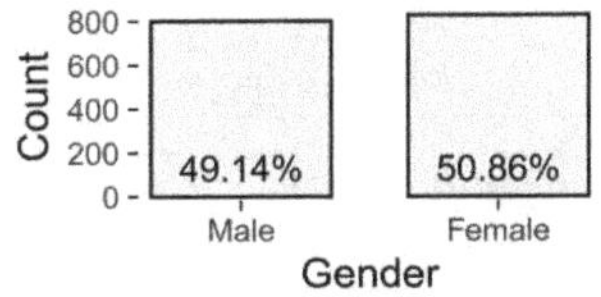	RIDGE	72.19±2.94*	71.41±5.46	73.02±4.30
			SVM	71.82 ± 3.66*	70.93 ± 5.17	72.70 ± 6.00
			LASSO	71.33 ± 3.03*	69.49 ± 4.23	73.19 ± 4.88
			GBT	70.35 ± 3.36*	70.91 ± 5.05	69.72 ± 6.20
			RF	68.63 ± 5.24*	68.67 ± 5.95	68.58 ± 7.14

LT	Subset	Target	Target distribution	Method	RMSE	R^2
2a	only ♀	TQ_distress (T0)	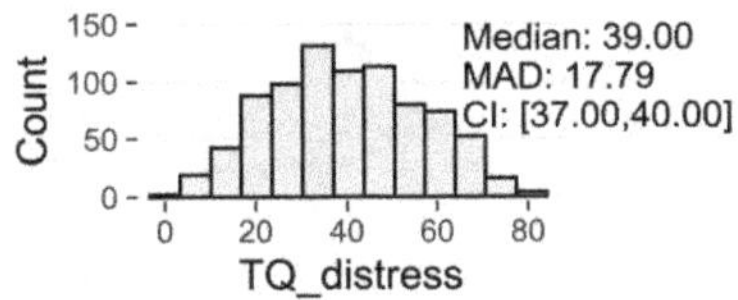	GBT	10.92±0.68*	0.55±0.04
				RF	11.38±0.74*	0.51±0.05
				LASSO	11.55±0.70*	0.50±0.04
				RIDGE	11.59±0.63*	0.50±0.04
				SVM	11.97±0.51*	0.46±0.03
2b	only ♂	TQ_distress (T0)	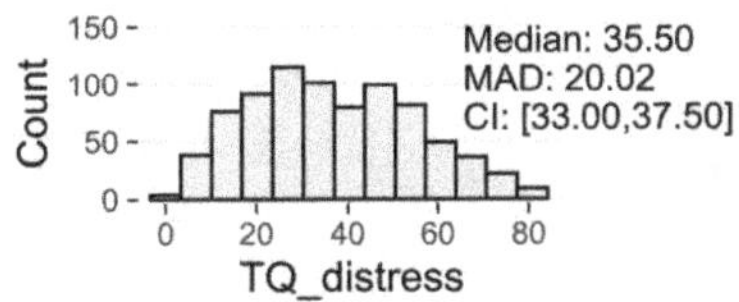	GBT	10.11±1.12*	0.68±0.06
				RF	10.58±1.01*	0.65±0.06
				LASSO	10.59±0.98*	0.65±0.05
				RIDGE	10.72±1.05*	0.64±0.06
				SVM	11.21±1.02*	0.61±0.06
3a	only ♀	ADSL_depression (T0)	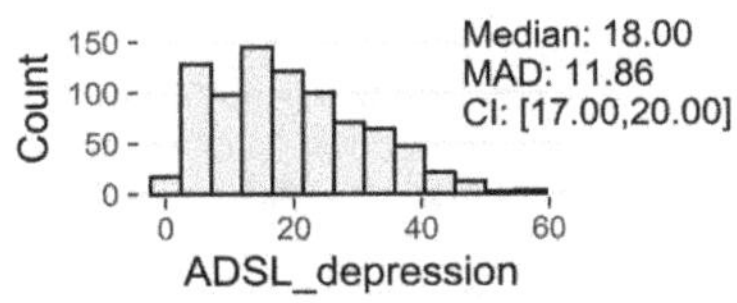	LASSO	5.80±0.73*	0.74±0.06
				GBT	5.88±0.65*	0.74±0.06
				RF	6.02±0.62*	0.72±0.05
				GBT	6.10±0.65*	0.72±0.06
				SVM	6.12±0.72*	0.71±0.06
3b	only ♂	ADSL_depression (T0)	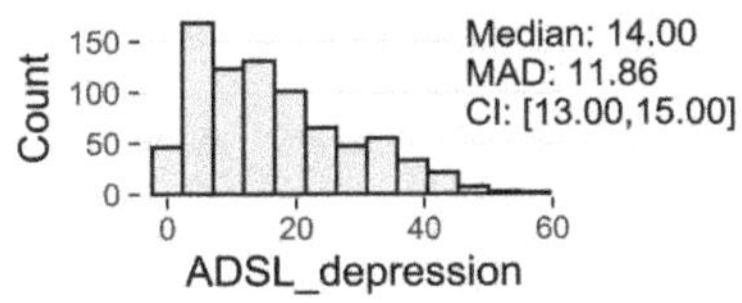	LASSO	5.10±0.38*	0.81±0.03
				RIDGE	5.14±0.38*	0.80±0.03
				GBT	5.16±0.42*	0.80±0.04
				SVM	5.29±0.38*	0.79±0.03
				RF	5.29±0.46*	0.79±0.04
4a	only ♀	Treatment effect TQ_distress (T0 → T1)	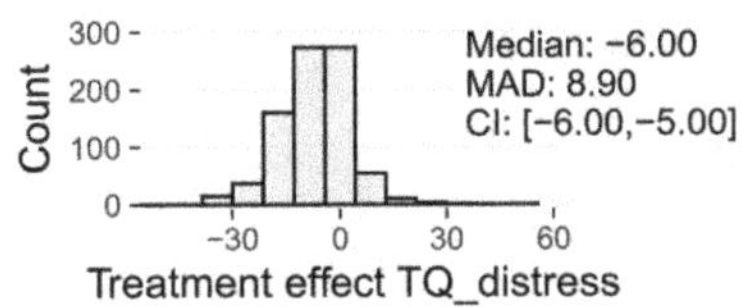	RF	9.55±0.84	0.02±0.09
				RIDGE	9.58±0.82	0.01±0.09
				GBT	9.59±0.82	0.01±0.08
				LASSO	9.61±0.82	0.01±0.08
				SVM	9.64±0.83	0.00±0.09
4b	only ♂	Treatment effect TQ_distress (T0 → T1)	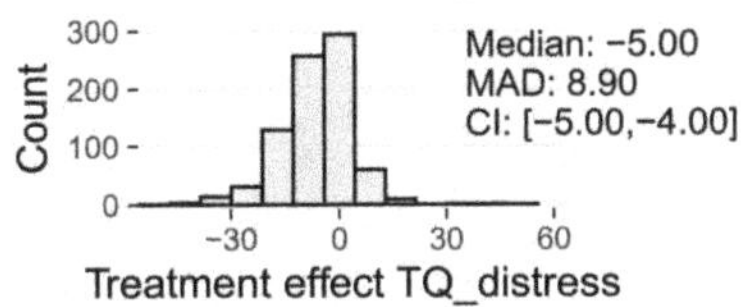	RF	9.34±1.31	0.04±0.14
				LASSO	9.41±1.34	0.03±0.14
				RIDGE	9.43±1.31	0.03±0.14
				GBT	9.54±1.32	0.00±0.14
				SVM	9.55±1.36	0.00±0.14
5a	only ♀	Treatment effect ADSL_depression (T0 → T1)	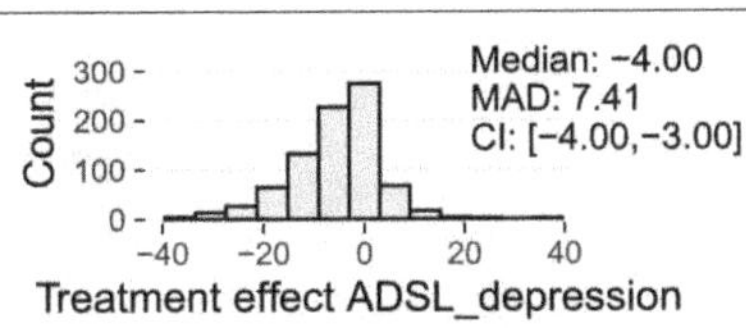	LASSO	8.21±0.77	0.14±0.09
				RIDGE	8.21±0.80	0.14±0.09
				RF	8.23±0.73	0.13±0.08
				SVM	8.26±0.84	0.13±0.10
				GBT	8.26±0.77	0.13±0.09
5b	only ♂	Treatment effect ADSL_depression (T0 → T1)	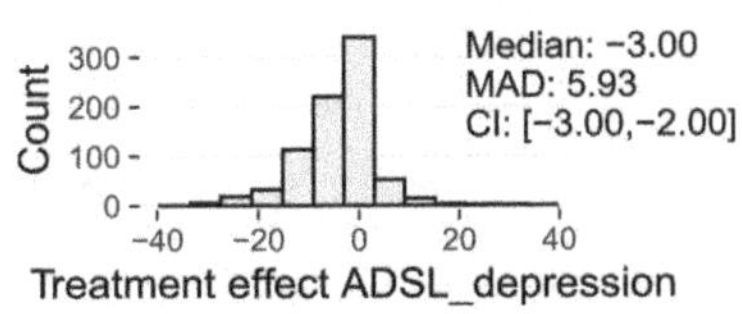	GBT	6.79±0.73	0.17±0.10
				RF	6.82±0.68	0.16±0.09
				RIDGE	6.84±0.73	0.16±0.10
				LASSO	6.85±0.71	0.15±0.10
				SVM	7.15±0.64	0.08±0.09

Performance values are cross-validation mean ± SD. Algorithms are sorted by primary performance measure, i.e., accuracy for LT1 and RMSE for LT2-5. Asterisks signify models with significantly better cross-validation performance compared to the baseline w.r.t. the primary performance measure (α = 0.05). A bar chart (LT1) and histograms (LT2-5) illustrate the distribution of the target variables. For the numerical targets, median, median absolute deviation (MAD), and 95% bootstrap confidence interval (CI) are depicted.

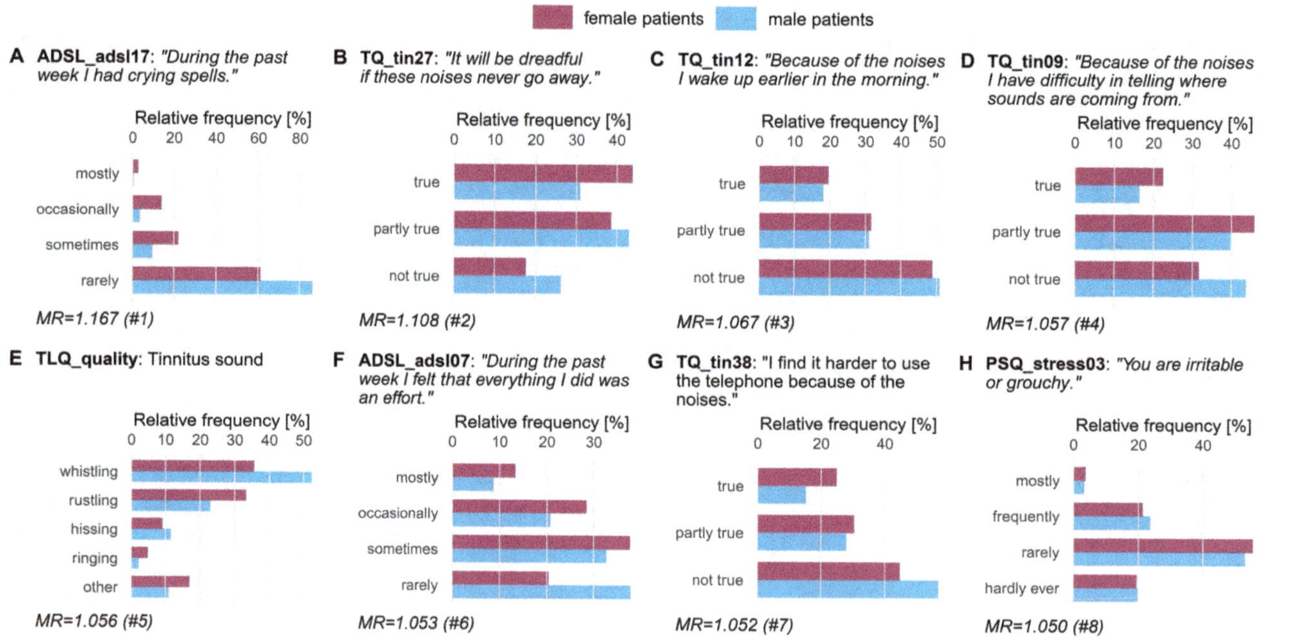

FIGURE 3 | Top-8 variables on gender (LT1). Gender-stratified item answer frequencies for the top-5% variables with the highest attribution toward model prediction quality according to model reliance (MR). ADSL: General Depression Scale–long form (Radloff, 1977; Hautzinger and Bailer, 2002); PSQ: Perceived Stress Questionnaire (Fliege et al., 2005); TLQ: Tinnitus Localization and Quality Questionnaire (Goebel and Hiller, 1992); TQ: German version of the Tinnitus Questionnaire (Goebel and Hiller, 1998).

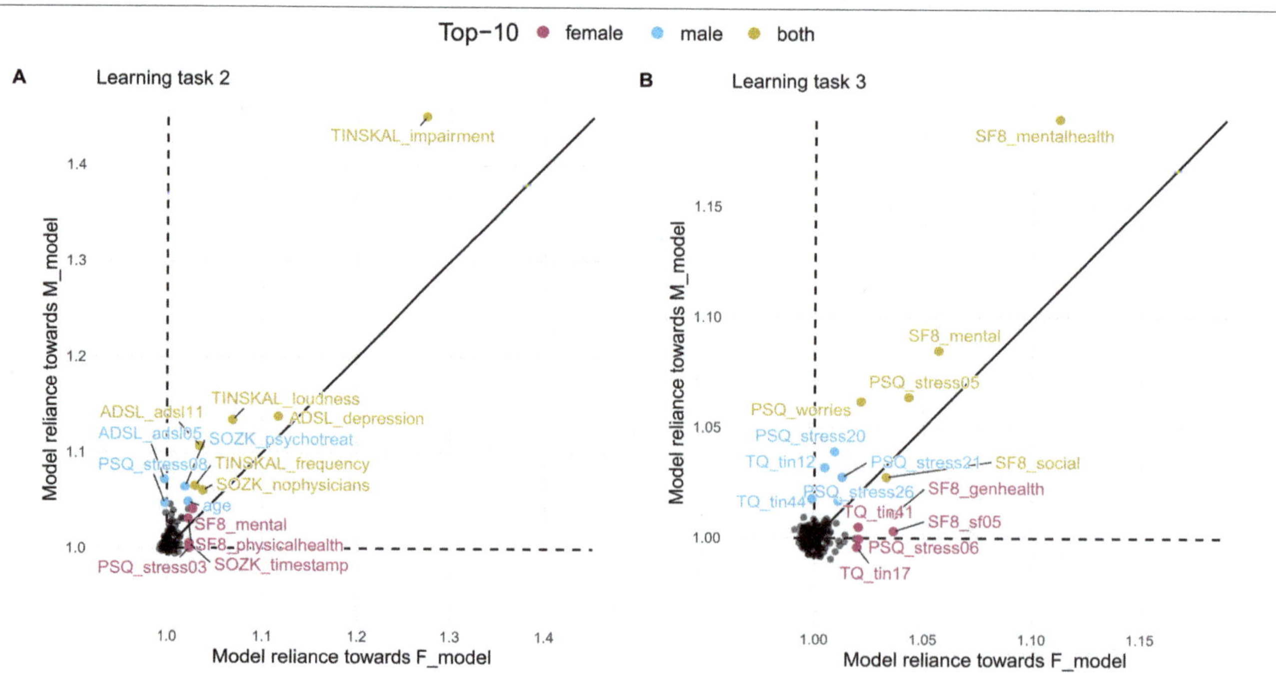

FIGURE 4 | Variable importance for models on tinnitus-related distress and depression. The position of a point represents the model reliance (MR) score of a variable with respect to the best model trained on the female patient subset (F_model; x-axis) and the best model trained on the male patient subset (M_model; y-axis) (cf. **Figure 2**). Variables among the top-10 highest-ranked variables according to MR in the F_model, M_model, or in both models are highlighted by color. **(A)** target variable: tinnitus-related distress; **(B)** target variable: depression severity. ADSL: General Depression Scale–long form (Radloff, 1977; Hautzinger and Bailer, 2002); PSQ: Perceived Stress Questionnaire (Fliege et al., 2005); TLQ: Tinnitus Localization and Quality Questionnaire (Goebel and Hiller, 1992); TQ: German version of the Tinnitus Questionnaire (Goebel and Hiller, 1998).

to the poor predictive quality, we decided not to study variable attributions of these models further.

4. DISCUSSION

We developed a data-driven workflow for the identification of gender-specific differences in patients with chronic tinnitus, solely based on self-report questionnaires measuring tinnitus-related distress, tinnitus frequency, loudness, localization and quality, physical and mental health status, depression severity, perceived stress, and socio-demographics that were extracted at baseline. In agreement with the findings of Seydel et al. (2013), female patients exhibited higher degrees of tinnitus distress and levels of stress than male patients. Although the trained classification models were not robust enough to separate male and female patients with very high confidence (accuracy of best model was 72%), we identified several features with a high attribution toward the model and significant differences between female and male patients, including levels of subjective stress, mood-related difficulties and tension which were higher in female patients, confirming the findings of Hébert et al. (2012), Seydel et al. (2013), and Schlee et al. (2017). Tinnitus quality was different between the genders: where the absolute majority of male patients reported their tinnitus to be a "whistling" sound more variation was observed in female patients. Notably, errors of models trained on the male subgroup were consistently lower across all learning tasks, possibly partly due to a higher variability in answers to questionnaire items in female patients. Gender-specific models exhibited similar indicators of tinnitus-related distress and depression, respectively. In particular, variables measuring similar constructs appeared to be highly relevant, e.g., the TINSKAL visual analogue scale score for tinnitus-related distress and the SF8 mental health score for depression severity. However, there were also differences in the description of tinnitus-related distress and stress experience.

In a previous study (Niemann et al., 2020), we investigated tinnitus-related distress without explicitly stratifying by gender. In agreement to the present study, TINSKAL_impairment as surrogate for TQ_distress and ADSL_depression were found to be the most important variables, gender-independent and specifically for each gender. As gender was not identified among the strongest predictors (Niemann et al., 2020), but possibly masked by other variables, we have emphasized in the present study on differences between female and male tinnitus patients on perceived tinnitus-related distress and depression. Seydel et al. (2013) provided evidence that both gender and age are the most important factors to describe tinnitus-related distress. We have confirmed differences between female and male patients with respect to tinnitus distress, tinnitus frequency, stress, mental, and physical health (cf. **Table 1**, **Figure 3**). For tinnitus-related distress as target variable, age exhibited the 9th (12th) highest model reliance score for the best male (female) model. Since our hypothesis-free approach did not pre-select any variables, we were able to identify other important variables such as TINSKAL_impairment for tinnitus-related distress and SF8_mentalhealth for depression severity.

A potential response bias [e.g., a social desirability bias (Kloostra et al., 2015; Strumila et al., 2017)], subjective judgment and differences in the experience of disorders may explain gender inconsistencies regarding self-assessment of tinnitus distress. These differences should always be considered while inspecting of results from questionnaires and may justify the development of gender-specific treatment strategies in the context of an individualized therapy. Gender differences in treatment effect with respect to tinnitus-related distress and depression severity were small but significant, despite the uniform therapy program. The treatment effect on tinnitus-related distress or depression severity could not be reliably predicted based on measurements in T0 only. Hence, future studies could investigate the potential of modular treatment procedures that combine basic, gender-specific, and individual components.

ETHICS STATEMENT

The studies involving human participants were reviewed and approved by ethics committee of the Charité Universitaetsmedizin Berlin (https://ethikkommission.charite.de/en/). The patients/participants provided their written informed consent to participate in this study.

AUTHOR CONTRIBUTIONS

UN designed and performed the data analysis and wrote the original draft. BB, PB, and BM curated the datasets. BB, PB, BM, and MS supervised the data analysis and reviewed and edited the manuscript. BM and MS led the project.

REFERENCES

Andersson, G. (2002). Psychological aspects of tinnitus and the application of cognitive-behavioral therapy. *Clin. Psychol. Rev.* 22, 977–990. doi: 10.1016/S0272-7358(01)00124-6

Andersson, G., and Lyttkens, L. (1999). A meta-analytic review of psychological treatments for tinnitus. *Br. J. Audiol.* 33, 201–210. doi: 10.3109/03005369909090101

Asher, M., Asnaani, A., and Aderka, I. M. (2017). Gender differences in social anxiety disorder: a review. *Clin. Psychol. Rev.* 56, 1–12. doi: 10.1016/j.cpr.2017.05.004

Boser, B. E., Guyon, I. M., and Vapnik, V. N. (1992). "A training algorithm for optimal margin classifiers," in *Proceedings of Workshop on Computational Learning Theory* (Pittsburgh, PA: ACM), 144–152. doi: 10.1145/130385.130401

Breiman, L. (2001). Random forests. *Mach. Learn.* 45, 5–32. doi: 10.1023/A:1010933404324

Brueggemann, P., Szczepek, A. J., Rose, M., McKenna, L., Olze, H., and

Mazurek, B. (2016). Impact of multiple factors on the degree of tinnitus distress. *Front. Hum. Neurosci.* 10:341. doi: 10.3389/fnhum.2016.00341

Bullinger, M., and Morfeld, M. (2008). "Der SF-36 health survey," in *Gesundheitsökonomische Evaluationen*, eds O. Schöffski, O. and J.-M. G. von der Schulenburg (Berlin; Heidelberg: Springer-Verlag), 387–402. doi: 10.1007/978-3-540-49559-8_15

Cima, R. F., Andersson, G., Schmidt, C. J., and Henry, J. A. (2014). Cognitive-behavioral treatments for tinnitus: a review of the literature. *J. Am. Acad. Audiol.* 25, 29–61. doi: 10.3766/jaaa.25.1.4

Cima, R. F., Maes, I. H., Joore, M. A., Scheyen, D. J., El Refaie, A., Baguley, D. M., et al. (2012). Specialised treatment based on cognitive behaviour therapy versus usual care for tinnitus: a randomised controlled trial. *Lancet* 379, 1951–1959. doi: 10.1016/S0140-6736(12)60469-3

DiCiccio, T. J., and Efron, B. (1996). Bootstrap confidence intervals. *Stat. Sci.* 189–212. doi: 10.1214/ss/1032280214

Eggermont, J. J., and Roberts, L. E. (2004). The neuroscience of tinnitus. *Trends Neurosci.* 27, 676–682. doi: 10.1016/j.tins.2004.08.010

Erlandsson, S. I., Hallberg, L. R., and Axelsson, A. (1992). Psychological and audiological correlates of perceived tinnitus severity. *Audiology* 31, 168–179. doi: 10.3109/00206099209072912

Fisher, A., Rudin, C., and Dominici, F. (2018). All Models are Wrong, but Many are Useful: Learning a Variable's Importance by Studying an Entire Class of Prediction Models Simultaneously. *J. Mach. Learn. Res.* 20, 1–81. Available online at: http://jmlr.org/papers/v20/18-760.html

Fliege, H., Rose, M., Arck, P., Walter, O. B., Kocalevent, R.-D., Weber, C., et al. (2005). The Perceived Stress Questionnaire (PSQ) reconsidered: validation and reference values from different clinical and healthy adult samples. *Psychosom. Med.* 67, 78–88. doi: 10.1097/01.psy.0000151491.80178.78

Friedman, J., Hastie, T., and Tibshirani, R. (2010). Regularization paths for generalized linear models via coordinate descent. *J. Stat. Softw.* 33, 1–22. doi: 10.18637/jss.v033.i01

Friedman, J. H. (2001). Greedy function approximation: a gradient boosting machine. *Ann. Stat.* 1189–1232. doi: 10.1214/aos/1013203451

Goebel, G., and Hiller, W. (1992). Psychische beschwerden bei chronischem tinnitus: erprobung und evaluation des tinnitus-fragebogens (TF). *Verhaltenstherapie* 2, 13–22. doi: 10.1159/000258202

Goebel, G., and Hiller, W. (1998). Tinnitus-Fragebogen:(TF); ein Instrument zur Erfassung von Belastung und Schweregrad bei Tinnitus; Handanweisung. Göttingen; Bern; Toronto, ON: hogrefe, Verlag für Psychologie. Availale online at: https://www.testzentrale.de/shop/handanweisung-49444.html

Halford, J. B., and Anderson, S. D. (1991). Tinnitus severity measured by a subjective scale, audiometry and clinical judgement. *J. Laryngol. Otol.* 105, 89–93. doi: 10.1017/S0022215100115038

Han, T. S., Jeong, J.-E., Park, S.-N., and Kim, J. J. (2019). Gender differences affecting psychiatric distress and tinnitus severity. *Clin. Psychopharmacol. Neurosci.* 17:113. doi: 10.9758/cpn.2019.17.1.113

Hautzinger, M., and Bailer, M. (2002). "ADS-allgemeine depressions skala," in *Diagnostische Verfahren in der Psychotherapie* (Beltz), eds E. Brähler, J. Schumacher, and B. Strauβ (Göttingen: Hogrefe) 25–27.

Hébert, S., Canlon, B., and Hasson, D. (2012). Emotional exhaustion as a predictor of tinnitus. *Psychother. Psychosom.* 81:324. doi: 10.1159/000335043

Hiller, W., and Goebel, G. (2006). Factors influencing tinnitus loudness and annoyance. *Arch. Otolaryngol. Head Neck Surg.* 132, 1323–1330. doi: 10.1001/archotol.132.12.1323

Hoerl, A. E., and Kennard, R. W. (1970). Ridge regression: biased estimation for nonorthogonal problems. *Technometrics* 12, 55–67. doi: 10.1080/00401706.1970.10488634

Jaussent, I., Dauvilliers, Y., Ancelin, M.-L., Dartigues, J.-F., Tavernier, B., Touchon, J., et al. (2011). Insomnia symptoms in older adults: associated factors and gender differences. *Am. J. Geriatr. Psychiatry* 19, 88–97. doi: 10.1097/JGP.0b013e3181e049b6

Kloostra, F. J., Arnold, R., Hofman, R., and Van Dijk, P. (2015). Changes in tinnitus after cochlear implantation and its relation with psychological functioning. *Audiol. Neurotol.* 20, 81–89. doi: 10.1159/000365959

Kuk, F. K., Tyler, R. S., Russell, D., and Jordan, H. (1990). The psychometric properties of a tinnitus handicap questionnaire. *Ear Hear.* 11, 434–445. doi: 10.1097/00003446-199012000-00005

Langguth, B., Kreuzer, P. M., Kleinjung, T., and De Ridder, D. (2013). Tinnitus: causes and clinical management. *Lancet Neurol.* 12, 920–930. doi: 10.1016/S1474-4422(13)70160-1

Langguth, B., Landgrebe, M., Kleinjung, T., Sand, G. P., and Hajak, G. (2011). Tinnitus and depression. *World J. Biol. Psychiatry* 12, 489–500. doi: 10.3109/15622975.2011.575178

Langguth, B., Salvi, R., and Elgoyhen, A. B. (2009). Emerging pharmacotherapy of tinnitus. *Expert Opin. Emerg. Drugs* 14, 687–702. doi: 10.1517/14728210903206975

Lugo, A., Trpchevska, N., Liu, X., Biswas, R., Magnusson, C., Gallus, S., et al. (2019). Sex-specific association of tinnitus with suicide attempts. *JAMA Otolaryngol. Head Neck Surg.* 145, 685–687. doi: 10.1001/jamaoto.2019.0566

Matud, M. P. (2004). Gender differences in stress and coping styles. *Pers. Individ. Differ.* 37, 1401–1415. doi: 10.1016/j.paid.2004.01.010

McCormack, A., Edmondson-Jones, M., Somerset, S., and Hall, D. (2016). A systematic review of the reporting of tinnitus prevalence and severity. *Hear. Res.* 337, 70–79. doi: 10.1016/j.heares.2016.05.009

McLean, C. P., Asnaani, A., Litz, B. T., and Hofmann, S. G. (2011). Gender differences in anxiety disorders: prevalence, course of illness, comorbidity and burden of illness. *J. Psychiatr. Res.* 45, 1027–1035. doi: 10.1016/j.jpsychires.2011.03.006

Meric, C., Gartner, M., Collet, L., and Chéry-Croze, S. (1998). Psychopathological profile of tinnitus sufferers: evidence concerning the relationship between tinnitus features and impact on life. *Audiol. Neurotol.* 3, 240–252. doi: 10.1159/000013796

Newman, C. W., Jacobson, G. P., and Spitzer, J. B. (1996). Development of the tinnitus handicap inventory. *Arch. Otolaryngol. Head Neck Surg.* 122, 143–148. doi: 10.1001/archotol.1996.01890140029007

Niemann, U., Boecking, B., Brueggemann, P., Mebus, W., Mazurek, B., and Spiliopoulou, M. (2020). Tinnitus-related distress after multimodal treatment can be characterized using a key subset of baseline variables. *PLoS ONE* 15:e228037. doi: 10.1371/journal.pone.0228037

Nolen-Hoeksema, S. (2001). Gender differences in depression. *Curr. Direct. Psychol. Sci.* 10, 173–176. doi: 10.1111/1467-8721.00142

Piccinelli, M., and Wilkinson, G. (2000). Gender differences in depression: critical review. *Br. J. Psychiatry* 177, 486–492. doi: 10.1192/bjp.177.6.486

Pinto, P. C. L., Sanchez, T. G., and Tomita, S. (2010). The impact of gender, age and hearing loss on tinnitus severity. *Braz. J. Otorhinolaryngol.* 76, 18–24. doi: 10.1590/S1808-86942010000100004

Radloff, L. S. (1977). The CES-D scale: a self-report depression scale for research in the general population. *Appl. Psychol. Meas.* 1, 385–401. doi: 10.1177/014662167700100306

Schlee, W., Hall, D. A., Edvall, N. K., Langguth, B., Canlon, B., and Cederroth, C. R. (2017). Visualization of global disease burden for the optimization of patient management and treatment. *Front. Med.* 4:86. doi: 10.3389/fmed.2017.00086

Seydel, C., Haupt, H., Olze, H., Szczepek, A. J., and Mazurek, B. (2013). Gender and chronic tinnitus: differences in tinnitus-related distress depend on age and duration of tinnitus. *Ear Hear.* 34, 661–672. doi: 10.1097/AUD.0b013e31828149f2

Strumila, R., Lengvenytė, A., Vainutienė, V., and Lesinskas, E. (2017). The role of questioning environment, personality traits, depressive and anxiety symptoms in tinnitus severity perception. *Psychiatr. Q.* 88, 865–877. doi: 10.1007/s11126-017-9502-2

Svensson, A. C., Fredlund, P., Laflamme, L., Hallqvist, J., Alfredsson, L., Ekbom, A., et al. (2012). Cohort profile: the stockholm public health cohort. *Int. J. Epidemiol.* 42, 1263–1272. doi: 10.1093/ije/dys126

Wilson, P. H., Henry, J., Bowen, M., and Haralambous, G. (1991). Tinnitus reaction questionnaire: psychometric properties of a measure of distress associated with tinnitus. *J. Speech Lang. Hear. Res.* 34, 197–201. doi: 10.1044/jshr.3401.197

21

Disrupted Intraregional Brain Activity and Functional Connectivity in Unilateral Acute Tinnitus Patients with Hearing Loss

Gang-Ping Zhou[1†], Xin-Yi Shi[2†], Heng-Le Wei[1], Li-Jie Qu[1], Yu-Sheng Yu[1], Qing-Qing Zhou[1], Xindao Yin[3], Hong Zhang[1] and Yue-Jin Tao[2*]*

[1] Department of Radiology, The Affiliated Jiangning Hospital of Nanjing Medical University, Nanjing, China, [2] Department of ENT, The Affiliated Jiangning Hospital of Nanjing Medical University, Nanjing, China, [3] Department of Radiology, Nanjing First Hospital, Nanjing Medical University, Nanjing, China

***Correspondence:**
Hong Zhang
jnyyfsk@126.com
Yue-Jin Tao
1125266270@qq.com

† These authors have contributed equally to this work

Purpose: The present study combined fractional amplitude of low-frequency fluctuations (fALFF), regional homogeneity (ReHo), and functional connectivity (FC) to explore brain functional abnormalities in acute tinnitus patients (AT) with hearing loss.

Methods: We recruited twenty-eight AT patients and 31 healthy controls (HCs) and ran resting-state functional magnetic resonance imaging (fMRI) scans. fALFF, ReHo, and FC were conducted and compared between AT patients and HCs. After that, we calculated correlation analyses among abnormal fALFF, ReHo, FC, and clinical data in AT patients.

Results: Compared with HCs, AT showed increased fALFF values in the right inferior temporal gyrus (ITG). In contrast, significantly decreased ReHo values were observed in the cerebellar vermis, the right calcarine cortex, the right precuneus, the right supramarginal gyrus (SMG), and the right middle frontal gyrus (MFG). Based on the differences in the fALFF and ReHo maps, the latter of which we defined as region-of-interest (ROI) for FC analysis, the right ITG exhibited increased connectivity with the right precentral gyrus. In addition, the right MFG demonstrated decreased connectivity with both the bilateral anterior cingulate cortex (ACC) and the left precentral gyrus.

Conclusion: By combining ReHo, fALFF, and FC analyses, our work indicated that AT with hearing loss had abnormal intraregional neural activity and disrupted connectivity in several brain regions which mainly involving the non-auditory area, and these regions are major components of default mode network (DMN), attention network, visual network, and executive control network. These findings will help us enhance the understanding of the neuroimaging mechanism in tinnitus populations. Moreover, these abnormalities remind us that we should focus on the early stages of this hearing disease.

Keywords: tinnitus, fMRI, fALFF, ReHo, FC, DMN

INTRODUCTION

Tinnitus, a common hearing disorder, is often described as a ringing, buzzing, or hissing sensation without any corresponding external auditory source (Jastreboff, 1990; Moller, 2007). It affects approximately 10–15% of the population, especially adults over the age of 65 (Eggermont and Roberts, 2004). Tinnitus can be divided into objective and subjective tinnitus. In rare cases, an objective source can be identified that is susceptible to treatment. However, in many of cases, tinnitus is subjective which is a kind of feeling that cannot be perceived by others. Moreover, tinnitus is related to hearing loss in the majority of cases, as both symptoms often occur together (Mühlnickel et al., 1998). People with tinnitus often suffer from sleep disorders, depression, and anxiety, conditions that reduce the quality of life (Reynolds et al., 2004; Baguley et al., 2013). The tinnitus symptoms can be acute or chronic. In clinical practice, we noticed that acute tinnitus patients (AT) are much more eager to seek for clinical help than chronic tinnitus patients. However, the underlying pathophysiology of tinnitus is still poorly understood.

According to previous studies, the central nervous system (CNS) is believed to play an important role in the pathophysiology of tinnitus (Lockwood et al., 2002; Eggermont, 2005; Bartels et al., 2007). Based on electrophysiological and neuroimaging studies (Lockwood et al., 1998; Kaltenbach et al., 2005), aberrant neural activity in the central auditory pathway may generate tinnitus by a range of mechanisms, such as altered neural synchrony, dysfunctional noise canceling, increased central noise, tonotopic map reorganization, upregulation of spontaneous firing rates, and aberrant neural connectivity between auditory and non-auditory structures. Specifically, the central auditory pathway appears to increase its gain to compensate for the reduced sensorineural input from the cochlea, which results in hyperactivity in the auditory pathway (Eggermont and Roberts, 2004). The neural synchrony increased after a noise-induced hearing loss, particularly for neurons representing the affected part of the tonotopic array, which tends to be spatially coincident with changes in the frequency tuning properties of the same affected neurons (Soleymani et al., 2011). A proposed model suggests that the tinnitus sensation might reach conscious awareness only when aberrant neuronal activity in the primary sensory cortex is connected to a broader cortical network involving frontal, parietal, and limbic regions (De Ridder et al., 2011a). Generally, the noise signal of tinnitus is identified by the limbic system and eliminated from perception ("tuned out") by feeding it back to the (inhibitory) thalamic reticular nucleus, which subtracts it from the afferent auditory signal. When the limbic regions become dysfunctional, noise-cancelation breaks down and the tinnitus signal permeates to the auditory cortex (Rauschecker et al., 2010). Additionally, the thalamic dysrhythmia, a disruption in the normal relay mechanism of the thalamus to the auditory cortex, also contributes the generation of the tinnitus percept (De Ridder et al., 2011b). As subjective tinnitus is an endogenous ongoing process, the neural network has been proven changing over time (Vanneste et al., 2011). Therefore, a better characterization of altered central neural processes in acute tinnitus can offer a better understanding of its physiopathology and may contribute to the development of therapeutic intervention procedures.

Since subjective tinnitus is characterized by highly subjective, intrinsic, and persistent sound hallucinations (Schecklmann et al., 2014), resting-state functional magnetic resonance imaging (rs-fMRI) has proven to be a powerful and non-invasive technique *in vivo* which reflected in the low-frequency (0.01–0.1 Hz) fluctuations in blood-oxygenation-level dependent (BOLD) signals (Mantini et al., 2007; Husain and Schmidt, 2014). Amplitude of low-frequency fluctuation (ALFF) reflects the intensity of regional neuronal activity by measuring intrinsic brain responses at the baseline state (Biswal et al., 1995). It has been proven as an effective method in assessing the altered neural activity of various neurological or psychiatric disorders (Hoptman et al., 2010; Zhang et al., 2010; Wang et al., 2011; Chen et al., 2012a). The pulsatile tinnitus patients have been reported significantly increased ALFF in bilateral precuneus and inferior frontal gyrus and decreased ALFF in multiple occipital area (Han et al., 2014). Another fMRI study using ALFF method reported significantly increased ALFF values within several selected regions which were correlated positively with tinnitus distress and duration (Chen et al., 2014). Compared with ALFF, fractional ALFF (fALFF) shows much more sensitive and specific in detecting regional spontaneous neural activity during the resting state by suppressing the physiological noise (Zou et al., 2008). Therefore, fALFF may be a useful index to reflect the abnormal neural activity in specific brain regions of tinnitus patients. Regional homogeneity (ReHo) is a robust algorithm that quantifies the local synchronization within neighboring voxels during resting state (Zang et al., 2004), which can be used to detect abnormal local neural activity coherence across the whole brain. Altered ReHo values may reflect the disequilibrium of spontaneous neural activity within and between corresponding brain regions. Indeed, aberrant ReHo values, indicative of disrupted local functionality, have been linked to several neurological impairments (Liu et al., 2006; He et al., 2007; Wu et al., 2009; Chen et al., 2012b). Therefore, ReHo measurement is a potentially powerful tool to detect aberrant resting-state brain activity. Based on the main brain regions involved in tinnitus, the ROI-based FC analysis is appropriate, which could accurately explore the characteristics of FC changes in brain regions directly related to tinnitus, and reflects the characteristics of brain network alterations. In previous studies, the auditory network, visual network, attention network, control network and default mode network (DMN) have been reported involving in tinnitus using ROI-based FC (Burton et al., 2012; Husain and Schmidt, 2014; Leaver et al., 2016; Chen et al., 2017a,b, 2018a). These studies have confirmed that FC is an effective method for studying the synchronization of functional activities in different brain regions of tinnitus, which could better reflect the abnormal FC changes in tinnitus brain regions. These three techniques can directly measure the intensity and consistency of neural activity and FC changes between brain regions and have high test-retest reliability. Thus, the combination of these three methods may detect more comprehensively local and regional neural functional changes than either method alone.

As we described above, chronic tinnitus patients showed altered resting-state brain networks including auditory network, visual network, attention network, control network, and DMN. However, the alterations of brain network in AT patients were poorly understood. To achieve this goal, we combined fALFF, ReHo, and FC to explore brain functional abnormalities in AT patients with hearing loss. The study focused on two main hypotheses: (1) altered fALFF, ReHo and FC would be observed between tinnitus patients and a healthy control group; (2)

the abnormal resting-state networks would be correlated with specific tinnitus characteristics.

MATERIALS AND METHODS

Subjects

This study included AT and a healthy control (HC) group with 59 right-handed subjects with at least 8 years of education. Patients were recruited at the Affiliated Jiangning Hospital, Nanjing Medical University from February 2018 to March 2019, including inpatients and outpatients. The selected patients had constant, unilateral tinnitus with sensorineural hearing loss (SHL) in one ear, duration <1 month. The healthy adults were recruited through community health screenings or newspaper advertisements and were matched with tinnitus patients with respect to age, sex, and education. The AT group had 28 (14 male) patients. Among them, 12 patients have tinnitus in the right ear and 16 patients with left ear tinnitus. The HC group consisted of 31 (19 male) subjects. Pure-tone audiometry (PTA) was performed to measure the hearing level at the frequencies of 125, 250, 500, 1000, 2000, 4000, and 8000 Hz. All patients were included if the mean PTA hearing threshold at the frequencies from 0.125 to 8 kHz was greater than 30 dB in one ear. All healthy control group subjects had normal hearing (defined as hearing loss of no more than 25 dB at any of the 7 frequencies). Additionally, individuals were excluded from the study if they had any of these situations, namely, Meniere's disease, pulsatile tinnitus, hyperacusis, a past history of severe alcoholism, smoking, head injury, stroke, Alzheimer's disease, Parkinson's disease, epilepsy, major depression or other neurological or psychiatric illness, major medical illness (e.g., cancer, anemia, and thyroid dysfunction), MRI contraindications or severe visual loss (Chen et al., 2018b). All the subjects provided written informed consent before their participation in the study protocol, which was approved by the Research Ethics Committee of the Nanjing Medical University.

All patients were required to accomplish the tinnitus handicap inventory (THI) questionnaire to assess the severity of their tinnitus (Newman et al., 1996). Higher total scores (from a range of 0 to 100) represent a higher impact of tinnitus on daily life. None of the participants had depression and anxiety according to the self-rating depression scale (SDS) and self-rating anxiety scale (SAS) (overall scores <50 for each). The detailed clinical characteristics and demographics of all participants were listed in **Table 1**.

MRI Data Acquisition

All patients were scanned before any drug treatment. The imaging data were acquired on a 3.0 T MRI scanner (Ingenia, Philips Medical Systems, Netherlands) with an 8-channel receiver array head coil. Head motion and scanner noise were reduced using foam padding and earplugs. All participants were asked to rest quietly with their eyes closed but to remain awake and were instructed not to focus their thoughts on anything in particular during the MR acquisition. First, a three-dimensional turbo fast echo (3D-TFE) T1 WI sequence with high resolution was performed to acquire structural images as follows: repetition time (TR)/echo time (TE) = 8.1/3.7 ms; slices = 170; thickness = 1 mm; gap = 0 mm; flip angle (FA) = 8°; acquisition matrix = 256 × 256; and field of view (FOV) = 256 mm × 256 mm. The structural sequence took 5 min and 29 s. Based on the anatomical images, functional images were obtained with a gradient echo-planar imaging sequence as follows: TR = 2000 ms; TE = 30 ms; slices = 36; thickness = 4 mm; gap = 0 mm; FOV = 240 mm × 240 mm; acquisition matrix = 64 × 64; and FA = 90°. The fMRI sequence took 8 min and 8 s. Finally, the conventional axial T2WI (TR = 4000 ms; TE = 107 ms; slices = 18; thickness = 5 mm; gap = 1.5 mm; FOV = 230 mm × 230 mm; acquisition matrix = 384 × 384; and FA = 90°) and sagittal T2WI FLAIR (TR = 10000 ms; TE = 120 ms; slices = 18; thickness = 5 mm; gap = 1.5 mm; FOV = 220 mm × 220 mm; acquisition matrix = 336 × 189) sequences are performed for excluding intracranial organic lesions.

MRI Data Analyses

Data Preprocessing

Data analyses were performed using the toolbox for Data Processing & Analysis for Brain Imaging (DPABI V3.1[1]) (Yan et al., 2016), which is based on Statistical Parametric Mapping (SPM8[2]). After removing the first 10 volumes, slice-timing, realignment for head motion correction, and nuisance covariate regression were performed. Afterward, the images were spatially normalized to the Montreal Neurological Institute template (resampling voxel size = 3 mm^3 × 3 mm^3 × 3 mm^3). Any subjects with a head motion of >2.0 mm translation or 2.0° rotation in any direction were excluded.

fALFF Analysis

After smoothing (FWHM = 4 mm), detrending and filtering (0.01–0.08 Hz), time courses were converted to the frequency

[1]http://rfmri.org/dpabi
[2]http://www.fil.ion.ucl.ac.uk/spm

TABLE 1 | Demographic and clinical characteristics of participants.

	ATs (*n* = 28)	HCs (*n* = 31)	*P* value
Age (years)	41.2 ± 11.61	45.4 ± 14.32	0.22
Genger (male/female)	14/14	12/19	0.40
Education (years)	13.6 ± 7.34	13.3 ± 3.31	0.81
Handedness (right/left)	28/0	32/0	1.00
Tinnitus laterality (right/left)	12/16	–	–
Duration (days)	7.79 ± 6.56	–	–
PTA of right ear (dB)	60.24 ± 13.56	14.2 ± 2.54	<0.001*
PTA of left ear (dB)	58.52 ± 14.21	14.6 ± 2.62	<0.001*
THI score	30.43 ± 11.89	–	–
SAS score	29.29 ± 4.67	27.32 ± 4.56	0.26
SDS score	27.71 ± 4.98	26.21 ± 4.63	0.33

*Data are presented as mean ± SD. PTA, pure-tone audiometry; THI, tinnitus handicap inventory; SAS, self-rating anxiety scale; SDS, self-rating depression scale. *P < 0.001 (independent-sample t-test, two-tailed), showed statistical difference in hearing threshold between ATs and HCs.*

domain using fast Fourier transform. Then, ALFF was computed by taking the square root of the power spectrum, then averaging and squaring across 0.01–0.08 Hz at each voxel. At last, fALFF was calculated as the ALFF divided by the value of the entire detectable frequency band. Two-sample *t*-tests were performed by using DPABI software (within a group mask) to calculate the fALFF difference between groups, with age, sex, education level, and gray matter (GM) volume as covariates. The result was determined by AlphaSim correction ($P < 0.001$ at the voxel level and $P < 0.01$ at the cluster level). Previous rs-fMRI study provided considerable evidences for abnormal intrinsic brain activity between patients with left-sided hearing impairment and those with right-sided hearing impairment (Xie et al., 2019), which makes this seem like a worthwhile question to explore. Thus, we presented unthresholded t-stat fALFF image for left and right-sided groups (uncorrected, $P < 0.05$, cluster size >20 voxels; Age, sex, education level, and GM volume were included as nuisance covariates).

ReHo Analysis

After bandpass filtering (0.01–0.08 Hz), Kendall's coefficient of concordance was performed to calculate the local synchronization of a given voxel with its 26 nearest neighbors (Zang et al., 2004). Then we standardized the ReHo value of each voxel by partitioning the primal value using the global mean ReHo value. After that, the normalized data were smoothed with a 4 mm full-width at half maximum (FWHM) Gaussian kernel for further statistical analysis. To explore between-group differences, a two-sample *t*-tests were performed under DPABI software. Age, sex, education level, and GM volume were included as nuisance covariates, to control for the possible influences of these factors on the results. A threshold was used by AlphaSim correction ($P < 0.001$ at the voxel level and $P < 0.001$ at the cluster level). As we described in fALFF analysis, the unthresholded t-stat ReHo image was also performed for left and right-sided groups (uncorrected, $P < 0.05$, cluster size >20 voxels; Age, sex, education level, and GM volume were included as nuisance covariates).

FC Analyses

Resting-state FC was also conducted under DPABI software. Based on the fALFF and ReHo findings in the brain regions between groups, we defined six ROIs including the right ITG, the vermis_8, the right calcarine cortex, the right precuneus, the right supramarginal gyrus (SMG), and the right middle frontal gyrus (MFG). The mean time series of each ROI was obtained for the reference time course. Then, Pearson's correlation coefficients were calculated between the mean signal change of each ROI and the time series of each voxel. Finally, a Fisher's *z*-transform was applied to improve the normality of the correlation coefficients (Lowe et al., 1998). Six head motion parameters and mean time series of global, white matter, and cerebrospinal fluid signals were included in the regression analysis to eliminate possible effects of such factors on the results. Two-sample *t*-tests were performed to explore the differences of the FC of each ROI between tinnitus patients and controls. Age, sex, education level, and GM volume were included as covariates. AlphaSim correction was used for the multiple comparisons ($P < 0.001$ at the voxel level and $P < 0.01$ at the cluster level).

Statistical Analysis

Independent two-sample *t* tests and Chi-square tests were performed using SPSS 22.0 software to compare general data and scale scores ($P < 0.05$ were considered to be significant). To explore the abnormalities of the fALFF, ReHo and FC maps between AT and HC group, two-sample *t* tests were analyzed by using DPABI software (within a Group mask). Additionally, we regressed out the impact of age, sex, education level, and GM volume. AlphaSim was used for the multiple comparisons (ReHo analysis: $P < 0.001$ at the voxel level and $P < 0.001$ at the cluster level; fALFF and FC analysis: $P < 0.001$ at the voxel level and $P < 0.01$ at the cluster level). The differences between left and right-sided group were conducted under two-sample *t* tests in DPABI software (within a Group mask), which was uncorrected ($P < 0.05$, cluster size >20 voxels). In addition, age, sex, education level, and GM volume were included as covariates. Pearson correlation analyses and Partial correlation analyses were then conducted between altered fALFF values, ReHo values, FC z-values and AT characteristics in the AT group using SPSS software. The Bonferroni correction for multiple comparisons was applied ($P < 0.05$ were considered statistically significant).

RESULTS

fMRI Data Analyses

Compared to the HCs, AT had significantly increased fALFF values in the right ITG (**Figure 1** and **Table 2**). We did not find any decreased regions between ATs and HCs in the fALFF map. At the same time, AT patients had lower ReHo values in the cerebellar vermis, the right calcarine cortex, the right precuneus, the right SMG, and the right MFG (**Figure 2** and **Table 2**). Moreover, no increased ReHo values were observed in the study. We also did not find any abnormal fALFF and ReHo values in auditory regions.

Compared with the right-sided acute tinnitus group, the left-sided group showed significantly higher fALFF values in the right cerebellar, bilateral middle temporal gyrus (MTG), left ITG, left triangular part inferior frontal gyrus, left superior frontal

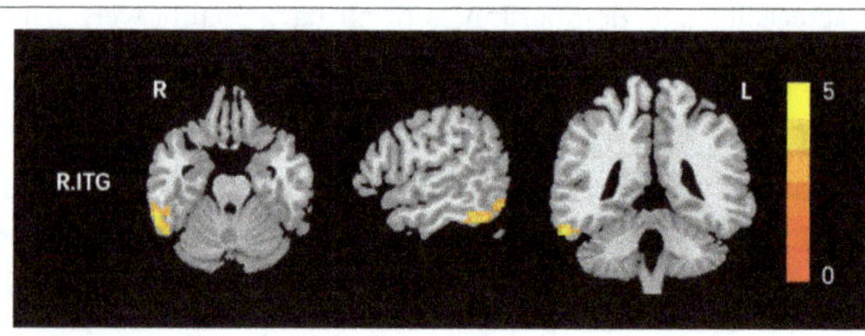

FIGURE 1 | Increased fALFF values between tinnitus patients and healthy controls (HCs). The threshold was determined by AlphaSim correction ($P < 0.001$ at the voxel and $P < 0.01$ at the cluster level). R, right; ITG, inferior temporal gyrus. Red to yellow means Increased fALFF values.

TABLE 2 | fALFF and ReHo differences between tinnitus and healthy controls.

	Brain region	Hemisphere	Peak MNI coordinates (x,y,z)	T score	Cluster size (voxels)
fALFF	Inferior temporal gyrus	R	60, −42, −24	4.8772	77
ReHo	Vermis_8	–	3, −69, −39	−6.089	27
	Calcarine cortex	R	27, −51, 6	−6.5194	22
	Precuneus	R	0, −57, 21	−5.2884	30
	Supramarginal gyrus	R	42, −42, 42	−5.2124	40
	Middle frontal gyrus	R	48, 12, 54	−5.7163	31

fALFF analysis: The threshold was determined by AlphaSim correction ($P < 0.001$ at the voxel and $P < 0.01$ at the cluster level); ReHo analysis: The threshold was determined by AlphaSim correction ($P < 0.001$ at the voxel and $P < 0.01$ at the cluster level). L, left; R, right; MNI, montreal neurological institute.

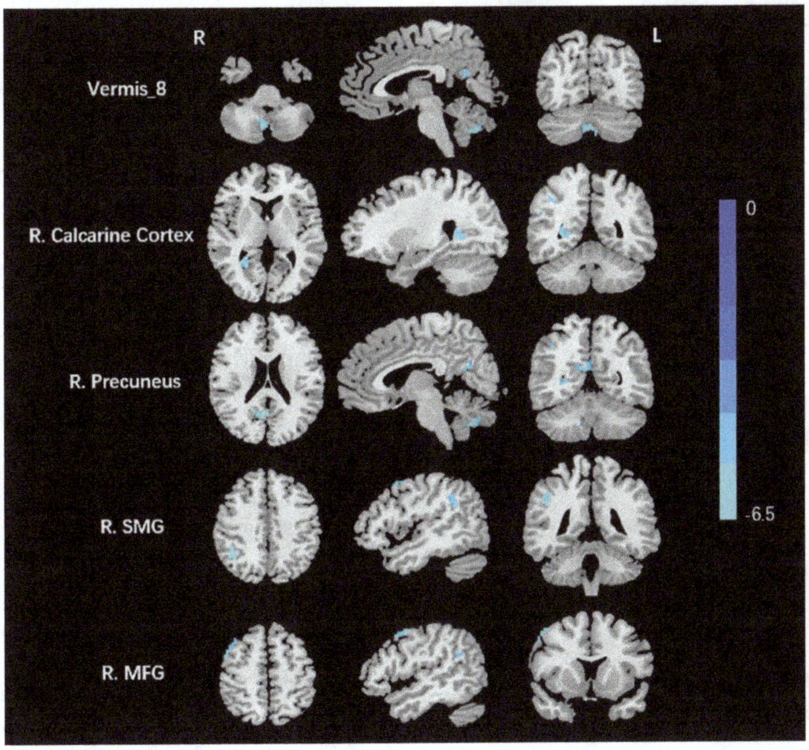

FIGURE 2 | Decreased ReHo values between tinnitus patients and HCs. The threshold was determined by AlphaSim correction ($P < 0.001$ at the voxel and $P < 0.01$ at the cluster level). R, right; SMG, supramarginal gyrus; MFG, middle frontal gyrus. Blue means decreased ReHo values.

gyrus (SFG), and left precentral gyrus; moreover, the left-sided acute tinnitus group showed significantly lower fALFF values in the left postcentral gyrus (**Supplementary Figure S1** and **Supplementary Table S1**). Compared with the right-sided acute tinnitus group, the left-sided group showed significantly higher ReHo values in the bilateral cerebellar, left fusiform gyrus, left MTG, left MFG, left medial superior frontal gyrus, right SMG, and right SFG; moreover, the left-sided acute tinnitus group showed significantly lower ReHo values in the left postcentral gyrus (**Supplementary Figure S2** and **Supplementary Table S1**). Unfortunately, there were no clusters survived under multiple comparison correction.

Based on the increased fALFF and decreased ReHo values in the tinnitus patients, six ROIs were defined for our connectivity analysis: the right ITG of the fALFF map, and the vermis_8, the right calcarine cortex, left precuneus, right SMG, and right MFG of the ReHo map. When we set the seed region in the vermis_8, the right calcarine cortex, the left precuneus, and the right SMG, and there were no significantly altered connectivity found after multiple comparisons correction by using AlphaSim. Compared to the control group, tinnitus patients showed significantly enhanced connectivity between the seed region in the right ITG and the right precentral gyrus (**Table 3** and **Figure 3**). Additionally, the seed region in the right MFG exhibited decreased connectivity with the bilateral anterior cingulate cortex (ACC) and the left precentral gyrus in AT patients (**Table 3** and **Figure 4**).

TABLE 3 | Regions showing seed-based FC differences between tinnitus patients and normal controls.

Seed region	Brain region	Hemisphere	Peak MNI coordinates (x,y,z)	T score	Cluster size (voxels)
R.MFG	Anterior cingulate cortex	B	9, 21, −6	−4.2742	118
	Precentral gyrus	L	−12, −27, 75	−4.5977	148
R.ITG	Precentral gyrus	R	51, −6, 7	4.7588	62

The threshold was determined by AlphaSim correction ($P < 0.001$ at the voxel and $P < 0.01$ at the cluster level). MNI, montreal neurological institute; L, left; R, right; B, bilateral; MFG, middle frontal gyrus; ITG, inferior temporal gyrus.

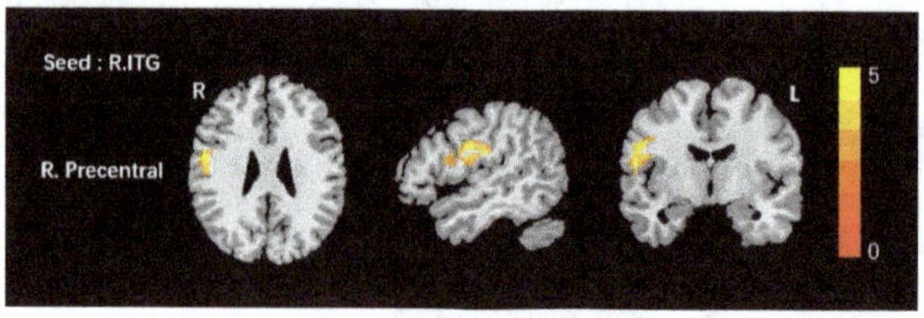

FIGURE 3 | Comparing to HCs, patients showed enhanced connectivity between the seed region in the right ITG and the right precentral gyrus. The threshold was determined by AlphaSim correction ($P < 0.001$ at the voxel and $P < 0.01$ at the cluster level). R, right; ITG, inferior temporal gyrus. Red to yellow means increased connectivity.

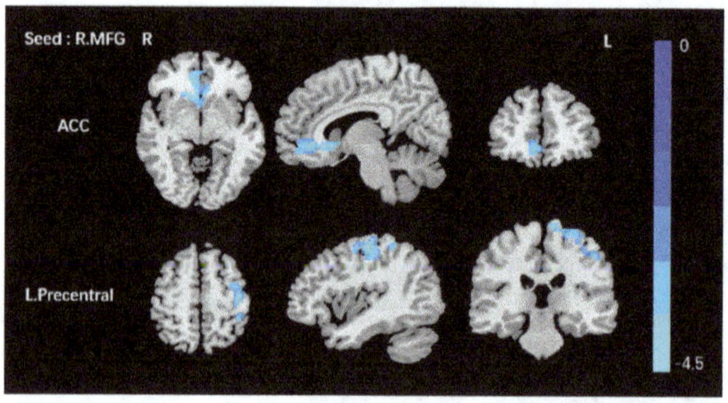

FIGURE 4 | Comparing to HCs, patients showed reduced connectivity between the seed region in the right MFG, and the bilateral ACC, left precentral gyrus. The threshold was determined by AlphaSim correction ($P < 0.001$ at the voxel and $P < 0.01$ at the cluster level). R, right; L, left; MFG, middle frontal gyrus; ACC anterior cingulate cortex. Blue means decreased connectivity.

Correlation Analyses

Surprisingly, in tinnitus patients, we did not find any significant correlations between fALFF values, ReHo values, FC, and tinnitus characteristics (including duration, THI, SAS, and SDS) neither controlled for age, sex, education, GM volume, average hearing thresholds nor the non-adjusted correlation analyses (**Table 4** and **Supplementary Table S2**). Even so, we found that the increased fALFF values in right ITG was almost negatively correlated with SDS scores ($r = -0.392$, $p = 0.052$, **Table 4**).

DISCUSSION

The present study focused on the early stage of tinnitus. The brain function abnormalities in patients with unilateral acute tinnitus and hearing loss were detected through fALFF, ReHo, and FC analysis. The results demonstrated abnormal spontaneous brain activity in certain brain regions, for instance, the right ITG, the vermis, the right calcarine cortex, the bilateral precuneus, the right SMG and the right MFG. Additionally, based on the different brain regions in fALFF and ReHo, FC analysis showed enhanced connectivity between the right ITG (seed region) and the right precentral gyri, along with reduced connectivity between the right MFG (seed region) and the bilateral ACC, left precentral gyrus. Thus, our work clearly exhibited intra- and interregional changes in the neural function of patients with unilateral acute tinnitus and hearing loss.

The middle frontal gyrus, an important part of the prefrontal cortex, is believed to principally participates in the neural mechanisms of inhibiting long-term disturbance (Konishi et al., 2005). A ^{18}F-fluoro-deoxyglucose positron emission tomography (FDG-PET) study indicated that tinnitus patients had enhanced FDG metabolism in the left MFG (Geven et al., 2014). Golm et al. (2013) demonstrated that the high neural activation in the left MFG was associated with tinnitus severity in chronic tinnitus patients based on a fMRI study. Structurally, Aldhafeeri et al. (2012) also found altered cortical thickness in the bilateral MFGs in patients with severe tinnitus. Therefore, it is believed that the neural activity in MFG in tinnitus may reflect the severity of the condition. Contrary to a previous study, our research found reduced ReHo values in the right MFG of AT. We speculated that it is probably related to the short duration of the tinnitus, as most of the tinnitus participants presented lower scores in the THI test. On the other hand, the various neuroimaging methods employed to study tinnitus (PET vs. fMRI) and the tinnitus patients' heterogeneity (with or without hearing loss) may lead to inconsistent results. Based on the FC analysis, we detected that tinnitus patients had decreased connectivity between the seed region in the right MFG and the bilateral ACC. The MFG and ACC are primary parts of the DMN. The DMN is usually active when people are in the resting state and is suppressed when the subject enters a task-based state (Raichle et al., 2001). We detected that tinnitus patients had decreased connectivity between the seed region in the right MFG and the bilateral ACC. The DMN is involved in episodic memory, self-evaluation, social functioning, foresight, and intrinsic expression (Andrews-Hanna, 2012). Chen et al. (2015b) and Zhang et al. (2015) found tinnitus patients

TABLE 4 | Correlation coefficients between altered fALFF, ReHo, FC values, and different tinnitus characteristics.

	Brain region	Duration	THI	SDS	SAS
fALFF	R.ITG	0.074/0.726	−0.175/0.404	−0.392/0.052	−0.056/0.792
ReHo	Vermis_8	−0.239/0.250	0.056/0.789	−0.121/0.566	−0.114/0.587
	R.Calcarine cortex	−0.142/0.499	0.177/0.397	0.003/0.989	−0.336/0.101
	R.Precuneus	−0.086/0.681	−0.152/0.468	−0.168/0.423	−0.257/0.216
	R.SMG	0.354/0.082	0.226/0.278	0.191/0.361	−0.142/0.497
	R.MFG	0.087/0.681	−0.168/0.422	−0.309/0.133	−0.206/0.322
FC	R.MFG-B.ACC	0.262/0.206	−0.018/0.933	0.196/0.348	−0.102/0.628
	R.MFG-L.Precentral gyrus	−0.004/0.984	0.352/0.084	0.137/0.512	0.091/0.664
	R.ITG-R.Precentral gyrus	−0.004/0.984	0.095/0.652	−0.271/0.190	−0.365/0.073

Partial correlations were controlled for age, sex, education level, GM volume, and mean hearing thresholds (data are represented as r/p). $P < 0.05$ was considered significant. L, left; R, right; B, bilateral; MFG, middle frontal gyrus; ITG, inferior temporal gyrus; ACC, anterior cingulate cortex.

had altered spontaneous neural activity or disrupted functional connection within the DMN which was associated with the severity of the tinnitus. Therefore, the auditory hallucinations discovered in tinnitus may be correlated with abnormalities of the DMN, and the abnormal or incoherent brain activity in this study may reflect this abnormal network. Additionally, we noticed that the right MFG had decreased connectivity with the left precentral gyrus, which was reported to be associated with the executive control network in tinnitus (Chen et al., 2017b).

The enhanced activity of the ITG observed in our study suggests that non-auditory pathways involved in tinnitus might reflect abnormal sensory integration and memory consolidation processes. Indeed, the ITG is involved in memory consolidation, visual processing and multimodal sensory integration (Mesulam, 1998). Many studies in EEG and PET have shown that tinnitus patients have hyperexcitability of the bilateral ITG compared to normal controls (Weiler et al., 2000; Ashton et al., 2007; Pawlak-Osinska et al., 2013; Adamchic et al., 2014; Song et al., 2015). This abnormal activation, confirmed by our results, might be related to a mechanism of maladaptive memory consolidation and/or abnormal sensory integration (Song et al., 2012). Additionally, the right ITG showed enhanced connectivity with the right precentral gyrus.

Traditionally, the cerebellum was considered to be restricted to motor control and coordination, but previous studies have indicated that it also showed an important role in the detection of auditory afferents and processing (Parsons et al., 2009; Salmi et al., 2009). Our present study found that AT patients had decreased ReHo values in the cerebellar vermis, and it is reported that the cerebellum is involved in receiving and processing information input from auditory-related cortices (Petacchi et al., 2005). We thus presume that the cerebellum may be related to the processing of tinnitus-related auditory hallucinations. Furthermore, an fMRI study found disrupted connectivity between the auditory cortex and the cerebellum (Maudoux et al., 2012a), which was in consistent with a salicylate tinnitus rat model study (Chen et al., 2015a). According to previous studies, we presumed that the cerebellum may participate in contrasting and integrating afferent signals from the cochlea and output signals from the auditory cortex in tinnitus patients, that is, acting as a selective gating control (Bauer et al., 2013), but further studies are needed for verification.

The calcarine cortex is also known as an important part of the primary visual cortex, which is the main site of input of signals coming from the retina. Our study indicated that AT showed decreased neural activity consistently in the right calcarine cortex. Chen et al. (2014) found decreased ALFF values in the visual area in chronic tinnitus patients. Anatomically, animal studies demonstrated an connection between auditory and visual regions (Iurilli et al., 2012), and the auditory cortex directly regulated the visual cortex (Ibrahim et al., 2016). Maudoux et al. (2012b) found functional connections between auditory and visual subnetworks in tinnitus patients. One interpretation of these results is that as patients attend to their phantom auditory sensation, they contemporaneously activate visual areas.

The supramarginal gyrus, a region associated with the attention network (Rushworth et al., 1997; Yamasaki et al., 2002), was found to have reduced ReHo value in AT patients. Previous EEG or PET studies also indicated that the SMG may play a role in tinnitus (Mirz et al., 1999; Weiler et al., 2000). Based on seed-FC analysis, Schmidt et al. (2013) demonstrated that the dorsal attention network (DAN) showed a declined relationship with the right SMG in tinnitus subjects. Hence, the decreased local neural activity in the SMG may change the connectivity in the DAN in tinnitus patients. This evidence indicates that the altered intraregional brain activity in the attention network might lead to abnormal local synchronization in tinnitus.

In the present study, we also found lower spontaneous brain activity in the precuneus. Prior studies showed that the precuneus is related to conscious and internal awareness (Cavanna and Trimble, 2006; Cavanna, 2007; Vanhaudenhuyse et al., 2011) and thus may play a role in tinnitus generation and persistence. Several hypotheses have suggested that conscious awareness is necessary for tinnitus perception. However, the percept can be effectively ignored if distractors are provided (Roberts et al., 2013). Tinnitus habituation may therefore be linked to networks of awareness, of which the precuneus plays a key role. Additionally, the precuneus is also an important structure of the DMN and it suggested that intrinsic alteration of DMN was involved in acute tinnitus.

Interestingly, almost all the alterations in ReHo, fALFF, and FC were lateralized to the right hemisphere in patients. A number of functional and structural studies in tinnitus demonstrated a lateralized effect (Smits et al., 2007; Schecklmann et al., 2013;

Chen et al., 2014, 2016, 2018b; Geven et al., 2014), some of them biased to the left and others to the right. We speculate that the cause of lateralization may due to the heterogeneity of tinnitus patients or the different neuroimaging methods used to investigate tinnitus. Therefore, the observed right-lateralization effect needs to be studied to determine whether it is related specifically to tinnitus or other factors.

In the correlation analyses, we failed to observe significant differences between fALFF values, ReHo values, FC and tinnitus characteristics. But we found that the increased fALFF values in right ITG was almost negatively correlated with SDS scores. We speculate that this might be associated with the short duration of the tinnitus in the patients. Furthermore, the method of neuroimaging we used may be insensitive to the early stages of tinnitus.

The present study has several constraints that must be acknowledged. First, because of the small sample size of tinnitus patients, we could not categorize the group into right/left side tinnitus to verify whether the bias of the tinnitus lead to the lateralization of functional activity. Although we performed the differences between left and right-side tinnitus in a exploratory way, it still needs specific work to verify. Second, due to the cross-sectional design, we could not study the changes on the brain impacted by disease and whether the neural tinnitus network will change over time. Therefore, a longitudinal study involving a larger number of participants will be needed for future research. Third, although we used earplugs to minimize noise effects in present study, the noise of the scanner could not be completely prevented. Thus, this limitation may reduce the differences in resting-state networks between tinnitus and control groups. Furthermore, although the seed-based FC method is a powerful tool to study the integration of distributed brain systems, it still raises concerns of double-dipping. Finally, in addition to functional alterations, more studies are needed to detect the potentially structural connectivity in acute tinnitus, in our knowledge, diffusion tensor imaging (DTI) may measure that more visually.

CONCLUSION

By combining ReHo, fALFF, and FC analyses, our work indicated that AT with hearing loss had abnormal intraregional neural activity and disrupted connectivity in several brain regions which mainly including the non-auditory area, and these regions are major components of DMN, attention network, visual network, and executive control network. These findings will help us enhance the understanding of the neuroimaging mechanism in tinnitus populations. Moreover, these abnormalities remind us that we should focus on the early stages of this hearing disease.

AUTHOR CONTRIBUTIONS

G-PZ and X-YS collected the fMRI data, performed the analysis, and wrote the manuscript. Y-SY helped with data collection. H-LW and L-JQ contributed to the fMRI data analysis and discussion. Q-QZ helped with data processing. XY revised this manuscript. HZ and Y-JT designed the MRI experiment and manuscript revision.

FUNDING

This work was supported by a grant from the National Natural Science Foundation of China (No. 81601477).

ACKNOWLEDGMENTS

We would like to thank all the tinnitus patients and healthy controls who participated in our research.

SUPPLEMENTARY MATERIAL

FIGURE S1 | Brain regions showed fALFF differences between left and right-sided acute tinnitus group (uncorrected, $P < 0.05$, cluster size >20 voxels). The regions with higher fALFF values were right cerebellar, bilateral MTG, left ITG, left triangular part inferior frontal gyrus, left SFG,and left precentral gyrus. The regions with lower fALFF values were left postcentral gyrus. MTG, middle temporal gyrus; ITG, inferior temporal gyrus; SFG, superior frontal gyrus. Yellow color means increased fALFF values and blue color means decreased fALFF values.

FIGURE S2 | Brain regions showed ReHo differences between left and right-sided acute tinnitus group (uncorrected, $P < 0.05$, cluster size >20 voxels). The regions with higher ReHo values were bilateral cerebellar, left fusiform gyrus, left MTG, left MFG, left medial superior frontal gyrus, right SMG, and right SFG. The regions with lower ReHo values were left postcentral gyrus. MTG, middle temporal gyrus; MFG, middle frontal gyrus; SMG, supramarginal gyrus. Yellow color means increased ReHo values and blue color means decreased ReHo values.

TABLE S1 | Brain regions showing fALFF and ReHo differences between left and right-sided tinnitus fALFF and ReHo analysis: $P < 0.05$ (uncorrected), cluster size >20 voxels; Age, sex, education level, and grey matter (GM) volume were included as nuisance covariates. L, left; R, right; B, bilateral. MNI, montreal neurological institute.

TABLE S2 | Pearson correlation analyses between altered fALFF, ReHo, FC values and different tinnitus characteristics Pearson correlation analyses were conducted without controlling for age, sex, education level, GM volume and mean hearing thresholds (Data are represented as r/p). $P < 0.05$ was considered significant. L, left; R, right; B, bilateral; MFG, middle frontal gyrus; ITG, inferior temporal gyrus; ACC, anterior cingulate cortex.

REFERENCES

Adamchic, I., Toth, T., Hauptmann, C., and Tass, P. A. (2014). Reversing pathologically increased EEG power by acoustic coordinated reset neuromodulation. *Hum. Brain Mapp.* 35, 2099–2118. doi: 10.1002/hbm.22314

Aldhafeeri, F. M., Mackenzie, I., Kay, T., Alghamdi, J., and Sluming, V. (2012). Neuroanatomical correlates of tinnitus revealed by cortical thickness analysis and diffusion tensor imaging. *Neuroradiology* 54, 883–892. doi: 10.1007/s00234-012-1044-6

Andrews-Hanna, J. R. (2012). The brain's default network and its adaptive role in internal mentation. *Neuroscientist* 18, 251–270. doi: 10.1177/1073858411403316

Ashton, H., Reid, K., Marsh, R., Johnson, I., Alter, K., and Griffiths, T. (2007). High frequency localised "hot spots" in temporal lobes of patients with intractable tinnitus: a quantitative electroencephalographic (QEEG) study. *Neurosci. Lett.* 426, 23–28. doi: 10.1016/j.neulet.2007.08.034

Baguley, D., McFerran, D., and Hall, D. (2013). Tinnitus. *Lancet* 382, 1600–1607. doi: 10.1016/s0140-6736(13)60142-7

Bartels, H., Staal, M. J., and Albers, F. W. (2007). Tinnitus and neural plasticity of the brain. *Otol. Neurotol.* 28, 178–184. doi: 10.1097/MAO.0b013e31802b3248

Bauer, C. A., Kurt, W., Sybert, L. T., and Brozoski, T. J. (2013). The cerebellum as a novel tinnitus generator. *Hear Res* 295, 130–139. doi: 10.1016/j.heares.2012.03.009

Biswal, B., Yetkin, F. Z., Haughton, V. M., and Hyde, J. S. (1995). Functional connectivity in the motor cortex of resting human brain using echo-planar MRI. *Magn. Reson. Med.* 34, 537–541. doi: 10.1002/mrm.1910340409

Burton, H., Wineland, A., Bhattacharya, M., Nicklaus, J., Garcia, K. S., and Piccirillo, J. F. (2012). Altered networks in bothersome tinnitus: a functional connectivity study. *BMC Neurosci.* 13:3. doi: 10.1186/1471-2202-13-3

Cavanna, A. E. (2007). The precuneus and consciousness. *CNS Spectr.* 12, 545–552. doi: 10.1017/s1092852900021295

Cavanna, A. E., and Trimble, M. R. (2006). The precuneus: a review of its functional anatomy and behavioural correlates. *Brain* 129(Pt 3), 564–583. doi: 10.1093/brain/awl004

Chen, H. J., Zhu, X. Q., Jiao, Y., Li, P. C., Wang, Y., and Teng, G. J. (2012a). Abnormal baseline brain activity in low-grade hepatic encephalopathy: a resting-state fMRI study. *J. Neurol. Sci.* 318, 140–145. doi: 10.1016/j.jns.2012.02.019

Chen, H. J., Zhu, X. Q., Yang, M., Liu, B., Zhang, Y., Wang, Y., et al. (2012b). Changes in the regional homogeneity of resting-state brain activity in minimal hepatic encephalopathy. *Neurosci. Lett.* 507, 5–9. doi: 10.1016/j.neulet.2011.11.033

Chen, Y. C., Chen, H., Bo, F., Xu, J. J., Deng, Y., Lv, H., et al. (2018a). Tinnitus distress is associated with enhanced resting-state functional connectivity within the default mode network. *Neuropsychiatr. Dis. Treat.* 14, 1919–1927. doi: 10.2147/ndt.S164619

Chen, Y. C., Liu, S., Lv, H., Bo, F., Feng, Y., Chen, H., et al. (2018b). Abnormal resting-state functional connectivity of the anterior cingulate cortex in unilateral chronic tinnitus patients. *Front. Neurosci.* 12:9. doi: 10.3389/fnins.2018.00009

Chen, Y. C., Feng, Y., Xu, J. J., Mao, C. N., Xia, W., Ren, J., et al. (2016). Disrupted brain functional network architecture in chronic tinnitus patients. *Front. Aging Neurosci.* 8:174. doi: 10.3389/fnagi.2016.00174

Chen, Y. C., Li, X., Liu, L., Wang, J., Lu, C. Q., Yang, M., et al. (2015a). Tinnitus and hyperacusis involve hyperactivity and enhanced connectivity in auditory-limbic-arousal-cerebellar network. *eLife* 4:e06576. doi: 10.7554/eLife.06576

Chen, Y. C., Zhang, J., Li, X. W., Xia, W., Feng, X., Qian, C., et al. (2015b). Altered intra- and interregional synchronization in resting-state cerebral networks associated with chronic tinnitus. *Neural Plast.* 2015:475382. doi: 10.1155/2015/475382

Chen, Y. C., Wang, F., Wang, J., Bo, F., Xia, W., Gu, J. P., et al. (2017a). Resting-state brain abnormalities in chronic subjective tinnitus: a meta-analysis. *Front. Hum. Neurosci.* 11:22. doi: 10.3389/fnhum.2017.00022

Chen, Y. C., Xia, W., Chen, H., Feng, Y., Xu, J. J., Gu, J. P., et al. (2017b). Tinnitus distress is linked to enhanced resting-state functional connectivity from the limbic system to the auditory cortex. *Hum. Brain Mapp.* 38, 2384–2397. doi: 10.1002/hbm.23525

Chen, Y. C., Zhang, J., Li, X. W., Xia, W., Feng, X., Gao, B., et al. (2014). Aberrant spontaneous brain activity in chronic tinnitus patients revealed by resting-state functional MRI. *Neuroimage Clin.* 6, 222–228. doi: 10.1016/j.nicl.2014.09.011

De Ridder, D., Elgoyhen, A. B., Romo, R., and Langguth, B. (2011a). Phantom percepts: tinnitus and pain as persisting aversive memory networks. *Proc. Natl. Acad. Sci. U.S.A.* 108, 8075–8080. doi: 10.1073/pnas.1018466108

De Ridder, D., van der Loo, E., Vanneste, S., Gais, S., Plazier, M., Kovacs, S., et al. (2011b). Theta-gamma dysrhythmia and auditory phantom perception. *J. Neurosurg.* 114, 912–921. doi: 10.3171/2010.11.Jns10335

Eggermont, J. J. (2005). Tinnitus: neurobiological substrates. *Drug Discov. Today* 10, 1283–1290. doi: 10.1016/s1359-6446(05)03542-7

Eggermont, J. J., and Roberts, L. E. (2004). The neuroscience of tinnitus. *Trends Neurosci.* 27, 676–682. doi: 10.1016/j.tins.2004.08.010

Geven, L. I., de Kleine, E., Willemsen, A. T., and van Dijk, P. (2014). Asymmetry in primary auditory cortex activity in tinnitus patients and controls. *Neuroscience* 256, 117–125. doi: 10.1016/j.neuroscience.2013.10.015

Golm, D., Schmidt-Samoa, C., Dechent, P., and Kroner-Herwig, B. (2013). Neural correlates of tinnitus related distress: an fMRI-study. *Hear. Res.* 295, 87–99. doi: 10.1016/j.heares.2012.03.003

Han, L., Zhaohui, L., Fei, Y., Ting, L., Pengfei, Z., Wang, D., et al. (2014). Abnormal baseline brain activity in patients with pulsatile tinnitus: a resting-state FMRI study. *Neural Plast.* 2014:549162. doi: 10.1155/2014/549162

He, Y., Wang, L., Zang, Y., Tian, L., Zhang, X., Li, K., et al. (2007). Regional coherence changes in the early stages of Alzheimer's disease: a combined structural and resting-state functional MRI study. *Neuroimage* 35, 488–500. doi: 10.1016/j.neuroimage.2006.11.042

Hoptman, M. J., Zuo, X. N., Butler, P. D., Javitt, D. C., D'Angelo, D., Mauro, C. J., et al. (2010). Amplitude of low-frequency oscillations in schizophrenia: a resting state fMRI study. *Schizophr. Res.* 117, 13–20. doi: 10.1016/j.schres.2009.09.030

Husain, F. T., and Schmidt, S. A. (2014). Using resting state functional connectivity to unravel networks of tinnitus. *Hear. Res.* 307, 153–162. doi: 10.1016/j.heares.2013.07.010

Ibrahim, L. A., Mesik, L., Ji, X. Y., Fang, Q., Li, H. F., Li, Y. T., et al. (2016). Cross-modality sharpening of visual cortical processing through layer-1-mediated inhibition and disinhibition. *Neuron* 89, 1031–1045. doi: 10.1016/j.neuron.2016.01.027

Iurilli, G., Ghezzi, D., Olcese, U., Lassi, G., Nazzaro, C., Tonini, R., et al. (2012). Sound-driven synaptic inhibition in primary visual cortex. *Neuron* 73, 814–828. doi: 10.1016/j.neuron.2011.12.026

Jastreboff, P. J. (1990). Phantom auditory perception (tinnitus): mechanisms of generation and perception. *Neurosci. Res.* 8, 221–254. doi: 10.1016/0168-0102(90)90031-9

Kaltenbach, J. A., Zhang, J., and Finlayson, P. (2005). Tinnitus as a plastic phenomenon and its possible neural underpinnings in the dorsal cochlear nucleus. *Hear. Res.* 206, 200–226. doi: 10.1016/j.heares.2005.02.013

Konishi, S., Chikazoe, J., Jimura, K., Asari, T., and Miyashita, Y. (2005). Neural mechanism in anterior prefrontal cortex for inhibition of prolonged set interference. *Proc. Natl. Acad. Sci. U.S.A.* 102, 12584–12588. doi: 10.1073/pnas.0500585102

Leaver, A. M., Turesky, T. K., Seydell-Greenwald, A., Morgan, S., Kim, H. J., and Rauschecker, J. P. (2016). Intrinsic network activity in tinnitus investigated using functional MRI. *Hum. Brain Mapp.* 37, 2717–2735. doi: 10.1002/hbm.23204

Liu, H., Liu, Z., Liang, M., Hao, Y., Tan, L., Kuang, F., et al. (2006). Decreased regional homogeneity in schizophrenia: a resting state functional magnetic resonance imaging study. *Neuroreport* 17, 19–22. doi: 10.1097/01.wnr.0000195666.22714.35

Lockwood, A. H., Salvi, R. J., and Burkard, R. F. (2002). Tinnitus. *N. Engl. J. Med.* 347, 904–910. doi: 10.1056/NEJMra013395

Lockwood, A. H., Salvi, R. J., Coad, M. L., Towsley, M. L., Wack, D. S., and Murphy, B. W. (1998). The functional neuroanatomy of tinnitus: evidence for limbic system links and neural plasticity. *Neurology* 50, 114–120. doi: 10.1212/wnl.50.1.114

Lowe, M. J., Mock, B. J., and Sorenson, J. A. (1998). Functional connectivity in single and multislice echoplanar imaging using resting-state fluctuations. *Neuroimage* 7, 119–132. doi: 10.1006/nimg.1997.0315

Mantini, D., Perrucci, M. G., Del Gratta, C., Romani, G. L., and Corbetta, M. (2007). Electrophysiological signatures of resting state networks in the human brain. *Proc. Natl. Acad. Sci. U.S.A.* 104, 13170–13175. doi: 10.1073/pnas.0700668104

Maudoux, A., Lefebvre, P., Cabay, J. E., Demertzi, A., Vanhaudenhuyse, A., Laureys, S., et al. (2012a). Auditory resting-state network connectivity in tinnitus: a functional MRI study. *PLoS One* 7:e36222. doi: 10.1371/journal.pone.0036222

Maudoux, A., Lefebvre, P., Cabay, J. E., Demertzi, A., Vanhaudenhuyse, A., Laureys, S., et al. (2012b). Connectivity graph analysis of the auditory resting state network in tinnitus. *Brain Res.* 1485, 10–21. doi: 10.1016/j.brainres.2012.05.006

Mesulam, M. M. (1998). From sensation to cognition. *Brain* 121(Pt 6), 1013–1052.

Mirz, F., Pedersen, B., Ishizu, K., Johannsen, P., Ovesen, T., Stodkilde-Jorgensen, H., et al. (1999). Positron emission tomography of cortical centers of tinnitus. *Hear. Res.* 134, 133–144. doi: 10.1016/s0378-5955(99)00075-1

Moller, A. R. (2007). Tinnitus: presence and future. *Prog. Brain Res.* 166, 3–16. doi: 10.1016/s0079-6123(07)66001-4

Mühlnickel, W., Elbert, T., Taub, E., and Flor, H. (1998). Reorganization of auditory cortex in tinnitus. *Proc. Natl. Acad. Sci. U.S.A.* 95, 10340–10343. doi: 10.1073/pnas.95.17.10340

Newman, C. W., Jacobson, G. P., and Spitzer, J. B. (1996). Development of the tinnitus handicap inventory. *Arch. Otolaryngol. Head Neck Surg.* 122, 143–148.

Parsons, L. M., Petacchi, A., Schmahmann, J. D., and Bower, J. M. (2009). Pitch discrimination in cerebellar patients: evidence for a sensory deficit. *Brain Res.* 1303, 84–96. doi: 10.1016/j.brainres.2009.09.052

Pawlak-Osinska, K., Kazmierczak, W., Kazmierczak, H., Wierzchowska, M., and Matuszewska, I. (2013). Cortical activity in tinnitus patients and its modification by phonostimulation. *Clinics* 68, 511–515. doi: 10.6061/clinics/2013(04)12

Petacchi, A., Laird, A. R., Fox, P. T., and Bower, J. M. (2005). Cerebellum and auditory function: an ALE meta-analysis of functional neuroimaging studies. *Hum. Brain Mapp.* 25, 118–128. doi: 10.1002/hbm.20137

Raichle, M. E., MacLeod, A. M., Snyder, A. Z., Powers, W. J., Gusnard, D. A., and Shulman, G. L. (2001). A default mode of brain function. *Proc. Natl. Acad. Sci. U.S.A.* 98, 676–682. doi: 10.1073/pnas.98.2.676

Rauschecker, J. P., Leaver, A. M., and Muhlau, M. (2010). Tuning out the noise: limbic-auditory interactions in tinnitus. *Neuron* 66, 819–826. doi: 10.1016/j.neuron.2010.04.032

Reynolds, P., Gardner, D., and Lee, R. (2004). Tinnitus and psychological morbidity: a cross-sectional study to investigate psychological morbidity in tinnitus patients and its relationship with severity of symptoms and illness perceptions. *Clin. Otolaryngol. Allied Sci.* 29, 628–634. doi: 10.1111/j.1365-2273.2004.00879.x

Roberts, L. E., Husain, F. T., and Eggermont, J. J. (2013). Role of attention in the generation and modulation of tinnitus. *Neurosci. Biobehav. Rev.* 37, 1754–1773. doi: 10.1016/j.neubiorev.2013.07.007

Rushworth, M. F., Nixon, P. D., Renowden, S., Wade, D. T., and Passingham, R. E. (1997). The left parietal cortex and motor attention. *Neuropsychologia* 35, 1261–1273. doi: 10.1016/s0028-3932(97)00050-x

Salmi, J., Rinne, T., Koistinen, S., Salonen, O., and Alho, K. (2009). Brain networks of bottom-up triggered and top-down controlled shifting of auditory attention. *Brain Res.* 1286, 155–164. doi: 10.1016/j.brainres.2009.06.083

Schecklmann, M., Landgrebe, M., and Langguth, B. (2014). Phenotypic characteristics of hyperacusis in tinnitus. *PLoS One* 9:e86944. doi: 10.1371/journal.pone.0086944

Schecklmann, M., Landgrebe, M., Poeppl, T. B., Kreuzer, P., Manner, P., Marienhagen, J., et al. (2013). Neural correlates of tinnitus duration and distress: a positron emission tomography study. *Hum. Brain Mapp.* 34, 233–240. doi: 10.1002/hbm.21426

Schmidt, S. A., Akrofi, K., Carpenter-Thompson, J. R., and Husain, F. T. (2013). Default mode, dorsal attention and auditory resting state networks exhibit differential functional connectivity in tinnitus and hearing loss. *PLoS One* 8:e76488. doi: 10.1371/journal.pone.0076488

Smits, M., Kovacs, S., de Ridder, D., Peeters, R. R., van Hecke, P., and Sunaert, S. (2007). Lateralization of functional magnetic resonance imaging (fMRI) activation in the auditory pathway of patients with lateralized tinnitus. *Neuroradiology* 49, 669–679. doi: 10.1007/s00234-007-0231-3

Soleymani, T., Pieton, D., Pezeshkian, P., Miller, P., Gorgulho, A. A., Pouratian, N., et al. (2011). Surgical approaches to tinnitus treatment: a review and novel approaches. *Surg. Neurol. Int.* 2:154. doi: 10.4103/2152-7806.86834

Song, J. J., De Ridder, D., Van de Heyning, P., and Vanneste, S. (2012). Mapping tinnitus-related brain activation: an activation-likelihood estimation metaanalysis of PET studies. *J. Nucl. Med.* 53, 1550–1557. doi: 10.2967/jnumed.112.102939

Song, J. J., Vanneste, S., Schlee, W., Van de Heyning, P., and De Ridder, D. (2015). Onset-related differences in neural substrates of tinnitus-related distress: the anterior cingulate cortex in late-onset tinnitus, and the frontal cortex in early-onset tinnitus. *Brain Struct. Funct.* 220, 571–584. doi: 10.1007/s00429-013-0648-x

Vanhaudenhuyse, A., Demertzi, A., Schabus, M., Noirhomme, Q., Bredart, S., Boly, M., et al. (2011). Two distinct neuronal networks mediate the awareness of environment and of self. *J. Cogn. Neurosci.* 23, 570–578. doi: 10.1162/jocn.2010.21488

Vanneste, S., van de Heyning, P., and De Ridder, D. (2011). The neural network of phantom sound changes over time: a comparison between recent-onset and chronic tinnitus patients. *Eur. J. Neurosci.* 34, 718–731. doi: 10.1111/j.1460-9568.2011.07793.x

Wang, Z., Yan, C., Zhao, C., Qi, Z., Zhou, W., Lu, J., et al. (2011). Spatial patterns of intrinsic brain activity in mild cognitive impairment and Alzheimer's disease: a resting-state functional MRI study. *Hum. Brain Mapp.* 32, 1720–1740. doi: 10.1002/hbm.21140

Weiler, E. W., Brill, K., Tachiki, K. H., and Wiegand, R. (2000). Electroencephalography correlates in tinnitus. *Int. Tinnitus J.* 6, 21–24.

Wu, T., Long, X., Zang, Y., Wang, L., Hallett, M., Li, K., et al. (2009). Regional homogeneity changes in patients with Parkinson's disease. *Hum. Brain Mapp.* 30, 1502–1510. doi: 10.1002/hbm.20622

Xie, X., Liu, Y., Han, X., Liu, P., Qiu, H., Li, J., et al. (2019). Differences in intrinsic brain abnormalities between patients with left- and right-sided long-term hearing impairment. *Front. Neurosci.* 13:206. doi: 10.3389/fnins.2019.00206

Yamasaki, H., LaBar, K. S., and McCarthy, G. (2002). Dissociable prefrontal brain systems for attention and emotion. *Proc. Natl. Acad. Sci. U.S.A.* 99, 11447–11451. doi: 10.1073/pnas.182176499

Yan, C. G., Wang, X. D., Zuo, X. N., and Zang, Y. F. (2016). DPABI: data processing & analysis for (resting-state) brain imaging. *Neuroinformatics* 14, 339–351. doi: 10.1007/s12021-016-9299-4

Zang, Y., Jiang, T., Lu, Y., He, Y., and Tian, L. (2004). Regional homogeneity approach to fMRI data analysis. *Neuroimage* 22, 394–400. doi: 10.1016/j.neuroimage.2003.12.030

Zhang, J., Chen, Y. C., Feng, X., Yang, M., Liu, B., Qian, C., et al. (2015). Impairments of thalamic resting-state functional connectivity in patients with chronic tinnitus. *Eur. J. Radiol.* 84, 1277–1284. doi: 10.1016/j.ejrad.2015.04.006

Zhang, Z., Lu, G., Zhong, Y., Tan, Q., Chen, H., Liao, W., et al. (2010). fMRI study of mesial temporal lobe epilepsy using amplitude of low-frequency fluctuation analysis. *Hum. Brain Mapp.* 31, 1851–1861. doi: 10.1002/hbm.20982

Zou, Q. H., Zhu, C. Z., Yang, Y., Zuo, X. N., Long, X. Y., Cao, Q. J., et al. (2008). An improved approach to detection of amplitude of low-frequency fluctuation (ALFF) for resting-state fMRI: fractional ALFF. *J. Neurosci. Methods* 172, 137–141. doi: 10.1016/j.jneumeth.2008.04.012

Permissions

All chapters in this book were first published by Frontiers; hereby published with permission under the Creative Commons Attribution License or equivalent. Every chapter published in this book has been scrutinized by our experts. Their significance has been extensively debated. The topics covered herein carry significant findings which will fuel the growth of the discipline. They may even be implemented as practical applications or may be referred to as a beginning point for another development.

The contributors of this book come from diverse backgrounds, making this book a truly international effort. This book will bring forth new frontiers with its revolutionizing research information and detailed analysis of the nascent developments around the world.

We would like to thank all the contributing authors for lending their expertise to make the book truly unique. They have played a crucial role in the development of this book. Without their invaluable contributions this book wouldn't have been possible. They have made vital efforts to compile up to date information on the varied aspects of this subject to make this book a valuable addition to the collection of many professionals and students.

This book was conceptualized with the vision of imparting up-to-date information and advanced data in this field. To ensure the same, a matchless editorial board was set up. Every individual on the board went through rigorous rounds of assessment to prove their worth. After which they invested a large part of their time researching and compiling the most relevant data for our readers.

The editorial board has been involved in producing this book since its inception. They have spent rigorous hours researching and exploring the diverse topics which have resulted in the successful publishing of this book. They have passed on their knowledge of decades through this book. To expedite this challenging task, the publisher supported the team at every step. A small team of assistant editors was also appointed to further simplify the editing procedure and attain best results for the readers.

Apart from the editorial board, the designing team has also invested a significant amount of their time in understanding the subject and creating the most relevant covers. They scrutinized every image to scout for the most suitable representation of the subject and create an appropriate cover for the book.

The publishing team has been an ardent support to the editorial, designing and production team. Their endless efforts to recruit the best for this project, has resulted in the accomplishment of this book. They are a veteran in the field of academics and their pool of knowledge is as vast as their experience in printing. Their expertise and guidance has proved useful at every step. Their uncompromising quality standards have made this book an exceptional effort. Their encouragement from time to time has been an inspiration for everyone.

The publisher and the editorial board hope that this book will prove to be a valuable piece of knowledge for researchers, students, practitioners and scholars across the globe.

List of Contributors

Annick Gilles
Department of Translational Neuroscience, Faculty of Medicine and Health Sciences, University of Antwerp, Wilrijk, Belgium
University Department of Otorhinolaryngology and Head and Neck Surgery, Antwerp University Hospital, Edegem, Belgium
Department of Human and Social Welfare, University College Ghent, Ghent, Belgium

Guy Van Camp
Center for Medical Genetics, Antwerp University Hospital and University of Antwerp, Antwerp, Belgium

Sarah Rabau and Paul Van de Heyning
Department of Translational Neuroscience, Faculty of Medicine and Health Sciences, University of Antwerp, Wilrijk, Belgium
University Department of Otorhinolaryngology and Head and Neck Surgery, Antwerp University Hospital, Edegem, Belgium

Erik Fransen
Center for Medical Genetics, Antwerp University Hospital and University of Antwerp, Antwerp Belgium
StatUa Center for Statistics, University of Antwerp, Antwerp, Belgium

Ryan J. Longenecker and Alexander V. Galazyuk
Department of Anatomy and Neurobiology, Northeast Ohio Medical University, Rootstown, OH, USA

Dominik Gollnast, Konstantin Tziridis and Holger Schulze
Experimental Otolaryngology, Department of Otorhinolaryngology, Head and Neck Surgery, Friedrich Alexander University Erlangen-Nürnberg (FAU), Erlangen, Germany

Patrick Krauss and Achim Schilling
Experimental Otolaryngology, Department of Otorhinolaryngology, Head and Neck Surgery, Friedrich Alexander University Erlangen-Nürnberg (FAU), Erlangen, Germany
Department of Physics, Center for Medical Physics and Technology, Biophysics Group, Friedrich-Alexander University Erlangen-Nürnberg (FAU), Erlangen, Germany

Ulrich Hoppe
Audiology, Department of Otorhinolaryngology, Head and Neck Surgery, Friedrich Alexander University Erlangen-Nürnberg (FAU), Erlangen, Germany

Veronika Vielsmeier, Thomas Steffens and Philipp R. O. Semmler
Department of Otorhinolaryngology, University of Regensburg, Regensburg, Germany
Interdisciplinary Tinnitus Center of the University of Regensburg, Regensburg, Germany

Peter M. Kreuzer, Winfried Schlee, Berthold Langguth and Martin Schecklmann
Interdisciplinary Tinnitus Center of the University of Regensburg, Regensburg, Germany
Department of Psychiatry and Psychotherapy, University ofRegensburg, Regensburg, Germany

Frank Haubner
Department of Otorhinolaryngology, University of Regensburg, Regensburg, Germany

Tobias Kleinjung
Department of Otorhinolaryngology, University of Zurich, Switzerland

Elisabeth Wallhäusser-Franke, Anna Glauner and Wolfgang Delb
Otorhinolaryngology, Phoniatrics and Audiology, Medical Faculty Mannheim, Heidelberg University, Mannheim, Germany

Roberto D'Amelio
Department of Internal Medicine IV and Neurocenter, Saarland University Medical Center, Saarland University, Homburg, Germany

Jérôme J. Servais and Ines Repik
Otorhinolaryngology, University Medical Centre Mannheim, Mannheim, Germany

Karl Hörmann
Otorhinolaryngology, Phoniatrics and Audiology, Medical Faculty Mannheim, Heidelberg University, Mannheim, Germany
Otorhinolaryngology, University Medical Centre Mannheim, Mannheim, Germany

Pia Lau, Andreas Wollbrink, Robert Wunderlich, Alva Engell, Alwina Löhe, Markus Junghöfer and Christo Pantev
Institute for Biomagnetism and Biosignalanalysis, University Hospital of Münster, Münster, Germany

Devon B. Palumbo, Ola A. Alsalman and Sven Vanneste
Lab for Clinical and Integrative Neuroscience, School of Behavioral and Brain Sciences, The University of Texas at Dallas, Dallas, TX, USA

Denise Tucker
Department of Communication Sciences and Disorders, University of North Carolina at Greensboro, Greensboro, NC, USA

Hong Yu
Laboratory of Experimental Audiology, Department of Physiology and Pharmacology, Karolinska Institutet, Stockholm, Sweden
Department of Otolaryngology, Head and Neck Surgery, First Hospital of JiLin University, Changchun, China

Kim Vikhe Patil, Barbara Canlon and Christopher R. Cederroth
Laboratory of Experimental Audiology, Department of Physiology and Pharmacology, Karolinska Institutet, Stockholm, Sweden

Chul Han and Shinichi Someya
Department of Aging and Geriatric Research, University of Florida, Gainesville, FL, USA

Brian Fabella
Howard Hughes Medical Institute and Laboratory of Sensory Neuroscience, The Rockefeller University, New York, USA

Anna K. Kähler
Department of Molecular Epidemiology and Biostatistics, Karolinska Institutet, Stockholm, Sweden

Patrick F. Sullivan
Department of Molecular Epidemiology and Biostatistics, Karolinska Institutet, Stockholm, Sweden
Department of Genetics, University of North Carolina, Chapel Hill, NC, United States
Department of Psychiatry, University of North Carolina, Chapel Hill, NC, United States

Jose A. Lopez-Escamez
Otology & Neurotology Group, Department of Genomic Medicine, Pfizer-Universidad de Granada-Junta de Andalucía Centre for Genomics and Oncology Research (GENyO), Granada, Spain
Department of Otolaryngology, Instituto de Investigación Biosanitaria ibs.GRANADA, Hospital Virgen de las Nieves, Universidad de Granada, Granada, Spain

Daniela Ivansic, Orlando Guntinas-Lichius, Boris Müller, Gerd F. Volk, Gerlind Schneider and Christian Dobel
Tinnitus-Centre, Department of Otorhinolaryngology, Jena University Hospital, Jena, Germany

Margarete Anna Ueberfuhr
German Center for Vertigo and Balance Disorders, University Hospital Munich, Ludwig-Maximilians Universität München, Munich, Germany
Graduate School of Systemic Neurosciences, Ludwig-Maximilians-Universität München, Martinsried, Germany

Lutz Wiegrebe
Graduate School of Systemic Neurosciences, Ludwig-Maximilians-Universität München, Martinsried, Germany
Division of Neurobiology, Department Biology II, Ludwig-Maximilians-Universität München, Martinsried, Germany

Eike Krause and Robert Gürkov
Department of Otorhinolaryngology, Head and Neck Surgery, Grosshadern Medical Centre, Ludwig-Maximilians Universität München, Munich, Germany

Markus Drexl
German Center for Vertigo and Balance Disorders, University Hospital Munich, Ludwig-Maximilians Universität München, Munich, Germany

Krysta J. Trevis, Neil M. McLachlan and Sarah J. Wilson
Psychological Sciences, The University of Melbourne, Melbourne, VIC, Australia

Winny Schlee
University Department of Psychology, University of Konstanz, Konstanz, Germany

Kristien Wouters
Department of Translational Neurosciences, Faculty of Medicine and Health Sciences, University of Antwerp, Wilrijk, Belgium
University Department of Scientific Coordination and Biostatistics, Antwerp University Hospital, Edegem, Belgium

Erik Fransen
Department of Medical Genetics, Faculty of Medicine and Health Sciences, University of Antwerp, Wilrijk, Belgium

Haúla F. Haider, Diogo Ribeiro and João C. Paço
ENT Department, Hospital Cuf Infante Santo, NOVA Medical School, Lisbon, Portugal

Marisa Flook and Graça Fialho
Deafness Research Group, BTR Unit, BioISI, Faculty of Sciences, University of Lisbon (FCUL), Lisbon, Portugal

Mariana Aparicio
Faculty of Sciences, University of Lisbon, Lisbon, Portugal

Marilia Antunes
Centro de Estatística e Aplicações, Faculty of Sciences, University of Lisbon, Lisbon, Portugal

Agnieszka J. Szczepek and Heidi Olze
Department of Otolaryngology, Charite University Hospital, Berlin, Germany

Derek J. Hoare
NIHR Nottingham Biomedical Research Centre, Division of Clinical Neuroscience, School of Medicine, University of Nottingham, Nottingham, United Kingdom

Helena Caria
Deafness Research Group, BTR Unit, BioISI, Faculty of Sciences, University of Lisbon (FCUL), Lisbon, Portugal
ESS/IPS- Biomedical Sciences Department, School of Health, Polytechnic Institute of Setubal, Setubal, Portugal

Alain Londero
Service ORL et CCF, Hôpital Européen G. Pompidou, Paris, France

Nicolas Charpentier
Faculté de médecine de Nancy, Université de Lorraine, Nancy, France

Damien Ponsot
Lycée Germaine Tillion, Académie de Lyon, Sain-Bel, France

Laurent Pezard
Laboratoire Neurosciences Intégratives et Adaptatives, UMR CNRS 7260, Fédération 3C, Aix-Marseille Université, Marseille, France

Dirk De Ridder
Department of Surgical Sciences, Section of Neurosurgery, Dunedin School of Medicine, University of Otago, Dunedin, New Zealand

Jae-Jin Song
Department of Otorhinolaryngology-Head and Neck Surgery, Seoul National University Bundang Hospital, Seongnam, South Korea

Michael Landgrebe
Department of Psychiatry and Psychotherapy, University of Regensburg, Regensburg, Germany
kbo Lech-Mangfall-Klinik Agatharied, Hausham, Germany

Susanne Staudinger
Interdisciplinary Tinnitus Center of the University of Regensburg, Regensburg, Germany

Hannah Frick
Department of Statistical Science, University College London, London, UK

Ulrich Frick
Department of Psychiatry and Psychotherapy, University of Regensburg, Regensburg, Germany
HSD University of Applied Sciences, Cologne, Germany

Petra Brüggemann, Benjamin Boecking and Birgit Mazurek
Tinnitus Center, Universitätsmedizin Berlin, Berlin, Germany

Matthias Rose
Department of Internal Medicine and Psychosomatics, Universitätsmedizin Berlin, Berlin, Germany

Laurence McKenna
Royal National Throat Nose and Ear Hospital, University College Hospitals, London, UK

Philippe Fournier and Arnaud J. Noreña
Laboratoire Neurosciences Intégratives et Adaptatives, UMR CNRS 7260, Fédération 3C, Aix-Marseille Université, Marseille, France
Centre National de la Recherche Scientifique, Aix-Marseille University, Marseille, France

Victoria Milloy, Daniel Benoit and Amineh Koravand
School of Rehabilitation Sciences, University of Ottawa, Ottawa, ON, Canada

Uli Niemann and Myra Spiliopoulou
Faculty of Computer Science, Otto von Guericke University Magdeburg, Magdeburg, Germany

Gang-Ping Zhou, Heng-Le Wei, Li-Jie Qu, Yu-Sheng Yu, Qing-Qing Zhou and Hong Zhang
Department of Radiology, The Affiliated Jiangning Hospital of Nanjing Medical University, Nanjing, China

Xin-Yi Shi and Yue-Jin Tao
Department of ENT, The Affiliated Jiangning Hospital of Nanjing Medical University, Nanjing, China

Xindao Yin
Department of Radiology, Nanjing First Hospital, Nanjing Medical University, Nanjing, China

Index

www.ingramcontent.com/pod-product-compliance
Lightning Source LLC
LaVergne TN
LVHW082221200926
848484LV00008B/2282

* 9 7 9 8 8 8 7 4 0 3 9 5 3 *